a LANGE medical book

Basic Histology
Examination and Board Review

Douglas F. Paulsen, PhD
Associate Professor of Anatomy
Morehouse School of Medicine
Atlanta, Georgia

APPLETON & LANGE
Norwalk, Connecticut/San Mateo, California

0-8385-3755-3

90 91 92 93 94 / 10 9 8 7 6 5 4 3 2 1

Prentice-Hall International (UK) Limited, *London*
Prentice-Hall of Australia Pty. Limited, *Sydney*
Prentice-Hall Canada Inc., *Toronto*
Prentice-Hall Hispanoamericana, S.A., *Mexico*
Prentice-Hall of India Private Limited, *New Delhi*
Prentice-Hall of Japan, Inc., *Tokyo*
Simon & Schuster Asia Pte. Ltd., *Singapore*
Editora Prentice-Hall do Brasil, Ltda., *Rio de Janeiro*
Prentice-Hall, *Englewood Cliffs, New Jersey*

ISBN 0-8385-3755-3
ISBN 1045-4586

Production Editor: Christine Langan
Designer: Steven Byrum

PRINTED IN THE UNITED STATES OF AMERICA

This book is dedicated to my students at the Morehouse School of Medicine for their dedication to providing quality primary care to the economically disadvantaged and the medically underserved.

Table of Contents

Preface

This book is intended to help you use your study time more effectively, both as you learn histology and as you review it for course or National Board (Part I or FLEX) exams. It is specifically designed as a companion to the sixth edition of *Basic Histology* by Junquiera, Carneiro, and Kelley. It contains many page references to this text that can help you find information quickly and easily. However, you can use this book successfully with any standard histology text.

Several distinctive features make this study guide useful and easy to understand. They include:

- A list of learning objectives for every chapter.
- A synopsis of each subject in outline format.
- A set of study-focusing questions for every chapter.
- A set of Boards-type multiple-choice questions and answers for every chapter.
- Four sets of Boards-type integrative multiple-choice questions and answers for related chapters.
- Page references to *Basic Histology,* sixth edition, for all of these questions.

Each chapter begins with a list of objectives that describe the most significant facts and concepts for that topic. The second section of each chapter is a synopsis of the topic presented in outline form.

The third section of each chapter consists of a set of study-focusing questions designed to direct your attention to the facts and concepts that most often appear on exams. Many of these questions can be answered with a word, phrase, list, or sketch. Others ask you to make comparisons and are best answered by making a chart or table and filling in the requested information. Every question asks for specific information and provides page references directing you to that information.

The last section of every chapter is a set of multiple-choice questions written in 4 of the formats commonly used by the National Board of Medical Examiners. In addition, this book contains 4 sets of integrative multiple-choice questions. The correct answers to all of the multiple-choice questions are included at the end of the book, along with page references to the sixth edition of *Basic Histology*. If you do not have this text, you can find the answers to these questions in any standard histology text by using the index. These page references will help you learn not only what the correct answers are, but why they are correct.

Douglas F. Paulsen, PhD
Atlanta, Georgia
August 1989

Part I: Fundamental Concepts

Methods of Study 1

Objectives

This chapter should help the student to:

- Know the mathematic relationships among the units of measure commonly used in analyzing histologic specimens.
- Name the instruments and techniques commonly used in the preparation and study of histologic specimens.
- Know the basic steps in preparing specimens for the various types of light and electron microscopy.
- Know the advantages and limitations of the various histologic instruments and techniques and choose the appropriate ones to reveal specific microscopic features of cells and tissues.

Synopsis

I. GENERAL FEATURES OF HISTOLOGY & ITS METHODS

A. Goals of Histology: The term *histology* means "the study of tissues." Histology is a largely visual science that relies on microscopy to reveal cell, tissue, and organ substructures. It's goals include:

1. Understanding cell, tissue, and organ structure at levels not visible to the unaided eye, including 3-dimensional relationships among their biochemical constituents.

2. Understanding the relationship between the substructure and the normal functions of cells, tissues, and organs.

3. Establishing a basis for learning histopathology—the relationship between abnormal tissue and organ structure and functional defects.

4. Providing a basis for treating diseased and injured tissues and organs. In medicine, this is the ultimate goal.

B. Histologic Methods: Histology is classed as a subdiscipline of anatomy ("cutting apart"), because its methods involve dividing tissues and organs into pieces and preparing them for microscopic examination and chemical analyses. These methods fall into 4 main groups:

1. Microscopy The purpose of histologic methods is analysis of histologic specimens with the aid of a microscope. The several types of microscopy are classified in 2 main groups, **light microscopy** (IV) and **electron microscopy (EM;** see V).

2. Tissue preparation for microscopy The optical characteristics of each type of microscope are attended by certain requirements in preparing a tissue for analysis (III). Examples of common preparative procedures include **sectioning** to produce thin, translucent tissue slices and **staining** with dyes and chemicals to reveal the otherwise transparent substructure of the slices.

3. Cell, tissue, and organ culture These methods allow observation of the effects of certain treatments on the structure and function of isolated cells, tissues, and organs (VI).

4. Cell fractionation This technique involves mechanically breaking cells and then separating their components by centrifugation for electron microscopic or biochemical analysis (VII).

C. Advantages and Limitations of Histologic Methods: Only by understanding the advantages and limitations of histologic methods can one properly interpret the information they provide. The advantages result from making small and complex structures and processes accessible to observation. The limitations result from the fact that the methods themselves, especially dividing an organism into pieces, often halt the very life processes we wish to analyze.

D. Structure and Function: Tissue structure and tissue function are so closely related that neither can be fully understood without an understanding of the other. Their relationship should be the main focus of both your initial study and your review.

II. UNITS OF MEASURE

A. Ångström unit (Å)* $= 10^{-10}$m $= 10^{-7}$mm $= 10^{-4}\mu$m $= 10^{-1}$nm
B. Nanometer (nm) $= 10^{-9}$m $= 10^{-6}$mm $= 10^{-3} = \mu$m $= 10$ Å
C. Micrometer (μm) $= 10^{-6}$m $= 10^{-3}$mm $= 10^{3}$ nm $= 10^{4}$Å

III. PREPARATION OF TISSUES FOR MICROSCOPIC EXAMINATION.

Light and electron microscopy share the basic types of preparative methods described below but differ in important details of preparation. The similarities and differences are summarized in Fig 1–1.

A. Fixation:

1. Purpose The purpose of fixation is to preserve the structural organization of the tissue. There are 2 main types of fixation: chemical fixation and freezing (physical fixation).

2. Advantages and limitations

a. Chemical fixation A good chemical fixative will prevent bacterial and enzymatic digestion, insolubilize tissue components to prevent diffusion, and protect against damage from subsequent steps in tissue processing. However, chemical fixation may cause changes in chemical composition and fine structure. The chemical changes may induce staining artifacts during sensitive histochemical procedures (see Chapter 2). The structural changes include denaturing and cross-linking certain tissue proteins.

b. Freezing Freezing is faster, because it eliminates several preparative steps (Fig 1–1). It also avoids dissolving lipids and denaturing fixative-sensitive proteins such as enzymes and antigens. However, frozen specimens do not last as long, and obtaining serial sections from them is difficult.

3. Chemical procedures The best fixation is achieved with rapid penetration of living tissue with fixative, by immersion or perfusion.

*This unit may be encountered in older publications, but it is now being replaced by the nanometer for structures in this size range.

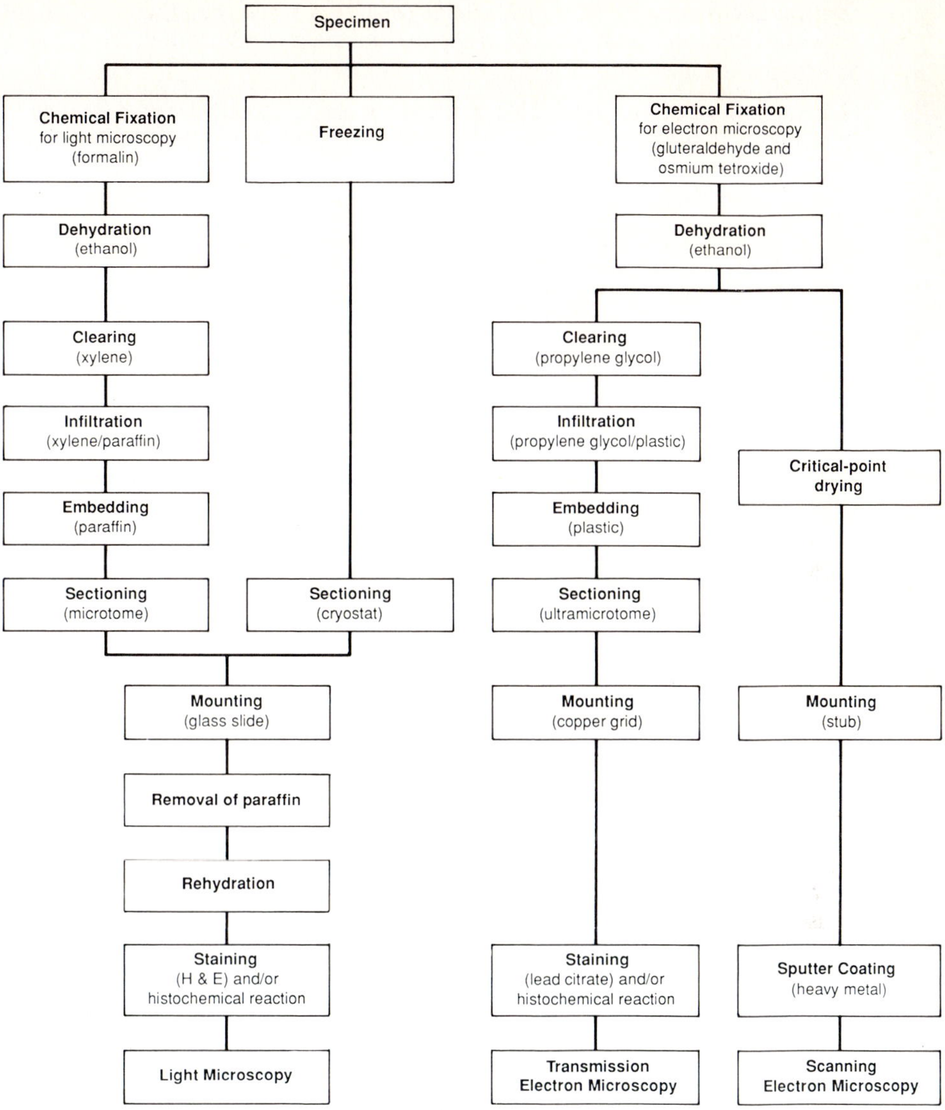

Figure 1-1. Steps in tissue preparation for microscopy. Common techniques and agents are shown in parentheses.

a. Immersion Small pieces of tissue may be fixed by simply immersing them in the fixative.

b. Perfusion Tissues and organs can be fixed before they are removed from the body by pumping fixative through the blood vessels that serve them. Perfusion is useful for fixing specimens too large to allow rapid fixative penetration by immersion (eg, in embalming).

4. Chemical fixatives

a. Aldehydes These react with amine groups, form cross-links among proteins, and cause coagulation (but not coarse precipitation) of tissue proteins. They may interfere with periodic acid-Schiff (PAS) and Feulgen staining specificity (see Chapter 2). Formalin (a solution of formaldehyde gas in water) is commonly used for light microscopy; glutaraldehyde is commonly used for electron microscopy.

b. Oxidizing agents These cross-link proteins and precipitate unsaturated lipids. Osmium tetroxide is an oxidizing agent often used with glutaraldehyde to fix tissues for electron microscopy. It reacts with lipids to form a black precipitate and doubles as a stain for cell membranes. Potassium permanganate and potassium dichromate are oxidizing agents sometimes used in light microscopy.

c. Protein-denaturing agents Normal protein shape is maintained largely by ionic interactions with water molecules. Acetic acid, methyl alcohol, ethyl alcohol, and acetone denature protein by removing the associated water molecules, changing the protein's shape. In the absence of cross-linking agents, rehydrating the tissue can sometimes restore proteins to their original conformation.

d. Other chemical fixatives Mercuric chloride and picric acid are useful light microscopy fixatives whose precise mechanism of action is unknown.

5. Fixative mixtures No single fixative is ideal for all the structural details of all tissues. Mixtures are used to exploit the advantages of a variety of fixatives while minimizing their disadvantages. Bouin's fluid, used for light microscopy, contains picric acid, formalin, acetic acid, and water; Zenker's formalin (Helley's fluid), also used for light microscopy, contains formalin, potassium dichromate, mercuric chloride, and water. Karnovsky's fixative, used for electron microscopy, contains paraformaldehyde and glutaraldehyde in a buffered salt solution.

6. Double fixation In this procedure, used for electron microscopy, the specimen is fixed in buffered glutaraldehyde, washed with phosphate buffer, and postfixed in buffered osmium tetroxide.

7. Physical procedures Tissue may be frozen to preserve its structure for either light or electron microscopy. Prior embedding in a cryoprotectant (eg, glycerin) and rapid freezing at low temperatures in liquid nitrogen helps prevent formation of large ice crystals and related artifacts. Freezing allows the tissue to be sectioned (or fractured; see III.F) without chemical fixation, dehydration, or clearing.

B. Dehydration:

1. Purpose The purpose of dehydration, or **substitution,** is to prepare chemically fixed tissue for infiltration with an embedding medium by replacing the water in the tissue with an organic solvent.

2. Procedure Ethyl alcohol is the most common dehydrating agent. Fixed tissue is immersed in a series of alcohol-water mixtures with increasing alcohol concentration until 100% alcohol is reached. Alcohol may denature proteins. Removal of water usually causes shrinkage.

C. Clearing and Infiltration:

1. Purpose In clearing, the dehydrating agent is replaced with a clearing agent (a solvent of the embedding medium), which renders the tissue transparent. Infiltration replaces the clearing agent with the embedding medium. Successful clearing and infiltration prevent bubbles from forming in the tissue. Clearing agents may denature proteins.

2. Procedures

a. Clearing The dehydrated tissue is immersed in a series of clearing agent-alcohol mixtures with increasing clearing-agent concentration, or it is placed directly in the clearing agent.

b. Infiltration The cleared tissue is immersed in a series of clearing agent-embedding medium mixtures with increasing embedding medium concentrations, at medium-high temperature. The clearing agent gradually evaporates and is replaced by the embedding medium.

3. Common clearing agents Xylene (a paraffin solvent) is most commonly used for light microscopy. Propylene glycol (a plastic solvent) is most commonly used for EM.

D. Embedding:

1. Purpose The purpose of embedding is to make the tissue firm and prevent crushing or other tissue disruption during sectioning. This permits thin, uniform sectioning.

2. Procedure The infiltrated tissue is positioned in a mold filled with the embedding medium. The medium hardens into a block, which is removed from the mold and attached to a chuck. When placed in the microtome, the chuck holds the block in place for sectioning.

3 Embedding media

a. For light microscopy Paraffin is the most common embedding medium. Others are celloidin, plastics (eg, methacrylate), and polyethylene glycol (water-soluble) wax.

b. For electron microscopy Plastics and epoxy resins (eg, Epon and Araldite) are most commonly used. These embedding media often require a catalyst to harden (polymerize) them after infiltration. Harder embedding media allow thinner sectioning, a requirement for electron microscopy.

E. Sectioning:

1. Purpose Most tissues are too thick and opaque to permit microscopic analysis of their internal structure. Cutting thin slices allows light or electrons to penetrate the specimen and form an image.

2. Instruments and procedures

a. For light microscopy A standard rotary **microtome** with a steel blade is used to cut sections (usually 3–8 μm thick) of specimens embedded in paraffin, celloidin, or polyethylene glycol. A microtome equipped with a glass or diamond knife may be used to cut sections (usually 1–5 μm thick) from plastic-embedded tissues. Frozen sections (10–30 μm thick) are cut with a freezing microtome, or in a cryostat, a standard microtome housed in a refrigerated chamber.

b. For electron microscopy An **ultramicrotome** with a glass or diamond knife is used to cut very thin sections (0.02–0.1 μm thick, or up to 0.5 μm thick for high-voltage electron microscopy). The instrument is equipped with a stereomicroscope for viewing the cutting.

F. Cryofracture and Freeze Etching:

1. Purpose Together, cryofracture and freeze etching permit EM examination of tissues without prior fixation and embedding, and thus, without fixative-related artifacts. These methods allow verification of results obtained by conventional EM techniques.

2. Procedures The tissue is frozen at very low temperatures and fractured with a sharp metal blade (cryofracture). The specimen is kept in a vacuum while the ice crystals sublimate, lowering the ice level from the specimen surface to reveal additional structures (freeze-etching). The etched tissue is coated with a layer of fine carbon particles to form a replica, which is then sprayed at an angle with heavy-metal (gold or platinum) particles to give a shadowed effect. The tissue and replica are returned to atmospheric pressure, the tissue is dissolved in strong acid, and the replica is mounted on a grid. EM examination of the replica produces a shadowed-relief image and provides a limited pseudo-3-D view of cell and tissue components. Resolution is limited by the size of the carbon particles and the thickness of the coating.

G. Mounting:

1. Purpose The purpose of mounting is to ease handling of and decrease damage to the specimen during microscopic examination.

2. Procedure

a. For light microscopy Specimens (usually sections) are placed on glass slides, which may be precoated with a thin layer of albumin, gelatin, or polylysine to improve tissue attachment. After staining, the sections are covered with coverslips to preserve them for repeated examination.

b. For electron microscopy Specimens are mounted on copper grids, because the electron beam cannot penetrate glass. Only portions of the specimen lying between the crossbars of the grid will be visible.

H. Staining:

1. Purpose Most tissue substructure is indistinguishable even at high magnification. Stains, ligands with specific binding affinities and optical properties, and radiolabels are used to localize and distinguish among various cell and tissue components. Knowledge of the specificities of such substances (Table 1–1) provides additional information about the structure and composition of a specimen. General staining procedures for light microscopy and electron microscopy are described here; more specific stains and techniques are described in Chapter 2.

2. Procedure for light microscopy After paraffin sections are attached to slides, the paraffin is dissolved and the tissue may be rehydrated prior to staining. Plastic-embed-

Table 1-1. Examples of common stains and their affinities.

Stain	Type	Affinity
Light microscopy Hematoxylin	Basic dye	Basophilic tissue components; eg, DNA, RNA, and polyanions such as sulfated glycosaminoglycans.
Toluidine blue		
Methylene blue		
Alcian blue		
Eosin	Acidic dye	Acidophilic tissue components; eg, basic proteins in the cytoplasm.
Orange G		
Acid fuchsin		
Oil red O	Lipid-soluble	Long-chain hydrocarbons (fats, oils, and waxes).
Sudan black		
Periodic acid-Schiff (PAS) reaction	Multicomponent histochemical reaction	Complex carbohydrates (glycosaminoglycans, glycogen).
Feulgen's reaction		Nuclear chromatin (DNA and associated protein).
Transmission electron microscopy Uranyl acetate	Heavy metal (electron-dense)	Nonspecific; adsorb to surfaces and enhance contrast.
Lead citrate		
Osmium tetroxide		Actually a fixative, but binds to phosphate groups of membrane phospholipids, enhancing contrast.
Ruthenium red		Polyanions; eg, complex carbohydrates such as oligosaccharides of the glycocalyx and glycosaminoglycans of the extracellular matrix.

ded sections are stained without removing the plastic. Most stain affinities are based on reciprocal acid-base characteristics of the stain and tissue components. Acidic stains such as eosin bind to basic, or **acidophilic,** structures and compounds (eg, cytoplasmic proteins and hemoglobin). Basic stains such as hematoxylin bind to acidic, or **basophilic,** tissue components (eg, the nucleoproteins in ribosomes). Stain mixtures reveal multiple cellular components. Hematoxylin and eosin (H&E), the most common stain mixture for light microscopy, distinguishes the nucleus from the cytoplasm.

3. Procedures for electron microscopy There are 2 types of electron microscopy (V.D):

a. Transmission electron microscopy procedures Most staining (contrasting) methods for transmission electron microscopy (TEM) are based on the stains' electron-absorbing or -scattering qualities and their affinities for particular cellular components. Heavy-metal salts such as lead citrate and uranyl acetate are most commonly used. The fixative osmium tetroxide interacts with lipids to form an electron-dense precipitate and thus doubles as a stain for cellular membranes.

b. Scanning electron microscopy procedures Specimens being prepared for scanning electron microscopy (SEM) do not require staining per se. Before mounting and sputter coating, SEM specimens are subjected to **critical point drying,** which prevents the development of artifacts related to surface tension. After dehydration, the specimens are soaked in a liquid miscible with CO_2 or Freon and placed in the critical point chamber. The chamber is heated to a critical temperature (31°C), causing the pressure to rise to a critical level (73 atm) at which the gaseous and liquid phases exist without surface tension and the liquid escapes the specimen without altering its structure. The specimen is then mounted on a stub and sputter-coated (sprayed) with a fine mist of heavy metal particles (eg, gold) before viewing.

I. Radioautography:

1. Purpose Radioautography allows localization of radioactive elements in cells or tissues. It is especially useful in tracing radiolabeled precursors and the molecules into which they are incorporated from one part of a tissue or cell to another.

2. Procedure The tissue is usually incubated with radiolabeled precursors prior to fixation, eg, with ^{3}H-thymidine for DNA, ^{3}H-uridine for RNA, ^{3}H- or ^{14}C-leucine for protein. Sections mounted on a slide are cleared of embedding medium, covered with photographic emulsion, and left in the dark. The emulsion becomes exposed (silver bromide is reduced to elemental silver) in areas in contact with the radiolabel; when it is developed, black grains (light microscopy) or curling particle tracks (electron microscopy) appear over labeled structures. The number of grains or tracks in the emulsion is directly proportionate to the amount of radiolabel present. For light microscopy, developed sections are often stained with hematoxylin to reveal tissue architecture.

J. Problems in Interpreting Tissue Sections:

Histologic techniques yield images that differ from the living state in certain predictable ways.

1. Artifacts Structural changes induced by histologic techniques are called artifacts. Some common artifacts caused by tissue preparation are discussed here; for lens-related artifacts, see IV.C.

a. Of fixation Fixation may cause precipitation of proteins normally in solution. It may also alter the chemistry of some tissue components, changing their staining properties.

b. Of dehydration and clearing Dehydration and clearing can cause cell and tissue components to shrink unevenly, according to their relative water content. This creates spaces between the cells and tissue layers that are not present in life.

c. Of sectioning Sectioning with a dull knife can result in crushed or pinched tissue sections. A burr or nick in the blade can tear the tissue. Chatter, or wavelike variations in the thickness of a section, can result from the knife vibrating during sectioning.

d. Of mounting During mounting, tissue sections may develop folds, so that some regions appear to have higher cell densities and darker staining properties than others.

e. Of staining Because the colors in stained tissue are artifacts of staining, it is best to focus more on structure than on the color of tissue components.

2. Conceptual problems Tissue sections can seduce the observer into thinking of 3-dimensional structures in terms of 2 dimensions. To overcome this problem, tissues and organs are sectioned in several planes to allow conceptual reassembly into 3-dimensional structures. In addition, analyzing **serial sections** in the order in which they were cut can help provide a 3-dimensional picture. Since even mixtures of stains are unable to stain every tissue component, adjacent sections are sometimes treated with different stains.

IV. LIGHT MICROSCOPY

A. Microscope Lenses:

1. The **condenser lens** is located between the light source and the specimen. It collects light from the source and projects a cone of illumination through the specimen.

2. The **objective lens,** consisting of one or more lenses (IV.C), is located between the specimen and the ocular lens. It enlarges and resolves the image of the specimen and projects it toward the ocular lens. Several objective lenses, each providing a different level of magnification, are generally mounted on a rotating turret.

3. The **ocular lens** is located between the objective lens and the observer or recording device. It further enlarges the image of the specimen and projects it onto the observer's retina, a screen, or a photographic emulsion.

B. Optical Properties of Lenses:

1. Magnification increases the apparent size of the specimen and makes it appear closer. It is a property of both objective and ocular lenses. The value for total magnification is obtained by multiplying the power of the objective by that of the ocular lens.

2. Resolution is a measure of how close together 2 objects can be and still appear separate; the smaller the value, the greater the resolution. The resolution of the human eye is 200 μm; of a light microscope, 0.2 μm; of an electron microscope, 0.001 μm. Increased magnification is virtually useless without increased resolution. The **resolving power** of a microscope, a measure of the resolution it provides, is independent of magnification and determines the clarity and richness of detail of the image. Resolving power (R) is calculated from the numerical aperture (NA) of the objective and the wavelength of illumination:

$$R = \frac{0.61\ \lambda}{NA}$$

The greater the value of R, the greater the resolution.

3. The **numerical aperture** of the objective lens is related to the width of the lens aperture. The lower the NA, the greater the resolving power of the microscope.

4. Refractive index is a measure of the comparative velocity of light in a medium. When there is air between the lens and the coverslip, some of the light projected through the specimen is refracted (bent) because of the change in refractive index at the air-glass interfaces. At high magnifications, the accompanying loss of resolution has a significant effect on image quality. Using immersion oil (which has the same refractive index as glass) between the coverslip and a special oil-immersion objective lens avoids the change in refractive index and thereby improves resolution.

C. Lens-Related Artifacts: Modern objective lenses contain a series of glass lenses. The first (frontal lens) is spheric or hemispheric and magnifies the image; the others correct for the following artifacts of lens curvature:

1. Chromatic aberration Spheric lenses bring light of shorter wavelength into focus closer to the retina than light of longer wavelength, resulting in multiple blurred images. This chromatic aberration can be avoided bv using **achromatic** or **apochromatic lenses.**

2. Spheric aberration Optical properties of the center of a spheric lens differ from those of the periphery. Apochromatic lenses completely correct for this spheric aberration.

3. Curvature of field Spheric lenses prevent simultaneous focusing on the entire field: either the center or the periphery is out of focus. **Planar lenses** correct this curvature of the field, providing flat-field focus.

D. Types of Light Microscope:

1. The **compound bright-field microscope** is the most common tool of histology and histopathology. It is described as compound (as opposed to simple) because it uses a series of lenses. It is called bright-field because the entire field is illuminated by means of an ordinary condenser lens. Specimens must be translucent and stained to provide contrast.

2. The **dark-field microscope** uses a special condenser lens to provide contrast in unstained material, allowing living specimens to be visualized. A disklike shield excludes the center of the light shaft projected by the condenser lens, so that the specimen is illuminated only from the sides. Only objects that deflect light into the objective lens are visible; these are bright on a dark background.

3. The **phase contrast microscope** uses a special lens system to transform invisible differences in phase retardation (light retardation) caused by the different refractive indexes of specimen components into visible differences in light intensity. This allows visualization of living specimens, because fixation and staining are not needed. The specimen must be thin and translucent. High resolution is difficult to obtain.

4. The **polarizing microscope** allows selective visualization of **birefringent** (anisotropic) **structures**—repetitive or crystalline structures such as collagen fibers or myofibrils. Staining is not necessary. Light from the light source passes through a polarizing filter, the condenser lens projects the polarized light onto the specimen, and birefringent structures in the specimen rotate the polarized light. The objective lens projects the image through the analyzer filter, which is oriented so that only light waves oscillating in a plane different from that of the original polarized light can pass to the ocular lens and be seen. Birefringent structures appear as bright, often colored objects on a dark background.

5. The **fluorescence microscope** allows localization of substances labeled with fluorescing compounds (fluorochromes). When stimulated by light of the proper wavelength, fluorochromes emit light of a longer wavelength. Fluorescence microscopes have a special light source and 2 special sets of filters. An ultraviolet light source is commonly used, and the emitted light is in the visible spectrum. An excitation filter between the light source and the specimen filters out all wavelengths except that needed to stimulate the desired fluorescence. A barrier filter between the objective and ocular lenses protects the eyes from ultraviolet rays.

6. The **interference microscope** provides contrast in unstained material, relying on differences in refractive index (IV.D.3). Unlike the phase contrast microscope, it quantitates the phase retardation induced by components of the specimen; it compares the refracted light with an unimpeded reference beam and provides an electronic readout of the data. Because refractive index and phase retardation are proportionate to mass, this instrument can be used to calculate the mass of cellular components.

V. ELECTRON MICROSCOPY

A. General Principles: The equation for resolution is the same as for light microscopy (IV.B.2). An electron beam (wavelength approximately 0.005 nm) is used instead of visible light (wavelength 397–723 nm), giving electron microscopes much greater resolution and allowing useful magnification up to 200 times that of light microscopes. Glass lenses are not transparent to wavelengths below 400 nm, but the negatively charged electron beam can be deflected and focused by electromagnets as it travels through a vacuum.

B. Major Components of Electron Microscopes:

1. **Cathode and anode** The cathode is a metallic filament that emits a spray of electrons when intensely heated in a vacuum by electric current. The anode is a positively charged metal plate with a small hole at its center. Because of the potential difference between the cathode and anode (60–100 kV), electrons accelerate toward the anode, and some of them pass through the hole in the anode to form the electron beam. Together, the cathode and anode are analogous to the light source of a light microscope.

2. **Condenser electromagnet** The condenser electromagnet induces an electromagnetic field that deflects the electron beam and focuses a cone of the beam at the object plane.

3. **Object** The specimen, or object, is typically an ultrathin section of tissue stained with electron-absorbing or -scattering substances to provide contrast. The image formed is actually the shadow of the contrast material.

4. **Objective electromagnet** The objective electromagnet induces an electromagnetic field that deflects the portion of the electron beam which has passed through the specimen, to form and magnify the image of the object.

5. **Projector electromagnet** The one or 2 projector electromagnets are analogous to the light microscope's ocular lenses. They further enlarge the image produced by the objective electromagnet and project it onto a fluorescent screen or photographic emulsion.

6. **Screen** The fluorescent screen is a plate coated with material that fluoresces as electrons strike it. Electrons deflected or absorbed by the specimen do not reach the screen, while those that pass through the specimen do. The result is a transmission image formed by shadows of the electron-dense components of the specimen.

C. Limitations:

1. Because the electron beam must travel to the specimen in a high vacuum, living tissue cannot be used.

2. Tissue sections must be very thin, or they will absorb or deflect the entire beam.

3. The electron beam may damage or alter specimen structure.

4. The image cannot be viewed directly but must be used to create a fluorescent or photographic image.

D. Types of Electron Microscope:

1. The **transmission electron microscope (TEM)** permits visualization of the internal ultrastructure of cells and tissues as well as extremely small structures within cells or in intercellular spaces. It operates as described above (V.B). Specimens are prepared as described in section III.

2. The **scanning electron microscope (SEM)** permits visualization of surface ultrastructure. After the specimen is coated with a thin layer of heavy metal (III.H.3.b), a narrow electron beam is directed across its surface in a point-by-point sequence, generating 2 major signals:

a. Secondary electrons are released from the specimen surface, collected on detectors, and converted electronically into an image that is displayed on a cathode ray tube. This image provides an apparently 3-dimensional representation of the specimen surface.

b. X-rays are generated when the electron beam strikes atoms heavier than sodium. Analysis of the x-ray signal can supply information regarding the concentration and distribution of certain elements in the specimen.

VI. CELL, TISSUE, & ORGAN CULTURE

A. Purpose: The purpose of cell, tissue, and organ culture is to study the function of living cells and tissues without the interference of the organism's normal homeostatic mechanisms. These methods permit easier control and manipulation of the cells' or tissue's environment. Cells and tissues isolated and grown in culture are referred to as **in vitro** (''in glass'') and those in the intact organism as **in vivo** (''in the living''). Cells may react differently to a particular treatment in vitro and in vivo.

B. Culture Types:

1. Cell culture In suspension culture, cells are suspended in culture medium, either free or attached to the surface of floating beads. In plate culture, cells are attached to plastic or glass tissue-culture dishes. The dishes may be coated with substances that improve attachment: gelatin, collagen, polylysine, serum albumin, or extracellular matrix extracts. Plate-cultured cells behave differently at different densities. They may be cultured in confluent monolayers (the entire culture surface is covered with cells in contact with one another) or at clonal densities (the cultures are seeded at low density to avoid cell-to-cell contact). The latter method allows growth of individual cell colonies, or clones.

2. Tissue and organ culture Fragments of tissues or organs are removed from the body and grown as intact explants, usually at the air-medium interface. This method is often used to study embryonic differentiation and morphogenesis away from the complex environment of the embryo.

C. Culture Medium: The medium consists of a buffered isotonic saline solution to which is added an array of essential nutrients (eg, amino acids, vitamins, hormones) or rigidly controlled composition. Recent advances in knowledge of cell and tissue growth requirements have decreased the use of serum and tissue extracts of less well-defined composition to supplement the medium. Antibacterial and antifungal agents are often added to the medium.

D. Isolation and Study of Pure Cell Strains: Individual cell types may be isolated and studied in vitro in order to examine their separate contributions to tissue and organ function. Cell suspensions are commonly obtained from tissues by enzymatic digestion (eg, with trypsin, collagenase, or hyaluronidase) of the cellular and intercellular components that hold cells together. Cell types may then be separated on the basis of size and mass through specialized forms of **centrifugation** (elutriation, density gradient centrifugation). Newer methods use specific antibodies to isolate particular cell types from a heterogeneous population in suspension. Some such methods exploit differential binding of cells by antibodies attached to a culture surface; others use a fluorescence-activated cell sorter, which separates cells labeled with fluorescent antibodies from unlabeled cells.

VII. CELL FRACTIONATION.

Cell fractionation is used to isolate and collect cellular components in quantity to study their contributions to cell function. This procedure begins with the mechanical **homogenization** of cells and tissues to break plasma membranes and release the cell components into suspension. The components (individual organelle types) are then separated on the basis of size and density, using either of 2 centrifugation methods.

In **differential centrifugation,** components are separated by their characteristic sedimentation rates, using different amounts of centrifugal force for varying periods of time. In **density gradient centrifugation,** the homogenate is layered on top of a gradient of solute and centrifuged until its components come to rest in portions of the gradient with densities similar to their own.

Study-Focusing Questions*

1. List, in order, the basic steps in the preparation of histologic sections for microscopy (1–3).
2. What is the purpose of fixation (1)?
3. What is the purpose of embedding a tissue or organ (2–3)?
4. What is the purpose of sectioning a tissue or organ (1)?
5. Why is it necessary to stain sections of tissues or organs for observation with a standard light microscope (3)?
6. Name the type of microscopy that best visualizes unstained living cells and tissues (5).
7. Compare light and electron microscopy in terms of:
    - **a.** Their methods of fixation (1–2), embedding (2–3), sectioning (3), and staining (3)
    - **b.** The thickness of their sections (3)
    - **c.** The support upon which their sections are mounted (3)
    - **d.** Their lenses (3–4, 7–8)
    - **e.** The type (7), source (3–4, 7), wavelength (5, 6), and path (4, 7–8) of their illuminating beams
    - **f.** Their magnification (7)
8. Compare transmission and scanning electron microscopy in terms of:
    - **a.** The methods of preparing tissue for observation (3, **HR**)
    - **b.** Their electron path (7, 9)
    - **c.** The image obtained (9)
9. What are some of the predictable artifacts associated with specimens prepared for microscopy (9; **HR**)?
10. What is cryofracture, and what are its advantages over conventional methods of preparing tissues for electron microscopy (9–10)?
11. What is radioautography, and what is unique about the type of information it can provide (10, 13)?
12. List the advantages of studying isolated cells, tissues, or organ rudiments in culture, as opposed to studying them in the intact organism (13–14).
13. How are suspensions of a single cell type isolated from a heterogeneous population of cells in an organ or tissue (14)?
14. What is the purpose of cell fractionation, and how is it accomplished (14, 16)?

Multiple-Choice Questions

For questions 1–1 and 1–2, select the single best answer.

1–1. The phase contrast microscope is an optical device used to:
- **A.** Convert invisible differences in refractive index into visible differences in light intensity
- **B.** Illuminate a specimen with a single wavelength of light

*The page references in this section refer to *Basic Histology,* 6th ed., Junqueira L, Carneiro J, Kelley R (editors), Appleton & Lange, 1989. **HR** (for Histology Review) is occasionally used instead of a page reference to indicate that the information referred to can be found in this book.

C. Obtain resolution greater than that of the electron microscope
D. Reveal birefringence of crystalline or fibrillar tissue components
E. Make quantitative measurements of light intensity

1-2. Which of the following is the electron microscope component that corresponds with the condenser lens of the light microscope?
A. Fluorescent screen
B. Cathode
C. Electromagnet
D. Anode
E. Electron beam

MATCHING (questions 1-3 through 1-19): Each choice may be used once, more than once, or not at all.

Questions 1-3 through 1-10:

A. Fixation
B. Dehydration
C. Clearing
D. Embedding
E. Sectioning
F. Staining
G. All of the above

1-3. Accomplished using a microtome
1-4. Impregnation of tissue with a solvent of the embedding medium
1-5. Preserves the morphology and chemical composition of the tissue
1-6. Removes water from cells and tissues
1-7. Agents used in this procedure often cause precipitation and coagulation of proteins and promote protein cross-linking
1-8. Paraffin, epoxy resins, and other plastic materials are commonly used for this process
1-9. Accomplished by immersing fixed tissue in a graded series of increasing concentrations of ethanol in water
1-10. Renders otherwise transparent cell and tissue components conspicuous and distinguishable from one another

Questions 1-11 through 1-19:

A. Radioautography
B. Cryofracture and freeze etch
C. Cell, tissue, and organ culture
D. Tissue homogenization
E. Differential centrifugation
F. Density gradient centrifugation

1-11. Permits electron microscopic examination of specimens without prior fixation or embedding
1-12. The actual specimen is destroyed with strong acid
1-13. Accomplished by grinding the specimen
1-14. Presence of silver grains in a photographic emulsion overlying an organelle reveals the presence of labeled precursors
1-15. Allows prolonged studies of living cells and tissues that are isolated from the organism
1-16. Releases cellular organelles into a solution by breaking plasma membranes
1-17. The term **in vitro** is applied to cells and tissues maintained in this manner
1-18. A replica of the dehydrated tissue surface is obtained by deposition of a thin layer of carbon followed by a layer of heavy metal
1-19. Homogenized cells and tissues are deposited on top of a solution whose solute concentration increases toward the bottom of the centrifuge tube

For questions 1–20 through 1–33, either, both, or neither of the answers may be correct. Select

A if only A is correct
B if only B is correct
C if both A and B are correct
D if neither A nor B is correct

Questions 1–20 through 1–29:

A. Light microscopy
B. Electron microscopy
C. Both
D. Neither

1–20. Paraffin is a common embedding medium
1–21. Only diamond or glass knives are used in sectioning
1–22. Tissue sections are mounted on copper grids
1–23. May be used with radioautography
1–24. Electromagnets are used as lenses
1–25. Tissues are commonly fixed, dehydrated, cleared, and embedded prior to sectioning
1–26. Greatest resolving power
1–27. Best choice for examining an entire tissue or organ
1–28. Best choice for examining individual organelles
1–29. The specimen is maintained in a vacuum during observation

Questions 1–30 through 1–33:

A. Acidophilia
B. Basophilia
C. Both
D. Neither

1–30. Staining property exploited in electron microscopy
1–31. Staining property detectable with H&E staining mixture
1–32. Staining property of acidic substances in cells and tissues
1–33. Staining property detectable with hematoxylin

For questions 1–34 through 1–38, one, more than one, or all of the answers may be correct. Select

A if only (1), (2), and (3) are correct
B if only (1) and (3) are correct
C if only (2) and (4) are correct
D if only (4) is correct
E if all answers are correct

1–34. One micrometer (μm) is equal to:
(1) 10^3 nm
(2) 0.001 mm
(3) 10,000 Å
(4) 0.0001 m

1–35. The techniques that were combined to produce the photomicrograph shown in Fig 1–2 include:
(1) Electron microscopy
(2) Cryofracture and freeze etching
(3) Radioautography
(4) Light microscopy

1–36. Techniques that permit the direct observation of living cells and tissues include:
(1) Phase contrast microscopy

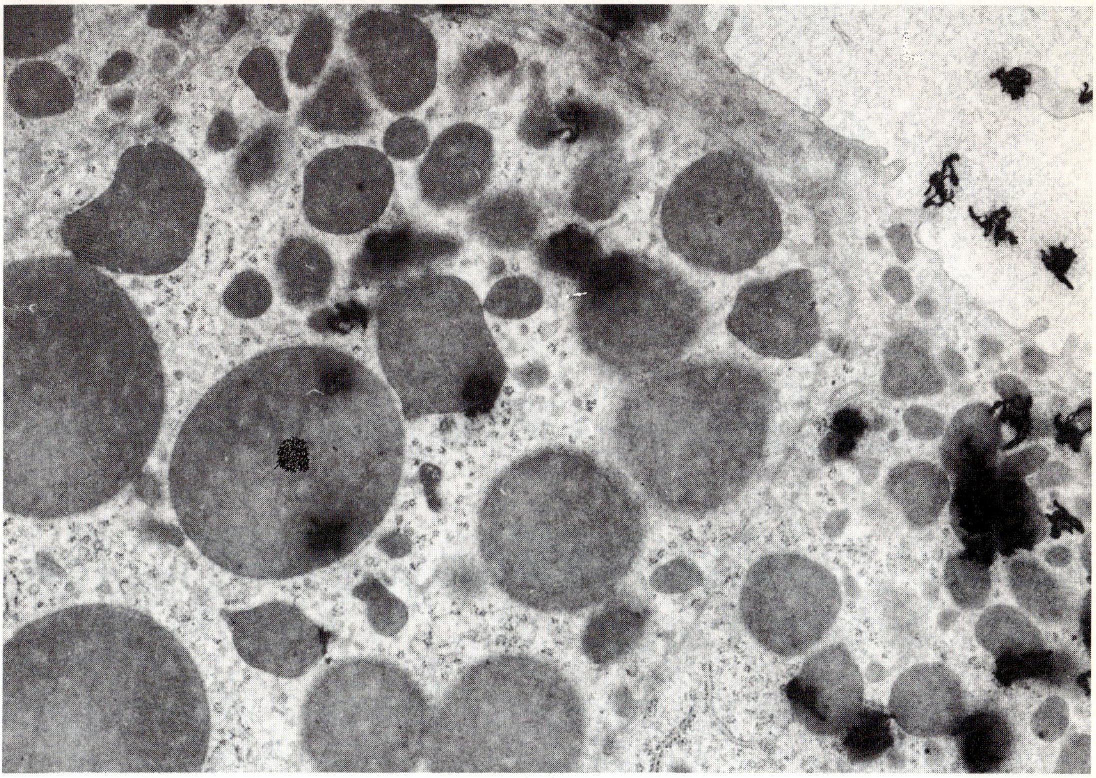

Figure 1-2.

(2) Homogenization
(3) Cell and tissue culture
(4) Transmission electron microscopy

1-37. Radioautography can reveal information concerning:
(1) The site of synthesis of various cellular components
(2) The biochemical composition of various cellular structures
(3) The intracellular movements of certain substances
(4) The rate of secretion of products of cellular synthesis

1-38. Fixation:
(1) Prevents autolysis
(2) Does not affect enzyme activity
(3) Is used to preserve structural detail
(4) Is a prerequisite for cryofracture

Histochemistry & Cytochemistry 2

Objectives

This chapter should help the student to:

- Describe the basic principles of histochemistry and cytochemistry.
- Know the substances of biologic interest that can be localized by histochemical and cytochemical techniques.

- Name the classes of histochemical and cytochemical techniques and describe the advantages and limitations of each.
- Choose appropriate techniques to reveal the location of specific substances in cells and tissues.

Synopsis

I. BASIC CRITERIA FOR HISTOCHEMICAL & CYTOCHEMICAL METHODS.

Histochemistry and cytochemistry marry the methods of histology and cytology with those of chemistry or biochemistry. The goal is to reveal the chemical and biochemical composition of tissues and cells beyond the acid-base distribution shown by standard staining methods (see Chapter 1) without disrupting the normal distribution of the chemicals. To achieve this goal, the following criteria must be met.

A. Preservation of Normal Chemical Distribution: The substance being analyzed must not diffuse away from its original site. Otherwise, standard chemical procedures would suffice.

B. Preservation of Normal Chemical Composition: The procedure must not block or denature the reactive chemical groups being analyzed or change normally unreactive groups into reactive groups.

C. Specificity of the Reaction: The method should be highly specific for the substance or chemical groups being analyzed, to avoid false-positive results.

D. Insolubility of the Reaction Product: The reaction product should be insoluble, so that it remains in close proximity to the substance it marks.

E. Visibility of the Reaction Product: The reaction product should be colored or electron-scattering, so that it can be visualized easily with a light or electron microscope.

II. SOME IMPORTANT BIOLOGIC SUBSTANCES & CLASSIC METHODS FOR DETECTING THEM

A. Ions: It is difficult to localize most ions accurately because of their small size and tendency to diffuse. However, certain ions are normally immobilized by their association with tissue proteins. Examples include the iron bound by hemoglobin in red blood cells (see Chapter 12) and the phosphate bound by collagen and other matrix proteins in mineralized bone (see Chapter 8).

1. Iron Incubating iron-containing tissue in potassium ferrocyanide and hydrochloric acid results in precipitation of dark blue ferric ferrocyanide (Perls' reaction). This reaction is used to identify cells involved in hemoglobin metabolism and to diagnose diseases characterized by iron deposits in tissues (hemosiderosis).

2. Phosphate Tissue phosphates react with silver nitrate to form silver phosphate, which reacts with hydroquinone to form a black precipitate of reduced silver. This reaction is used primarily in studies of calcium phosphate deposition during bone formation.

B. Lipids: Lipids are usually dissolved away by organic fixatives or clearing agents, leaving gaps in the tissue, but they are preserved in frozen sections. For light microscopy, lipids are best demonstrated by dyes that are more soluble in lipid than in the dye solvents (eg, Sudan IV, Sudan black, and oil red O). EM specimens are treated with reagents that react with lipids to form insoluble precipitates (eg, osmium tetroxide). Such methods are used to show normal lipid distribution and disease-related lipid accumulation (eg, fatty change in the liver).

C. Nucleic Acids: The nucleic acids, **DNA** and **RNA,** can be localized by specific and nonspecific methods. DNA is found mainly in nuclei, and its amount is much the same in every cell. RNA is found both in nuclei and in cytoplasm, and its amount varies widely, depending on a cell's functional state.

1. Feulgen's reaction Hydrochloric acid is used to partially hydrolyze DNA, promoting the formation of free aldehydes. These then react with Schiff's reagent (bleached fuchsin) to form an insoluble magenta precipitate in amounts proportionate to the amount of DNA present.

2. Acridine orange Complexes of acridine orange and nucleic acids emit a fluorescence whose intensity is proportionate to the amount of nucleic acid present. The fluorescence is yellow-green if the complex contains DNA and red-orange if it contains RNA. Neoplastic and other rapidly growing cells contain more RNA than slower-growing cells and may thus be distinguished from them.

3. Basic dyes Both DNA and RNA stain nonspecifically with basic dyes. Because of the strong affinity of RNA for such dyes, its distribution in cells and tissues may be studied by subtraction. In this procedure, one of 2 adjacent sections is treated with ribonuclease (RNase) to remove RNA; then both are stained with basic dyes (eg, toluidine blue, methylene blue). Basophilic structures present in the untreated section (eg, ribosomes) but absent in the RNase-treated section contain RNA.

D. Proteins and Amino Acids: Most older methods of protein identification are nonspecific for proteins but specific for particular amino acids. ***Examples:*** Millon reaction for tyrosine, Sakaguchi reaction for arginine, tetrazotized benzidine reaction for tryptophan. Specific classes of enzymes can be detected by the techniques of enzyme histochemistry (III). Specific proteins can now be localized through the methods of immunohistochemistry (IV).

E. Carbohydrates: Complex carbohydrates, ie, **polysaccharides** and **oligosaccharides,** can be localized by the histochemical techniques described below. In addition, some carbohydrates are immunogenic owing to their large size or their presence as covalently linked components of **glycoconjugates** (proteoglycans, glycoproteins, glycolipids); these can be analyzed by immunohistochemical methods.

1. PAS reaction The periodic acid-Schiff (PAS) reaction is the most common technique for demonstrating polysaccharides, particularly **glycogen.** Periodic acid reacts with the 1,2-glycol groups of sugars to form aldehydes. Schiff's reagent then reacts with the aldehydes to form an insoluble magenta pigment (compare II.C.1). Because the PAS reaction stains many polysaccharides and oligosaccharides, the specific localization of glycogen requires enzymatic subtraction of glycogen from an adjacent section; this is done with amylase. This method is used to distinguish among types of glycogen-storage diseases.

2. Alcian blue Alcian blue is a nonspecific basic stain at neutral pH, but it is specific for sulfate groups when staining is carried out at pH 1. It is used to demonstrate sulfated **glycosaminoglycans** (eg, chondroitin sulfate) that are abundant in the extracellular matrix of cartilage.

3. Ruthenium red Ruthenium red binds nonspecifically to polyanions and forms an electron-scattering precipitate useful in EM demonstration of polysaccharides.

4. Lectins Lectins are highly specific sugar-binding proteins found in plants and animals. Fluorescently labeled lectins can show the distribution of specific terminal sugar residues on oligosaccharides, such as those in the glycocalyx of cell membranes. ***Examples:*** Concanavalin A binds to mannose; peanut agglutinin and *Ricinus communis* agglutinin bind to galactose; and wheat germ agglutinin binds to N-acetyl-D-glucosamine.

F. Catecholamines: The catecholamines, including **epinephrine** and **norepinephrine,** fluoresce in the presence of dry formaldehyde vapor at 60–80 °C. This reaction is used in studies of catecholamine distribution in nerve tissue.

III. ENZYME HISTOCHEMISTRY.

The techniques of enzyme histochemistry, which relate structure and function, can be used to locate many enzymes, including **acid phosphatase, dehydrogenases,** and **peroxidases.** Because fixation and clearing typically inactivate enzymes, frozen sections are commonly used. The sections are incubated in solutions containing substrates for the enzymes of interest and reagents that yield insoluble colored or electron-dense precipitates at the sites of enzyme activity.

A. Acid Phosphatase: In the Gomori method for detecting acid phosphatase, the tissue is incubated with glycerophosphate and lead nitrate. The enzyme liberates phosphate, which combines with lead to produce lead phosphate, a colorless precipitate. The tissue is then immersed in a solution of ammonium sulfide, which reacts with lead phosphate to form lead sulfide, a black precipitate.

B. Dehydrogenases: Dehydrogenases can be localized by incubating tissue sections in a solution containing an appropriate substrate and tetrazole. The enzyme transfers hydrogen ions from the substrate to tetrazole, reducing tetrazole to formazan, a dark precipitate. Specific dehydrogenases can be targeted by choosing specific substrates.

C. Peroxidases: Peroxidases are most often demonstrated by incubating tissue with 3,3′-diaminobenzidine (DAB) and hydrogen peroxide. The enzyme transfers hydrogen from DAB to the peroxide, and the oxidized DAB forms an electron-dense dark brown to black precipitate at the site of enzyme activity. This reaction is useful for both light and electron microscopy.

IV. IMMUNOHISTOCHEMISTRY & IMMUNOCYTOCHEMISTRY.

Immunohistochemistry and immunocytochemistry utilize labeled **antibodies** to localize specific cell and tissue **antigens** and are among the most sensitive and specific histochemical and cytochemical techniques. Because many targeted antigens are proteins whose structure might be altered by fixation and clearing, frozen sections are commonly used. In some cases, water-soluble plastics and waxes can be used for embedding.

A. Raising Antibodies: Repeated injection of antigens (proteins, glycoproteins, proteoglycans, and some polysaccharides) causes the injected animal's B lymphocytes to differentiate into plasma cells and produce antibodies. Members of a lymphocyte **clone** (descendents of a single lymphocyte) produce a single type of antibody, which binds to a specific antigenic site, or **epitope.**

1. Polyclonal antibodies Large complex antigens may have multiple epitopes and give rise to several antibody types. Mixtures of different antibodies to a single antigen (obtained through fractionation of the injected animal's serum) are called polyclonal antibodies and are commonly raised in rabbits and goats.

2. Monoclonal antibodies Antibodies specific for a single epitope and produced by a single clone are called monoclonal antibodies and are commonly raised in mice.

Lymphocytes from the spleen of an antigen-injected mouse are mixed with myeloma cells (lymphocyte-derived tumor cells) under conditions that cause the lymphocytes and myeloma cells to fuse. Each resulting **hybridoma** cell has the myeloma's capacity for rapid cell division in culture and the lymphocyte's capacity for unique antibody secretion. An isolated hybridoma gives rise to a large clone that produces large quantities of pure antibody.

B. Labeling Antibodies: Antibodies are not visible with standard microscopy and must be labeled in a manner that does not interfere with their binding specificity. Common labels include fluorochromes (eg, fluorescein, rhodamine); enzymes demonstrable via enzyme histochemical techniques (eg, peroxidase, alkaline phosphatase); and electron-scattering compounds for use in electron microscopy (eg, ferritin, colloidal gold).

C. Antigen Localization in Tissues:

1. Direct method **In direct immunochemistry,** antigen-containing tissue is incubated in a solution containing labeled antibody. The antibody binds directly to the antigen, and the label appears at the antigenic site.

2. Indirect method **In indirect immunochemistry,** antigen-containing tissue is incubated in a solution containing unlabeled antibody. This **primary antibody,** which binds directly to the antigen in the tissue, is named according to its antibody class and the animal that produced it (eg, mouse IgG). The tissue is then incubated with a labeled **secondary antibody** (an antibody to the primary antibody, eg, rabbit anti-mouse IgG). Several labeled secondary antibodies bind to each primary antibody, so more label can accumulate at the antigenic site than with the direct method. The indirect method is thus more sensitive. It also avoids the risk of altering the primary antibody's binding specificity by attaching a label directly.

V. IN SITU HYBRIDIZATION. In situ hybridization is a new method of analyzing the presence and distribution of particular nucleotide sequences in DNA (eg, specific genes) and RNA (eg, specific mRNAs). **Hybridization** refers to the binding of complementary nucleotide sequences to one another with high specificity. Recombinant DNA technology permits copies of selected single-strand nucleotide sequences to be synthesized in large numbers. Synthetic sequences complementary to the RNA or DNA sequence an investigator wishes to localize are termed **probes** and can be labeled during synthesis with radioisotopes (eg, ^{32}P) or after synthesis with biotin. Radiolabeled probes are demonstrated with enzymes (eg, peroxidase) or fluorochromes covalently linked to avidin, a molecule with high affinity for biotin. Labeled probes were first used to analyze nucleic acids isolated from cell or tissue homogenates. The term **in situ** refers to the application of this technique to tissue sections or smears of cells: when such specimens are incubated with labeled probes, the probes bind to and reveal their complementary sequences.

Study-Focusing Questions*

1. List the principles of histochemistry and cytochemistry (18).
2. List the major classes of chemical and biochemical substances in cells and tissues that can be identified by histochemical and cytochemical techniques (18–24).
3. Name a technique that can be used for identification of each substance listed in answer to question 2; indicate which of the criteria listed in answer to question 1 is met by each technique (18–24).

*The page references in this section refer to *Basic Histology,* 6th ed., Junqueira L, Carneiro J, Kelley R (editors), Appleton & Lange, 1989. **HR** (for Histology Review) is occasionally used instead of a page reference to indicate that the information referred to can be found in this book.

4. The periodic acid-Schiff (PAS) reaction allows the localization of what class of substances in cells and tissues (20)?
5. Describe a typical enzyme histochemical reaction (22–23) in terms of:
   a. How the site of activity of a particular enzyme is marked
   b. Any special considerations necessary in preparing tissue for sectioning
6. Name 3 types of markers used to make antibodies visible with a microscope, allowing localization of specific antigens in cells and tissues (24, 25).
7. Compare the direct and indirect methods of immunohistochemistry in terms of procedure and sensitivity (25–26).

Multiple-Choice Questions

For questions 2–1 through 2–3, select the single best answer.

2–1. Basic histochemical and cytochemical principles include all of the following *except:*
- **A.** The method should be specific for the substance or chemical groups being studied
- **B.** The reaction product should be soluble
- **C.** The substance being analyzed must remain at its original site
- **D.** The reaction product should be colored or electron-scattering
- **E.** Tissue preparation must not denature or block the reactive groups

2–2. Of the following techniques, the one most commonly used to locate glycogen in cells is:
- **A.** Methylene blue staining
- **B.** Feulgen's reaction
- **C.** PAS reaction
- **D.** Enzyme histochemistry
- **E.** Immunohistochemistry

2–3. The most sensitive and specific method for localizing proteins in cells and tissues is:
- **A.** The direct method of immunohistochemistry
- **B.** The PAS reaction
- **C.** The Millon reaction
- **D.** The indirect method of immunohistochemistry
- **E.** Feulgen's reaction

MATCHING (questions 2–4 through 2–11): Each choice may be used once, more than once, or not at all.

- **A.** PAS technique
- **B.** Hematoxylin
- **C.** Enzyme histochemistry
- **D.** Immunohistochemistry
- **E.** None of the above

2–4. Used to locate the intracellular site of peroxidase activity
2–5. Commonly used to locate carbohydrates (eg, polysaccharides)
2–6. Technique useful in distinguishing lysosomes from other cytoplasmic granules and organelles
2–7. Commonly used to locate lipids
2–8. Commonly used to visualize nuclei
2–9. Highly specific method for localizing nonenzymatic proteins
2–10. Often used with fluorescent substances
2–11. Commoly used to locate ribosomes

For questions 2–12 through 2–16, one, more than one, or all of the answers may be correct. Select

A if only (1), (2), and (3) are correct
B if only (1) and (3) are correct
C if only (2) and (4) are correct
D if only (4) is correct
E if all answers are correct

2–12. Histochemical cytochemical techniques can be used to localize:
(1) Proteins
(2) Lipids
(3) Carbohydrates
(4) Specific ions

2–13. Histochemical techniques useful in the localization of nucleic acids include:
(1) Toluidine blue staining
(2) Feulgen's reaction
(3) Acridine orange staining
(4) Sudan IV or Sudan black staining

2–14. Markers commonly coupled to antibodies for use in immunohistochemistry include:
(1) Fluorescent compounds
(2) Enzymes
(3) Electron-scattering compounds
(4) Glycoconjugates

2–15. To prevent alteration or removal of targeted substances by fixatives and clearing agents, frozen sectioning may be required in preparing tissues for:
(1) Immunohistochemistry
(2) Demonstration of lipids
(3) Enzyme histochemistry
(4) Demonstration of catecholamines

2–16. In situ hybridization can be used to:
(1) Localize specific genes in cells and tissues
(2) Demonstrate the presence of specific nucleotide sequences in nucleic acids
(3) Localize specific mRNAs in cells and tissues
(4) Demonstrate the presence of specific amino acid sequences in proteins

The Cell 3

Objectives

This chapter should help the student to:

- Perceive the inseparability of structure and function in living organisms.
- Know the names and functions of the various structural components (organelles and cellular inclusions) of cells.
- Know the important subunits of each cellular component and the relationship of each subunit to the component's function.
- Name the general and specialized functions of cells, and know the role of the various cellular components in each function.
- Recognize a cell's structural components in a light or electron photomicrograph and from this predict the cell's function(s).
- Predict which structures will be present in a cell from its function.

- Predict the functional deficit(s) that would occur in a cell as a result of specific structural aberrations.
- Predict the cell component(s) most likely to be involved in a particular functional deficit.
- Understand and give examples of cell differentiation.

Synopsis

I. GENERAL FEATURES OF CELLS

A. Subunits of Life: Cells are the structural and functional units of life (and of disease processes) in all tissues, organs, and organ systems. Therefore, students of histology must perceive that a cell's capabilities and limitations are implicit in its structure and functions.

B. Prokaryotes and Eukaryotes: There are 2 basic cell types. Prokaryotic cells are typically small, single-celled organisms (eg, bacteria) that lack a nuclear envelope, histones, and membranous organelles. Eukaryotic cells exist primarily as components of multicellular organisms. This chapter covers the basic structural and functional features of eukaryotic cells. Specific human cell types are described in later chapters.

C. Cellular Components: Eukaryotic cells have 3 major components:

1. The **cell membranes** (II) separate a cell from its environment and form distinct functional compartments (nucleus, organelles) in the cell. The outer cell membrane is called the **plasma membrane,** or **plasmalemma.**

2. The membrane-bound **nucleus** (IV) contains a cell's DNA, which encodes the genetic information needed for protein synthesis and thus for all the activities of the cell. It also has components that help determine which parts of the genetic code are used and that deliver coded information to the cytoplasm.

3. The **cytoplasm** (III) surrounds the nucleus and is enclosed by the plasma membrane. It contains the structures and substances needed to decode the instructions of DNA and carry on the activities of the cell.

D. Cellular Functions: The 3 major activities characteristic of most living organisms are nourishment, growth and development, and reproduction. Basic functions directed toward these activities are described in this chapter. Other cell functions will receive more detailed treatment in later chapters.

II. CELL MEMBRANES

A. Biochemical Components:

1. Lipids Lipids are present in cell membranes as **phospholipids, sphingolipids,** and **cholesterol.** Phospholipids (eg, lecithin) are by far the most abundant. Each phospholipid molecule has a polar (hydrophilic) phosphate-containing head group and a nonpolar (hydrophobic) pair of fatty-acid tails. Membrane phospholipids are arranged in a bilayer with their tails directed toward one another at the center of the membrane. In electron micrographs of osmium-stained tissue, a single membrane, or **unit membrane,** has 2 dark outer lines with a lighter layer between them. This trilaminar appearance may be due to the deposition of reduced osmium on the hydrophilic head groups.

2. Protein Protein may comprise over 50% of membrane weight. Most membrane proteins are globular and belong to one of the following 2 groups:

a. Integral membrane proteins are tightly lodged in the lipid bilayer; detergents are required to extract them. They are folded, with their hydrophilic amino acids in contact with the phosphate groups of the membrane phospholipids and their hydrophobic amino acids in contact with the fatty-acid tails. Some protrude from only one membrane surface, while others, called **transmembrane proteins,** penetrate the entire membrane and protrude from both sides. Some transmembrane proteins, such as **protein-3-tetramer,** may serve as hydrophilic channels for the passage of water and water-soluble materials through hydrophobic regions.

b. Peripheral membrane proteins are more loosely associated with the inner or outer membrane surface; some are globular, some filamentous. In erythrocytes, examples on the cytoplasmic surface include **spectrin,** which helps maintain membrane integrity, and **ankyrin,** which links spectrin to the portion of protein-3-tetramer facing the cytoplasm.

3. Carbohydrates Carbohydrates occur on plasma membranes mainly as oligosaccharide moieties of membrane glycoproteins and glycolipids. Membrane oligosaccharides have a characteristic branching structure and project from the cell's outer surface, forming a superficial coat called the **glycocalyx** that participates in cell adhesion and recognition.

B. Membrane Organization: The widely accepted **fluid mosaic model** describes biologic membranes as "protein icebergs in a lipid sea." Integral proteins exhibit lateral mobility and may undergo rearrangement determined by their association with peripheral proteins, cytoskeletal filaments within the cell (III.I), membrane components of adjacent cells, and components of the extracellular matrix. Integral proteins not anchored by such associations sometimes diffuse to and accumulate in one membrane region, a process termed **capping.**

C. Membrane Functions:

1. Selective permeability The cell membrane forms an effective seal between a cell or organelle's internal and external environment, preventing intrusion of harmful substances, dispersion of macromolecules, and dilution of enzymes and substrates. However, membranes display selective permeability, essential to maintaining the functional steady state, or **homeostasis,** required for cell survival. Homeostatic mechanisms attributable to the cell membrane maintain optimal intracellular concentrations of ions, water, enzymes, and substrates. Three mechanisms allow passage of selected molecules.

a. Passive diffusion Certain substances (eg, water) can cross the membrane in either direction, following a concentration gradient. Passive diffusion does not require energy expenditure.

b. Facilitated diffusion Certain molecules (eg, glucose) cannot freely diffuse across membranes but must be helped across by a membrane component. This facilitated diffusion is often unidirectional, but it follows a concentration gradient and requires no energy.

c. Active transport Some nondiffusible molecules can move into or out of a cell either along or against a concentration gradient. Such movement requires energy, usually as ATP. An example of this active transport is the sodium pump (Na^+/K^+-ATPase), which can expel sodium ions from a cell even when the external sodium concentration is higher than the internal one.

2. Transduction of signals Receptors with strong binding affinities for extrinsic signals such as hormones are located at the cell surface. The signal molecule to which a receptor binds specifically is called its **ligand.** Once receptors bind their signal molecules, they may transmit the signal to the cell interior (a phenomenon called transduction of signals) by one of a variety of mechanisms:

a. Receptors may transmit the signal through their association with cytoskeletal components at the inner surface of the membrane.

b. Receptors may interact with other membrane components to produce second-messenger molecules, which then transmit the message to the cell's interior.

c. Signal-receptor complexes may be moved into the region of a coated pit and be endocytosed (see below), carrying the signal into the cell.

d. The receptor itself may have enzyme activity (stimulated by binding the signal molecule) and transmit the signal by enzymatically altering intracellular proteins.

3. Endocytosis Cells engulf extracellular substances and bring them into the cytoplasm in membrane-limited vesicles by mechanisms described collectively as endocytosis.

a. In **phagocytosis** ("cell eating"), the cell engulfs insoluble extracellular substances, such as large macromolecules or entire bacteria. The vesicles formed are termed **phagosomes.**

b. In **pinocytosis** ("cell drinking"), the cell engulfs small amounts of intercellular fluid, which may contain a variety of solutes. Pinocytotic vesicles are usually smaller than phagosomes.

c. In **receptor-mediated endocytosis,** the cell engulfs foreign substances along with their own surface receptors. Binding of ligand to receptor induces the collection of ligand-receptor complexes in **coated pits,** shallow membrane depressions with **clathrin** protein coats lining their cytoplasmic surfaces. Invagination and pinching off of the pit creates a **coated vesicle,** which carries the ligand-receptor complexes into the cell. The clathrin coating is released from the vesicle, now termed an **endosome,** and the ligands dissociate from the receptors. The later endosome, or CURL (*c*ompartment of *u*ncoupling of *re*ceptor and *l*igand), becomes more tubular and divides into 2 portions, segregating the receptors from the ligands. The receptors are returned to the plasma membrane, and the ligands are directed to lysosomes.

4. Exocytosis Exocytosis removes substances from the cell. Cells use this process both for secretion and for excretion of undigested material. A membrane-limited vesicle or secretory granule fuses with the plasma membrane and releases its contents into the extracellular space, without disrupting the plasma membrane.

5. Compartmentalization Membranes selectively inhibit the passage of most water-soluble substances. The cytoplasm has many membrane-limited compartments (organelles), each with a different internal environment with respect to concentrations of solutes. This compartmentalization prevents dilution of metabolic intermediates and cofactors in multistep biochemical reactions, and it protects sensitive reactions from intrusion of extraneous substances.

6. Spatiotemporal organization of metabolic processes Some cellular membranes (eg, the inner mitochondrial membrane and the Golgi complex) contain series of enzymes arranged so that intermediates in multistep metabolic processes are passed from one enzyme to the next. The spatial arrangement of enzymes maintains the chronologic order of such processes, and it sets rate limitations by maintaining particular concentrations of intermediates.

7. Storage, transport, and secretion Membrane-limited vesicles serve to isolate certain substances during intracellular processes. Substances in vesicles may be kept for later use (storage), shuttled from one compartment to another for further processing (transport; see Membrane Flow), or expelled from the cell (secretion, II.C.4).

D. Membrane Flow: The movement of membrane from one organelle to another is called membrane flow and is a general feature of organelle function. Membranes bud as vesicles from an organelle and fuse with another membrane, allowing the amount of membrane in a particular organelle to change without membrane synthesis or breakdown.

III. CYTOPLASM.

Cytoplasmic structures can be divided into 3 groups. **Organelles** are membrane-bound, enzyme-containing, permanent subcellular compartments (eg, mitochondria). Each type of organelle has a distinctive structure and performs unique functions. **Cytoplasmic inclusions** are structures, membrane-bound or not, that are generally more transient than organelles and less actively involved in cell metabolism (eg, lipid droplets). Organelles and inclusions are discussed in sections III.A–III.H. The **cytoskeleton (III.I)** is composed of proteinaceous elements that form a supporting network within the cytoplasm; some of these elements (microtubules) also form discrete cytoplasmic structures such as centrioles.

A. Mitochondria:

The largest of the cytoplasmic organelles, mitochondria are the energy providers (''powerhouses'') of the cell.

1. Structure Mitochondria are comparable in size to bacteria (usually 2–6 μm in length and 0.2 μm in diameter but quite variable) and have various shapes: spheric, ovoid, filamentous. Each mitochondrion is bounded by 2 unit membranes.

a. The **outer mitochondrial membrane** has a smooth contour and forms a continuous but relatively porous covering. It is freely permeable to various small molecules.

b. The **inner mitochondrial membrane** is less porous and is therefore semipermeable. It has numerous infoldings, or **cristae,** that project into the mitochondrion's interior. The mitochondrial cristae of most cells are shelflike, but those in steroid-secreting cells are typically more tubular. The inner surface of the inner membrane is covered by **inner membrane subunits,** also called **F1 subunits** (or lollipops, because of their shape); these are the sites of mitochondrial **ATPase** activity. Mitochondrial ribosomes are also associated with the inner surface. Intercalated within the inner membrane are components of the **electron transport system,** including enzymes and cofactors with important roles in mitochondrial function (eg, cytochromes, dehydrogenases, flavoproteins).

c. The mitochondrial membranes create 2 membrane-limited spaces. The **intermembrane space** is located between the inner and outer membranes and is continuous with the **intracristal space** that extends into the cristae. The **intercristal space,** or **matrix space,** is enclosed by the inner membrane and contains the mitochondrial matrix.

d. The **mitochondrial matrix** contains water, solutes, and large **matrix granules,** believed to be concerned with mitochondrial calcium-ion concentrations. It also contains **circular DNA** and **mitochondrial ribosomes** similar to those of bacteria. The matrix contains numerous soluble enzymes involved in such specialized mitochondrial functions as the **Krebs cycle** (citric acid cycle, tricarboxylic acid cycle), **β-oxidation** of lipids, and mitochondrial DNA synthesis.

2. Function Mitochondria provide the cell with the energy for chemical and mechanical work by storing energy generated from cellular metabolites in the high-energy bonds of ATP. The ATP leaves the mitochondrion and releases its stored energy at a variety of intracellular sites. Mitochondria synthesize their own DNA and some proteins. They grow and reproduce by fission or budding and can undergo rapid movement and shape changes.

3. Location Mitochondria are found in nearly all eukaryotic cells, and in most they are dispersed throughout the cytoplasm. However, they accumulate in the highest concentrations in cell types and intracellular regions with the highest energy requirements. Cardiac muscle cells are notable for the abundance of their mitochondria. Epithelial cells lining the kidney tubules have abundant mitochondria interdigitated between basal plasma membrane infoldings where active transport of ions and water occurs.

B. Ribosomes:

The ribosomes are protein-synthesizing organelles. There are 2 basic types. Mitochondrial (like prokaryotic) ribosomes are smaller (20 nm) than the cytoplasmic ribosomes of eukaryotes (25 nm).

1. Structure Each type of ribosome has 2 unequal **ribosomal subunits,** named for their sedimentation rates during ultracentrifugation (but often called simply ''large'' and "small"). Mitochondrial ribosomes have a 50S and a 30S subunit; cytoplasmic ribosomes (80S overall) have a 60S and a 40S subunit. Cytoplasmic ribosomes are composed of **ribosomal RNA (rRNA)** synthesized in the nucleolus and associated proteins synthesized in the cytoplasm. They are intensely basophilic. Light microscopy reveals cytoplasmic accumulations of ribosomes as basophilic patches, formerly termed **ergastoplasm** in glandular cells and **Nissl bodies** in neurons. In electron micrographs, ribosomes appear as small, electron-dense cytoplasmic granules.

2. Location and function Cytoplasmic ribosomes occur in 2 forms. **Free ribosomes** are individual ribosomes dispersed in cytoplasm. **Polyribosomes,** or **polysomes,** are groups of ribosomes evenly distributed along a single strand of messenger RNA (mRNA), an arrangement that permits synthesis of multiple copies of a protein from the same message. Polysomal ribosomes read (translate) the mRNA code and thus play a critical role in assembling amino acids into specific proteins. Polysomes are found free in the cytoplasm (free polysomes) and attached to membranes of the rough endoplasmic reticulum (polysomes of the endoplasmic reticulum). Free polysomes are involved in the synthesis of structural proteins and enzymes for intracellular use. Polysomes of the rough endoplasmic reticulum are involved in synthesizing proteins that are secreted or isolated.

C. Endoplasmic Reticulum: The endoplasmic reticulum (ER) is a complex organelle involved in the synthesis, packaging, and processing of various cell substances. It is a freely anastomosing network (reticulum) of membranes that form **vesicles,** or **cisternae;** these may be elongated, flattened, rounded, or tubular. **Transfer vesicles** (transitional vesicles) are small, membrane-limited vesicles that bud from the ER and cross the intervening cytoplasm to reach the Golgi complex for further processing or packaging of their contents. In fully differentiated cells, ER occurs in 2 forms, called rough and smooth.

1. Rough endoplasmic reticulum

a. Structure The rough endoplasmic reticulum (RER), also called granular endoplasmic reticulum, is studded with ribosomes, many of them in polysomal clusters. RER cisternae are typically parallel, flattened, and elongated, especially in cells specialized for protein secretion (eg, pancreatic acinar cells, plasma cells), in which RER is particularly abundant. The ribosomes give RER basophilic staining properties. The fine structure of RER (membranes and individual ribosomes) is visible only with the electron microscope. Proteins unique to RER membranes include **docking protein,** which functions as a receptor, and **ribophorins I and II.**

b. Function RER is mainly concerned with the synthesis of proteins for sequestration from the rest of the cytoplasm, ie, secretory proteins such as collagen, proteins for incorporation into cell membranes, and lysosomal enzymes (separated from the rest of the cytoplasm to prevent **autolysis**). Ribosomes or free polysomes begin reading at the 5′ end of mRNAs and move toward the 3′ end. The 5′ end of mRNAs for secretory and sequestered proteins carries the code for a 20- to 25-amino acid **signal sequence.** The signal sequence is translated first on a free polysome and interacts with a **signal recognition particle (SRP),** which is 6 polypeptides plus a 7S RNA molecule. SRP inhibits further translation until the SRP-polyribosome complex binds to the RER docking protein; then the SRP is released and translation continues. Ribophorins I and II mediate the attachment of the large ribosomal subunit to the RER membrane. They may also provide a hydrophilic channel for **vectorial discharge** (unidirectional passage) of nascent protein into the RER lumen, where the signal sequence is cleaved by **signal peptidase** and the remainder of the nascent protein is folded and modified. One important posttranslational modification is **core glycosylation:** Oligosaccharides, usually high in mannose residues, are transferred from a lipid carrier (eg, dolichol phosphate) to amino acids, especially asparagine. The oligosaccharides may "address" proteins for transport to intracellular destinations.

c. Location The RER is suspended in the cytoplasm and shows continuity at various points along the outer membrane of the nuclear envelope. RER in protein-secreting epithelial cells often lies in the basal cytoplasm, between the basal plasma membrane and the nucleus.

2. Smooth endoplasmic reticulum

a. Structure The smooth endoplasmic reticulum (SER) lacks ribosomes and thus appears smooth in electron micrographs. SER cisternae are more tubular or vesicular than those of RER. SER stains poorly, if at all, so with the light microscope it is indistinguishable from the rest of the cytoplasm.

b. Function Because it lacks ribosomes, the SER cannot synthesize proteins. It has many enzymes, important in lipid metabolism, steroid hormone synthesis, glycogen synthesis (glucose-6-phosphatase), and detoxification. The last occurs via enzymatic conjugation, oxidation, and methylation of potentially toxic substances.

c. Location The SER is suspended in the cytoplasm of many cells and is especially abundant in cells that synthesize steroid hormones (eg, cells of the adrenal cortex and the gonads). It is also abundant in liver cells (hepatocytes), where it is involved in glycogen synthesis and drug detoxification. Specialized SER termed **sarcoplasmic reticulum** is found in striated muscle cells, where it helps to regulate muscle contraction by sequestering and releasing calcium ions.

D. Golgi Complex: The **Golgi complex** (Golgi apparatus) participates in many activities, particularly those associated with secretion. It has an essential role in coordinating membrane flow and vesicle traffic among organelles.

1. Structure This membranous organelle is composed of 3 major compartments: (1) a conspicuous stack of 3–10 discrete, slightly curved, flattened cisternae; (2) numerous small vesicles peripheral to the stack; and (3) a few large vacuoles, sometimes called **condensing vacuoles,** at the concave surface of the stack. The ***cis* face** (convex face, forming face) of the stack is usually closest to adjacent dilated ER cisternae and is surrounded by transfer vesicles. Its cisternae stain more darkly with osmium. The ***trans* face** (concave face, maturing face) often harbors several condensing vacuoles and generally faces away from the nucleus.

2. Functions

a. Polysaccharide synthesis The Golgi complex contains various **glycosyltransferases** that initiate or lengthen polysaccharide or oligosaccharide chains, adding one sugar at a time.

b. Modification of secretory products Golgi enzymes are involved in the glycosylation of proteins and lipids and the sulfation of glycosaminoglycans (GAGs). The Golgi complex is thus important in the synthesis of secretory glycoproteins, proteoglycans, glycolipids, and sulfated GAGs.

c. Packaging of secretory products Products synthesized by the ER are packaged in vesicles by the Golgi complex. These secretory vesicles, or **secretory granules,** are transported to the plasma membrane for exocytosis.

d. Concentration and storage of secretory products The Golgi complexes of some cells concentrate and store secretory products prior to secretion. Such concentration is a major function of the condensing vacuoles on the *trans* face of the Golgi complex, which also often serve as precursors to secretory granules.

3. Location The Golgi complex is typically near the nucleus (juxtanuclear) and is often found near centrioles (which may also have an important role in directing vesicle traffic). Golgi complexes are best developed in neurons and glandular cells, which are specialized for secretion.

4. Flow of materials through the Golgi complex Secretory materials have long been thought to follow a one-way route through the Golgi complex. In this scheme, transfer vesicles bud from the ER and fuse with the forming (*cis*) face. The vesicle contents are then modified as they pass successively from cisterna to cisterna toward the maturing (*trans*) face, which buds off the secretory vesicles containing the final product. However, this view is now being challenged as an oversimplification. The role of the Golgi complex in packaging lysosomal enzymes is also controversial; some think that the main site for packaging such enzymes is the **GERL** (*G*olgi, *E*ndoplasmic *R*eticulum, *L*ysosome). The GERL consists of elements of the endoplasmic reticulum located near the *trans* face of the Golgi complex and contains lysosomal enzymes.

E. Phagosomes: Phagosomes are membrane-limited vesicles of varying size containing material destined for lysosomal digestion. Two major types are known. **Heterophagosomes** contain the products of **heterophagy,** ie, material of extracellular origin ingested by phagocytosis. **Autophagosomes** contain the products of **autophagy,** ie, material of intracellular origin such as worn or damaged organelles. The digestion of phagosomal contents begins when a phagosome fuses with one or more primary lysosomes to form a secondary lysosome, as described below. (***Note:*** Some authors use the term heterophagosome to refer to secondary lysosomes.)

F. Lysosomes: Lysosomes are spheric, membrane-limited vesicles that may contain more than 50 enzymes each and function as the cellular digestive system. Their characteristic enzyme activities distinguish them from other cellular granules. The enzyme most widely exploited for their identification is **acid phosphatase,** because it occurs almost exclusively in lysosomes. Other enzymes common in lysosomes are ribonucleases, deoxyribonucleases, cathepsins, sulfatases, β-glucuronidase, and phospholipases and other proteases, glucosidases, and lipases. Lysosomal enzymes usually occur as glycoproteins and are most active at an acidic pH. Lysosomes occur in various sizes and electron densities, depending on their level of activity.

1. Primary lysosomes are small (5–8 nm in diameter), with electron-dense contents; they appear as black circles in electron micrographs. They are the storage form of lysosomes, and their enzymes are mostly inactive. Lysosomal enzymes synthesized and core-glycosylated in the RER are transferred to the Golgi complex for further glycosylation; it is uncertain whether their final packaging as primary lysosomes occurs in the Golgi complex or in GERL. The primary lysosomes disperse through the cytoplasm. They are found in most cells but are most abundant in phagocytic cells (eg, macrophages, neutrophils).

2. Secondary lysosomes are larger and less electron-dense and have a mottled appearance in electron micrographs. They are formed by the fusion of one or more primary lysosomes with a phagosome. Their primary function is the digestion of products of heterophagy and autophagy; when the lysosomal enzymes mix with the phagosome contents, they become active. Digestion produces usable metabolites for cell maintenance and growth (small usable molecules diffuse into the surrounding cytoplasm) and aids in the turnover of organelles. Lysosomal enzymes also catabolize certain products of cell synthesis, thus regulating the quality and quantity of secretory material. Secondary lysosomes occur throughout the cytoplasm in many cells, in numbers that reflect the cell's lysosomal and phagocytic activity.

3. Residual bodies are membrane-limited inclusions of varying size and electron density associated with the terminal phases of lysosome function. They contain undigestible materials such as pigments, crystals, and certain lipids. Some cells (eg, macrophages) expel residual bodies as waste, but long-lived cells (eg, nerve, muscle) tend to accumulate them. In the latter, waste-containing residual bodies reflect cellular aging and may be referred to as "**wear-and-tear pigment,**" or **lipofuscin granules.** These granules appear yellowish brown with light microscopy and as electron-dense particles in electron micrographs.

G. Peroxisomes: Peroxisomes are membrane-limited, enzyme-containing vesicles somewhat larger than primary lysosomes. In some animals (not humans), they are distinguishable from lysosomes by an electron-dense, granular **nucleoid** of urate oxidase. Peroxisomes function in hydrogen peroxide metabolism. They contain urate oxidase, hydroxyacid oxidase, and D-amino acid oxidase, which produce hydrogen peroxide capable of killing bacteria; they also contain catalase, which oxidizes various substrates and uses the hydrogen removed in the process to convert the toxic hydrogen peroxide to water. Peroxisomes also participate in gluconeogenesis by assisting in the β-oxidation of fatty acids. They are found dispersed in the cytoplasm or in association with the SER.

H. Other Cytoplasmic Inclusions: Prominent among inclusions serving as storage depots are spheric **lipid droplets,** which differ in appearance depending upon the type of histologic preparation. **Glycogen granules** are inclusions that are PAS-positive in light microscopy and appear in electron micrographs as rosettes of electron-dense particles. Both lipid droplets and glycogen granules lack a limiting membrane. **Melanin** is a brownish pigment widely distributed in vertebrates, often found in electron-dense, membrane-limited granules termed **melanosomes.** It is particularly abundant in epidermal cells and in the pigment layer of the retina.

I. Cytoskeleton: The cytoskeleton, a mesh of filamentous elements called **microtubules, microfilaments,** and **intermediate filaments,** provides structural stability for the maintenance of cell shape. It is important in cell movement and in the rearrangement of cytoplasmic components. In one model of cytoplasmic organization, organelles and cytoplasmic inclusions are embedded in a delicate meshwork termed the **microtrabecular lattice,** which incorporates the cytoskeleton, enzymes, and other cytoplasmic constituents previously considered soluble and randomly dispersed in an amorphous **cytosol.** This hypothetic lattice may provide a framework for coordinated arrays of enzymes involved in multistep reactions, as do some membranes (II.C.6). However, recent evidence suggests that the latticelike appearance of the cytoplasm is a fixation artifact.

1. Microtubules

a. Structure Microtubules are the thickest components of the cytoskeleton, with diameters of 24 nm. They are fine tubular structures of variable length, with dense walls (5 nm thick) and a clear internal space (14 nm in internal diameter). The walls are composed of subunits called **tubulin heterodimers,** each of which consists of one α-tubulin and one β-tubulin protein molecule. The tubulin heterodimers are arranged in **protofilaments.** Thirteen of these threadlike polymers of α- and β-tubulin align parallel to one another to form the wall of each microtubule. Microtubules increase in length by adding new heterodimers to one end, called the **nucleation site.** This polymerization can be controlled experimentally by regulating calcium ion concentration or by treating cells with antimitotic alkaloids. **Colchicine** blocks the process by binding to the nucleation site. **Vinblastine** disrupts microtubules by binding to tubulin.

b. Function Microtubules have roles in maintenance of cell shape, axoplasmic transport in neurons, melanin dispersion in pigment cells, chromosome movements during mitosis, and the shuttling of vesicles within the cell. Unlike microfilaments, microtubules are unable to contract. Shortening occurs via depolymerization.

c. Location Microtubules are found throughout the cytoplasm of most cells and in highly organized groupings in centrioles, cilia, flagella, basal bodies, and the mitotic spindle apparatus.

1. Centrioles

(a.) Structure A centriole is a cylindric group of microtubules, 150 nm in overall diameter and 350–500 nm long, containing 9 microtubule **triplets** in a pinwheel array. Each microtubule in a triplet shares a portion of the wall of the neighboring microtubule. An interphase (nondividing) cell has a pair of adjacent centrioles with perpendicular long axes, each surrounded by several electron-dense satellites, or **pericentriolar bodies.** Other cytoplasmic microtubules originate from the pericentriolar bodies and radiate into the cytoplasm.

(b.) Function Centrioles are the structural organizers of the cell. Centriole duplication is a prerequisite for cell division, and during mitosis the centrioles organize the microtubules of the mitotic spindle. Even in vitro, isolated centrioles can control microtubule polymerization; in the cell, centrioles may transmit unknown physical organizing forces via the microtubules originating from pericentriolar bodies. Through their effects on microtubules, centrioles may have some control over organelle, vesicle, and granule organization and movements within the cell. Centrioles give rise to basal bodies (see below).

(c.) Location Between cell divisions, centrioles are near the nucleus, often surrounded by Golgi complexes. The centrioles and associated Golgi complexes constitute the cell **cytocenter,** which appears as a clear zone near the nucleus. During the S phase of interphase, each centriole duplicates by giving rise to a **procentriole** that grows at right angles to the original. During mitosis, the new centriole pairs migrate to opposite cell poles to organize the spindle.

(2.) Basal bodies In cells bearing cilia or flagella, centrioles migrate to the apical plasma membrane and give rise to basal bodies in a manner similar to centriole self-duplication. Basal bodies are structurally similar to centrioles, with 9 microtubule triplets. They occur in the cytoplasm, one at the base of each cilium or flagellum, and serve as the anchoring points and microtubule organizers for these structures.

(3.) Cilia A ciliated cell usually has hundreds of cilia, motile 5–10 μm long, 0.2 μm wide, cell-surface evaginations covered by plasma membrane. Each cilium contains a core, or **axoneme,** composed of 9 peripheral microtubule **doublets** surrounding a pair of unjoined microtubules (the "9 + 2" arrangement). Partners in a doublet are called subfibers A and B. Subfiber A is a complete microtubule, having 13 tubulin **protofilaments.** Subfiber B has 10 or 11 protofilaments and is completed by sharing part of its partner's wall. A pair of arms made of **dynein** (a protein with ATPase activity) extends from the wall of each subfiber A toward the adjacent doublet. Protein bridges called **nexins** link adjacent doublets, and **radial spokes** link the doublets to the sheath surrounding the central microtubule pair. Each axoneme is organized by and anchored in a basal body.

(4.) Flagella A flagellum is like a cilium, but it is longer, and there is usually only one or 2 flagella on a cell. In humans and other mammals, flagella occur only in the tails of spermatozoa, which are typically 50–55 μm long and 0.2–0.5 μm thick along most of their length. The axoneme of a flagellum is identical to that of a cilium.

(5.) Mitotic spindle apparatus The spindle-shaped microtubule array called the mitotic spindle apparatus occurs between 2 pairs of centrioles at opposite poles of mitotic cells. Some spindle microtubules (continuous fibers) extend from centriole to centriole. Others (chromosomal fibers) extend from one centriole to the centromere of a chromosome. The spindle apparatus is crucial for chromosome separation during mitosis.

2. Microfilaments

a. Structure Microfilaments are the thinnest cytoskeletal components (5–7 nm wide). They are usually composed of one of several types of **actin** protein. In striated muscle cells, actin filaments form a stable paracrystalline array in association with filaments of myosin. Actin filaments in other cells are less stable and can dissociate and reassemble. These changes are regulated in part by calcium ions and cyclic AMP and by **actin-binding proteins** in the cytoplasm.

b. Function Microfilaments are contractile, but to contract, they usually must interact with myosin. In muscle cells, myosin forms thick filaments. In nonmuscle cells, it exists in soluble form. Treatment with **cytochalasins** disrupts microfilament organization and interferes with the following functions: endocytosis; exocytosis; contraction of microvilli; cell movement; movement of organelles, vesicles, and granules; cytoplasmic streaming; maintenance of cell shape; and equatorial constriction of dividing cells.

c. Location In nonmuscle cells, microfilaments are generally distributed as an irregular meshwork throughout the cytoplasm. In addition, local accumulations may be present as a thin sheath beneath the plasma membrane called the **terminal web,** as parallel strands in cores of microvilli, in the cytoplasm at the leading edge of various types of pseudopods, in association with organelles or other cytoplasmic components, or as a belt ("purse string") around the equator of dividing cells.

3. Intermediate filaments

a. Structure Intermediate filaments are intermediate in thickness (10–12 nm) between microtubules and microfilaments. They are composed of proteins that are structurally related to nuclear lamins and differ depending on the cell type. Examples of intermediate filament proteins: **cytokeratins** in epithelial cells, **vimentin** in mesenchymally derived cells (eg, fibroblasts, chondrocytes), **desmin** in muscle cells, **glial fibrillary acidic protein** inglial cells, **neurofilaments** (intermediate filament bundles) in neurons.

b. Function The function of intermediate filaments is currently being investigated. They are probably involved in maintenance of cell shape, possibly as components of the microtrabecular lattice. The significance of their relationship to nuclear lamins is not clear.

c. Location Most intermediate filament types are distributed throughout the cytoplasm. Their apparently random distribution may represent a highly ordered arrangement that is not yet understood. One example of an ordered arrangement of intermediate filaments is the cytokeratin-containing tonofilaments of desmosomes, discussed in Chapter 4.

IV. NUCLEUS

A. General Considerations: Nuclei vary in appearance from tissue to tissue and cell to cell, but they generally have a nuclear envelope, chromatin, nucleoplasm, and one to several nucleoli. Although certain mature cells (eg, erythrocytes) lack nuclei, at least one nucleus is present at some stage in all eukaryotic cells. The nucleus contains a linear code (DNA) for the synthesis of cell components and products, conferring upon the cell a range of adaptability to changing environmental conditions and to extrinsic signals such as hormones. The microscopic appearance of the nucleus is important in identifying and classifying both normal and diseased cells and tissues. Nuclei display wide variations in (1) size, both absolute and relative to the amount of cytoplasm (nucleocytoplasmic ratio); (2) number per cell, allowing classification of cells as enucleate, mononucleate, binucleate, or multinucleate; (3) chromatin pattern, ie, the amount and distribution of heterochromatin; and (4) location, eg, basal, central, eccentric.

B. Nuclear Envelope: The nuclear contents are set apart from the cytoplasm by a double membrane called the nuclear envelope and a narrow (40–70 nm) intermembrane space called the **perinuclear cisterna,** or perinuclear space. The nuclear envelope is often considered an extension of the RER, because its outer surface is often peppered with ribosomes and shows occasional continuities with the RER. The inside of the inner membrane is lined with the **fibrous lamina,** a layer consisting of proteins called **lamins.** The envelope is perforated by many **nuclear pores,** each of which has a diameter of about 70 nm and is bounded by 8 globular subunits called **annular proteins,** which present an octagonal appearance in some preparations. Each pore is covered by a proteinaceous **diaphragm** that is thinner than the envelope. The pores provide a channel for the movement of important molecules between the nucleus and cytoplasm; these molecules include nucleic acids synthesized in the nucleus and used in the cytoplasm (mRNA, rRNA, tRNA) and proteins synthesized in the cytoplasm and used in the nucleus (histones, polymerases).

C. Chromatin: Nuclear chromatin is an intensely basophilic substance consisting of DNA and associated histone and nonhistone proteins.

1. Nucleosomes Isolated chromatin appears in electron micrographs as thin strands studded with beadlike particles at regular intervals. Each strand is a double-helical molecule of DNA, and the particles are the repeating structural subunits of chromatin termed nucleosomes. Each nucleosome is composed of 166 base pairs of the DNA strand coiled tightly around a core of 8 **histones** (2 copies each of H2A, H2B, H3, and H4). The portion of the strand between 2 nucleosomes contains an additional 48 base pairs and is called the linker region. Another histone (usually H1) is bound to the outside of the nucleosome and to the linker. The beaded strand coils into a superhelix with 6 nucleosomes per turn (selenoid) to form the condensed form of chromatin, ie, heterochromatin.

2. Chromatin types Nuclei containing highly coiled chromatin, termed **heterochromatin,** stain darkly with basic dyes. Because the DNA of chromatin must uncoil to be transcribed, cells with dark-staining (heterochromatic) nuclei are less active in DNA transcription than other cells, using a smaller portion of their total genome. Uncoiled chromatin, termed **euchromatin,** stains poorly and is difficult to distinguish even with electron microscopy. Large, pale-staining (euchromatic) nuclei usually indicate greater transcriptional activity and faster cell division.

3. Chromatin pattern Differences in the amount and distribution of nuclear chromatin are often used to identify cell types, especially in cells with no characteristic cytoplasmic staining properties. Even in mostly euchromatic nuclei, a rim of heterochromatin is often found on the inner surface of the nuclear envelope in association with the fibrous lamina. This envelope-associated heterochromatin allows resolution of the nuclear boundary with the light microscope.

4. Chromosomes The chromosomes, the most highly condensed form of chromatin, are visible during mitosis. To form chromosomes, selenoids fold further and wind on a central nonhistone protein scaffold. Of the 23 chromosome pairs in human somatic cells, 22 (somatic chromosomes) consist of 2 structurally similar chromosomes. The other pair (sex chromosomes) consists of structurally dissimilar chromosomes (XY) in males and similar ones (XX) in females. In females, only one X chromosome (either of the 2) is used by each cell; the inactive X chromosome is often visible as a clump of heterochromatin termed **sex chromatin,** or the **Barr body.** In most cells, the Barr body is attached to the inner surface of the nuclear envelope. In a neutrophilic leukocyte, it may appear as a drumstick-shaped appendage of the lobulated nucleus.

5. Karyotyping A cell's **karyotype** is its chromosome inventory or a picture of its chromosomes arranged by chromosome type. Preparing such a picture is called karyotyping. Cells in culture are stimulated to enter mitosis with phytohemagglutinin (a plant-derived mitogen). The dividing cells are treated with colchicine to arrest them in metaphase, when the chromosomes are highly coiled and visible. Lysis of the cells with a hypotonic solution causes the chromosomes to spread out on the slide with little or no overlapping. The chromosome spread is photographed, and pictures of the chromosomes are cut out, paired, and assembled into a specific sequence. Karyotyping allows cataloging of chromosomes for detection of structural abnormalities and deleted or excess chromosomes.

D. Nucleolus: During interphase (between mitoses), each nucleus usually has at least one (or 2) intensely basophilic body called a nucleolus. Nucleoli are the synthesis sites for most ribosomal RNA (rRNA). They are usually distinguishable from heterochromatin but may be obscured in very dark nuclei. They are largest and most numerous in embryonic cells, cells actively synthesizing proteins, and rapidly growing malignant tumor cells. A small amount of heterochromatin is attached to the nucleolus; the significance of this **nucleolus-associated chromatin** is unknown. The nucleolus disappears in preparation for mitosis and reappears after mitosis is completed. Distinct nucleolar components can be seen with the electron microscope.

1. The name **pars amorpha** refers to the pale-staining nucleolar region(s) containing **nucleolar organizer DNA,** which carries the code for rRNA. Five chromosome pairs have nucleolar organizer regions in humans. Thus, up to 10 nucleoli per cell are possible, but fusion of the organizers into fewer, larger nucleoli is more common. Newly synthesized rRNA appears first in this region.

2. The term **nucleolonema** is used by light microscopists to refer to a threadlike basophilic substructure of the nucleolus. The nucleolonema contains 2 rRNA-rich components distinguishable by electron microscopy.

a. The **pars fibrosa** consists of densely packed ribonucleoprotein fibers, 5–10 nm in diameter. These fibers consist of the newly synthesized primary transcripts of the rRNA genes and associated proteins. Newly synthesized rRNA appears second in this region.

b. The **pars granulosa** contains dense granules, 15–20 nm in diameter, that represent maturing ribosomal subunits during assembly for export to the cytoplasm. Newly synthesized rRNA appears third in this region.

E. Nucleoplasm: The nucleoplasm is the matrix in which the other intranuclear components are embedded. It is composed of enzymatic and nonenzymatic proteins, metabolites, ions, and water. It includes the **nuclear matrix**—a fibrillar "nucleoskeletal" structure that appears to bind certain hormone receptors—and newly synthesized DNA.

V. CELL FUNCTIONS.

Cells are both empowered and constrained by their available resources. The amounts and types of energy and raw materials at their disposal, the information encoded in their genes, and the intrinsic and extrinsic factors that control their access to that information are the major determinants of cell function. Cells in tissues undergoing growth or repair use a large part of their resources in preparing for, and carrying out, cell division. Fully differentiated cells typically concentrate on more specialized functions such as secretion and contraction. Maintaining a constant internal environment (homeostasis), even in apparently quiescent cells, requires the expenditure of significant amounts of energy and other resources.

A. Cellular Reproduction: The reproductive cycle of a cell is termed the **cell cycle.** Each complete cycle ends with cell division **(mitosis)** and results in the production of 2 daughter cells, each about half the size of the parent.

1. Mitosis and interphase Early views of cellular reproduction focused on easily detected structural changes during mitosis. The apparently inactive phase between successive mitoses seemed a resting period and was dubbed **interphase.** Yet, even in rapidly dividing cells, the time spent in mitosis is very brief compared to that spent in interphase. We now know that cells carry out many important activities during interphase, including those needed to recover from the previous, and to prepare for the next, mitosis. Both mitosis and interphase are now viewed as complex and important components of the cell cycle and have each been divided into a series of steps to facilitate our understanding of cellular reproduction.

2. The steps in cell division (mitosis) Mitosis is a brief, continuous process. Structural changes observed during this complex process have been used to divide it into 4 successive phases: prophase, metaphase, anaphase, and telophase.

a. During **prophase,** the chromatin coils extensively to form chromosomes. As the nucleolar organizer DNA is coiled into its respective chromosomes, the nucleoli disperse and begin to disappear. The nuclear membrane remains intact. The 2 pairs of centrioles migrate to opposite poles of the cell, and the mitotic spindle apparatus begins to assemble between the centriole pairs.

b. During **metaphase,** the nucleolus and the nuclear envelope disappear. The chromosomes line up at the cell equator between the centriole pairs, and each chromosome splits lengthwise to form a pair of **sister chromatids.** Each chromosome has a **centromere (kinetochore),** to which microtubules of the spindle apparatus attach.

c. During **anaphase,** sister chromatids separate and move to opposite poles of the now-elliptical cell along the mitotic spindle. The centromere leads, with the chromatin dragging behind, often in a V shape. The separation mechanism is unknown, but the chromatids appear to be pulled by the spindle microtubules.

d. During **telophase,** the chromosomes begin to uncoil. Nucleoli and nuclear envelopes appear as components of 2 separate nuclei at opposite ends of the cell. A **purse-string constriction,** formed by bands of microfilaments beneath the plasma membrane, appears at the equator. Tightening of the constriction eventually divides the cytoplasm and organelles between the daughter cells.

B. The Cell Cycle: The cell cycle model takes into account important but less visible changes in the cell between divisions. It retains the 4 phases of mitosis but focuses on the timing of DNA synthesis and divides interphase into 3 phases; G_1, S, and G_2.

1. The **G_1 (gap 1)** phase of interphase follows telophase of mitosis. A gap is a period during which no DNA synthesis occurs, as shown by the fact that no radiolabeled thymidine (^{3}H-thymidine) is incorporated into the cell's DNA. RNA and protein synthesis do occur during the gap phases, and each daughter cell grows to about the size of the parent. G_1, usually the longest phase of the cycle, is also the most variable in length among different cell types. In rapidly dividing cells, G_1 is short and the transition to subsequent phases is continuous. More highly differentiated cells may pull out of the cycle and enter a phase called G_0, in which preparations for mitosis are suspended in favor of specialized functions. G_0 cells unable to reenter the cycle (eg, muscle and nerve cells) are **terminally differentiated.** Other cells in G_0 (eg, hepatocytes and fibroblasts) can reenter the cell cycle in response to injury.

2. During the **S (synthesis)** phase, DNA synthesis and replication occur, as shown by ^{3}H-thymidine uptake. The centrioles often self-duplicate during this stage.

3. During **G_2 (gap 2),** the final preparations for cell division occur, including synthesis of tubulin for the spindle apparatus and accumulation of ATP for the energy-expensive mitosis. Very little synthesis occurs during mitosis.

C. Cellular Differentiation: Refinements in cell structure and function accompany embryonic and fetal development, as well as maturation and aging. This process of cellular differentiation generally results in a cell's having fewer but more efficient capabilities than an embryonic cell. The functions of a differentiated cell can be roughly gauged by the organelles it contains. For example, cells specialized for protein secretion contain abundant RER and a well-developed Golgi complex. While differentiation can result in dramatic changes, it does not occur suddenly. It is accomplished in a series of steps, often separated by one or more passes through the cell cycle, and involves interactions between the cell's environment, the metabolic machinery in its cytoplasm, and the information in its DNA.

D. Intercellular Communication: Tissues, organs, and organ systems are collections of cells and cell products that must act in concert to carry out their complex functions. The embryonic cells that ultimately form a tissue develop communication strategies early in embryogenesis. Many types of intercellular communication occur—some direct, some indirect.

1. Direct communication In some tissues, especially the epithelia, cells have direct contact with their neighbors over large areas of their surface membranes. These areas of contact are often marked by specialized plasma membrane structures called junctional complexes (see Chapter 4). Some components of junctional complexes are specialized for attachment (physical communication), whereas others (gap junctions) provide cytoplasmic channels for transmission of electrical and chemical signals.

2. Indirect communication Signals can also be transmitted from one cell to another even without the cells being in contact. In proximal communication, the signal traverses a short distance, eg, hormones or other signal molecules may be produced by one cell type and have effects on another cell type in the same tissue. In cell-to-cell recognition or in contact inhibition of cell division, signal transmission may require temporary physical contact. In distal communication, the signal travels farther, eg, when hormone-producing cells in one tissue ellicit responses from targets in different tissues.

Study-Focusing Questions*

1. Compare prokaryotic and eukaryotic cells (28) in terms of:
   a. The presence of a membrane-limited nucleus
   b. The presence of histones
   c. The presence of membranous organelles in the cytoplasm
   d. Their size
2. Compare organelles and cytoplasmic inclusions (28, 30) in terms of:
   a. The presence of limiting membranes
   b. Their content of enzymes
   c. The level of their participation (active or passive) in cell function
   d. The permanence of their residence in the cytoplasm
3. List several functions of cell membranes (30).
4. List the major biochemical constituents of cell membranes (30–31) and sketch their organization as described in the fluid mosaic model of membrane structure (32).
5. Explain why a membrane's phospholipid bilayer appears as a trilaminar structure in transmission electron micrographs (30).
6. Compare peripheral and integral membrane proteins (31, 32) in terms of:
   a. Their location in association with lipid bilayers of membranes
   b. The methods required to isolate them from membranes
7. Compare phagocytosis (33) and pinocytosis (32) in terms of the:
   a. Way vacuoles or vesicles are formed
   b. Types of materials endocytosed
   c. Relative size of the vacuoles and vesicles
8. List the steps involved in receptor-mediated endocytosis, beginning with the association of a ligand with its cell-surface receptor and ending with the return of the receptor to the cell surface (32–33).
9. What is the major function of mitochondria (33)?
10. Sketch a mitochondrion (29) and label or show the location of the following:
    a. Outer mitochrondrial membrane (34)
    b. Inner mitochondrial membrane (34)
    c. Cristae (34)
    d. Inner membrane (F1) subunits (29, 34)
    e. Intramembrane space (34)
    f. Intracristal space (34)
    g. Intercristal space (34)
    h. Matrix (34)
    i. Matrix granules (34)
    j. ATPase (34)
    k. Krebs cycle enzymes (34–35)
    l. Electron transport system (35)
11. Which substances and structures in the mitochondrial matrix are similar to those found in prokaryotic cells and duplicate eukaryotic cell components found elsewhere in the cell (34)?
12. Compare the mitochondrial cristae of most cells with those of steroid-secreting cells and cells with a high rate of metabolism (34).
13. What is the primary function of ribosomes (35)?
14. List the biochemical and structural components of ribosomes, and name the sites of their synthesis and association (35).
15. Compare the appearance of ribosomes in light and electron microscopy (35).
16. How are individual ribosomes held together to form a polyribosome (35)?
17. What is the difference between the functions of free polyribosomes and polyribosomes found attached to the rough endoplasmic reticulum (35)?

*The page references in this section refer to *Basic Histology,* 6th ed., Junqueira L, Carneiro J, Kelley R (editors), Appleton & Lange, 1989. **HR** (for Histology Review) is occasionally used instead of a page reference to indicate that the information referred to can be found in this book.

18. Compare rough and smooth endoplasmic reticula in terms of:
   a. The presence of ribosomes (36, 37)
   b. The shapes of their cisternae (36, 37)
   c. Their functions (36, 37)
   d. The cell types in which each is particularly abundant, including examples (36, 37)
19. List the steps in RER-associated protein synthesis and subsequent posttranslational modification, beginning with attachment of mRNAs for proteins destined for secretion and ending with budding of transfer vesicles for transport to the Golgi complex (37).
20. List the functions of the Golgi complex (39).
21. Sketch a Golgi complex (29, 37–39) and label the following:
   a. Cisternae
   b. *Cis* face
   c. *Trans* face
   d. Transfer vesicles
   e. Associated GERL
   f. Condensing vacuoles and secretory granules
   g. Site of selective osmium deposition
22. Compare primary lysosomes with secondary lysosomes in terms of their:
   a. Size (39, 40)
   b. Appearance (39, 40)
   c. Contents (39, 40)
23. Compare lysosomes and peroxisomes in terms of their:
   a. Size (39, 40, 43)
   b. Contents (39, 43)
   c. Appearance (39, 40, 43)
   d. Function (39, 43)
24. Compare the contents of autophagosomes and heterophagosomes (40, 42).
25. Trace the steps in the ingestion and digestion of extracellular materials, beginning with endocytosis (32–33) and ending with the formation of residual bodies (40, 42)
26. How would an inherited deficiency or complete lack of a particular lysosomal enzyme affect the intracellular concentration of substrates of that enzyme (43)?
27. Compare microfilaments and microtubules in terms of:
   a. Their diameter (43, 48)
   b. Their major protein components (43, 48)
   c. Their functions (45, 48)
   d. The polymerization of their subunits (44, 48)
   e. Their contractile capability (45, 48)
   f. Their location in the cell (45, 47, 48)
28. Compare centrioles, basal bodies, and cilia and flagella in terms of the number and organization of their microtubules (47).
29. What role do centrioles play in cell function (47)?
30. Compare cilia and flagella (47) in terms of:
   a. Their structure
   b. Their length
   c. The typical number of each per cell
31. Give the diameter of intermediate filaments in nanometers and angstroms (48).
32. List 5 types of intermediate filaments and the cell types in which each may be found (48–49).
33. Name the components of the microtrabecular lattice, and describe their organization and probable functions (50–51).
34. List the 4 major structural components of the nucleus (51).
35. Why is the term "nuclear envelope" more appropriate than "nuclear membrane" (51)?
36. List the substances and structures associated with the internal and external surfaces of the nuclear envelope (51–52).
37. List several important macromolecules that must traverse the nuclear pores for basic cell functions to be carried out (35, 53–56).
38. Compare and contrast euchromatin and heterochromatin in terms of their:
   a. Appearance in light and electron microscopy (53)

  - **b.** Degree of coiling (53–54)
  - **c.** Activity (54, 56)

39. List the components of a nucleosome (53, 55).
40. List the parts of a nucleolus (56–57).
41. What is the major function of the nucleolus (35)?
42. What types of cells would you expect to have particularly large nucleoli (57)?
43. List in order the phases of mitosis, and sketch the appearance and location of the chromosomes during each phase (58–60).
44. Describe what happens to the following during mitosis (58–60):
  - **a.** Nucleolus
  - **b.** Nuclear envelope
  - **c.** Centrioles
  - **d.** Spindle apparatus
  - **e.** Golgi apparatus
  - **f.** Chromatin

45. During which phase(s) of mitosis does each of the changes described in your answer to question 44 occur (58–60)?
46. Give examples of tissues characterized by a rapid mitotic rate and of those with a slow mitotic rate (60).
47. List in order the phases of interphase (60).
48. Which phase(s) of interphase (60) is associated with:
  - **a.** Most extensive protein and RNA synthesis
  - **b.** Restoration of cell volume
  - **c.** Exit from the cell cycle into G_0
  - **d.** DNA synthesis and replication
  - **e.** Duplication of the centrioles
  - **f.** Production and accumulation of energy (ATP) to be used during mitosis
  - **g.** Increased synthesis of tubulin

49. Beginning with transcription in the nucleus, trace the steps in the synthesis and secretion of a glycoprotein and relate the steps to the organelles involved.

Multiple-Choice Questions

For questions 3–1 through 3–15, select the single best answer.

3–1. Because of the frequent presence of ribosomes on its outer surface, the nuclear envelope may be considered a specialized portion of the:
  - **A.** Golgi complex
  - **B.** Smooth endoplasmic reticulum
  - **C.** Plasma membrane
  - **D.** Rough endoplasmic reticulum
  - **E.** Nucleolus

3–2. Which of the following organelles would show the highest concentration of label after being subjected to enzyme histochemical methods designed to detect the location of acid phosphatase?
  - **A.** Plasma membrane
  - **B.** Lysosomes
  - **C.** Ribosomes
  - **D.** Smooth endoplasmic reticulum
  - **E.** Microtubules

3–3. The electron microscopic appearance of a unit membrane is best described as:
  - **A.** A porous structure
  - **B.** A lipid bilayer
  - **C.** A trilaminar structure
  - **D.** A pentalaminar structure
  - **E.** None of the above

3–4. Which of the following is composed primarily of actin or actinlike proteins?
  - **A.** Basal bodies

B. Microtubules
C. Intermediate filaments
D. Cilia
E. Microfilaments

3–5. The cytoplasmic half of a freeze-fractured membrane usually contains most of the intramembrane particles and is called the:
A. Replica
B. *Trans* face
C. P face
D. *Cis* face
E. E face

3–6. In hepatocytes, the crystalline nucleoid (dense core) of peroxisomes is believed to be composed of:
A. Hydrogen peroxide
B. Urate oxidase
C. Acid phosphatase
D. Divalent cations
E. None of the above

3–7. The average diameter of intermediate filaments if approximately:
A. 250 μm
B. 100–120μm
C. 100–120 nm
D. 10–12 nm
E. 250 nm

3–8. The synthesis of all proteins appears to be initiated on:
A. Free ribosomes
B. Rough endoplasmic reticulum
C. Golgi complex
D. Nucleosomes
E. Ribophorin

3–9. For continually dividing cells, which phase would not be present?
A. Prophase
B. G_0
C. G_1
D. G_2
E. S

3–10. A secondary lysosome:
A. Contains a mixture of hydrolytic enzymes and phagocytosed material
B. May become a residual body
C. Is an organelle formed by fusion of primary lysosomes and phagosomes
D. All of the above
E. None of the above

3–11. The cryofracture preparation shown in Fig 3–1 is of a:
A. Lysosome
B. Golgi complex
C. Nucleolus
D. Gap junction
E. Nuclear envelope

3–12. The structure indicated by the arrows in Fig 3–2 is a:
A. Mitochondrion
B. Primary lysosome
C. Peroxisome
D. Secondary lysosome
E. Ribosome

3–13. The electron micrograph in Fig 3–3 shows:
A. A smooth endoplasmic reticulum
B. A rough endoplasmic reticulum
C. A Golgi complex
D. Glycogen granules
E. A plasma membrane

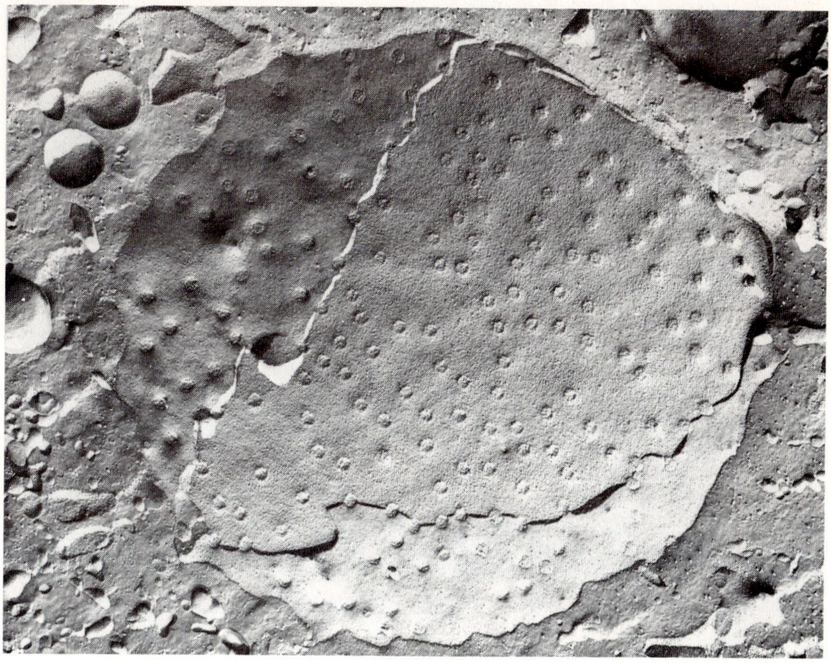

Figure 3-1.

3-14. The structure indicated by the arrow in Fig 3-4 is:

- **A.** A heterophagosome
- **B.** A primary lysosome
- **C.** A peroxisome
- **D.** An autophagosome
- **E.** None of the above

3-15. The cell shown in Fig 3-5 is in which phase of cell division?

- **A.** Interphase
- **B.** Prophase

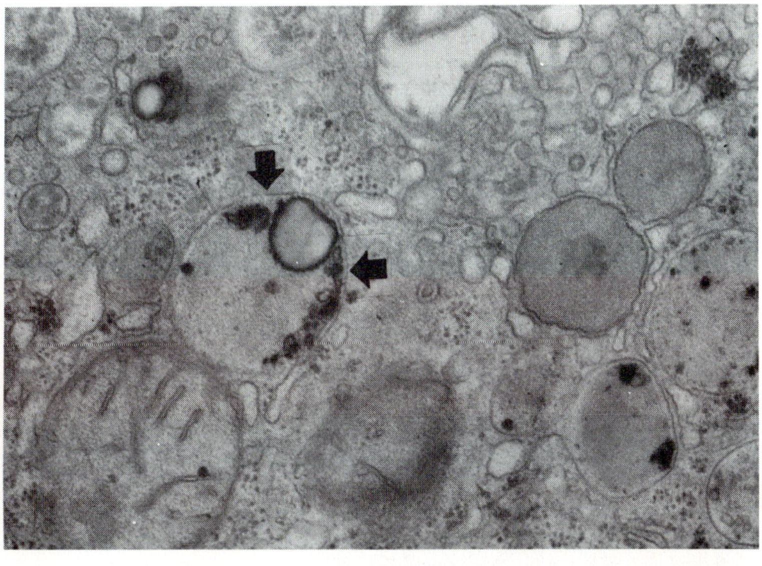

Figure 3-2.

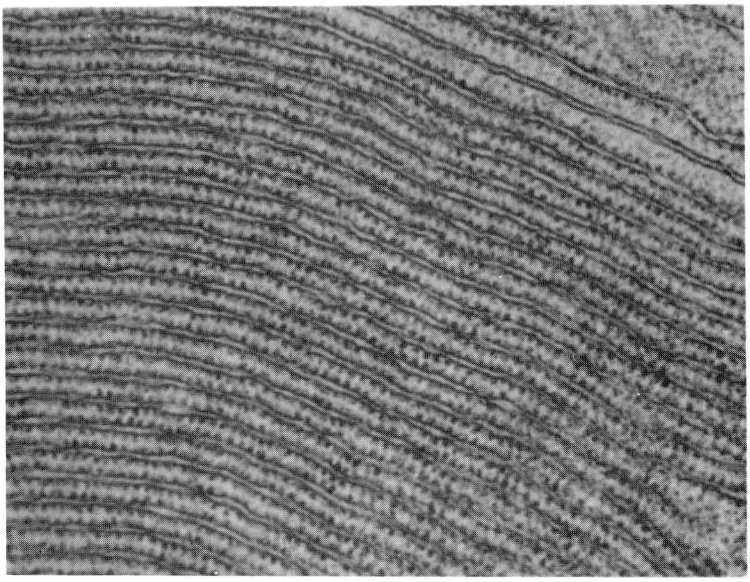

Figure 3-3.

C. Metaphase
D. Anaphase
E. Telophase

MATCHING (questions 3-16 through 3-40): Each choice may be used once, more than once, or not at all.

Questions 3-16 through 3-21:

A. Mitochondrial matrix
B. Mitochondrial matrix granule
C. Inner mitochondrial membrane
D. Outer mitochondrial membrane
E. None of the above

3-16. Location of Krebs cycle enzymes
3-17. Site of calcium ion sequestration
3-18. Location of electron transport system
3-19. Forms shelflike or tubular projections (cristae) into the matrix
3-20. Location of mitochrondrial DNA
3-21. Location of globular structures with ATPase activity

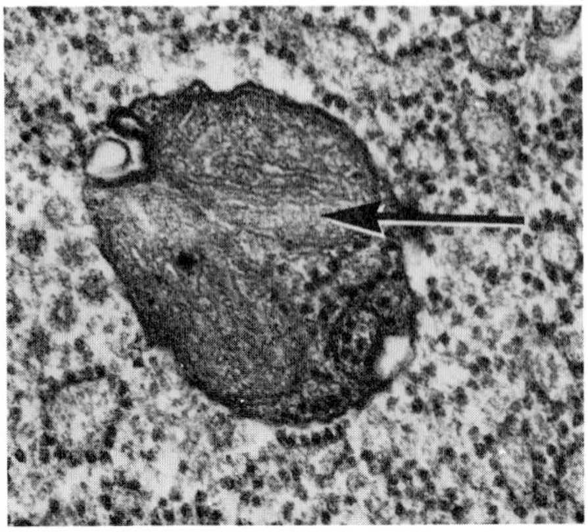

Figure 3-4.

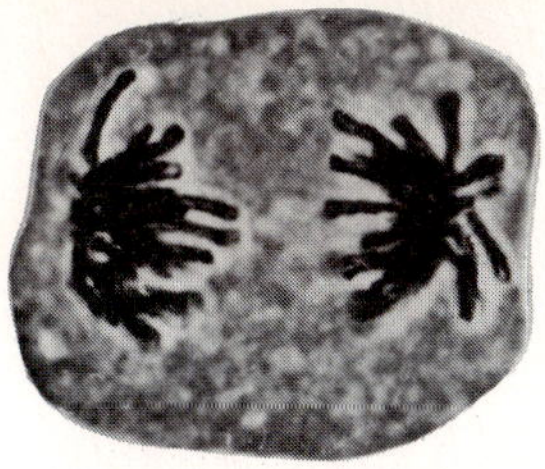

Figure 3-5.

Questions 3-22 through 3-32:

A. Ribophorin
B. Lipofuscin
C. Colchicine
D. Melanin
E. Euchromatin
F. Nexin
G. Clathrin
H. Heterochromatin
I. Lamin
J. Dynein
K. Vimentin
L. None of the above

3-22. Helps attach ribosomes to rough endoplasmic reticulum
3-23. Found in greater abundance with increasing age in nerve cells
3-24. Forms the coating of coated pits and vesicles
3-25. Inactive hereditary material
3-26. Inhibits microtubule polymerization
3-27. ATPase activity in axonemes
3-28. Links adjacent microtubule doublets in axonemes
3-29. Polypeptide associated with the inner surface of the nuclear envelope
3-30. Intermediate filament protein
3-31. Pigment normally associated with the epidermis of the skin and the pigment layer of the retina
3-32. More abundant in interphase nuclei of rapidly dividing cells

Questions 3-33 through 3-40:

A. Centriole
B. Free polysomes
C. Mitochondria
D. Rough endoplasmic reticulum
E. Smooth endoplasmic reticulum
F. Golgi complex

3-33. Site of synthesis of protein for secretion
3-34. Site of synthesis of actin and tubulin
3-35. Site of drug detoxification
3-36. Site of intense ATP production
3-37. Site of steroid hormone synthesis
3-38. Primary site of packaging of secretory products
3-39. Site of core glycosylation of secretory proteins
3-40. Site of sulfation of sulfated glycosaminoglycans

For questions 3–41 through 4–47, more than one answer may be correct.

A. Carbohydrates
B. Lipids
C. Nucleic acids
D. Proteins
E. All of the above

3–41. Synthesized on polyribosomes
3–42. Can be hydrolyzed by enzymes found in lysosomes
3–43. Synthesized by the nucleolus
3–44. Project from the cell surface in branching chains and confer a chemical identity upon the cell
3–45. Added to proteins in the Golgi complex
3–46. Composition of the nucleolar organizer
3–47. Most numerous molecules in cellular membranes

For questions 3–48 through 3–66, select the one correct answer.

Questions 3–48 through 3–60:

A. Microtubules
B. Microfilaments
C. Both
D. Neither

3–48. Are polymers of protein subunits
3–49. Are composed of actin
3–50. Are considered components of the cytoskeleton
3–51. Are composed of tubulin heterodimers
3–52. Can increase or decrease in length depending on cytoplasmic conditions
3–53. Form the "purse-string" constriction in mitotic cells
3–54. May be composed of desmin or vimentin
3–55. Are important components of centrioles
3–56. Form protofilaments
3–57. Important components of axonemes
3–58. Have an outer diameter of about 24 nm
3–59. Usually require myosin for contraction
3–60. Important components of cilia and flagella

Questions 3–61 through 3–66:

A. Organelles
B. Cytoplasmic inclusions
C. Both
D. Neither

3–61. More likely to be membrane-limited
3–62. Often act as storage depots for metabolic precursors
3–63. More active participants in cell functions
3–64. Usually located in the cytoplasm
3–65. More likely to contain enzymes
3–66. Regarded as more temporary occupants of the cell

For questions 3–67 through 3–77, one, more than one, or all of the answers may be correct. Select

A if only (1), (2), and (3) are correct
B if only (1) and (3) are correct
C if only (2) and (4) are correct

D if only (4) is correct
E if all answers are correct

3-67. Functions of the Golgi complex include:
(1) Packaging of secretory materials
(2) Synthesis of polysaccharides
(3) Concentration of secretory products
(4) Sulfation of polysaccharides

3-68. Functions of biologic membranes include:
(1) Compartmentalization of the cytoplasm
(2) Homeostasis
(3) Transduction of extracellular signals
(4) Selective uptake of nutrients into the cell

3-69. Which of the following are components of intermediate filaments?
(1) Desmin
(2) Actin
(3) Vimentin
(4) Tubulin

3-70. Centrioles are involved in a variety of functions including:
(1) Mitosis
(2) Organization of the Golgi apparatus
(3) Cell motility
(4) Movements of cytoplasmic vesicles

3-71. The structures dispersed and then reorganized during each pass through the cell cycle include the:
(1) Spindle apparatus
(2) Nucleolus
(3) Nuclear envelope
(4) Golgi complex

3-72. A phagosome:
(1) Contains densely-packed, inactive hydrolytic enzymes
(2) Can fuse with a lysosome
(3) Is surrounded by a membrane derived directly from the Golgi apparatus
(4) Contains material engulfed during phagocytosis

3-73. Ribosomes are not found in mature red blood cells. From this, one can deduce that mature red blood cells:
(1) Contain no endoplasmic reticulum
(2) Cannot manufacture enzymes
(3) Never had a nucleolus at any point in their development
(4) Are incapable of protein synthesis, even if they contain mRNA

3-74. Substances that must pass through the nuclear pores to assume their normal roles in cell functions include:
(1) Histones
(2) Messenger RNA (mRNA)
(3) Ribosomal subunits
(4) Ribosomal proteins

3-75. The microtrabecular lattice:
(1) Is a component of the cytoplasm
(2) Contains microfilaments and microtubules
(3) May be involved in coordinating movements of organelles and multistep metabolic processes
(4) Contains intermediate filaments

3-76. Nucleosomes:
(1) Are chromatin subunits
(2) Include 8 histones each
(3) All have equal amounts of DNA
(4) Can coil further to form superhelical selenoids

3-77. Ribosomal RNA (rRNA) is synthesized by:
(1) The rough endoplasmic reticulum
(2) Free polyribosomes
(3) The smooth endoplasmic reticulum
(4) The nucleolus

Part II: The 4 Basic Tissue Types

Epithelial Cells & Tissues 4

Objectives

This chapter should help the student to:

- Know the structural and functional characteristics of epithelial tissues that distinguish them from the 3 other basic tissue types.
- Know the various types of epithelial tissues and give examples of body sites where each may be found.
- Know the functional capabilities of each type of epithelial tissue and relate them to the tissue's structure.
- Describe the specialized functions of the various types of epithelial cells and give examples of body sites where each type may be found.
- Recognize the various epithelial types in photomicrographs or slides and predict their function from their structure.
- Know the criteria used to classify glands.
- Know the names of the types of glands commonly found in humans and give examples of body sites where each may be found.
- Recognize specific glands in photomicrographs or diagrams and identify the gland type.

Synopsis

I. THE 4 BASIC TISSUE TYPES. A tissue is a complex assemblage of cells and cell products having a common function. The many body tissues are grouped according to their cells and cell products into 4 basic types: **epithelial, connective, muscular,** and **nervous tissues.**

II. GENERAL FEATURES OF EPITHELIAL TISSUES. **Epithelial tissues** usually occur as structurally minor but functionally important components of complex organs. **Glands,** derived from the invagination and ingrowth of lining epithelia into underlying connective tissue, are composed mainly of epithelial cells in adults and are considered a type of epithelial tissue.

A. Diversity: Epithelial tissues are very diverse in form and function. They range from one to several cell layers in thickness, forming sheets, solid organs, or glands. Their functions range from protection to secretion and absorption.

B. Metaplasia: When faced with a chronic change of environmental conditions, epithelia are capable of metaplasia, ie, they may change from one type to another.

C. Lining and Covering: Epithelia cover or line all body surfaces and cavities except articular cartilage in joint cavities. Their function is analogous to that of cell membranes: (1) They separate self from nonself; (2) they divide the body interior into functional compartments; and (3) they form passive and active barriers that monitor, control, and modify substances that traverse them.

D. Basal Lamina: Epithelia rest on an extracellular basal lamina (or basement membrane) that separates them from an underlying connective tissue layer, the **lamina propria.**

E. Renewal: Epithelia are continuously renewed and replaced. The epithelial cells closest to the basal lamina undergo continuous mitosis, and their progeny replace the surface cells.

F. Avascularity: Blood vessels in the subjacent connective tissue rarely penetrate the basal lamina to invade epithelia.

G. Cell Packing: Epithelial tissues have very little intercellular substance. The cells are usually densely packed, closely apposed, and joined by specialized junctions.

H. Derivation: Ectoderm, mesoderm, and endoderm can all give rise to epithelia.

III. CLASSIFICATION OF EPITHELIAL TISSUES

A. Classifying Principles: Epithelia are classified and named according to the number of their cell layers and the shape of the cells in the surface layer.

1. Number of cell layers

a. Simple epithelia have one cell layer.

b. Stratified epithelia have 2 or more cell layers.

c. Pseudostratified epithelia have all their cells resting on the basal lamina, but not all the cells extend to the surface. The nuclei lie at different depths, giving the appearance of multiple cell layers.

2. Shape of the surface cells

a. Squamous cells are flat and platelike.

b. Cuboidal cells are polygonal and about as tall as they are wide.

c. Columnar cells are polygonal and taller than they are wide.

B. Specific Epithelial Types:

1. Simple squamous epithelium is a single layer of flat, platelike cells that usually functions as a semipermeable barrier between compartments. It lines blood vessels (endothelium) and body cavities (mesothelium) and forms the parietal layer of the renal corpuscles of the kidney.

2. Simple cuboidal epithelium is a single layer of blocklike cells. It forms the walls of conduits that carry secretory and excretory products, and it regulates ion and water concentration in certain specialized (striated) salivary ducts. It may act as a protective barrier in some locations. It lines the kidney tubules and the smaller (intercalary and interlobular) ducts of many glands, and it covers the free surface of the ovary and the inner surface of the lens capsule.

3. Simple columnar epithelium is a single layer of roughly cylindric cells whose apical (free) surfaces may be covered with cilia or microvilli. It functions in secretion, absorption, and propulsion of mucus (if ciliated) and often as a protective barrier. It lines the stomach, intestines, rectum, uterus, and oviducts, as well as the larger ducts of certain glands and the papillary ducts of the kidneys.

4. Pseudostratified columnar epithelium is a single layer of cells of variable shape and height, with nuclei at 2 or more levels (III.A.1.c). Cells reaching the surface are often ciliated. This epithelium forms a protective barrier and, when ciliated, moves surface mucus and trapped debris. Ciliated pseudostratified columnar epithelium, or respiratory epithelium, lines the larger diameter respiratory passageways. Pseudostratified columnar epithelium also lines some parts of the male reproductive tract, where its apical surfaces are often covered with nonmotile stereocilia (IV.A.4).

5. Stratified squamous epithelium occurs in 2 forms:

a. The **keratinized** (cornified) type is a multilayered sheet of cells. The superficial cells are squamous, dead, and filled with the scleroprotein keratin; they lack nuclei. Deeper layers have polygonal cells in progressive stages of keratinization. The deepest layer has cuboidal to columnar cells and lies on the basal lamina. Keratinized stratified squamous epithelium is found mainly in the skin and forms a highly specialized barrier against friction, abrasion, infection, and water loss.

b. The **nonkeratinized** (noncornified) type is similar in structure but is thinner and lacks heavily keratinized cells. Its surface cells are flattened but nucleated. Nonkeratinized stratified squamous epithelium, also called **mucous membrane,** forms a protective barrier that is less resistant to water loss than the keratinized type. It lines wet cavities subject to abrasion (eg, mouth, esophagus, vagina, and anal canal, vocal folds).

6. Stratified cuboidal epithelium usually has 2–3 layers of cuboidal cells. This relatively rare epithelium lines the ducts of some glands (eg, salivary, sweat).

7. Stratified columnar epithelium is similar to stratified cuboidal, but its superficial cells are columnar and may be ciliated. Also rare, it lines the larger ducts of some large glands, forms the conjunctiva, and occurs in small, isolated patches in some mucous membranes. It sometimes covers the respiratory surface of the epiglottis.

8. Transitional epithelium is a stratified epithelium that forms the lining of most urinary passages (renal pelvis, ureters, bladder, proximal portions of the urethra). Its surface cells are large and often binucleate. When the bladder is empty, the surface cells appear domelike, giving the epithelium a "cobblestone" appearance. When the bladder is full, the surface cells stretch and flatten.

IV. POLARITY & SPECIALIZATIONS OF EPITHELIAL CELLS.

Polarity (structural and functional asymmetry) is characteristic of most epithelial cells. It is best seen in simple epithelia, where each cell has 3 types of surfaces: an apical (free) surface, a variable number of lateral surfaces that abut neighboring cells, and a basal surface attached to the basal lamina.

A. Specializations of the Apical Surface:

The cell's apical surface is on the organ's external or internal (lumen) surface. It is specialized to carry out functions that occur at these interfaces, including secretion, absorption, and movement of luminal contents.

1. Cilia (see Chapter 3) typically occur in tufts, or covering the entire apical surface. They beat in waves, often moving a surface coat of mucus and trapped materials. Ciliated epithelia include ciliated pseudostratified columnar (respiratory) epithelium and the ciliated simple columnar epithelium of the oviducts.

2. Flagella (see Chapter 3) are also concerned with movement. Spermatozoa, derived from seminiferons epithelia, are the only human flagellated cells.

3. Microvilli are plasma membrane-covered extensions of the cell surface. Their cores (unlike those of cilia and flagella) are composed of numerous parallel actin microfilaments; these are anchored in a dense mat of filaments in the apical cytoplasm called the **terminal web.** By interacting with cytoplasmic myosin, the microfilaments can contract, shortening the microvilli. The apical surface of absorptive cells is usually covered with microvilli, which greatly increase the apical surface area when extended. Microvillus-covered epithelia, said to exhibit a **striated border,** or **brush border,** include the absorptive simple columnar epithelium lining the small intestines and the absorptive simple cuboidal epithelium lining the proximal tubules of the kidney.

4. Stereocilia are not true cilia but very long microvilli. They are found in the male reproductive tract (epididymis, ductus deferens), where they have an absorptive function, and in the internal ear (hair cells of the maculae and organ of Corti), where they have a sensory function.

B. Specializations of the Lateral Surfaces: Epithelial cells are usually tightly attached to one another by specialized **intercellular junctions** composed of opposing membranes and some intra- and extracellular material. Junctions occur in 3 major forms: **Zonulae** are bandlike and completely encircle the cell; **maculae** are disklike and attach 2 cells at a single spot; **gap junctions** are similar in shape to maculae but differ in composition and function. A **junctional complex** (formerly called a terminal bar) is any combination of intercellular junctions close to the cell apex that looks dark in the light microscope.

1. Zonula occludens Zonulae occludentes (tight junctions, occluding junctions) are located near the cell apex and seal off the intercellular space, allowing the epithelium to isolate certain body compartments (eg, they help keep intestinal bacteria and toxins out of the bloodstream). Their structure, best seen in freeze-fracture preparations, results from the fusion of 2 trilaminar membranes to form a pentalaminar structure (as seen in transmission electron microscopy [TEM]); this fusion may require specific "tight-junction proteins." In some tissues, tight junctions can be disrupted by removing calcium ions or treating with protease.

2. Zonula adherens Zonulae adherentes (sometimes called belt desmosomes) are usually just basal to the tight junctions. The membranes of the adhering cells are typically 20–90 nm apart at a zonula adherens; the gap may be wider there than in nonjunctional areas. An electron-dense plaque containing myosin, tropomyosin, alpha actinin, and vinculin is found on the cytoplasmic surface of each of the membranes participating in the junction. Actin-containing microfilaments arising from each cell's terminal web insert into the plaques and appear to stabilize the junction.

3. Macula adherens A macula adherens, or **desmosome,** consists of 2 dense, granular **attachment plaques** composed of several proteins and borne on the cytoplasmic surfaces of the opposing cell membranes. Transverse thin electron microscopic (EM) sections show dense arrays of **tonofilaments** (cytokeratin intermediate filaments) that insert into the plaques or make hairpin turns and return to the cytoplasm. The gap between the attached membranes is often over 30 nm. Sometimes fibrillar or granular material (probably glycoprotein) is seen as a dense central line in the intercellular space. Desmosomes, distributed in patches along the lateral membranes of most epithelial cells, form particularly stable attachments but do not hamper the flow of substances between the cells.

4. Gap junction A gap junction (nexus) is a disk- or patch-shaped structure, best appreciated by viewing both freeze-fracture and transverse thin EM sections. The intercellular gap is 2 nm, and the membrane on each side contains a circular patch of **connexons.** Each connexon is a protein hexamer with a central 1.5-nm hydrophilic pore. The connexons in one membrane link with those in the other to form continuous pores that bridge the intercellular gap, allowing passage of ions and small molecules ($<$ 800 daltons). As sites of electrotonic coupling (reduced resistance to ion flow), gap junctions are important in intercellular communication and coordination; they are found in most tissues.

C. Specializations of the Basal Surface: The basal surface contacts the basal lamina. Because it is the surface closest to the underlying blood supply, it often contains receptors for blood-borne factors such as hormones.

1. A **basal lamina** underlies all true epithelial tissues.

a. Structure The basal lamina is a sheetlike structure, usually composed of **type IV collagen, proteoglycan,** and **laminin,** a glycoprotein that aids in adhesion of the basal lamina to the cells. The basal lamina exhibits electron-lucent and electron-dense regions termed the **lamina lucida** (lamina rara) and the **lamina densa,** respectively. The lamina densa is composed of a 20- to 100-nm-thick fibrillar network; the amount of lamina lucida is variable. Basal lamina components are contributed by the epithelial cells, the underlying connective tissue cells, and (in some locations) muscle, adipose, and Schwann cells. In some sites, a layer of type III collagen fibers (reticular fibers), produced by the connective tissue cells and termed the **reticular lamina,** underlies the basal lamina. Basal laminae accompanied by reticular laminae are often thick enough to be seen with the light microscope as PAS-positive layers and are sometimes termed **basement membranes.**

b. Functions The basal lamina forms a sievelike barrier between the epithelium and connective tissue. It aids in tissue organization and cell adhesion and (through transmembrane linkages with cytoskeletal components) helps maintain cell shape. It has a role in maintaining specific cell functions, probably through its effect on shape. Muscle basal laminae are critical in establishing neuromuscular junctions.

2. Hemidesmosomes are located on the inner surface of basal plasma membranes in contact with the basal lamina. Essentially half desmosomes, they help to attach epithelial cells to the basal lamina. The best examples are found in the basal layers of stratified squamous epithelium.

3. Sodium-potassium ATPase is a plasma membrane-bound enzyme localized preferentially in the basal and basolateral regions of epithelial cells. It transports sodium out of and potassium into the cell (VI.A.1).

D. Intracellular Polarity: The nucleus and organelles are often found in characteristic regions of epithelial cells, a feature particularly important to glandular cells. For example, in protein-secreting cells, the rough endoplasmic reticulum is preferentially located in the basal cytoplasm, the nucleus in the basal to middle region just above the rough endoplasmic reticulum, and the Golgi complex just above the nucleus. Mature secretory vesicles collect in the apical cytoplasm.

V. GLANDS.

Glands are single cells or groups of cells specialized for secretion.

A. Exocrine and Endocrine Glands: All glands arise in early development from lining or covering epithelia. Exocrine glands, described below, are those that keep their connection with the epithelium in the form of a **duct.** Endocrine glands (ductless glands) lose their connection with the surface and release their secretions into the bloodstream. Endocrine glands are compared with exocrine glands in Table 4–1; they are described in more detail in Chapters 20 and 21.

B. Classification of Exocrine Glands: Exocrine glands may be classified according to their structure, acretory product, or mode of secretion.

1. By structure Structural classification (Table 4–2) is based on the number of cells, the type of duct system, and the shape of the secretory portion of the gland.

a. Number of cells **Unicellular glands** are single secretory cells scattered among other cell types in epithelia (eg, mucus-secreting goblet cells). **Multicellular glands** occur in 2 forms: Sheet glands, which empty their secretions directly into the lumen of a hollow organ (eg, glands of the trachea), and solid glands, whose secretions are carried by ducts to the body surface (eg, sweat glands) or to a lumen (eg, salivary glands).

b. Duct system The duct system may be **simple** (unbranched), or **compound** (branched). Simple ducts may be **straight** or **coiled.**

Table 4-1. Some Comparisons of Exocrine and Endocrine Glands

Category	Exocrine Glands	Endocrine Glands
Transport of secretions	Typically **by ducts.**	Typically **by the bloodstream.** No ducts.
Cell number	May be **unicellular** (eg, goblet cells) or **multicellular** (eg, salivary glands).	May be **unicellular** (eg, DNES cells) or **multicellular** (eg, thyroid gland).
Secretory products	Include **proteins** (eg, digestive enzymes), **glycoproteins** (eg, mucus), and some mixtures containing **lipids** (eg, sebum, bile, apocrine sweat, and milk).	**Hormones** of 2 main types: **peptide hormones** (eg, insulin) and **steroid hormones** (eg, adrenocorticoids). **Plasma proteins** produced by the liver (eg, serum albumin and clotting factors) are also considered endocrine secretory products.
Mode of secretion	**Merocrine** (ie, by exocytosis, no loss of cytoplasm); **apocrine** (loss of apical cytoplasm); **holocrine** (entire cell released into duct).	**Merocrine only.**

c. Secretory portion The secretory portion of the gland may be **tubular** (test tube-shaped); **alveolar,** or **acinar** (flask-shaped); or **tubuloacinar** (with acini branching off the straight tubular portion).

2. By secretory product

a. Mucous secretion, or **mucus,** is a thick secretion containing proteins, chiefly highly glycosylated glycoproteins called **mucins** or mucin precursors called **mucinogens.** Other glycoproteins (eg, membrane glycoproteins) commonly have short, N-linked oligosaccharides attached to asparagine. Mucous glycoproteins have longer, O-linked oligosaccharide chains attached to hydroxyl groups of serine or threonine. This attachment is mediated by special glycosyltransferases in the Golgi complex of the mucus-secreting cells. Examples of mucus-secreting glands include goblet cells and the sublingual salivary glands.

b. Serous secretion is a watery secretion containing proteins and glycoproteins. The exocrine pancreas and parotid salivary glands produce serous secretions.

c. Seromucous secretion is a mixed secretion of intermediate thickness. The submandibular salivary gland contains both serous and mucous secretory cells and produces seromucous secretions.

3. By mode of secretion

a. In **merocrine secretion** (eccrine secretion), the secretory product exits by exocytosis, with no loss of cytoplasm or membrane. Most secretory cells release their products in this manner. Specific examples include the pancreas and pituitary.

Table 4-2. Examples of Structural Classifications of Multicellular Exocrine Glands

Duct System	Secretory Portion	Example
Simple	Tubular	Intestinal crypts of Lieberkühn
Simple	Coiled tubular	Eccrine sweat glands of the skin
Simple	Branched tubular	Fundic glands of the stomach
Simple	Branched acinar	Sebaceous glands of the skin
Compound	Tubular	Cardiac glands of the stomach
Compound	Tubuloacinar	Submandibular salivary glands
Compound	Acinar	Exocrine pancreas

b. In **apocrine secretion,** the secretory product collects in the cell apex, and the entire apex is released, with some loss of cytoplasm and membrane. Apocrine sweat glands of the skin and mammary glands both employ this type of secretion.

c. In **holocrine secretion,** storage of large amounts of secretory products in the cytoplasm is followed by cell lysis. The entire cell is released into the duct. The skin's sebaceous glands are the classic examples for this mode of secretion.

VI. MAJOR TYPES OF EPITHELIAL CELLS

A. Epithelial Cells Specialized for Transport:

1. Ion-transporting cells Some epithelial cells are specialized for **transcellular transport,** ie, they can pump ions across their entire thickness, apex to base. Sheets of such cells form active barriers that control ion and water concentrations in body compartments. Tight junctions are often found between the cells and appear to prevent backflow. Ion-transporting cells typically have highly infolded basal plasma membranes that interdigitate with numerous mitochondria. Commonly, the ion pump is specific for sodium (ie, it is Na^+/K^+-ATPase), and chloride ions and water follow the sodium-ion flow passively. Some ion-transporting epithelia exploit this mechanism to concentrate other solutes by moving water from one compartment to another. Important ion-transporting epithelia are found in the kidney tubules, the striated ducts of the salivary glands, the gallbladder, the choroid plexus and the ciliary body of the eye.

2. Cells that transport by pinocytosis Epithelial cells specialized for pinocytosis have tight junctions and abundant pinocytotic vesicles. The vesicles transport substances across the cell from the luminal surface to the basal surface, where the vesicle contents are released. The best example is the endothelial cells lining the blood vessels, where transcellular transport is rapid (2–3 minutes).

B. Epithelial Cells Specialized for Absorption:

Specialized absorptive cells lining the digestive tract (especially the small intestine) have numerous microvilli on their apical surfaces to increase the exposed area. Small nutrient molecules diffuse into the microvilli, and contraction of the microfilaments shortens the microvilli, bringing the nutrients into the cytoplasm. Other nutrients are pinocytosed between microvilli. Absorptive cells with similar specializations occur in the proximal tubules of the kidney.

C. Epithelial Cells Specialized for Secretion:

1. Protein-secreting cells Cells that synthesize proteins for segregation and secretion have abundant basophilic rough endoplasmic reticulum, a well-developed Golgi complex, and, frequently, an accumulation of secretory granules in the cell apex. Proteins secreted by epithelial cells include the digestive enzymes, produced by pancreatic acinar cells and the chief cells of the stomach; serum albumin, produced by liver hepatocytes; and protein hormones, eg, parathyroid hormone produced by the chief cells of the parathyroid gland.

2. Polypeptide-secreting cells Secreted polypeptides have fewer amino acids than the secreted proteins just mentioned. Polypeptide-secreting cells have a small amount of rough endoplasmic reticulum, a supranuclear Golgi complex, and an accumulation of 100- to 400-nm secretory granules in their bases. These **APUD cells** (*a*mine *p*recursor *u*ptake and *d*ecarboxylation) characteristically concentrate important bioactive amines such as epinephrine, norepinephrine, and serotonin in their cytoplasm. They may absorb these amines from the bloodstream or synthesize them from amino acid precursors by means of amino acid decarboxylases, also found in high concentrations in these cells. Most APUD cells are unicellular glands scattered among other epithelial cells. The number, variety, and wide distribution of cells with these characteristics has generated the concept of the ***d*iffuse *n*euro*e*ndocrine *s*ystem (DNES).** DNES is becoming the preferred designation, but DNES and APUD refer to the same polypeptide-secreting cells. Some

APUD polypeptide hormone cells have **paracrine** effects on neighboring cells; others are released into the bloodstream and have endocrine effects on distant cells. Some important APUD polypeptides are glucagon, from pancreatic islet A cells; insulin, from pancreatic islet B cells; gastrin, from the stomach, small intestine, and pancreatic islet G cells; and somatostatin, from the stomach, small intestine, and pancreatic islet D cells. Tumors composed of APUD cells are called **apudomas.**

3. Mucous cells Mucus-secreting cells occur as unicellular, sheet, or solid glands. Histologic features of these cells include a light-staining, foamy appearance caused by numerous large mucus-containing vesicles concentrated near the cell apex; PAS-positive staining from an abundance of oligosaccharide residues; predominantly acidophilic staining with H&E; a large supranuclear Golgi complex with distinctive glycosyltransferases (V.B.2.a); and nuclei and sparse rough endoplasmic reticulum in the base of the cell. Goblet cells and mucous cells of the sublingual salivary glands are examples of unicellular and multicellular mucous glands, respectively.

4. Serous cells Cells that produce serous secretions have characteristics of protein-secreting cells. They are usually smaller, darker-staining, and more basophilic than mucus-secreting cells. Serous cells include pancreatic acinar cells and secretory cells of the parotid salivary glands.

5. Steroid-secreting cells Endocrine cells specialized to secrete steroid hormones are polygonal or rounded, with a central nucleus and pale-staining, acidophilic cytoplasm that often contains numerous lipid droplets. Their abundant smooth endoplasmic reticulum contains enzymes for cholesterol synthesis and for converting steroid hormone precursors (eg, pregnenolone) into specific hormones (eg, androgens, estrogens, and progesterone). Their numerous mitochondria typically have tubular rather than shelflike cristae and contain enzymes that convert cholesterol to pregnenolone. Steroid hormones include testosterone, produced by interstitial cells of the testes; estrogen, from follicle cells of the ovaries; progesterone, from granulosa lutein cells of the corpus luteum; and cortisone and aldosterone, from cells of the adrenal cortex.

D. Contractile Epithelial Cells: Contractile epithelial cells, or **myoepithelial cells,** are located between the basal lamina and the bases of the epithelial cells of secretory acini and ducts. They are stellate or spindle-shaped, flattened epithelial cells, with fingerlike processes that embrace the acinus or duct. Their cytoplasm contains abundant actin microfilaments, myosin, tropomyosin, and intermediate filaments (cytokeratin). Several myoepithelial cells may surround a single acinus or duct, and their contraction helps expel the products of exocrine glands. Gap junctions between myoepithelial and other cells facilitate synchronous contraction. Myoepithelial cells are found in lacrimal, salivary, mammary, and sweat glands and around the seminiferous tubules in the testis.

Study-Focusing Questions*

1. List the principal functions of epithelial tissues (64).
2. From which embryonic germ layer(s) are epithelial tissues derived? Give examples of epithelia derived from each (64).
3. List the structural and functional characteristics of epithelial tissues that distinguish them from other tissue types. Consider:
   a. Cell polarity (77)
   b. Specializations of the apical (71–72), lateral (66–71), and basal (66) surfaces
   c. Nutrition (77–78)

*The page references in this section refer to *Basic Histology,* 6th ed., Junqueira L, Carneiro J, Kelley R, (editors), Appleton & Lange, 1989. **HR** (for Histology Review) is occasionally used instead of a page reference to indicate that the information referred to can be found in this book.

   d. Innervation (78)
   e. Mitotic rate (78)
4. Describe the basal lamina in terms of its:
   a. Location (66)
   b. Composition (66)
   c. Staining properties (66)
5. What structures (66, 71) and molecules (66) specifically aid in the attachment of epithelial cells to their basal laminae?
6. Compare basal laminae and basement membranes (66).
7. Name 4 types of junctions found between epithelial cells (67–71).
8. Which junction(s) named in the answer to question 7 is associated with:
   a. A disklike structure (68, 71)
   b. A bandlike structure (67)
   c. Areas of fusion of the outer leaflets of the plasma membranes of adjacent cells (67)
   d. A sealing effect (67)
   e. Cytokeratins (71)
   f. Dense attachment plaques (71)
   g. Connexons (69)
9. What type of cellular junction is more important in cell-to-cell communication than in cell-to-cell adhesion (68–69)?
10. Compare microvilli, stereocilia, cilia, and flagella in terms of:
    a. Their width and length (72)
    b. The presence of plasma-membrane covering (72)
    c. The presence of microtubules or microfilaments (72)
    d. Their motility (72)
    e. The presence of axonemes and basal bodies (72, 73)
    f. Their function and location in the body (72)
11. List the types of simple epithelia and give examples of body sites where each may be found (72–74).
12. List the types of stratified epithelia and give examples of body sites where each may be found (73–74).
13. Compare endocrine and exocrine glands in terms of:
    a. Their embryonic origin (75)
    b. The way their products are transported (75)
14. What structural criteria are used to classify exocrine glands (76)?
15. Compare the merocrine, holocrine, and apocrine modes of secretion in terms of the portion of the cell that is released, and give an example of each type of gland (76–77).
16. How do exogenous chemical messengers that do not readily cross the plasma membrane control the intracellular events involved in secretion (78)?
17. Name the structural modifications and staining properties of epithelial cell types specialized for the following and give examples of each type:
    a. Transport of ions and water (78–79)
    b. Synthesis and secretion of proteins (80–85)
    c. Synthesis and secretion of mucus (86)
    d. Synthesis and secretion of steroids (88–89)
18. Compare neurocrine, paracrine, and endocrine cells in terms of the distances their products must travel to reach their targets, and give examples of each type of cell (80).
19. Describe DNES (APUD) cells (85) in terms of:
    a. What the acronyms DNES and APUD stand for
    b. Their embryonic origin
    c. Their structure
    d. The type of their secretory product
    e. Their distribution in the body
20. Give examples of DNES (APUD) cells, and name the substance produced by each (85).
21. Compare serous and mucous cells in terms of appearance and secretory product (86).

Multiple-Choice Questions

For questions 4–1 through 4–5, select the single best answer.

4–1. The epithelial type shown in Fig 4–1 is:
- **A.** Stratified squamous, keratinized
- **B.** Simple ciliated columnar
- **C.** Stratified columnar
- **D.** Pseudostratified ciliated columnar
- **E.** Simple cuboidal

4–2. The epithelial type lining the ducts shown in Fig 4–2 is:
- **A.** Simple cuboidal
- **B.** Stratified squamous, nonkeratinized
- **C.** Stratified cuboidal
- **D.** Simple ciliated columnar
- **E.** Pseudostratified columnar

4–3. The intercellular junction (∗) shown in Fig 4–3 is a:
- **A.** Gap junction
- **B.** Zonula occludens
- **C.** Desmosome
- **D.** Zonula adherens
- **E.** Hemidesmosome

4–4. In pseudostratified columnar epithelium:
- **A.** All nuclei lie at the same depth from the surface
- **B.** All cells border on the lumen
- **C.** All cells touch the basal lamina
- **D.** The cells are always of ectodermal origin
- **E.** All of the above

4–5. The cytokeratin filaments associated with desmosomes and zonulae adherentes are a form of:
- **A.** Microfilaments
- **B.** Intermediate filaments
- **C.** Microtubules
- **D.** Actin filaments
- **E.** Myosin filaments

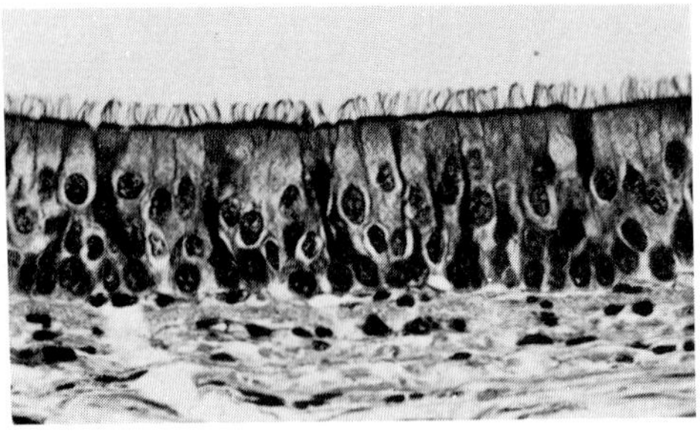

Figure 4–1.

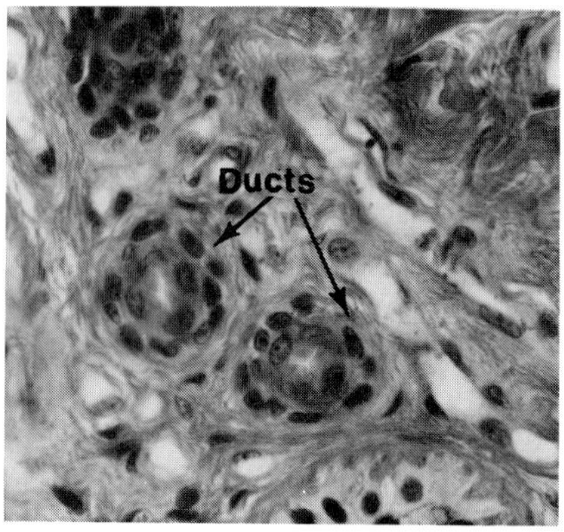

Figure 4–2.

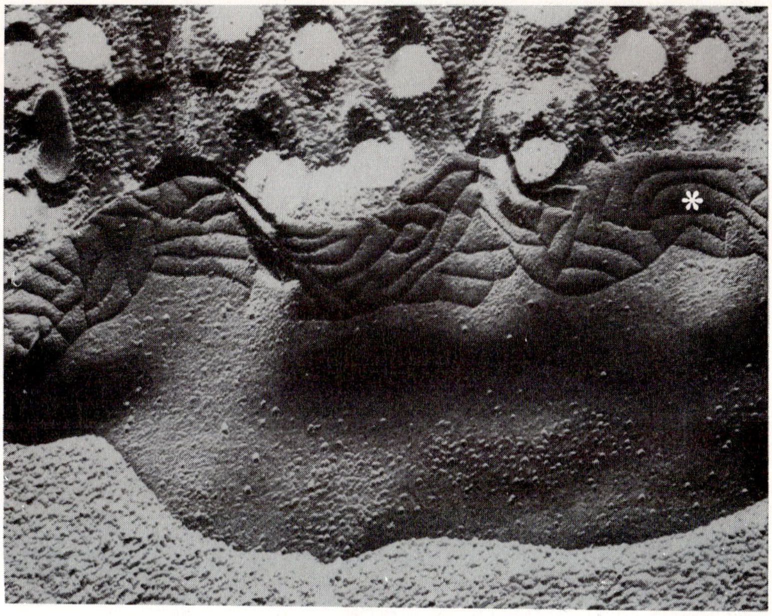

Figure 4-3.

MATCHING (questions 4-6 through 4-29): Each choice may be used once, more than once, or not at all.

Questions 4-6 through 4-10:

A. Stratified squamous, keratinized
B. Pseudostratified columnar
C. Transitional
D. Simple columnar
E. Simple squamous
F. Simple cuboidal

4-6. Epidermis of the skin
4-7. Lining of the urinary bladder
4-8. Lining of the capillaries
4-9. Lining of the trachea
4-10. Lining of the small intestine
4-11. Covering of the ovaries (germinal epithelium)

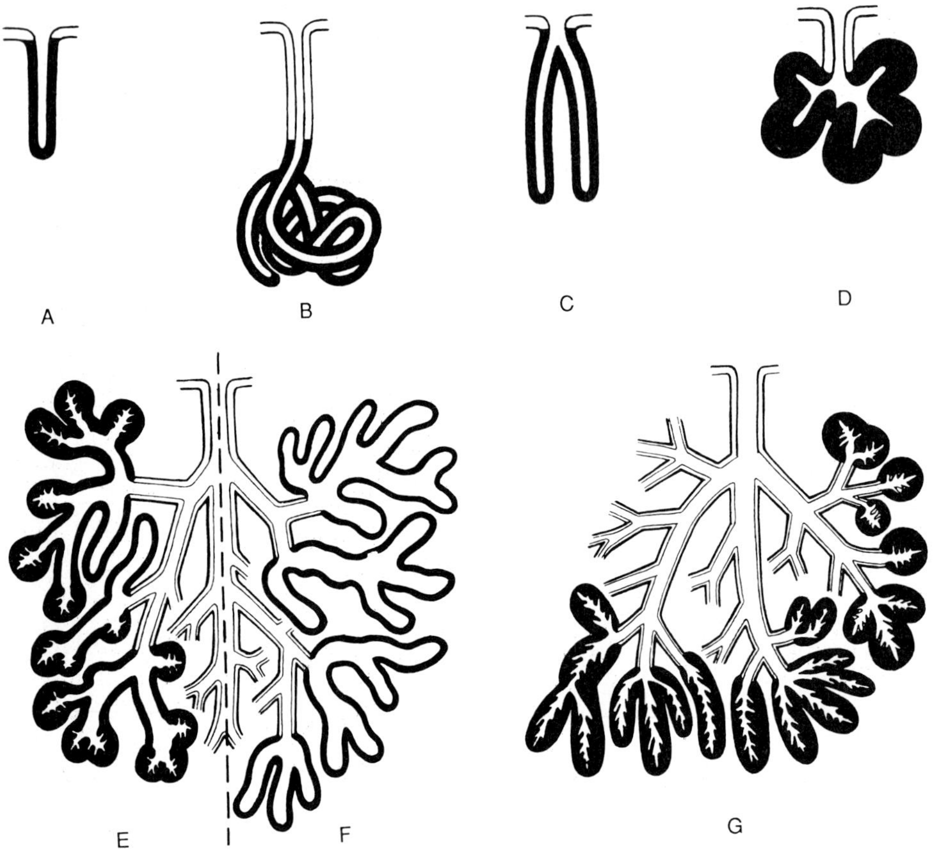

Figure 4–4.

Questions 4–12 through 4–18 use the letters in Fig 4–4.

4–12. Simple branched acinar gland
4–13. Compound tubuloacinar gland
4–14. Simple coiled tubular gland
4–15. Simple branched tubular gland
4–16. Compound acinar gland
4–17. Compound tubular gland
4–18. Simple tubular gland

Questions 4–19 through 4–23:

A. Ion-transporting cells
B. Protein-secreting cells
C. Mucus-secreting cells
D. Steroid-secreting cells
E. All of the above

4–19. Best characterized by abundant rough endoplasmic reticulum
4–20. Best characterized by abundant smooth endoplasmic reticulum
4–21. Apices of cells contain numerous large light-staining secretory granules filled with glycoproteins
4–22. Often contain mitochondria with tubular cristae
4–23. Contain abundant basal mitochondria between infoldings of the basal plasma membrane

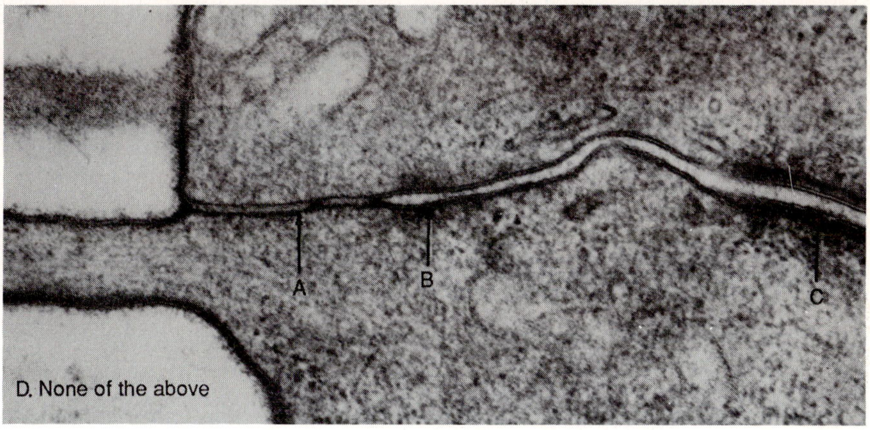

Figure 4-5.

Questions 4–24 through 4–29 use the letters in Fig 4–5.

4–24. Zonula occludens
4–25. Zonula adherens
4–26. Gap junction
4–27. Macula adherens
4–28. Hemidesmosome
4–29. Desmosome

For questions 4–30 through 4–38, select the one correct answer.

A. Cilia
B. Microvilli
C. Both
D. Neither

4–30. Covered by plasma membrane
4–31. Core contains microfilaments
4–32. Core contains microtubules
4–33. Anchored in basal bodies
4–34. Anchored in the terminal web
4–35. Core contains an axoneme
4–36. Usually only one per cell
4–37. Associated with absorptive epithelia
4–38. May be a specialization of the apical membrane of columnar cells

For questions 4–39 through 4–46, one, more than one, or all of the answers may be correct. Select

A if only (1), (2), and (3) are correct
B if only (1) and (3) are correct
C if only (2) and (4) are correct
D if only (4) is correct
E if all answers are correct

4–39. General features of epithelial tissues include:
(1) Epithelia rest on a basal lamina
(2) Epithelia are capable of metaplasia
(3) Epithelia are avascular
(4) All epithelia are derived from ectoderm

4-40. Criteria used in naming types of epithelia include:
- **(1)** Shape of cells in the surface layer
- **(2)** Presence of cilia
- **(3)** Number of layers of epithelial cells
- **(4)** Number of gap junctions per cell

4-41. The zonula occludens:
- **(1)** Is characterized by the fusion of the outer leaflets of adjacent trilaminar unit membranes into a single pentalaminar unit
- **(2)** Is characterized by the presence of abundant cytokeratin filaments in the vicinity of the junction
- **(3)** Surrounds the entire cell in the apical region of the lateral plasma membrane (in columnar cells)
- **(4)** Is characterized by a dense intracellular plaque

4-42. Stereocilia:
- **(1)** Are structurally most similar to cilia
- **(2)** Are nonmotile
- **(3)** Contain an axoneme
- **(4)** Are structurally most similar to microvilli

4-43. A simple branched tubular gland:
- **(1)** Is an exocrine gland
- **(2)** Has a branched duct
- **(3)** Has a tubular secretory portion
- **(4)** Has an acinar secretory portion

4-44. Holocrine secretion:
- **(1)** Occurs in sebaceous glands
- **(2)** Occurs only in endocrine glands
- **(3)** Involves cell death
- **(4)** Involves little or no loss of cytoplasm

4-45. Merocrine glands:
- **(1)** May be endocrine glands
- **(2)** May be exocrine glands
- **(3)** Contain a well-developed Golgi apparatus
- **(4)** Lose the apical portion of the secretory cell cytoplasm during secretion

4-46. Components of a basement membrane may include:
- **(1)** Laminin
- **(2)** Proteoglycan
- **(3)** Type IV collagen
- **(4)** Type III collagen (reticular fibers)

5 Connective Tissue

Objectives

This chapter should help the student to:

- List the structural and functional characteristics of connective tissue that distinguish it from the other basic tissue types.
- Know the functions carried out by connective tissues.
- Know the 3 fundamental components found in all connective tissues.
- Know the biochemical composition and the sites of synthesis of the components of extracellular matrix and how they associate with one another.

- Know the structure and function of the various cell types found in connective tissue.
- Compare the different types of connective tissues in terms of the types, relative amounts, and arrangement of cells, fibers, and ground substance.
- Relate the composition of the various connective tissue types to their specific functions.
- Name body sites where each connective tissue type may be found and relate these locations to the tissue's function.
- Recognize the types of connective tissues and connective tissue cells in a photomicrograph or slide of a tissue or organ and describe their probable function.
- Predict the functional consequences of a given structural defect in a connective tissue.

Synopsis

I. GENERAL FEATURES OF CONNECTIVE TISSUES

A. Functions: The functions of connective tissues, determined chiefly by their mechanical properties, include the binding together, compartmentalization, support, and physical and immunologic protection of other tissues and organs, as well as storage. For further detail, see IV.A.

B. Types: The connective tissues specifically described in this chapter (III) are loose and dense collagenous connective tissue (connective tissue proper), reticular connective tissue, elastic connective tissue, and mucous connective tissue. Adipose tissue, cartilage, and bone are specialized connective tissues considered in Chapters 6, 7, and 8, respectively. Questions pertaining to all these connective tissues (see Integrative Multiple Choice Questions: Connective Tissues) are included at the end of Chapter 8. Blood, often considered a highly specialized type of connective tissue, is discussed in Chapters 12 and 13.

C. Three Fundamental Components: The types of connective tissue differ in microscopic appearance, but all consist of **cells, fibers,** and **ground substance.** Connective tissue types and subtypes are classified according to the amounts, types, and proportions of these components.

D. Extracellular Matrix: The fibers and ground substance constitute the extracellular matrix. Connective tissues contain abundant matrix, which largely determines their mechanical properties. The fibers are of 2 types, collagen fibers and elastic fibers. The ground substance, in which the fibers and cells are embedded, is composed mainly of **glycosaminoglycans (GAGs)** dissolved in **tissue fluid.** Matrix viscosity and rigidity are determined by the amount and types of GAGs, the association of GAGs with core proteins to form proteoglycans, GAG-fiber associations, and GAG-GAG associations. Components of the fibers and ground substance are synthesized and secreted by connective tissue cells (mostly by fibroblasts), and the fibers are assembled in the extracellular space.

E. Embryonic Origin: All connective tissue cell types derive from cells of the embryonic mesenchyme. Mesenchyme derives from embryonic mesoderm, except head mesenchyme, which derives from the neural crest (mesectoderm).

II. COMPONENTS OF CONNECTIVE TISSUE

A. Collagen Fibers: The protein collagen is the most abundant in the body. There are many collagen types, some of which form fibers. Collagen fibers often collect to form fiber bundles ranging from 0.5–15 μm in diameter.

1. Synthesis and assembly

a. Intracellular steps Free polysomes reading collagen mRNA attach to the rough endoplasmic reticulum (see Chapter 3), and **protocollagen** polypeptides are deposited in the cisternae. Each protocollagen chain, or **alpha chain,** has a molecular weight of about 28,000 daltons and about 250 amino acids; every third amino acid is **glycine.** Proline and lysine residues within the chains are then hydroxylated by proline and lysine hydroxylases (possibly in smooth endoplasmic reticulum) to form **hydroxyproline** and **hydroxylysine,** unusual amino acids present in relatively large amounts in collagen. Core sugars (galactose and glucose) attach to the hydroxylysine residues in the endoplasmic reticulum. With the aid of **registration peptides** at the ends of the alpha chains, 3 chains coil around one another to form a triple helical molecule called **procollagen.** Further glycosylation may occur in the Golgi complex, where procollagen is packaged for secretion. Golgi vesicles release procollagen into the extracellular space by exocytosis.

b. Extracellular steps In the extracellular space, the enzyme **procollagen peptidase** cleaves the registration peptides from procollagen, converting it to **tropocollagen.** Tropocollagen molecules become aligned in staggered fashion to form collagen fibrils, possibly under the control of the adjacent cell.

2. Collagen types Not all collagen types are well characterized. A few examples of collagens whose biochemical structure, function, and location have been studied in some detail are described here.

a. Type I collagen, the most abundant and widespread, forms large fibers and fiber bundles. It is found in tendons, ligaments, bone, dermis, organ capsules, and loose connective tissue.

b. Type II collagen is found in adults only in the cartilage matrix (some occurs in the embryonic notochord) and forms only thin fibrils.

c. Type III collagen is similar to type I, but it is more heavily glycosylated and stains with silver. Often found in association with type I, type III forms networks of thin fibrils that surround and support soft flexible tissues (adipocytes, smooth muscle cells, nerve fibers). It is the major fiber component of hematopoietic tissues (eg, bone marrow, spleen) and of the reticular laminae underlying epithelial basal laminae.

d. Type IV collagen is the major collagen type in basal laminae. It does not form fibers or fibrils.

e. Type V collagen is present in placental basement membranes and blood vessels and in small amounts elsewhere. Its structure and function are poorly characterized.

f. Type X collagen is found in the matrix surrounding hypertrophic chondrocytes of degenerating growth plate cartilage in sites of future bone formation (see Chapter 8).

3. Histologic appearance

a. Light microscopy Collagen occurring in large or small bundles of fibrils or as individual fibrils exhibits acidophilic staining properties in H&E-stained sections. In sections stained with Masson's trichrome, collagen fibers stain green. Thin fibers (eg, type III) stain darkly with silver stains, but thicker bundles do not. Collagen molecules that do not form fibers or fibrils (eg, type IV) cannot be distinguished from the surrounding ground substance except by immunohistochemistry.

b. Electron microscopy All collagen fibrils and fibers have stripes at intervals of 64 nm along their length. This periodicity reflects the staggering of tropocollagen molecules.

4. Mechanical properties Collagen fibers' most important mechanical property is their tensile strength, which is (weight for weight) greater than that of steel.

5. Location Collagen fibers are found in all connective tissues and in the reticular laminae of certain basement membranes. In bone, its lacunar regions (spaces between overlapping tropocollagen units) may act as nucleation sites for the hydroxyapatite crystals of bone matrix.

B. Reticular Fibers: Reticular fibers are chemically identical to collagen, but they are thinner (0.1–1.5 μm) and form delicate silver-staining networks instead of thick bundles. The networks serve as supportive lattices that allow motile cells to move about in loosely arranged tissues such as hematopoietic tissues. Reticular fibers are composed mainly of type III collagen and some glycoproteins.

C. Elastic Fibers: Elastic fibers consist of an amorphous albuminoid protein called **elastin** and numerous proteinaceous **microfibrils** that become embedded in the elastin. They range in diameter from 0.1–10 μm.

1. Synthesis and assembly

a. Intracellular steps Microfibrillar proteins and proelastin are synthesized on ribosomes of the RER and secreted separately. Proelastin contains large amounts of the hydrophobic amino acids glycine, proline, and valine, accounting for elastin's insolubility. Microfibrillar protein contains mostly hydrophilic amino acids.

b. Extracellular steps Proelastin molecules polymerize extracellularly to form elastin chains. **Lysyl oxidases** then catalyze the conversion of certain lysine residues of elastin to aldehydes, 3 of which condense with a fourth, unaltered lysine residue to form **desmosine** and **isodesmosine.** These amino acids, very rare except in elastin, cross-link individual elastin chains. Elastin then associates with numerous microfibrils to form a branching and anastomosing network of elastic fibers.

2. Histologic appearance Elastin contains few charged amino acids, so it stains poorly with standard ionic dyes. Special stains, such as Verhoeff's stain or Weigert's resorcin-fuchsin stain, are used in light microscopic preparations. In EM preparations, both amorphous elastin and microfibrils can be visualized.

3. Mechanical properties Elastic fibers are extremely pliable and elastic. They can be stretched to 150% of their length without breaking and then return to their original length.

4. Location Elastic fibers are found where their mechanical properties are necessary to allow tissues to stretch or expand and then return to their original shape, eg, in arterial walls, interalveolar septa, bronchi and bronchioles of the lungs, vocal ligaments, and ligamenta flava of the vertebral column.

D. Ground Substance: The ground substance consists mostly of glycoconjugates of 2 classes, proteoglycans and glycoproteins. Tissue fluids and salts are also present.

1. Proteoglycans are composed of a **core protein** to which GAGs are attached. The GAGs of proteoglycans are straight-chain polymers of repeating sugar heterodimers made up of hexosamine (glucosamine or galactosamine) and uronic acid (glucuronic or iduronic acid). Five major classes of GAGs, differing in their sugars, exist in connective tissues: **hyaluronic acid** (which does not form proteoglycans), **chondroitin sulfate, dermatan sulfate, keratan sulfate,** and **heparan sulfate.** Proteoglycans are discussed further in Chapter 7.

2. Glycoproteins are proteins to which shorter, branched oligosaccharide chains are covalently bound. Glycoproteins of ground substance are much smaller than proteoglycans. ***Examples:*** **fibronectin,** which mediates the attachment of cells to the extracellular matrix; **laminin,** a component of basal laminae that mediates attachment of epithelial cells; and **chondronectin,** a component of cartilage matrix that mediates the attachment of chondrocytes to their matrix.

E. Cells: Connective tissue cells are grouped into 2 classes, fixed and wandering.

1. Fixed cells are native to the tissue in which they are found.

a. Mesenchymal cells These are the precursors of most cells indigenous to connective tissues, including fibroblasts and adipose cells. Embryonic mesenchyme consists of a loose network of stellate mesenchymal cells and abundant intercellular fluid. Some mesenchymal cells remain undifferentiated in adult connective tissue and constitute a reserve population of stem cells called **adventitial cells,** which are difficult to distinguish from some fibroblasts.

b. Fibroblasts These are the predominant connective tissue cells and are ubiquitous in connective tissue proper (III.A). They synthesize, secrete, and maintain all the major components of the extracellular matrix. Structurally, fibroblasts are of 2 types, one of which resembles mesenchymal cells. This type is stellate, with long cytoplasmic processes and a large, ovoid, pale-staining nucleus. The cytoplasm contains abundant rough endoplasmic reticulum and Golgi complexes, and this cell type is important in the production of collagen and other matrix components. Cells of the second type are less active and are sometimes termed **fibrocytes,** because they are believed to be more mature. Fibrocytes are smaller and spindle-shaped, with a dark, elongate nucleus and fewer cytoplasmic organelles. They can revert to the fibroblast state and participate in tissue repair.

c. Reticular cells These reticular connective tissue (III.B) cells make up a functionally diverse yet morphologically similar group. They produce the reticular fibers (II.B) that form the netlike stroma of hematopoietic and lymphoid tissues. Some apparently can phagocytose antigenic material and cellular debris. Others (antigen-presenting cells) collect antigens on their surfaces and help activate immunocompetent cells to mount an immune response. Reticular cells are typically stellate wth long, thin cytoplasmic processes. Each has a central, pale, irregularly rounded nucleus and a prominent nucleolus. In the cytoplasm, the number of mitochondria and the degree of development of the Golgi complex and rough endoplasmic reticulum is variable. Some reticular cells, particularly those with less developed organelles, may be stem cells of various blood types.

d. Adipose cells Adipose cells, or **adipocytes,** are mesenchymal derivatives specialized as storage depots for lipids (see Chapter 6).

2. Wandering cells are immigrant cells, usually from blood or bone marrow (for further information, consult Chapters 12–14). Some retain their original characteristics and may eventually leave the connective tissue; others undergo differentiation and take up permanent residence there.

a. Mast cells These derive from bone marrow precursors and are characterized by abundant basophilic cytoplasmic granules. At the EM level, these granules appear as electron-dense granules. Other features of mast cells at this level are many small plasma membrane folds and a well-developed Golgi complex. The granules, which usually obscure the small central nucleus, contain heparin, histamine, and eosinophil chemotactic factor of anaphylaxis (ECF-A). Mast cells have surface receptors for IgE antibodies and are involved in the inflammatory response of the immune system.

b. Macrophages These are large, stellate cells derived from cells of the blood monocyte lineage that infiltrate connective tissue and develop into phagocytes. Resident macrophages can proliferate and form additional macrophages. Dye particles injected into the body are engulfed by these cells and accumulate in cytoplasmic granules. Macrophages contain many lysosomes, which aid in digesting phagocytosed materials, and a well-developed Golgi complex. They help maintain the integrity of connective tissues by removing foreign substances and cellular debris, and they participate in the immune response by presenting phagocytosed antigens to lymphocytes. To remove large foreign objects such as splinters, macrophages may fuse to form **multinuclear giant cells.** Monocyte-derived phagocytes, which together constitute the **mononuclear phagocyte system,** include the macrophages (lymphoid organs, lungs, serous cavities, and connective tissue), as well as Kupffer cells (liver), osteoclasts (bone) and microglial cells (central nervous system).

c. Plasma cells These differentiate from antigen-stimulated B lymphocytes and are the primary producers of circulating antibodies. They are sparsely distributed throughout the body but abundant in areas susceptible to penetration by bacteria. Plasma cells are large and ovoid, with an eccentric nucleus and abundant rough endoplasmic reticulum. The characteristic "clock face" of the nucleus results from a large, central nucleolus and several large heterochromatin clumps regularly spaced inside the nuclear envelope. These cells usually exhibit a clear juxtanuclear area (cytocenter) containing a well-developed Golgi complex and centrioles.

d. Other blood-derived connective tissue cells Many wandering cell types originate in the bone marrow and are carried to connective tissue by the blood and lymph. Blood-derived cells found in connective tissues include the leukocytes (white blood cells, ie, **lymphocytes, monocytes, neutrophils, eosinophils,** and **basophils**) which have roles in the immune response and are described in detail in Chapters 12–14.

III. CONNECTIVE TISSUE TYPES

A. Connective Tissue Proper: Connective tissue proper, found in most organs, is characterized by a predominance of fibers (mainly type I collagen) in the extracellular matrix. Its varied functions are chiefly related to binding cells and tissues into organs and organ systems. Its subclasses are based on the type, density, and orientation of its fibers.

1. Loose connective tissue Loose connective tissue or **areolar tissue,** generally appears very disorganized. It consists of a loosely arranged network of different types of fibers, upon which many kinds of fixed and wandering cells are suspended. The ground substance is abundant and only moderately viscous. (The types of cells and fibers and the composition of the ground substance are summarized in Table 5–1.) This flexible yet delicate tissue surrounds and suspends vessels and nerves as they traverse most organs, underlies and supports most epithelia, and fills spaces between other tissues (eg, between muscle fibers and their dense connective tissue sheaths). It also supports the serous membranes (mesothelia) of the pleura, pericardium, and peritoneum. Always well vascularized, areolar tissue conveys oxygen and nutrients to avascular epithelia. Its cells function in immune surveillance for foreign substances entering the body through the blood or epithelia.

2. Dense connective tissue Collagen fibers are the predominant component of dense connective tissue. Nearly all the fibers are of type I collagen. The cells are predominantly mature fibroblasts (fibrocytes). The ground substance is essentially identical to that of areolar tissue but is present in lesser quantities (Table 5–1). There are 2 types of dense connective tissue: regular, with a ropelike arrangement of fiber bundles, and irregular, with a fabriclike arrangement.

a. Dense regular connective tissue The fibers of this tissue are tightly packed into parallel bundles, between which are a few highly attenuated, spindle-shaped fibroblasts. The small, cigar-shaped nuclei of the fibroblasts are oriented parallel to the fibers; the cytoplasm is difficult to distinguish with the light microscope. There is little room for the ground substance, which nevertheless permeates the tissue. The tensile strength of the packed collagen fibers makes them ideal for transmitting mechanical force over long distances using a minimum of material and space, while resisting mechanical forces from other directions. This tissue therefore serves to transmit the force of muscle contraction, to attach bones to one another, and to protect other tissues and organs. It is found in tendons, ligaments, periosteum, perichondrium, deep fascia, and some organ capsules.

b. Dense irregular connective tissue The components of this tissue are identical to those found in dense regular connective tissue (Table 5–1). At first glance, dense irregular connective tissue seems poorly organized, but its collagen bundles have a complex woven pattern that provides resistance to tensile stress from any direction. Its functions include covering the more fragile tissues and organs and protecting them from multidirectional mechanical stresses. It is found in the reticular layer of the dermis and in most organ capsules.

Table 5-1. Characteristics of Connective Tissue (CT) Types

Connective Tissue	Tissue Type	Cells	Fibers	Ground Substance	Organization	Functions	Locations
Embryonic CT	Mesenchyme	Mesenchymal cells.	Relatively few. Collagen and I and III.	Watery. Mainly tissue-fluid. Some glycoprotein and glycosaminoglycan.	Loose array of stellate cells. Large intercellular spaces filled with ground substance.	Embryonic connective tissue. Forms all connective tissue listed below.	Throughout all vertebrate embryos. That in head and neck derives from neural crest (ectoderm), rest from mesoderm.
	Mucous CT	Mesenchymal cells and fibroblasts.	Small number. Mainly collagen. Few elastic and reticular.	Syrupy to jelly-like. Mainly hyaluronic acid and glycoproteins.	Cells and fibers distributed randomly in abundant ground substance.	Forms an elastic cushion to protect nearby structures from pressure.	Wharton's jelly of umbilical cord. Pulp of developing teeth. Nucleus pulposus of intervertebral disks.
CT Proper	Loose (Areolar) CT	Fibroblasts, fibrocytes, mesenchymal cells, mast cells, macrophages, adipocytes, plasma cells, and leukocytes (basophils, eosinophils, lymphocytes, and neutrophils).	Collagen (type I), elastic and reticular (type III collagen).	Moderately viscous. Hyaluronic acid, glycoproteins, sulfated glycosaminoglycans, and proteoglycans.	More cellular than dense CT. Cells suspended in what appears to be a disorganized network of loosely interwoven fibers whose interstices are filled with ground substance.	Suspends, supports, and protects vessels, nerves, and epithelia.	Around vessels and nerves. Under covering and lining epithelia (ie, lamina propria). Supports serous membranes (eg, peritoneum, pericardium, pleura). Fills potential spaces between other tissues.
	Dense Regular CT	Predomniantly mature fibroblasts (fibrocytes). Other types listed for loose CT may be present, but not in abundance.	Almost all type I collagen. Some elastic and reticular fibers are often present.	Similar to that for loose CT, but in smaller quantities.	Fibers predominate. Large collagen fibers packed into parallel bundles. Cells (fibrocytes) scattered between fiber bundles with their long axes oriented parallel to that of the fibers.	Transmits mechanical force of muscles. Binds bones to one another. Forms protective cover for some organs.	Tendons, ligaments, periosteum, perichondrium, joint capsules, deep fascia, and some organ capsules.
	Dense Irregular CT				Fiber bundles of differing sizes woven into a dense collagenous mat or fabric.	Resists tensile stress from all directions. Protects fragile organs.	Reticular layer of dermis. Most organ capsules.

Connective Tissue	Tissue Type	Cells	Fibers	Ground Substance	Organization	Functions	Locations
Specialized CT	Reticular CT	Reticular cells. Presence of other types depends on location.	Reticular fibers (type III collagen).	Very little. Composition unclear.	Delicate 3-D fiber network. Reticular cells attach to and cover fibers with long, thin cell processes. Other cells suspended in spaces.	Support for motile cells. Important in filtration of blood.	Mainly hematopoietic tissues (eg, bone marrow, spleen, and lymph nodes).
	Elastic CT	Fibroblasts predominate. Other types listed for loose CT may be present but not in abundance.	Elastic fibers predominate. Some collagen.	Sparse. Composition similar to that of dense CT.	Fibers predominate and collect in parallel wavy bundles separated by collagen and fibroblasts. Resembles dense regular CT, but fibers are wider and more retractile.	Flexible support.	Ligamenta flava of vertebral column, vocal ligament, and suspensory ligament of the penis.

B. Reticular Connective Tissue: The reticular fibers (type III collagen) of this tissue form a delicate 3-dimensional, netlike scaffolding upon which cells, the predominant element, are suspended. Reticular cells are firmly attached to the fibers, which may be mostly covered by the long attenuated reticular cell processes. Other cell types, such as lymphocytes, are suspended in the spaces of the network (Table 5–1). There is very little ground substance. Reticular connective tissue functions in the support of motile cells and filtration of body fluids. It is found mainly in hematopoietic tissues such as bone marrow, spleen, and lymph nodes.

C. Elastic Connective Tissue: In H&E-stained sections, elastic tissue closely resembles dense regular (collagenous) connective tissue. Fibers are the predominant element; most of these fibers are elastic, while some are collagen. The elastic fibers are collected into thick, wavy bundles oriented parallel to one another. The bundles are separated by loose collagenous tissue and occasional fibroblasts with attenuated cytoplasm and condensed, oblong nuclei. Other connective tissue cells may be present in small numbers (Table 5–1). The ground substance is sparse and similar to that of other dense connective tissues. Elastic connective tissue provides flexible support and is limited in distribution to the ligamenta flava of the vertebral column and the suspensory ligament of the penis.

D. Mucous Connective Tissue: This tissue has small numbers of cells and fibers distributed randomly in the abundant ground substance, which has a syrupy to jellylike consistency and is composed chiefly of hyaluronic acid (Table 5–1). Mucous tissue yields readily to pressure but can return to its original shape, so it is useful for protecting underlying structures from excess pressure. It is the predominant component (Wharton's jelly) of the umbilical cord, of the nucleus pulposis of the intervertebral disks, and of the pulp of young teeth.

IV. HISTOPHYSIOLOGY OF CONNECTIVE TISSUE

A. Functions:

1. Support Structural support is the major function of connective tissue, which forms the framework upon which all other body tissues are assembled. Its physical properties allow it to bind, to fill spaces, and to separate functional units of other tissues and organs. It thus maintains functional units in their proper 3-dimensional relationships, allowing maintenance and coordination of all body functions.

2. Defense

a. Physical The viscosity of the extracellular matrix, due largely to hyaluronic acid, slows the progress of many bacteria and foreign particles. Sheets of tightly packed and often interwoven collagen fibers, as in organ capsules, help to confine local infections. However, some bacteria secrete enzymes that break down matrix components; eg, staphylococci, clostridia, streptococci, and pneumococci secrete **hyaluronidase** and *Clostridium perfringens* secretes **collagenase.**

b. Immunologic Foreign bodies that successfully penetrate epithelia are intercepted by immunoresponsive cells that inhabit the underlying connective tissue (II.E.2). These cells not only activate a local immune response (inflammation) but mobilize the immune system to supply additional cells via the bloodstream. Recruited cells migrate through capillary and venule walls into the connective tissue, a process called **diapedesis.**

3. Repair Rapidly closing any breaches in the body's protective barriers is an important function of connective tissue. Injury stimulates invasion of the site by immunocompetent cells and the proliferation of fibroblasts. Macrophages remove clotted blood, damaged tissue, and foreign material, while fibroblasts secrete extracellular matrix materials to fill the breach. Rapidly formed collagenous matrices that close wounds are often less well organized than the original tissues and form scars. Small scars may eventually be completely remodeled; larger scars are only partially remodeled.

4. Storage Reserves of water and electrolytes, especially sodium, are stored in the extracellular matrix, owing to the high polyanionic charge density of glycosaminoglycans. Energy reserves in the form of lipids are stored in adipocytes.

5. Transport Except in the central nervous system, most blood and lymphatic vessels are surrounded by loose connective tissue, which is thus a crossroads for transporting substances to and from other tissues.

B. Edema:

The water in tissue fluid comes from the arterial ends of capillaries in capillary beds, forced out by **hydrostatic pressure** (arterial pressure). Loss of fluid to the tissues increases the blood solute concentration at the venous end of the capillary; this increased **colloid osmotic pressure,** along with the lower hydrostatic pressure at the venous end, draws most of the lost fluid back into the blood. Any excess fluid remaining in the tissue is normally drained away by lymphatic capillaries, so that there is no net change in the amount of blood or tissue fluid. Edema, or accumulation of excess tissue fluid, accompanies pathological conditions that cause:

1. Increased hydrostatic pressure in capillaries by obstructing venous blood flow (eg, congestive heart failure);

2. Decreased colloid osmotic pressure in the blood caused by lack of blood proteins (eg, starvation);

3. Increased hydrostatic pressure in the tissue caused by blockage of lymphatic drainage by parasites or tumor cells; and

4. Increased colloid osmotic pressure in the tissue caused by excessive accumulation of glycosaminoglycans in the matrix. Edema caused by this condition is called **myxedema.**

C. Hormonal Effects:

Cortisol (hydrocortisone), produced by the adrenal glands under the influence of pituitary adrenocorticotropic hormone (ACTH), inhibits connective tissue fiber synthesis by fibroblasts and retards local inflammatory and immune responses by other connective tissue cells. Cortisol or synthetic cortisone therefore reduce local heat, redness, and tenderness but delay and impair wound healing. Insufficient levels of thyroid hormone (hypothyroidism) cause accumulation of excess glycosaminoglycans in the connective tissue matrix, leading to myxedema.

D. Nutritional Factors: As a cofactor of proline hydroxylase (II.A.1.a), **vitamin C** (ascorbic acid) is required for normal collagen synthesis. Vitamin C deficiency leads to a condition called **scurvy,** characterized by weakening of all connective tissue. Proline hydroxylase activity also requires iron, molecular oxygen, and α-ketoglutarate. The importance of vitamins to connective tissues is also discussed in Chapter 8.

E. Collagen Renewal: Collagen is a very stable protein, and its turnover is quite slow—slowest in tendons and other dense connective tissues, fastest in loose connective tissue. Macrophages and neutrophils release collagenase, which breaks down old collagen, and new collagen is synthesized by fibroblasts. As humans age, their extracellular collagen becomes increasingly cross-linked, and its turnover slows in all connective tissues.

Study-Focusing Questions*

1. List the 3 major classes of connective tissue components (91).
2. List the general functions of connective tissues (91).
3. Name the germ layer(s) from which connective tissue cells are derived and the embryonic tissues composed of undifferentiated connective tissue cells (91).
4. List the 2 major classes of macromolecules that constitute the ground substance (91).
5. List the types of glycosaminoglycans commonly found in the ground substance and give examples of body sites where each type may be found (92-93).
6. Name 3 important structural glycoproteins found in connective tissue ground substance and describe their functions (93).
7. Name the 2 forces (pressures) that act on the water in capillaries, affecting the amount of fluid in connective tissue (94).
8. Give some common causes of edema and describe the effect of each on the pressures named in answer to question 7 (95).
9. Name the 3 main fiber types found in connective tissues (96) and compare them in terms of:
    - **a.** Their protein composition (95, 100–101)
    - **b.** The arrangement of their protein subunits (97–101)
    - **c.** Their characteristic amino acids (96, 100–101)
    - **d.** Their degree of glycosylation (100)
    - **e.** The arrangement and appearance of fibers in their tissues (95, 100–101)
    - **f.** Their diameter (100; **HR**)
    - **g.** Their physical properties and function (100–101)
    - **h.** Their staining properties (100–101)
    - **i.** Their location in the body (95, 98, 100–101, 113–118)
10. Name the major types of collagen (95-96) and compare them in terms of:
    - **a.** Their protein composition
    - **b.** Their tendency to form fibers or fibrils
    - **c.** Their tissue distribution
    - **d.** The cell type responsible for their synthesis
11. Describe collagen synthesis and assembly and indicate the intracellular or extracellular location where each step of the process occurs (96, 98, 99). It might be helpful to draw a diagram of a cell with numbered steps.

*The page references in this section refer to *Basic Histology,* 6th ed., Junqueira L, Carneiro J, Kelley R (editors), Appleton & Lange, 1989. **HR** (for Histology Review) is occasionally used instead of a page reference to indicate that the information referred to can be found in this book.

12. What is the difference between procollagen and tropocollagen (98)?
13. Describe the roles played by the following enzymes in connective tissue fiber synthesis, assembly, and turnover:
    a. Collagenase (98, 120)
    b. Elastase (101)
    c. Signal peptidase (36)
    d. Lysyl oxidase (98)
    e. Procollagen peptidase (98)
    f. Proline hydroxylase (96, 120)
14. List the cell types found in connective tissues and indicate which type is most common (104).
15. Compare fibroblasts and fibrocytes (104–105) in terms of:
    a. Their cell shape
    b. The morphologic characteristics of their nuclei
    c. Their mitotic activity
    d. Their synthetic activity
16. List the important substances synthesized and secreted by fibroblasts and the organelles necessary for their synthesis and secretion (104–105).
17. From which type of circulating blood cells are macrophages derived (104)?
18. Name the organelles characteristically found in abundance in macrophages and the major function for which they are needed (105–107).
19. Describe mast cells in terms of:
    a. Their shape and size (107)
    b. Their staining properties (107)
    c. The contents of their cytoplasmic granules (108)
    d. The cause of their degranulation (release of granule contents) (109–110)
    e. The effects of their degranulation (110)
    f. Their role in allergic reactions (109–110)
20. Describe plasma cells (110–112) in terms of:
    a. Their shape
    b. Their staining properties
    c. The appearance of their nuclei
    d. Their major cytoplasmic organelles
    e. Their major secretory product
    f. Their role in immunity
    g. The specific blood cell type from which they derive
21. List the types of leukocytes commonly found in connective tissue (112–113) and describe each in terms of:
    a. The presence of cytoplasmic granules
    b. Their staining properties
    c. The morphologic characteristics of thin nuclei
    d. Their major functions
22. Name 3 types of connective tissue proper and compare them in terms of general function and location in the body (113, 116–117).
23. Compare loose (areolar) and dense connective tissue (113–117) in terms of:
    a. Their abundance
    b. The types and proportions of their matrix components
    c. The number of their cells
    d. Their flexibility and resistance to stress
    e. Their rate of collagen turnover (120)
24. Compare dense regular and dense irregular connective tissue in terms of the arrangement of their collagen bundles and their locations in the body (113, 116–117).
25. Describe elastic connective tissue (117–118) in terms of its:
    a. Composition
    b. Predominant cell type
    c. Color in the fresh state
    d. Location in the body
26. Describe reticular connective tissue (118) in terms of:
    a. Its characteristic appearance
    b. The types of organs in which it is commonly found
    c. Its predominant cell type
    d. Its function

27. Describe mucous connective tissue (118) in terms of its:
   a. Predominant matrix component
   b. Consistency
   c. Predominant cell type
   d. Location

28. Discuss the active (immunologic) and passive (physical) roles of connective tissue in defending the body against the invasion of pathogens (119–120).

29. Name 2 enzymes produced and released by pathogenic bacteria that digest specific components of connective tissue extracellular matrix (120).

30. Which connective tissue cells specifically contribute to the repair of wounds by removing (107) and replacing (104, 120) damaged tissue?

31. Discuss the role of loose (areolar) connective tissue as a "crossroads" and defensive barrier between blood vessels and the tissues they supply (113, 119).

32. List the effects of the following (120) on connective tissue structure and function:
   a. Hydrocortisone
   b. ACTH
   c. Hypothyroidism
   d. Ascorbic acid

Multiple-Choice Questions

For questions 5–1 through 5–9, select the single best answer.

5–1. The ground substance of connective tissue includes all of the following components *except:*
   A. Hyaluronic acid
   B. Proteoglycans
   C. Fibronectin
   D. Collagen fibers
   E. Glycosaminoglycans

5–2. The cell type mainly responsible for producing and maintaining all the components of connective tissue extracellular matrix is the:
   A. Mesothelial cell
   B. Fibroblast
   C. Mast cell
   D. Lymphocyte
   E. Macrophage

5–3. Collagen synthesis is initiated:
   A. On a polyribosome
   B. With the reading of the code for the registration peptide
   C. On the rough endoplasmic reticulum
   D. On the smooth endoplasmic reticulum
   E. In the extracellular matrix

5–4. Dense regular connective tissue:
   A. Is composed primarily of fibroblasts
   B. Is composed primarily of ground substance
   C. Is the predominant tissue type in most organ capsules
   D. Contains more mast cells than any other type of connective tissue
   E. May be found in tendons

5–5. The 3 basic components of all types of connective tissue are:
   A. Cells, fibers, and ground substance
   B. Arteries, veins, and capillaries
   C. Fibroblasts, reticular fibers, and proteoglycan aggregates
   D. Type II collagen, hyaluronate, and fibronectin
   E. Mast cells, lymphocytes, and adipocytes

5–6. All of the following substances are glycosaminoglycans *except:*
   A. Keratan sulfate
   B. Hyaluronic acid
   C. Chondroitin sulfate

D. Heparan sulfate
E. Fibronectin

5–7. The fiber type most commonly associated with the formation of a fine supportive network in the soft tissues of the body is:
A. Type I collagen
B. Elastic fibers
C. Reticular fibers
D. Purkinje fibers
E. Type II collagen

5–8. The tissue type shown in Fig 5–1 is:
A. Dense regular connective tissue
B. Dense irregular connective tissue
C. Elastic connective tissue
D. Loose (areolar) connective tissue
E. Reticular connective tissue

5–9. The tissue type shown in Fig 5–2 is:
A. Dense regular connective tissue
B. Dense irregular connective tissue
C. Elastic connective tissue
D. Loose (areolar) connective tissue
E. Reticular connective tissue

MATCHING (questions 5–10 through 5–21): each choice may be used once, more than once, or not at all.

Questions 5–10 through 5–13:

A. Desmosine
B. Hydroxyproline
C. Hydroxylysine
D. Glycine
E. None of the above

5–10. Every third amino acid in collagen
5–11. Glycosylated during collagen synthesis
5–12. Characteristic of elastic fibers
5–13. Absent in areolar tissue

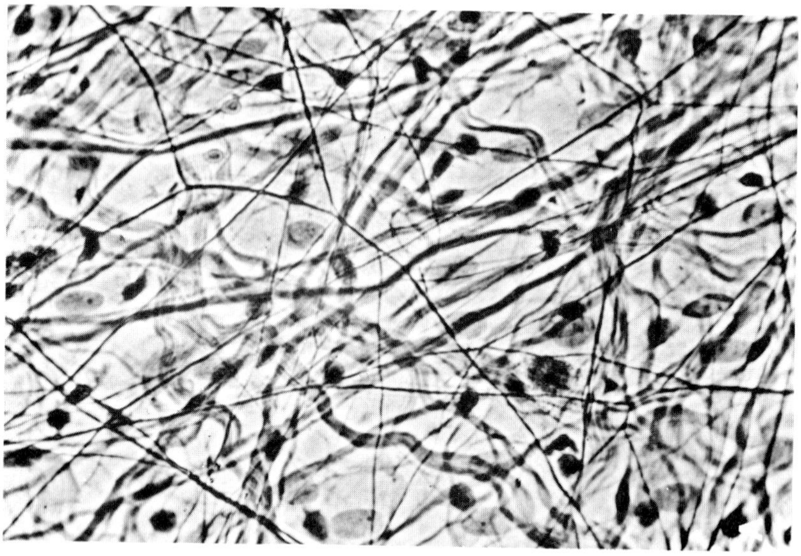

Figure 5–1.

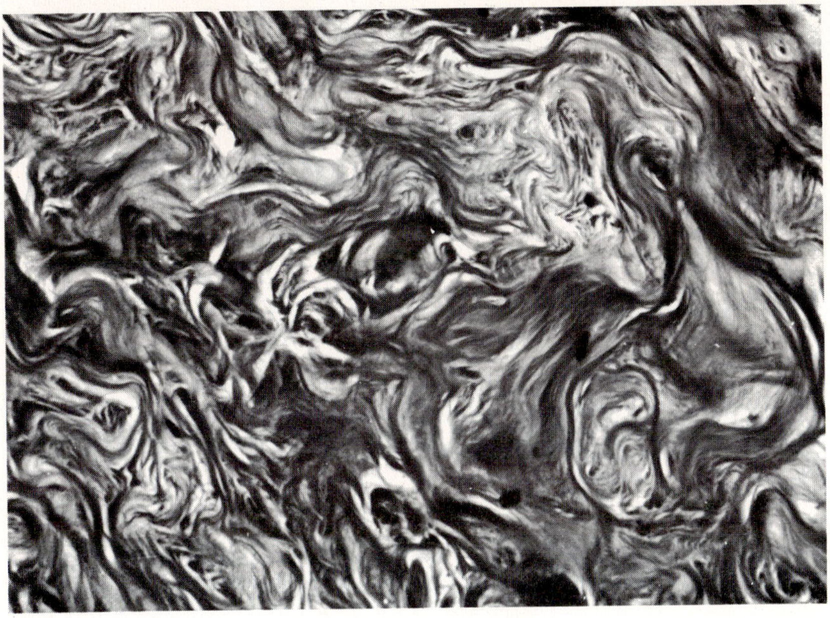

Figure 5-2.

Questions 5-14 through 5-21:

- **A.** Fibroblasts
- **B.** Lymphocytes
- **C.** Mast cells
- **D.** Plasma cells
- **E.** Macrophages

5-14. Primary function is synthesis and secretion of immunoglobulins (antibodies)
5-15. Predominant cell type in connective tissue proper
5-16. Contain granules filled with heparin and histamine
5-17. Have a rounded heterochromatic nucleus and very little cytoplasm
5-18. Contain more lysosomes than the other listed cells
5-19. Binding of antigen to IgE on the cell surface causes degranulation
5-20. Nucleus exhibits a "clock face" pattern of heterochromatin
5-21. Mature cells exhibit an elongated fusiform (spindle-shaped) structure

For questions 5-22 through 5-25, select the one correct answer.

- **A.** Tropocollagen
- **B.** Procollagen
- **C.** Both
- **D.** Neither

5-22. Includes registration peptides
5-23. Form secreted by fibroblasts
5-24. Found in the extracellular matrix
5-25. Also referred to as an alpha chain

For questions 5-26 through 5-30, one, more than one, or all of the answers may be correct. Select

A if only (1), (2), and (3) are correct
B if only (1) and (3) are correct
C if only (2) and (4) are correct
D if only (4) is correct
E if all answers are correct

5-26. Functions of connective tissue include
- **(1)** Immunologic protection
- **(2)** Tissue repair after injury
- **(3)** Structural support
- **(4)** Fuel storage

5-27. Fibroblasts secrete:
- **(1)** Proelastin
- **(2)** Procollagen
- **(3)** Glycosaminoglycans
- **(4)** Fibronectin

5-28. The synthesis and assembly of collagen fibers involves the:
- **(1)** Rough endoplasmic reticulum
- **(2)** Golgi apparatus
- **(3)** Transfer vesicles
- **(4)** Extracellular space

5-29. Mucous connective tissue:
- **(1)** Has a thick syrupy ground substance
- **(2)** Is sometimes referred to as Wharton's jelly
- **(3)** Cushions and protects the umbilical vessels
- **(4)** Is composed primarily of hyaluronic acid

5-30. Elastic fibers:
- **(1)** Can be stretched to 150% of their length and spring back to their original size
- **(2)** Are ensheathed by microfibrillar proteins
- **(3)** Contain the scleroprotein elastin
- **(4)** Are found only in elastic connective tissue

6 Adipose Tissue

Objectives

This chapter should help the student to:

- Relate the various functions of adipose tissue to its structural characteristics.
- Describe adipose tissue as a connective tissue in terms of the relative amount and types of its cells, fibers, and ground substance.
- Know the differences and similarities between the 2 types of adipose tissue.
- Recognize the type of adipose tissue present in a photomicrograph or slide of a tissue or organ.

Synopsis

I. GENERAL FEATURES OF ADIPOSE TISSUE

A. A Tissue and an Organ: Adipose tissue, or fat, is a connective tissue specialized to store fuel. If we were not equipped to store fuel, all of our time would have to be spent obtaining food. The cytoplasm of fat cells, or **adipocytes,** contains large triglyceride deposits in the form of one or more lipid droplets with no limiting membranes. Together, the clusters of adipocytes scattered throughout the body constitute an extremely important metabolic organ that varies widely in size and distribution, depending on such factors as age, sex, and nutritional status.

B. General Organization: Clusters of adipocytes are separated into lobes and lobules by septa of collagenous connective tissue of variable density. Individual cells are surrounded by a network of reticular fibers. The ground substance is sparse.

C. Two Types: There are 2 basic types of adipose tissue, termed white adipose tissue, or **white fat,** and brown adipose tissue, or **brown fat.** A white fat adipocyte has a single large lipid droplet; a brown fat adipocyte has many small droplets.

II. WHITE ADIPOSE TISSUE

A. Distinguishing Features: White adipose tissue, the more abundant of the 2 types, is also termed **unilocular adipose tissue,** a reference to the single fat droplet in each of its cells. In mature adipocytes, the droplet is so large that it displaces the nucleus and remaining cytoplasm to the cellular periphery. Cell diameter varies from 50 to 150 μm. Adipocytes in histologic sections have a **signet-ring** appearance because most of the lipid is washed away during preparation, leaving only a flattened nucleus and a thin rim of cytoplasm. The cytoplasm near the nucleus contains a Golgi apparatus, mitochondria, a small amount of rough endoplasmic reticulum, and free ribosomes. The cytoplasm in the thin rim contains smooth endoplasmic reticulum and pinocytotic vesicles. This tissue is sometimes termed yellow adipose tissue or **yellow fat;** dietary carotenoids accumulate in the lipid droplets, making the tissue yellow. White fat is richly vascularized but not as richly as brown fat.

B. Distribution:

1. Subcutaneous fat Subcutaneous fat (hypodermis) is the layer of white adipose tissue found just beneath the skin except in the eyelids, penis, scrotum, and most of the external ear. (There is some fat in the earlobe.) In infants, it forms a continuous thermal insulating layer of uniform thickness covering the entire body and is termed the **panniculus adiposus.** In adults it becomes thicker or thinner in selected areas, depending upon the person's age, sex, and dietary habits. Where it becomes thinner, the tissue takes on the appearance of areolar tissue. In males, the fat layer thickens over the nape of the neck, deltoids (shoulders), triceps brachii (back of the upper arm), lumbosacral region (lower back), and buttocks. In females, additional fat is deposited in the breasts and buttocks and over the epitrochanteric region (hips) and anterior aspect of the thighs.

2. Intra-abdominal fat Fat deposits of varying sizes surround blood and lymphatic vessels in the omentum and mesenteries suspended in the abdominal cavity. Additional accumulations occur in retroperitoneal areas, such as around the kidneys on the posterior abdominal wall.

3. Other locations Other prominent accumulations of fat are found within the eye orbits and surrounding major joints (eg, knees). Such accumulations also form pads in the palms and soles.

C. Functional Characteristics: Adipocytes store fatty acids in triglycerides (esters of glycerol and 3 fatty acids). The triglycerides stored in both white and brown fat undergo continuous turnover. Their released fatty acids serve as a source of chemical energy for cells (the predominant source in resting muscle) and as a source of the raw materials for making phospholipids (the predominant component of biologic membranes). Turnover is regulated by several histophysiologic factors, which shift the equilibrium toward fat uptake or fat mobilization, depending on the body's level of, and need for, circulating fatty acids.

1. Factors influencing lipid uptake (lipogenic influences)

a. Dietary abundance Dietary fats can be absorbed by intestinal epithelial cells and carried by lymphatic vessels to the blood in particles called **chylomicrons** (see Chapter 15). Chylomicron triglycerides are hydrolyzed by lipoprotein lipases in the capillaries of adipose tissue; the released fatty acids are absorbed by adipocytes and resynthesized into triglycerides for storage. Dietary glucose can be converted in the liver to fatty acids, which the blood then carries to adipocytes in the triglycerides of **very low density lipoproteins (VLDL).** Glucose can also be directly absorbed from the blood and converted into triglycerides by the adipocytes themselves.

b. Hormones Insulin dramatically increases the uptake of glucose by adipocytes and enhances the synthesis of triglycerides from carbohydrates.

2. Factors influencing lipid mobilization (lipolytic influences) When the blood levels of fatty acids and glucose fall below homeostatic levels, eg, during starvation or prolonged exercise, adipocytes release stored fatty acids into the blood. Lipid mobilization occurs first from subcutaneous, mesenteric, and retroperitoneal adipose tissue and last from deposits in the hands, feet, and retro-orbital fat pads.

a. Hormone-sensitive lipases Peptide hormones and norepinephrine increase cyclic AMP levels (see Chapter 20) in adipocytes. Hormone-sensitive lipases in the adipocyte cytoplasm are activated by cyclic AMP and cleave fatty acids from stored triglycerides.

b. Hormones Adrenocorticotropic hormone (ACTH), released by the anterior pituitary, stimulates the release of free fatty acids from adipocytes. Other hormones with varying degrees of lipolytic ability are glucagon, growth hormone, and thyroid hormone. A sex-dependent regional sensitivity of adipose tissue to circulating androgens and estrogens exerts a major influence on sex-dependent differences in the uptake and mobilization of fatty acids by adipocytes.

c. Innervation Interruption of the autonomic nerve supply to adipose tissue decreases fat loss from the affected region, so it would appear that the autonomic nervous system is important in fatty acid mobilization. Autonomic fibers to white fat terminate only on the walls of blood vessels, but in brown fat they also make direct contact with the adipocytes. The addition of exogenous norepinephrine can double the blood levels of free fatty acids by its effect on adipose tissue.

D. Histogenesis: The unilocular adipocytes of white fat derive from mesenchymal precursor cells that resemble fibroblasts. The appearance of numerous small lipid droplets in the cytoplasm signals the transformation of these cells into **lipoblasts.** As lipid accumulation continues, the small droplets fuse until a single large lipid droplet forms.

III. BROWN ADIPOSE TISSUE

A. Distinguishing Features: Brown fat is called **multilocular adipose tissue** because of the multiple small lipid droplets in its adipocytes. Brown adipocytes are smaller than white adipocytes and have a spheric, centrally located nucleus. They contain large numbers of mitochondria; the tan to reddish-brown tissue color is due chiefly to mitochondrial cytochromes. Loose connective tissue septa give brown adipose tissue a lobular appearance like that of a gland in histologic section. The vascular supply (partly responsible for the color) is very rich, as is the autonomic nerve supply. Many unmyelinated nerve fibers contact the adipocytes.

B. Distribution: Brown fat is less abundant than white at all ages. Young and middle-aged adults have little or none, but fetuses, newborns, and the elderly have accumulations in the axilla, the posterior triangle of the neck (near the carotid artery and thyroid gland), and around the renal hilus.

C. Functional Characteristics: Brown fat has essentially the same functional capabilities as white, but its metabolic activity is more intense and can lead to generation of heat. Under conditions of excessive cold, autonomic stimulation can cause oxidative phosphorylation in the numerous mitochondria to be uncoupled from adenosine triphosphate (ATP) synthesis, and the released energy dissipates as heat. The numerous vessels supplying this tissue carry the heat to the body. Brown fat is important in hibernating animals and in human infants before other thermoregulatory mechanisms are well developed.

D. Histogenesis: The multilocular adipocytes of brown fat derive from mesenchymal precursors that assume an epithelial shape and arrangement. The multiple small fat droplets that appear during development do not coalesce during maturation.

Study-Focusing Questions*

1. Explain why the body must store fuel (121).
2. List the functions of unilocular (white, yellow) adipose tissue (121).
3. Name the locations in the body notable for their complete lack of unilocular adipose tissue (121).
4. Describe the distribution of collagen and reticular fibers in adipose tissue (122).
5. Compare unilocular and multilocular adipose tissue in terms of:
    a. The size of their predominant cell type (121–122, 125)
    b. The distribution of lipid in their cytoplasm (121)
    c. The shape and location of their nuclei (122, 125)
    d. The number of their mitochondria (122, 125)
    e. The distribution of their other organelles (122, 125)
    f. Their precursor cell (type and appearance) (124, 125)
    g. The functional capabilities of their tissues (122, 125)
    h. The richness of their vascular supplies (121, 122, 125)
    i. The distribution of their autonomic nerve fibers (124)
    j. Their abundance (125)
    k. Their location (121, 125)
6. Name the chief biochemical constituent of the lipid droplets found in adipocytes (122).
7. List the factors that lead to:
    a. Increased lipid storage and synthesis by adipocytes (lipogenic factors) (123)
    b. Increased mobilization of lipid by adipocytes (lipolytic factors) (123)
8. Under circumstances of bodily need, which of the body's lipid deposits begin mobilization first and which last (123)?
9. What accounts for the color of brown adipose tissue (125) and of yellow adipose tissue (121)?
10. List the structural and functional characteristics of adipose tissue that distinguish it from other types of connective tissue. (Consider the types and proportions of cells, fibers, and ground substance. How do the functions listed in the answer to question 2 differ from the functions of, for example, dense regular connective tissue?)

Multiple-Choice Questions

For questions 6–1 and 6–2, select the single best answer.

6–1. Adipocytes release stored fat in response to:
   A. Increased insulin levels in the blood
   B. Increased dietary uptake of glucose

*The page references in this section refer to *Basic Histology,* 6th ed., Junqueira L, Carneiro J, Kelley R (editors), Appleton & Lange, 1989. **HR** (for Histology Review) is occasionally used instead of a page reference to indicate that the information referred to can be found in this book.

C. Interruption of the autonomic nerve supply to adipose tissue
D. Increased triglyceride levels in the blood
E. Norepinephrine

6–2. The fat in this location is among the *last* to be mobilized during prolonged starvation:
A. Subcutaneous fat deposits
B. Fat pads of the hands and feet
C. Retroperitoneal fat deposits
D. Mesenteric fat deposits

MATCHING (questions 6–3 through 6–9): Each choice may be used once, more than once, or not at all.

A. Chylomicrons
B. Glucose
C. Triglycerides
D. Free fatty acids
E. Glycerol

6–3. Esters of fatty acids and glycerol
6–4. Large, fat-containing particles formed by the intestinal epithelium
6–5. Transported in the blood by albumin
6–6. Central core of triglycerides and cholesteryl esters surrounded by a layer of cholesterol and phospholipids
6–7. Can be used by adipocytes as a precursor molecule in the synthesis of either fatty acids or glycerol
6–8. Primary form of stored lipid in adipocytes
6–9. Broken down by hormone-sensitive lipase

For questions 6–10 through 6–22, select the one correct answer.

A. Unilocular adipose tissue
B. Multilocular adipose tissue
C. Both
D. Neither

6–10. Brown fat
6–11. White or yellow fat
6–12. Of the tissues listed, the most widely distributed in adults
6–13. Of the tissues listed, the most widely distributed in newborns
6–14. Highly vascular
6–15. Functions in the generation of heat
6–16. Cells have a "signet-ring" appearance in histologic sections
6–17. More important in heat retention (insulation) than in heat production
6–18. Of the 2 types listed, this has the smaller cells
6–19. Exhibits a glandlike appearance
6–20. Derived from mesenchyme
6–21. Color primarily due to carotenoids dissolved in fat droplets
6–22. Color largely due to mitochondrial cytochromes

For questions 6–23 through 6–25, one, more than one, or all of the answers may be correct. Select

A if only (1), (2), and (3) are correct
B if only (1) and (3) are correct
C if only (2) and (4) are correct
D if only (4) is correct
E if all answers are correct

6–23. Hormones that affect the metabolism or distribution of adipose tissue include:
- **(1)** The sex hormones
- **(2)** Thyroid hormone
- **(3)** Insulin
- **(4)** Growth hormone

6–24. During fat mobilization, which of the following are released into the bloodstream by adipocytes?
- **(1)** Fatty acids
- **(2)** Norepinephrine
- **(3)** Glycerol
- **(4)** Chylomicrons

6–25. The effects of insulin on adipocytes include:
- **(1)** Activation of hormone-sensitive lipase
- **(2)** Accelerated synthesis of fatty acids from glucose
- **(3)** Uncoupling of oxidative phosphorylation
- **(4)** Increased uptake of glucose

Cartilage 7

Objectives

This chapter should help the student to:

- Know the differences and similarities among the 3 types of cartilage.
- Know the functions of the 3 types of cartilage and relate them to their structural characteristics and location in the body.
- Know the steps in the histogenesis and growth of cartilage.
- Relate the ultrastructure of the chondrocyte to its functional role in the synthesis and maintenance of the extracellular matrix.
- Recognize the type of cartilage present and identify its components (eg, chondrocytes, perichondrium, capsular matrix) in a photomicrograph or slide of a tissue or organ.

Synopsis

I. GENERAL FEATURES OF CARTILAGE. Cartilage is a **skeletal connective tissue** characterized by firmness and resiliency. It forms most of the fetal skeleton and persists in locations where its mechanical properties are needed. Most fetal cartilage eventually becomes bone.

A. Composition: Like all connective tissues, cartilage is composed of cells, fibers, and ground substance. The extracellular matrix predominates and determines cartilage's mechanical properties. Type II collagen is a characteristic cartilage matrix component, and the abundant ground substance is firm and gellike. Cartilage cells are termed **chondrocytes.**

B. Vascular Supply: Most cartilage is enveloped by a layer of dense connective tissue, the **perichondrium,** which contains the vascular supply and fibroblastlike stem cells from which additional chondrocytes may arise. Few blood vessels (or nerves) are found within cartilage, thus the composition of the ground substance is crucial to the percolation of nutrients and oxygen to chondrocytes from the surrounding vessels.

C. Cells: Under the light microscope, chondrocytes are generally rounded, with an eccentric nucleus, a prominent nucleolus, and basophilic cytoplasm. With EM, chondrocyte surfaces exhibit characteristic projections and infoldings. The rough endoplasmic reticulum and Golgi complex are well developed; the Golgi complex increases in size as the cell grows, and its cisternae fill with secretory material. A few lipid droplets are typically found in the cytoplasm. Chondrocytes synthesize and secrete the fibers and ground substance of the extracellular matrix: collagen is synthesized on the rough endoplasmic reticulum, and GAGs are assembled and sulfated in the Golgi complex. Because of their meager oxygen supply, chondrocytes produce much of their energy by anaerobic glycolysis.

II. THE 3 TYPES OF CARTILAGE.

Hyaline cartilage, elastic cartilage, and **fibrocartilage** differ in appearance and mechanical properties, owing to differences in the composition of their extracellular matrix. These differences are summarized in Table 7–1 and discussed below. Generally, no distinction is made among the cells present in the different cartilage types.

A. Hyaline Cartilage: Hyaline cartilage, the most common type in both fetus and adult, is white and translucent in the fresh state, with a firm, gellike consistency.

1. Composition

a. Fibers Hyaline cartilage matrix is characterized by type II collagen in the form of thin fibrils rather than bundles. Their small size and their refractive index (close to that of the ground substance) make them difficult to distinguish with the light microscope. Type II collagen contains a higher proportion of hydroxylysine than type I.

b. Ground substance This, the predominant tissue component, is composed of:

(1) GAGs, mostly chondroitin sulfates and hyaluronic acid, with smaller amounts of keratan sulfate and heparan sulfate;

(2) Proteoglycans, core proteins with GAG side chains;

(3) Proteoglycan aggregates, proteoglycans covalently linked to long chains of hyaluronic acid by link protein;

(4) Glycoproteins, which attach various matrix components to one another and cells to the matrix, including link protein, fibronectin, chondronectin; and

(5) Tissue fluid; an ultrafiltrate of blood plasma.

2. Organization The consistency of hyaline cartilage results from extensive cross-linking among its components. **Link protein** (see above) attaches the core proteins of proteoglycans to long chains of hyaluronic acid to form **proteoglycan aggregates.** The GAG side chains of the proteoglycans associate with type II collagen fibrils. The chondrocytes are embedded in the matrix either singly or in **isogenous groups** of 2–8 cells derived from one parent cell. The potential space occupied by each chondrocyte, called a **lacuna,** is visible only after the cell's death or after shrinkage during tissue processing. The chondrocytes at the core of a tissue mass are usually spheric; those at the periphery are flattened or elliptic. The matrix immediately surrounding the chondrocytes, called the **capsular (territorial) matrix,** is more intensely basophilic and PAS-positive than the **intercapsular (interterritorial) matrix** because of the higher concentration of sulfated GAGs and lower concentration of collagen in the capsular region. Except for articular (joint) cartilage, all hyaline cartilage is surrounded and nourished by perichondrium. Articular cartilage is nourished by the synovial fluid in the joint cavity (see Chapter 8).

Table 7-1. Characteristics of Cartilage Types

	Cell Type	Fiber Type	Ground Substance	Organization	Functions	Locations
Hyaline cartilage	Chondrocytes	Type II collagen	Predominant tissue component. Includes glycosaminoglycans (GAGs, mainly chondroitin sulfate, smaller amounts of keratan and heparan sulfates). Proteoglycan aggregated. Glycoprotein (fibronectin, chondronectin, and link protein).	Cells and fibers embedded in abundant ground substance. Notable lack of capillaries. Cells may occur in isogenous groups. Fibers difficult to distinguish from ground substance. Extensive cross-linking among ground substance components (proteoglycan aggregates) and between fibers and ground substance.	Useful as fetal skeleton owing to ability to provide support and grow rapidly. Maintains airways in respiratory passages. Cushions and provides low-friction surface in joints.	Fetal skeleton; articular and costal cartilages; laryngeal, tracheal, and bronchial cartilages.
Elastic cartilage	Chondrocytes	Elastic fibers, type II collagen	Same as hyaline.	Organization identical to that of hyaline cartilage except for presence of a dense network of elastic fibers.	Flexible support. Semirigid; returns to original shape after being deformed.	External ear, auditory tubes, epiglottis, corniculate and cuneiform cartilages of larynx.
Fibrocartilage	Chondrocytes	Type I collagen, type II collagen	Similar to that of hyaline but with equal amounts of chondroitin and dermatan sulfates.	Cross between cartilage and dense regular connective tissues. Chondrocytes usually in rowlike isogenous groups surrounded by typical hyaline matrix. Nests of chondrocytes lie between densely packed bundles of large type I collagen fibers.	Attaches bone to bone and provides restricted mobility under great mechanical stress.	Annulus fibrosus of intervertebral disks, pubic symphysis, and bone-ligament functions. Always found in association with dense connective tissue.

3. Histogenesis All cartilage is derived from embryonic mesenchyme. During the development of hyaline cartilage, mesenchymal cells retract their cytoplasmic extensions and assume a rounded shape, becoming **chondroblasts;** at the same time they become more tightly packed, forming a **mesenchymal condensation,** or precartilage condensation. The increased cell-to-cell contact stimulates cartilage differentiation, which progresses from the center outward. Chondroblasts at the core of the condensation are the first to secrete cartilaginous matrix materials, which separate the cells from one another again. When it is completely surrounded by cartilage matrix, a chondroblast is termed a chondrocyte. Peripheral mesenchyme condenses around the developing cartilage mass to form the fibroblast-containing, dense regular connective tissue of the perichondrium.

4. Growth Cartilage continues to grow by 2 distinct processes. In both types of growth, the newly formed chondrocytes deposit matrix around themselves. Matrix synthesis is enhanced by growth hormone, thyroxine, and testosterone and is inhibited by estradiol and excess cortisone.

a. Interstitial growth results from the division of existing chondrocytes and gives rise to the isogenous groups. It is important in the formation of the fetal skeleton and continues in the epiphyseal plates and articular cartilages (see below).

b. Appositional growth results from the differentiation into chondrocytes by chondroblasts and stem cells on the inner surface of the perichondrium. It is responsible for continued increase in the girth of the cartilage masses.

5. Repair Repair of cartilage fractures involves invasion of the breach by mesenchymal stem cells from the perichondrium, which then differentiate into chondrocytes. If the gap is large, a dense connective tissue scar may form.

6. Function and location Its ability to grow rapidly while maintaining its rigidity makes hyaline cartilage an ideal fetal skeletal tissue. As fetal cartilage is replaced by bone, hyaline cartilage remains in the **epiphyseal plates** at the ends of long bones, allowing these bones to grow in length between birth and adulthood. At all ages, hyaline cartilage without a perichondrium (articular cartilage) covers the articular surfaces of bone, where its resistance to compression and its smooth texture make it a good cushion and low-friction surface. Hyaline cartilage is the most abundant and widely distributed cartilage type in the body. The costal (rib) cartilages, most of the laryngeal cartilages, the cartilaginous rings supporting trachea, and the irregular cartilage plates in the walls of the bronchi are hyaline cartilage.

B. Elastic Cartilage: Elastic cartilage is yellowish when fresh. It is more flexible than hyaline cartilage.

1. Composition and organization Elastic cartilage is structurally identical to hyaline cartilage except that it contains, in addition to type II collagen fibers, a dense network of branching and anastomosing elastic fibers. This network is densest at the core of the cartilage mass and when stained with elastic stains (eg, Verhoeff's or Weigert's) may obscure the organization of the tissue. The chondrocytes characteristically occur in isogenous groups. A perichondrium surrounds the elastic cartilage mass.

2. Histogenesis and growth Elastic cartilage develops from a primitive connective tissue containing wavy bundles of fibrils that differ in protein composition from both elastin and collagen. Fibroblasts eventually secrete elastin, and the fiber bundles are transformed into branching elastic fibers by an unknown mechanism. The development of chondrocytes and production of the other matrix materials is the same as in hyaline cartilage. Further growth resembles that of hyaline cartilage.

3. Function and location Elastic cartilage provides flexible support. It occurs alone and with hyaline cartilage; the 2 may grade into each other in a single cartilage mass. In humans, elastic cartilage is found in the auricle of the external ear, the walls of the external auditory canals and auditory tubes, the epiglottis, and the corniculate and cuneiform cartilages of the larynx.

C. Fibrocartilage: Fibrocartilage is intermediate in character between hyaline cartilage and dense connective tissue.

1. Composition and organization Fibrocartilage is characterized by an abundance of type I collagen fibers; when seen through a microscope at low power, it closely resembles dense connective tissue. The ground substance contains equal amounts of dermatan sulfate and chondroitin sulfate (Table 7–1). The matrix immediately surrounding the chondrocytes resembles that of hyaline cartilage and contains some type II collagen. The chondrocytes are distributed in columnar isogenous groups between the densely packed collagen bundles. There is no distinguishable perichondrium.

2. Histogenesis and growth At sites where strong mechanical stresses occur, fibrocartilage develops from dense regular connective tissue through the transformation of fibroblasts or fibroblastlike precursors into chondrocytes. Fibrocartilage growth has not been closely examined.

3. Function and location Fibrocartilage is always found in association with dense connective tissue, and the border between the 2 is usually indistinct. Its combination of cartilaginous ground substance and dense collagen bundles allows fibrocartilage to resist deformation under great stress; it is important in attaching bone to bone and providing restricted mobility. Sites in humans include the annulus fibrosus of the intervertebral disks, the symphysis pubis, and certain bone-ligament junctions.

III. INTERVERTEBRAL DISKS. The intervertebral disks act as cushions between the vertebrae, allowing limited movement of the vertebral column. They are bound to the vertebrae by ligaments. Each disk is composed of 2 parts.

A. Annulus Fibrosus: This is the outer ring, composed mainly of fibrocartilage and covered on its outer surface by the dense connective tissue of associated ligaments. The fibrocartilage is arranged in concentric layers, with the collagen bundles of each layer oriented at right angles to those in the next. This organization appears as a ''herringbone'' pattern when seen through a light microscope at low power.

B. Nucleus Pulposus: This structure forms the center of the disk and is derived from the embryonic notochord. It is composed of mucous connective tissue, with a few fibers and rounded cells embedded in syrupy, hyaluronic acid-rich ground substance. The nucleus pulposus is smaller in adults than in children, because it is partially replaced by fibrocartilage.

Study-Focusing Questions*

1. Compare the 3 types of cartilage in terms of:
   a. The type, amount, and arrangement of their cells (129, 132, 133), fibers (129, 132–133), and ground substance (129, 132, 133)
   b. Their location in the body (127, 132–135)
   c. Their histogenesis (131, **HR**)
   d. Their function (127, 132, 133)
2. Sketch a typical proteoglycan aggregate of cartilage ground substance (129–130). Label the following components and indicate which of them are glycosaminoglycans:
   a. Hyaluronic acid
   b. Link protein
   c. Core protein
   d. Chondroitin sulfate
   e. A proteoglycan molecule
3. Compare the territorial (capsular) matrix and the interterritorial matrix (129) in terms of their:
   a. Location
   b. Composition
   c. Staining properties
4. Describe the structure and function of the perichondrium (127, 129).
5. List the functions of chondrocytes and name the organelles involved in each function (127, 130).
6. List the factors known to increase or decrease the synthesis and secretion of sulfated glycosaminoglycans (eg, chondroitin sulfate) by chondrocytes (130).
7. Beginning with undifferentiated mesenchymal tissue, list the steps in the histogenesis of hyaline cartilage (131).
8. Name the 2 types of growth that occur in hyaline cartilage (131) and compare them in terms of:

*The page references in this section refer to *Basic Histology,* 6th ed., Junqueira L, Carneiro J, Kelley R (editors), Appleton & Lange, 1989. **HR** (for Histology Review) is occasionally used instead of a page reference to indicate that the information referred to can be found in this book.

a. The location of their dividing cells
b. Their importance in growth in girth, replacement of worn articular cartilage, and growth in length at the epiphyseal plate

9. What is the major structural difference between articular cartilage and hyaline cartilage found in other locations (127)?
10. How are the chondrocytes of articular cartilage supplied with nutrients and oxygen? (127)
11. What process, in addition to cell division, is important to the increase in cartilage mass during growth (131)?
12. When a cartilage is fractured, where do the additional chondrocytes that fill in and repair the fracture come from (132)?
13. Describe an intervertebral disk (135) in terms of
    a. Its location
    b. Its function
    c. The tissue composition of the annulus fibrosus
    d. The tissue composition of the nucleus pulposus
    e. The embryonic origin of the nucleus pulposus

Multiple-Choice Questions

For questions 7–1 through 7–7, select the single best answer.

7–1. Which of the following characteristics of cartilage distinguishes it from most other connective tissues?
- **A.** Its extracellular matrix contains collagen
- **B.** Its predominant cell type is a mesenchymal derivative
- **C.** Its predominant cell type secretes both fibers and ground substance
- **D.** It lacks blood vessels
- **E.** It functions in mechanical support

7–2. Which of the following is most important in the synthesis and sulfation of glycosaminoglycans by chondrocytes?
- **A.** Rough endoplasmic reticulum
- **B.** Polyribosomes
- **C.** Smooth endoplasmic reticulum
- **D.** Transitional (transfer) vesicles
- **E.** Golgi complex

7–3. The area of cartilage that is characteristically collagen-poor and sulfated glycosaminoglycan-rich is the:
- **A.** Perichondrium
- **B.** Capsular matrix
- **C.** Epiphyseal plate
- **D.** Annulus fibrosus
- **E.** Intercapsular matrix

7–4. Articular cartilage differs from most hyaline cartilage in that it:
- **A.** Contains isogenous groups of chondrocytes
- **B.** Lacks blood vessels
- **C.** Lacks a perichondrium
- **D.** Contains type II collagen
- **E.** Is derived from embryonic mesenchyme

7–5. The tissue shown in Fig 7–1 is:
- **A.** Hyaline cartilage
- **B.** Elastic cartilage
- **C.** Fibrocartilage
- **D.** None of the above

7–6. Which of the following occurs first in cartilage histogenesis?
- **A.** Appositional growth
- **B.** Secretion of the matrix
- **C.** Formation of mesenchymal condensations

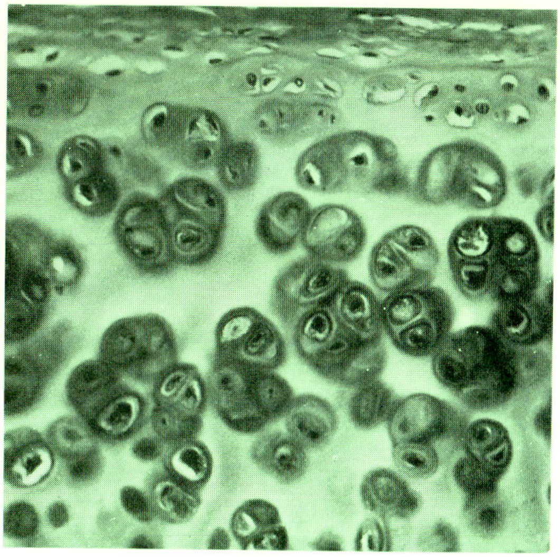

Figure 7-1.

D. Interstitial growth
E. Differentiation of chondroblasts into chondrocytes

7-7. The link protein of proteoglycan aggregates attaches:
A. The core protein to hyaluronic acid
B. Chondroitin sulfate to the core protein
C. Chondroitin sulfate to hyaluronic acid
D. The core protein to collagen
E. Chondroitin sulfate to collagen

MATCHING (questions 7-8 through 7-20): Each answer may be used once, more than once, or not at all.

A. Hyaline cartilage
B. Elastic cartilage
C. Fibrocartilage
D. All of the above
E. None of the above

7-8. Primary skeletal tissue in the fetus
7-9. Contains predominantly reticular fibers
7-10. No identifiable perichondrium
7-11. Most widely distributed cartilage type in the body
7-12. Contains abundant type I collagen
7-13. Has a yellowish appearance in the fresh state
7-14. Articular cartilage
7-15. Predominant cartilage type in the external ear (auricle)
7-16. Found in the annulus fibrosus of intervertebral disks
7-17. Contains type II collagen
7-18. Chondrocytes differentiate from fibroblasts or fibroblastlike cells
7-19. Cartilage of epiphyseal plates
7-20. Derived from mesenchyme

For questions 7-21 through 7-26, select the one correct answer.

A. Interstitial growth
B. Appositional growth
C. Both
D. Neither

7–21. Accounts for increase in cartilage size
7–22. Division of preexisting chondrocytes
7–23. Differentiation of peripheral perichondrial cells into chondroblasts
7–24. Most likely to result in the formation of isogenous groups
7–25. Predominant type of growth in epiphyseal plates
7–26. Involves only cell division

For questions 7–27 through 7–29, one, more than one, or all of the answers may be correct. Select

A if only (1), (2), and (3) are correct
B if only (1) and (3) are correct
C if only (2) and (4) are correct
D if only (4) is correct
E if all answers are correct

7–27. Fibrocartilage:
- **(1)** Contains large numbers of elastic fibers
- **(2)** Often contains isogenous groups of cells
- **(3)** Is the type of cartilage found in the epiphyses of the long bones of young children
- **(4)** Is structurally intermediate between dense connective tissue and cartilage

7–28. Chondrocytes normally synthesize and secrete:
- **(1)** Type II collagen
- **(2)** Hyaluronic acid
- **(3)** Sulfated glycosaminoglycans
- **(4)** Type I collagen

7–29. The synthesis of glycosaminoglycans by chondrocytes can be accelerated by:
- **(1)** Cortisone
- **(2)** Thyroxine
- **(3)** Estradiol
- **(4)** Growth hormone

8 Bone

Objectives

This chapter should help the student to:

- Describe bone as a connective tissue in terms of its cells, fibers, and ground substance.
- Compare the various types of bone cells in terms of their origin, structure, and primary functions.
- List the functions and physical properties of bone tissue and relate them to specific components of the tissue.
- List the different types of bone tissue and name sites in the body where each may be found.
- Compare the 2 processes of bone tissue formation in terms of embryonic tissue of origin, intermediate steps, and structure of the resulting mature tissue, and location in the body.
- Compare growth in length with growth in girth of bones.
- Compare the steps in bone histogenesis with those in fracture repair.

- Know the alterations in tissue structure that occur during bone remodeling.
- Explain the effects of nutritional and hormonal factors on the structure and function of bone tissue.
- Recognize the type of bone, the cell types, and the named structures of bone (eg, periosteum, spicules, haversian canals) in a photomicrograph or slide of bone tissue.
- List the types of joints, name sites in the body where each is found, and compare them in terms of their structural composition and mobility.

Synopsis

I. GENERAL FEATURES OF BONE. Bone is the main constituent of the adult skeletal system. Like cartilage, it is a skeletal connective tissue specialized for support and protection.

A. Composition: All mature bone tissue has cells (osteocytes, osteoblasts, and osteoclasts) fibers (type I collagen), and ground substance. It differs from other connective tissues primarily in having large quantities of inorganic salts in its matrix, accounting for its hardness.

B. Functions: Bone is second only to cartilage in its ability to withstand mechanical stress and second only to enamel in hardness. It supports and protects the more fragile tissues and organs, harbors the hematopoietic tissue (bone marrow; see Chapter 13), and forms a system of levers and pulleys that multiply and focus the contractile forces of muscle. The constant turnover of bone tissue results from a balance between the activities of the bone-forming osteoblasts and the bone-resorbing osteoclasts and allows bone matrix to function as an important storage site for calcium and other essential minerals. Some bone functions are discussed in more detail in section III.D.

C. Types of Bone Tissue: Bone tissue is classified according to its gross architecture as spongy or compact and according to its fine structure as primary (woven) or secondary (lamellar). All bone tissue begins as primary bone, but nearly all is eventually replaced by secondary bone. An additional distinction between intramembranous and endochondral bone is based on the histogenesis of the primary bone tissue, but this difference in origin is difficult to detect microscopically in mature bone.

D. Terminology: The study of bone is complicated by the multiple connotations of certain terms applied to its structure and development. The term "bone" itself refers both to bone tissue and to an individual named element of the adult skeleton—a bone. A bone is an organ composed largely of bone tissue but also containing other connective tissues, as well as bone marrow, blood vessels, and nerves (II). Other confusing usages are pointed out in this chapter. Confusion can be avoided by careful attention to context.

II. BONES. The adult skeleton consists of more than 200 bones that, with cartilage and ligaments, form the supportive framework of the body.

A. Shape: Bones are classified by their overall shape (eg, long bones, flat bones) and the process by which they form (endochondral bones, membrane bones). Most exhibit protuberances that serve as attachment sites for muscles, tendons, and ligaments.

B. Surfaces: The outer surfaces of bones are covered by a double-layered coat of connective tissue, the **periosteum.** The outer layer of the periosteum is dense connective tissue; the inner or osteogenic layer, is a looser tissue containing bone-cell precursors. **Sharpey's fibers** are periosteal collagen fibers that penetrate bone matrix and anchor the periosteum to the bone. The internal surfaces of bones are covered by a thinner, condensed reticular connective tissue (see Chapter 5) called endosteum that contains bone and blood cell precursors.

C. Parts of Long Bones: Most bones of the arms and legs (eg, the femur) are termed long bones, and the terms describing their parts are important to the study of regional differences in bone histology. The **diaphysis** is the shaft of a long bone, and the **epiphysis** is its bulbous end. In adults, the diaphysis is a cylindric structure with walls composed of compact bone (III.B.2) and a central marrow cavity lined with endosteum. Each of the 2 epiphyses contains mostly spongy bone. Where bones contact other bones to form movable joints (V.B), their surfaces are covered by articular cartilage.

III. BONE TISSUE

A. Composition: Like other connective tissues, bone is composed of cells, fibers, and ground substance. **Bone matrix,** containing abundant mineral salts, is the predominant tissue component. The hardness of bone makes it difficult to section. Special techniques for obtaining thin sections include grinding bone slices until they become translucent and demineralizing fixed bone by immersion in solutions of dilute acid or calcium-chelating agents (eg, EDTA). Demineralized bone can be sectioned and stained by standard histologic methods.

1. Bone cells

a. Osteoprogenitor cells are stem cells found in the endosteum and periosteum. These spindle-shaped cells have ovoid to elongate nuclei and unremarkable cytoplasm. There are 2 types, distinguishable only with the electron microscope: one type gives rise to osteoblasts, the other to osteoclasts. Osteoblast precursors derive from embryonic mesenchyme and have sparse rough endoplasmic reticular and Golgi complexes. Osteoclast precursors derive from blood monocyles and have abundant free ribosomes and mitochondria.

b. Osteoblasts, the major bone-forming cells, are typically cuboidal, each with a large, round nucleus and basophilic cytoplasm. They form one-cell-thick sheets resembling simple cuboidal epithelium on surfaces where new bone is being deposited. Osteoblasts exhibit high alkaline phosphatase activity and have the well-developed rough endoplasmic reticulum and Golgi complex typical of protein-secreting cells. They synthesize and secrete all the organic components of bone matrix (see below) and may also be involved in bone mineralization. Once surrounded by matrix, osteoblasts are considered mature and called osteocytes.

c. Osteocytes are terminally differentiated bone cells found in cavities in the bone matrix called **lacunae.** Their long, thin cytoplasmic processes, called **filopodia,** radiate from the cell body in fine extensions of the lacunar cavity called **canaliculi.** Osteocytes are isolated from one another by the impermeable bone matrix and contact one another through the tips of their filopodia, which are often joined by gap junctions. This arrangement provides limited cytoplasmic continuity between the cells and explains how osteocytes obtain nutrients and oxygen and dispose of wastes at relatively great distances from the blood vessels. While incapable of mitosis, osteocytes retain some synthetic and resorptive capacity whereby they turn over and maintain nearby bone matrix. The death of osteocytes results in bone breakdown, or resorption (see below). Osteocytes recently derived from osteoblasts are located near the bone surface in rounded lacunae; older cells are found farther from the surface in flattened lacunae.

d. Osteoclasts are bone-resorbing cells that lie on bony surfaces in shallow depressions termed **Howship's lacunae.** They are typically large and multinucleated (2–50 nuclei per cell), with acidophilic cytoplasm containing abundant lysosomes and mitochondria and a well-developed Golgi complex. The osteoclast surface facing the depression exhibits a **ruffled border** of plasma-membrane infoldings, which form many isolated compartments between the cell and the bone surface. The cells release acid, collagenase, and other lytic enzymes into the compartments; these break down bone matrix and release minerals, a process called **bone resorption.** Osteoclasts respond to parathyroid hormone (III.D.1.a) by enlarging their ruffled borders and increasing their activity, resulting in increased blood calcium levels. The effect of PTH may be indirect and mediated by a signal from the osteoblasts. Calcitonin (III.D.1.b), which decreases blood calcium, reduces surface ruffling and osteoclast activity. While their immediate precursors are found in the endosteum and periosteum, osteoblasts ultimately derive from the fusion of blood monocyte derivatives and are considered components of the mononuclear phagocyte system.

2. Bone matrix Bone matrix contains organic components, or **osteoid,** and inorganic components, or **bone mineral.**

a. Organic components Osteoid constitutes about 50% of bone volume and 25% of bone weight. It is composed of fibers and unmineralized ground substance.

(1) Fibers Type I collagen fibers constitute 90–95% of the osteoid. The overlapping pattern of staggered tropocollagen (see Chapter 5) results in periodic gaps (lacunar regions), which may contain up to 50% of the hydroxyapatite crystals (mineral) in bone.

(2) Ground substance Hydroxyapatite crystals and collagen fibers are embedded in the highly acidic ground substance, which is composed of proteins, carbohydrates, and small amounts of proteoglycans and lipids. The proteins are glycoproteins, phosphoproteins, sialoproteins (eg, osteopontin), and γ-carboxyglutamic acid-containing proteins. The carbohydrates (glycosaminoglycans) include chondroitin sulfates and keratan sulfate. Some ground substance components may be nucleation sites for hydroxyapatite crystals.

b. Inorganic components Bone mineral comprises about 50% of bone volume and 75% of bone weight. It is composed primarily of calcium and phosphate, with some bicarbonate, citrate, magnesium, and potassium and trace amounts of other metals. Calcium and phosphate form needlelike crystals of **hydroxyapatite,** $Ca_{10}(PO_4)_6(OH)_2$. Hydrated ions at the crystal surface form an enveloping **hydration shell,** through which ions are exchanged between the crystal and surrounding body fluids (III.D.1.a).

B. Organization: Adult bone occurs in 2 basic organizational types, spongy and compact. The 2 are similar in composition and microscopic appearance but differ in their overall architecture.

1. Spongy bone, also called **cancellous bone,** forms a fine 3-dimensional lattice containing many open spaces. The branching and anastomosing slips of bone between the spaces, termed **trabeculae** or **spicules,** are aligned along the lines of stress to which the bones are subjected, maximizing the weight-bearing capacity of this bone tissue. Spongy bone is found at the core of the epiphyses of mature long bones, at the core of short bones (eg, phalanges), and between the thick plates, or tables, of the flat bones of the skull, where it is called the diploe. It may be composed of either primary or secondary bone (III.C.1, III.C.2).

2. Compact bone, also called **dense bone** or **cortical bone,** does not have large spaces or trabeculae. It forms the thick diaphyseal cylinder of long bones, a thin covering over the epiphyses, and the tables of the flat bones of the skull. Compact bone is always composed of secondary bone.

C. Histogenesis, Remodeling, Growth, and Repair:

1. Primary bone The first bone tissue to appear during the formation of new bone or in the repair of fractures is termed primary bone, or **woven bone.** This immature bone, which is always spongy, is replaced by secondary bone except in a few sites, eg, near the skull sutures and in alveolar bone of the mandible and maxilla. Its matrix is less organized than that of secondary bone, ie, the collagen fibers do not form concentric rings (III.C.2). It is less mineralized than secondary bone, making it more radiolucent (penetrable by x-rays), and it has a higher osteocyte-to-matrix ratio. Primary bone can form by either of 2 separate mechanisms, intramembranous bone formation or endochondral bone formation.

a. **Intramembranous bone formation** occurs within sheetlike **mesenchymal condensations,** of membranes. The cells in such a connective tissue membrane differentiate into osteoblasts and begin to synthesize and secrete osteoid, which later becomes mineralized. The osteoblasts surround themselves with bone matrix, forming spicules that eventually fuse into a spongy latticework of primary bone. Only a few human bones are formed entirely in this way; most of these are flat and called **membrane bones.** Membrane bones of the skull are the frontal and parietal bones, the mandible, and the maxilla. The term "membrane bone" is also applied to the tissue type formed by this mechanism. Membrane bone constitutes portions of some bones, such as the temporal and occipital bones of the skull and the periosteal bone collar of endochondral bones.

b. **Endochondral bone formation** involves the replacement of cartilage by bone and occurs in all bones except membrane bones. It is thus easier to know which bones are membrane bones and that the remainder are **endochondral bones** (or "cartilage bones").

(1) Basic steps in the formation of an endochondral bone

(a) Cartilage model In the embryo, a hyaline cartilage model is laid down which closely resembles the bone to be formed.

(b) The periosteal bone collar Capillaries invade the perichondrium, and mesenchymal cells on its inner surface become osteoprogenitor cells. Some of these differentiate into osteoblasts and secrete bone matrix, creating primary bone spicules just inside the perichondrium (now periosteum). The spicules eventually fuse to form a thin periosteal bone collar of membrane bone around the cartilage model. Thus, the first bone tissue in an endochondral bone forms by intramembranous ossification.

(c) Proliferation While the periosteal bone collar is forming, structural and functional changes begin occurring in the cartilage model. The chondrocytes near the collar begin rapid proliferation, forming long columns (isogenous groups) of flattened cells oriented parallel to the long axis of the bone.

(d) Hypertrophy The chondrocytes hypertrophy rapidly into large, rounded cells that are not separated by matrix. The result is tubelike superlacunae filled with columns of hypertrophic chondrocytes, which secrete type X collagen.

(e) Calcification As hypertrophy progresses, the long strips of cartilage matrix between the tubular cavities begin to calcify. Thus, oxygen, nutrients, and cellular wastes can no longer diffuse through the matrix, and the hypertrophic chondrocytes die.

(f) Formation of the primary marrow cavity Dead chondrocytes and some of the calcified cartilage matrix are removed by **chondroclasts** (large, multinucleated cells resembling osteoclasts). Tunnels at the center of the developing bone, created by the proliferation and hypertrophy of chondrocytes and enlarged by chondroclasts, become the bone's **primary marrow cavity.**

(g) The periosteal bud The periosteal bud, a small cluster of blood vessels and perivascular tissue from the periosteum, penetrates the primary marrow cavity. This bud and its branches come to occupy the tunnels left by the dead chondrocytes. Osteoprogenitor cells and bone marrow stem cells, delivered by the invading blood vessels, are deposited on the surface of the calcified cartilage matrix.

(h) Ossification Ossification is another term whose interpretation requires attention to context. In its broadest sense, ossification is synonymous with bone formation. Here, in a more restricted connotation, it refers to the final steps in the process, including the deposition and mineralization of the osteoid. The osteoprogenitor cells divide and differentiate into osteoblasts, which deposit primary bone on the surface of the calcified cartilage matrix strips. The primary bone and the residual calcified cartilage are later resorbed and replaced by secondary bone (III.C.2).

(2) Ossification centers The above steps may occur more than once in forming a bone. In long bones, the process occurs first near the middle of the diaphysis, forming the **primary ossification center.** The **secondary ossification centers** form later, by the same process, in the epiphyses. The region between a primary and a secondary ossification center is termed a **metaphysis.** The ossification centers enlarge until all that is left between them is a thin plate with resting cartilage at its center, the **epiphyseal plate.** The primary and secondary ossification centers of primary bone should not be confused with primary and secondary bone formation. Some bones later form **tertiary ossification centers,** which form the bony tubercles and ridges to which large muscle groups or ligaments attach. In humans, the first bone to ossify is the clavicle.

c. Histologic appearance of forming endochondral bone The microscopic structure of the metaphyses of developing endochondral bones is characterized by 5 overlapping zones:

(1) The **zone of resting cartilage** is composed of typical hyaline cartilage and is farthest from the primary marrow cavity.

(2) The **zone of proliferation** contains columns (isogenous groups) of flattened chondrocytes.

(3) In the **zone of hypertrophy,** the chondrocytes in the columns are enlarged and rounded.

(4) The **zone of calcification,** in H&E-stained sections, is characterized by an intensely basophilic matrix. There is often a significant overlap between zones 3 and 4, which are sometimes referred to as a single **zone of hypertrophy and calcification.**

(5) The **zone of ossification** borders directly on the primary marrow cavity. It is characterized by intensely acidophilic osteoid, osteocytes within the bone matrix, and a monolayer of basophilic osteoblasts on the surface of the newly formed primary bone.

2. Secondary bone In adults, both dense and spongy bone are composed of **secondary bone,** or **lamellar bone.**

a. Secondary bone formation (remodeling) Osteoclasts erode the primary bone matrix; blood vessels, nerves, and lymphatics invade the cavity formed by the erosion; and osteogenic cells in the perivascular connective tissue are deposited on the walls of the cavity. Osteoblasts descended from these cells along with osteocytes released from their lacunae during resorption deposit the secondary bone in concentric layers, or **lamellae,** the oldest of which are farthest from the vessels. Owing to its greater organization, secondary bone is more efficient than the primary bone it replaces. Remodeling helps reshape growing bones to adapt to changing stresses and loads. It occurs continuously, even in adults, as secondary bone is eroded and replaced by new secondary bone.

b. Microscopic appearance of secondary bone Secondary bone appears as a collection of densely packed bony cylinders, each with a central endosteum-lined **haversian canal** containing lymphatic and blood vessels, nerves, and some loose connective tissue. The cylinder surrounding each canal is composed of a series of concentric lamellae. The collagen fibers in each lamella are oriented parallel to one another and nearly perpendicular to those in adjacent lamellae, an arrangement that lends added strength to the tissue. Osteocytes lie between the lamellae in rows of lacunae; their filopodia are in canaliculi extending radially from each lacuna. A haversian canal, its contents, and the surrounding system of osteocytes and lamellae are termed a **haversian system,** or **osteon.** Vascular connections between osteons are established by **Volkmann's canals,** which run perpendicular to haversian canals and cut across the lamellae. Osteons may bifurcate, but they lie roughly parallel to one another and are held together by **cementing substance,** which fills in the spaces between the tightly packed cylinders. Often an old osteon is only partially eroded before a new one begins to form, so that wedge-shaped portions of old lamellae appear between recently formed osteons. The lamellae of partially eroded osteons are called **interstitial lamellae.**

3. Bone growth Bones increase in size from birth into early adulthood. During this growth, the bone tissue is continuously remodeled. Growth occurs in 2 directions.

a. Growth in length of long bones is primarily due to the proliferation of chondrocytes in the resting cartilage and in the zone of proliferation of the epiphyseal plates, under the influence of growth hormone. Childhood levels of growth hormone cause cartilage to be produced in the epiphyseal plates as fast as it can be replaced by endochondral bone formation. At puberty, growth hormone levels decline and endochondral bone gradually overtakes and replaces the remaining cartilage, a process termed **closure of the epiphyseal plates.**

b. Growth in girth occurs by proliferation and differentiation of osteoprogenitor cells in the inner layer of the periosteum and deposition of new ossified tissue on the outer surface of the bone.

4. Bone repair Bone fractures tear vessels in the periosteum, endosteum, and haversian and Volkmann's canals, causing local hemorrhage and clot formation between the broken ends of the bone. The periosteum and endosteum provide macrophages and fibroblasts; the former remove the clot, and the latter fill the breach with fibrous connective tissue. Some of the connective tissue cells differentiate into chondrocytes, and the connective tissue eventually becomes a **callus** containing islands of fibrocartilage and hyaline cartilage that serves as a model for bone formation. The presence of cartilage in the callus is characteristic of endochondral bones (eg, long bones), while flat membrane bones (eg, the mandible) typically heal without cartilage formation. Beginning in the subperiosteal region (as soon as 2 days after the injury in young people), the callus is gradually replaced by primary bone, which is subsequently remodeled and replaced by secondary bone. The time required for complete healing depends on the site and extent of the injury and is longer in older people.

D. Histophysiology of Bone:

1. Calcium reserve The skeleton contains 99% of the body's calcium, which serves as a critical cofactor for many enzyme systems and is important in muscle contraction, transmission of nerve impulses, blood clotting, and cell adhesion. Blood and tissue calcium concentrations are normally maintained within narrow limits, and bone serves as the calcium reservoir, storing excess calcium and releasing it when it is needed.

a. Calcium mobilization The release, or mobilization, of calcium occurs by 2 mechanisms. **Rapid mobilization** is simply the physical transfer of ions between hydroxyapatite crystals and the interstitial fluid along a concentration gradient. This occurs most readily where bone has a high surface-to-volume ratio, ie, around spicules of primary bone and in spongy secondary bone. The second mechanism involves **parathyroid hormone (PTH)** and is also rapid, although slower than the first. Cells of the parathyroid gland (see Chapter 21) sense a decrease in blood calcium concentration and release PTH, which increases the number of osteoclasts and activates existing ones. The result is increased breakdown, or **resorption,** of bone and release of its calcium to the blood. PTH also inhibits bone deposition by osteoblasts and reduces calcium excretion by the kidneys (see Chapter 19). Excessive production of PTH (hyperparathyroidism) results in the depletion of bone calcium, elevation of blood calcium, and abnormal deposition of calcium in soft tissues, especially the kidneys and arterial walls.

b. Calcium deposition The storage, or deposition, of calcium is promoted by **calcitonin,** a hormone secreted by the parafollicular C cells of the thyroid gland (see Chapter 21). Calcitonin has effects opposite those of PTH: it enhances matrix synthesis by osteoblasts as well as deposition of calcium. The rapid ion exchange described for calcium mobilization is also involved in calcium deposition.

2. Osteoporosis This condition is caused by decreased bone formation or increased bone resorption. Most often seen in chronically immobilized patients and postmenopausal women, it is characterized by decreased bone mass and a normal mineral-to-matrix ratio. Do not confuse osteoporosis with osteomalacia (see below), in which the mineral-to-matrix ratio is below normal.

3. Nutritional factors

a. Protein deficiency causes reduced collagen synthesis, which inhibits bone growth and maintenance.

b. Calcium deficiency leads to incomplete calcification of the bone matrix and, if prolonged, to bone resorption. In growing children, this causes **rickets,** ie, bone deformities, including bowing of the legs. In adults, it causes **osteomalacia,** ie, insufficient calcification of newly deposited bone, which weakens but does not deform the bones. Such bones are more susceptible to fracture and slower to repair. Osteomalacia may be exacerbated by pregnancy, because of the fetus's demand for calcium. In this disease, the mineral-to-matrix ratio is below normal.

c. Vitamin D deficiency results in reduced blood calcium concentration, because vitamin D aids in the intestinal absorption of dietary calcium. The effects are the same as those in dietary calcium deficiency.

d. Vitamin A deficiency slows bone growth and affects the distribution of the bone cells. Poor coordination between the rates of skull and brain growth may cause abnormally high pressure on the brain and damage to the central nervous system.

e. Vitamin A excess slows cartilage growth and accelerates ossification. An excess before birth, especially during the formation of the cartilage models, causes skeletal deformities and deletions. Excess in childhood or adolescence causes bone formation to overtake cartilage formation, resulting in premature closure of the epiphyses and small stature.

f. Vitamin C deficiency inhibits bone growth and slows fracture repair, because ascorbic acid is required for normal collagen synthesis.

4. Hormonal factors

a. PTH and calcitonin See III.D.1.a and III.D.1.b.

b. Growth hormone This hormone, produced by the anterior pituitary (see Chapter 20), stimulates overall growth, especially that of the epiphyseal cartilage of long bones. During childhood, growth hormone deficiency causes **pituitary dwarfism** and an excess causes **gigantism.** Excess growth hormone production in adults causes **acromegaly,** which involves excessive bone thickening.

c. Sex steroids The effects of the sex steroids (androgens and estrogens) on bone formation are complex but, in general, stimulatory. They influence the time of appearance of the ossification centers and of the closure of epiphyses. Precocious sexual maturity owing to increased sex hormone synthesis by tumors may cause early closure of epiphyses and short stature. Conversely, sex hormone deficiency may delay puberty and closure of the epiphyses, resulting in tall stature.

IV. JOINTS.

Joints, or **arthroses,** are complex connective tissue structures that join individual bones together to form the skeletal system.

A. Synarthroses:

These joints permit little or no movement. There are 3 subclasses:

1. In **synostoses,** the individual bones are fused and immobilized. ***Example:*** between the bones of the skull in the elderly.

2. In **synchondroses,** the individual bones are joined by cartilage and permit slight movement. ***Example:*** between the ribs and sternum, in the pubic symphysis.

3. In **syndesmoses,** the individual bones are joined by dense connective tissue. These joints permit slight movement. ***Example:*** between the bones of the skull in younger people and at the inferior tibiofibular articulation.

B. Diarthroses:

These are movable joints, like those found between long bones. The articulating surfaces of the bones are covered by **articular cartilage** (hyaline cartilage without a perichondrium), providing a smooth surface. The ends of the bones are joined by a 2-layered **joint capsule** made of connective tissue that seals off the **articular cavity** from the surrounding tissues. The outer or **fibrous layer** of the capsule is composed of dense connective tissue and lends support to the junction. The inner layer is a **synovial membrane** containing cells that produce the **synovial fluid** of the articular cavity. This fluid is viscous, owing to the presence of hyaluronic acid, and lubricates the articular cartilage, further reducing friction. Some diarthroses (eg, the knee) are reinforced by ligaments inside or outside the articular cavity (cruciate or collateral ligaments, respectively), and most are stabilized by surrounding muscles and tendons.

Study-Focusing Questions*

1. List the functions of bone (136).
2. Describe 2 common means of preparing bone tissue for microscopy that are necessitated by its hardness (137). Which most resembles a step in bone resorption (137, 141)?
3. List the functions of osteoblasts and name the organelle(s) involved in each function (137, 139).
4. Describe the staining properties of osteoblast cytoplasm and name the cytoplasmic components responsible (137, 139).
5. Describe the relationship of osteoprogenitor cells, osteoblasts, and osteocytes (156).
6. Compare osteocytes with osteoblasts in terms of:
   - **a.** Their shape (137, 139)
   - **b.** The length of their filopodia (137, 139)
   - **c.** The amount of rough endoplasmic reticulum in their cytoplasm (139)
   - **d.** Which ones are found in lacunae (139)
   - **e.** Which ones are found on bone surfaces (137)
   - **f.** Their rate of matrix synthesis (137, 139)
7. Nutrients, oxygen, and wastes cannot diffuse through calcified bone matrix, so how are osteocytes located far from capillaries able to survive (139)?
8. Describe osteoclasts in terms of:
   - **a.** Their size (139)
   - **b.** The number of their nuclei (140)
   - **c.** The precursor cell from which they originate (140)
   - **d.** The staining properties of their cytoplasm (140)
   - **e.** The organelles present (141)
   - **f.** Their major function (136, 141)
   - **g.** The substances they secrete (141)
   - **h.** The location and function of their ruffled border (140)
   - **i.** Their reaction to parathyroid hormone (155)
   - **j.** Their reaction to calcitonin (155)
9. List the major inorganic components of bone matrix. Which 2 are most abundant in the matrix (141–142)?
10. Describe the composition of the organic matter (osteoid) of bone matrix in terms of fiber type and ground substance (142).
11. Compare the endosteum and periosteum (142) in terms of:
    - **a.** Their location
    - **b.** Their thickness
    - **c.** The number of their layers
    - **d.** The cell types present
12. Compare compact and spongy bone (143–144) in terms of:
    - **a.** The presence of cavities and trabeculae
    - **b.** Their histologic structure when seen under high-power magnification
    - **c.** Their location
13. Compare primary and secondary bone in terms of:
    - **a.** Their relative permanence (144)
    - **b.** The type prevalent in adults (144)
    - **c.** The orientation of their collagen fibers (144–145)

*The page references in this section refer to *Basic Histology,* 6th ed., Junqueira L, Carneiro J, Kelley R, R, (editors), Appleton & Lange, 1989. **HR** (for Histology Review) is occasionally used instead of a page reference to indicate that the information referred to can be found in this book.

d. Their cellularity (cell-to-matrix ratio) (144)
e. The presence of lamellae (144)
f. Their relative mineral content (144)

14. Sketch an osteon (haversian system) in cross section (140, 144–145) and label the following:
    a. Haversian canal
    b. Endosteum
    c. Blood vessel
    d. Nerve
    e. Lymphatic vessel
    f. Lamellae
    g. Lacunae
    h. Osteocytes
    i. Filopodia
    j. Canaliculi
15. Compare haversian and Volkmann's canals (143, 144) in terms of their:
    a. Contents
    b. Orientation
    c. Encirclement by bony lamellae
16. Beginning with embryonic mesenchymal tissue, list the steps in intramembranous bone formation (145, 147).
17. Beginning with embryonic mesenchymal tissue, list the steps in endochondral bone formation (131, 147–150)
18. Compare your answers to questions 16 and 17. At what point do the 2 processes diverge? At what point do they reconverge? What is the major difference between these 2 types and bone formation?
19. Beginning with the zone of resting cartilage and ending with the zone of ossification, name in order the zones of endochondral bone formation seen in an epiphyseal plate (148). In which zone are there large isogenous groups of chondrocytes (148)?
20. Compare calcified cartilage matrix and bone matrix in terms of their staining properties (148, 150)
21. How do long bones grow in length and width (151–153)?
22. Describe the steps in the repair of a long bone fracture (153–154). Compare this to your answer to question 17.
23. Using what you have learned about the mechanisms of bone growth and remodeling, describe the cellular events that must occur in the bony alveolus (socket) of a tooth to allow a permanent reorientation of that tooth through the application of braces (154).
24. Describe the effects of the following on bone tissue:
    a. Increased circulating levels of parathyroid hormone (154–155)
    b. Increased circulating levels of calcitonin (155)
    c. Lower than normal levels of calcium in the blood (154–155)
    d. Higher than normal levels of calcium in the blood (154–55)
    e. Dietary deficiency of protein and vitamin C (155)
    f. Vitamin D deficiency (155)
    g. Vitamin A deficiency (155)
    h. Vitamin A excess (155)
    i. Insufficient growth hormone production in children (155)
    j. Excess growth hormone production in children (155)
    k. Excess growth hormone production in adults (155)
25. Compare osteomalacia and osteoporosis (155) in terms of their:
    a. Cause
    b. Effect on the mineral-to-matrix ratio in bone
26. Compare synarthroses and diarthroses in terms of the amount of movement they permit (157).
27. Compare synostoses, synchondroses, and syndesmoses in terms of the type of tissue that intervenes between the bones being united. Give examples of body sites where each may be found (157).
28. Draw a schematic diagram of a diarthrosis (157) and label the following:
    a. Articular cartilage
    b. Bone

- **c.** Periosteum
- **d.** Joint (articular) capsule
- **e.** Fibrous layer of the capsule
- **f.** Synovial membrane
- **g.** Joint cavity

29. Describe the synovial fluid (157–158) in terms of:
- **a.** Its location
- **b.** The tissue that produces it
- **c.** The cell type that produces its hyaluronic acid
- **d.** Its composition
- **e.** Its functions

Multiple-Choice Questions

For questions 8–1 through 8–4, select the single best answer.

8–1. The cell type in bone most probably derived from blood monocytes is the:
- **A.** Osteocyte
- **B.** Periosteal fibroblast
- **C.** Osteoblast
- **D.** Osteoclast
- **E.** Endothelial cell

8–2. All the following facilitate the distribution of nutrients and oxygen to osteocytes *except:*
- **A.** Gap junctions
- **B.** Filopodia
- **C.** Bone matrix
- **D.** Haversian canals
- **E.** Canaliculi

8–3. The first bone to begin to ossify in humans is the:
- **A.** Femur
- **B.** Hard palate
- **C.** Clavicle
- **D.** Parietal diploe
- **E.** Seventh cervical vertebra

8–4. All the following statements are true of Volkmann's canals *except* that they:
- **A.** Are surrounded by concentric bony lamellae
- **B.** Form connections between haversian canals
- **C.** Carry blood vessels
- **D.** Are found in compact bone
- **E.** May be found in the diaphyses of adult long bones

MATCHING (questions 8–5 through 8–34): Each answer may be used once, more than once, or not at all.

Questions 8–5 through 8–21 use the letters in Fig 8–1.

8–5. Osteoblast
8–6. Osteocyte
8–7. Mesenchyme
8–8. Osteoid
8–9. Osteoclast
8–10. Calcified bone matrix
8–11. Uncalcified bone matrix
8–12. Most basophilic cell type
8–13. Most acidophilic cell type
8–14. Direct precursor of osteocyte
8–15. Site of bone marrow development

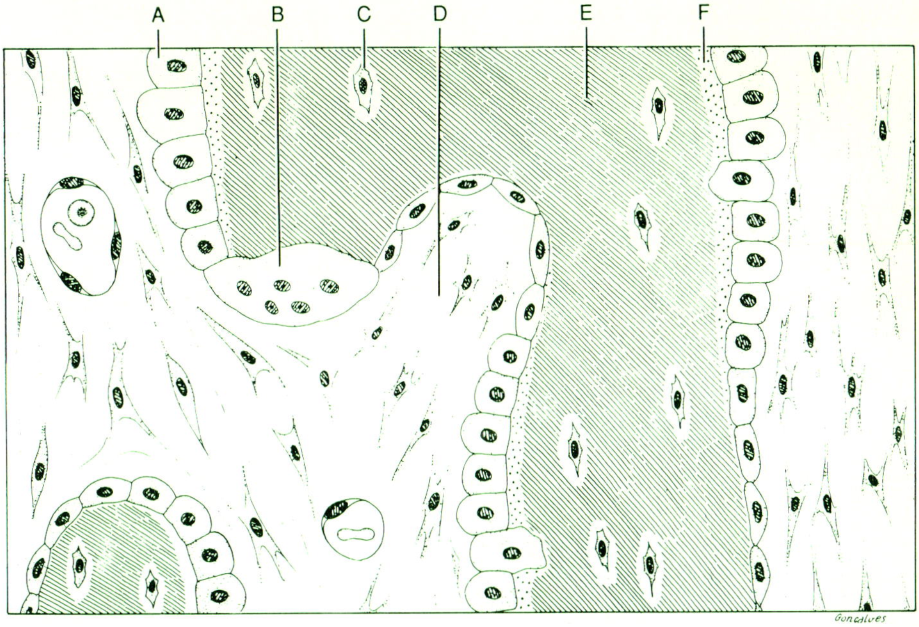

Figure 8-1.

8-16. Most active in synthesis of osteoid
8-17. Contains abundant lysosomes
8-18. Cell most responsible for bone resorption
8-19. Cell with most abundant rough endoplasmic reticulum
8-20. Activity stimulated by parathyroid hormone
8-21. Characteristically exhibits a ruffled border

Questions 8-22 through 8-26:

A. Lacuna
B. Filopodium
C. Canaliculus
D. Spicule (trabecula)
E. Howship's lacuna

8-22. Contains the thin cytoplasmic processes of osteocytes
8-23. Thin bony process formed during primary bone formation
8-24. Cavity in bone in which cell bodies of osteocytes are located
8-25. Cytoplasmic process terminating in a gap junction whereby osteocytes communicate with neighboring cells
8-26. Depression in bone in which active osteoclasts are located

Questions 8-27 through 8-34:

A. Synostosis
B. Synchondrosis
C. Syndesmosis
D. Diarthrosis
E. A, B, and C only

8–27. Synarthrosis
8–28. Allows great mobility
8–29. Allows no movement at all
8–30. Bones united by hyaline cartilage
8–31. Bones united by bone
8–32. Bones separated by a joint cavity
8–33. Bones united by connective tissue (no joint cavity)
8–34. Elbow joint is an example

For questions 8–35 through 8–81, select the one correct answer.

Questions 8–35 through 8–42:

A. Endosteum
B. Periosteum
C. Both
D. Neither

8–35. Composed of 2 layers, osteogenic and fibrous
8–36. Continuous with the joint capsule
8–37. Attached to bone by Sharpey's fibers
8–38. Contains cells with latent osteogenic capabilities
8–39. Lines the marrow cavity
8–40. Contains osteocytes
8–41. Contains blood vessels
8–42. Important in the growth and repair of bone

Questions 8–43 through 8–50:

A. Spongy bone
B. Compact bone
C. Both
D. Neither

8–43. Predominant bone tissue in the epiphyses of adult long bones
8–44. Predominant bone tissue in the diaphyses of adult long bones
8–45. Forms the diploe
8–46. Can be either primary or secondary bone
8–47. Secondary bone only
8–48. Not found in adults
8–49. Cancellous bone
8–50. Haversian bone (characteristically contains osteons)

Questions 8–51 through 8–59:

A. Primary bone
B. Secondary bone
C. Both
D. Neither

8–51. First bone tissue to appear during either intramembranous or endochondral bone formation
8–52. First bone to appear during fracture repair
8–53. Product of bone remodeling
8–54. May appear as either spongy or compact bone
8–55. Collagen fibers exhibit an irregular "woven" appearance
8–56. Collagen fibers are regularly arranged in layers of parallel bundles, and the bundles in adjacent layers spiral in opposite directions
8–57. Lamellar bone
8–58. Haversian bone
8–59. Lower mineral content

Questions 8–60 through 8–70:

A. Intramembranous bone formation
B. Endochondral bone formation
C. Both
D. Neither

8–60. Often forms flat bones, such as those in the skull
8–61. Source of long bones, such as those in the limbs
8–62. Replacement of a cartilage model by bone occurs by this process
8–63. Periosteal bone collar formation occurs by this process
8–64. Involves zones of proliferation, hypertrophy, and calcification
8–65. Ultimate origin is from a mesenchymal condensation
8–66. Begins at a primary ossification center
8–67. Forms epiphyseal plates between primary and secondary ossification centers
8–68. May have a role in fracture repair
8–69. Forms most of the bony skeleton in humans
8–70. Its osteoid is synthesized by osteoblasts

Questions 8–71 through 8–75:

A. Parathyroid hormone
B. Calcitonin
C. Both
D. Neither

8–71. Stimulates bone deposition
8–72. Stimulates bone resorption
8–73. Regulates blood calcium concentration
8–74. Activates and increases the number of osteoclasts
8–75. Excess blood levels may result in calcium deposition in soft tissues such as the kidneys and arterial walls

Questions 8–76 through 8–81:

A. Osteomalacia
B. Osteoporosis
C. Both
D. Neither

8–76. Excessive calcium in bones
8–77. Depletion of calcium from bone with little loss of osteoid
8–78. Depletion of bone mass (loss of calcium and osteoid)
8–79. This condition in adults corresponds to rickets in children
8–80. More often seen in immobilized patients and postmenopausal women
8–81. Condition resulting from a nutritional deficiency in calcium that may be aggravated by pregnancy

For questions 8–82 through 8–85, one, more than one, or all of the answers may be correct. Select

A if only (1), (2), and (3) are correct
B if only (1) and (3) are correct
C if only (2) and (4) are correct
D if all answers are correct

8–82. The epiphyseal plate:
(1) Is responsible for the growth in length of long bones
(2) Forms only after the formation of the secondary ossification center
(3) Will ossify prematurely in children who lack sufficient growth hormone
(4) Is composed of fibrocartilage

8-83. Components of bone matrix include:
- **(1)** Osteoid
- **(2)** Type I collagen
- **(3)** Hydroxyapatite
- **(4)** Glycosaminoglycans

8-84. Interstitial lamellae:
- **(1)** Never border directly on a haversian canal
- **(2)** Are remnants of primary bone in secondary bone
- **(3)** Are the result of bone remodeling
- **(4)** Are remnants of calcified cartilage in primary bone

8-85. The capsule surrounding a diarthrosis:
- **(1)** Has an outer fibrous layer continuous with the periosteum
- **(2)** Contains phagocytic A cells, which help clear the articular cavity of debris formed as a result of friction between the articular cartilages
- **(3)** Is covered on its inner surface by a synovial layer
- **(4)** Produces a viscous fluid that reduces friction and nourishes the articular chondrocytes

INTEGRATIVE MULTIPLE-CHOICE QUESTIONS: CONNECTIVE TISSUES

For questions CT–1 through CT–5, select the single best answer.

CT–1. Cells capable of uncoupling oxidative phosphorylation with consequent production of heat are:
- **A.** Chondrocytes
- **B.** Multilocular adipocytes
- **C.** Mast cells
- **D.** Unilocular adipocytes
- **E.** Osteoclasts

CT–2. Which of the following conditions has an effect on connective tissue structure and function and cannot be remedied or prevented by attention to diet?
- **A.** Scurvy
- **B.** Osteomalacia
- **C.** Myxedema
- **D.** Rickets
- **E.** None of the above (all can be prevented by attention to diet)

CT–3. Factors that decrease the regenerative capacity of connective tissues include all of the following *except:*
- **A.** Hydrocortisone
- **B.** Insufficient dietary vitamin C
- **C.** Calcitonin
- **D.** Adrenocorticotropic hormone (ACTH)
- **E.** Insufficient iron in the diet

CT–4. The silver-stained connective tissue type shown in the photomicrograph in Fig CT–1 is:
- **A.** Loose (areolar) connective tissue
- **B.** Spongy bone
- **C.** Reticular connective tissue
- **D.** Dense irregular connective tissue
- **E.** Elastic connective tissue

CT–5. The connective tissue type shown in the photomicrograph in Fig CT–2 is:
- **A.** Dense regular connective tissue
- **B.** Dense (compact) bone

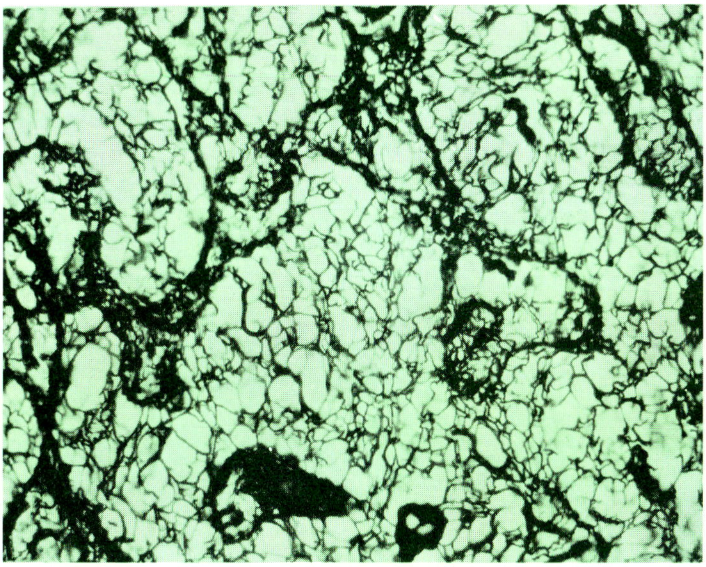

Figure CT–1.

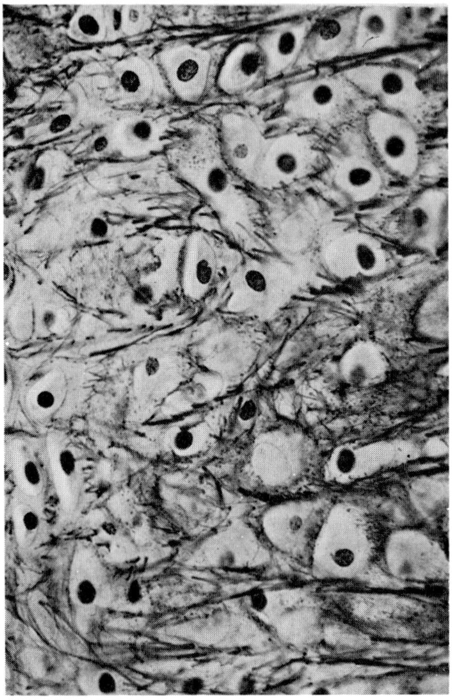

Figure CT-2.

C. Elastic connective tissue
D. Elastic cartilage
E. Fibrocartilage

MATCHING (questions CT-6 through CT-42): Each may be used once, more than once, or not at all.

Questions CT-6 through CT-12:

A. Collagen fibers
B. Elastic fibers
C. Reticular fibers
D. A and B only
E. A and C only
F. A, B, and C
G. None of the above

CT-6. Found in some types of connective tissue proper
CT-7. Found in significant amounts in some types of cartilage
CT-8. Found in significant amounts in adipose tissue
CT-9. Component of connective tissue ground substance
CT-10. Include microfibrillar proteins as a component of their structure
CT-11. Have subunits formed from 3 alpha chains
CT-12. Major fibrous component of bone matrix

Questions CT-13 through CT-21:

A. Type I collagen
B. Type II collagen
C. Type III collagen
D. Type IV collagen
E. Type V collagen.

CT–13. Predominant fiber type in hyaline cartilage
CT–14. Predominant fiber type in bone
CT–15. Predominant fiber type in most basal laminae
CT–16. Predominant fiber type in hemopoietic organs
CT–17. Predominant fiber type in the dermis
CT–18. Reticular fibers
CT–19. Predominant fiber type in fibrocartilage
CT–20. Predominant fiber type in placental basement membranes
CT–21. $[\alpha\ 1\ (II)]_3$

Questions CT–22 through CT–36:

A. Connective tissue proper
B. Reticular connective tissue
C. Elastic connective tissue
D. Mucous connective tissue
E. Adipose tissue
F. Cartilage
G. Bone
H. All of the above

CT–22. Supporting tissue for the spleen
CT–23. Annulus fibrous
CT–24. Functions in the storage of fuel
CT–25. Comprises tendons
CT–26. Least vascular
CT–27. Most vascular
CT–28. Wharton's jelly
CT–29. Predominant cells have characteristic signet-ring appearance
CT–30. Covers articular surfaces in diarthroses
CT–31. Contains widest variety of connective tissue cell types
CT–32. Composed of cells, fibers, and ground substance
CT–33. Found in greatest concentration in the yellow ligament (ligamentum flavum) of the vertebral column
CT–34. Functions as a calcium depot
CT–35. Fetal skeletal tissue
CT–36. Derived from embryonic mesenchyme

Questions CT–37 through CT–42 use the letters in Fig CT–3.

CT–37. Hyaluronic acid
CT–38. Proteoglycan
CT–39. Core protein
CT–40. Link protein
CT–41. Sulfated glycosaminoglycan
CT–42. Nonsulfated glycosaminoglycan

For questions CT–43 through CT–46, one, more than one, or all of the answers may be correct. Select

A if only (1), (2), and (3) are correct
B if only (1) and (3) are correct
C if only (2) and (4) are correct
D if only (4) is correct
E if all answers are correct

CT–43. Connective tissue cell types believed to be derived from blood monocytes and thus considered a part of the mononuclear phagocyte system include:
(1) Neutrophils
(2) Osteoclasts
(3) Plasma cells
(4) Macrophages

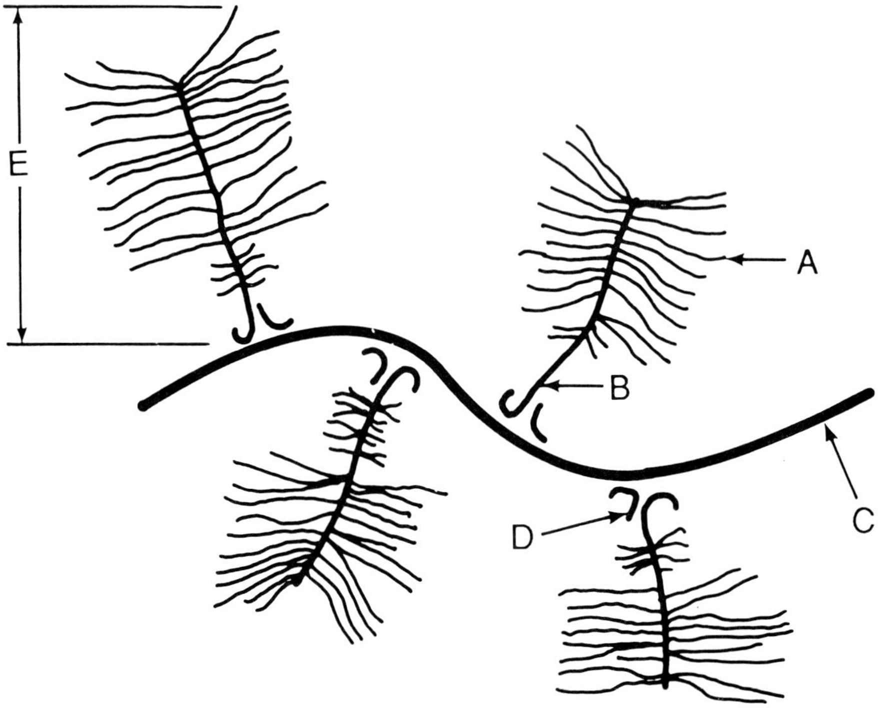

Figure CT-3.

CT-44. Cells that characteristically synthesize and secrete some form of collagen include:
- **(1)** Fibroblasts
- **(2)** Chondroblasts
- **(3)** Osteoblasts
- **(4)** Reticular cells

CT-45. Connective tissue cell types capable of synthesizing and secreting glycosaminoglycans include:
- **(1)** Fibroblasts
- **(2)** Osteoblasts
- **(3)** Chondroblasts
- **(4)** Mast cells

CT-46. Cell types that require large numbers of lysosomes to carry out their specialized functions in connective tissues include:
- **(1)** Osteoclasts
- **(2)** Neutrophils
- **(3)** Macrophages
- **(4)** Mast cells

Nerve Tissue 9

Objectives

This chapter should help the student to:

- List the structural and functional characteristics of nerve tissue that distinguish it from the other basic tissue types.
- Know the structure, function, and embryonic origin of the various types of cells in nerve tissue and give examples of body sites where each may be found.
- Relate the structural and functional characteristics of the cells in nerve tissue to overall nerve tissue function and predict the functional effects of a given structural deficit in nerve tissue.
- Describe in detail how neurons receive, propagate, and transmit signals.
- Know the role of the organelles and cytoplasmic inclusions of neurons in the transmission of nerve impulses and in the repair of damage.
- Know in which parts of the neuron (cell body, axon, dendrites) each organelle or inclusion is found.
- Know the structural components, function, and various classes of synapses.
- Describe in general terms the divisions, location, organization, function, and distinguishing features of the autonomic nervous system.
- Describe the structure and functions of the protective coverings (meninges) of the central nervous system.
- Describe the source, composition, and circulation of the cerebrospinal fluid.
- Recognize the type of nerve tissue and identify the individual cells and cell processes in a photomicrograph or slide of a tissue or organ.
- Describe the response of nerve tissue to injury.

Synopsis

I. GENERAL FEATURES OF NERVE TISSUE & THE NERVOUS SYSTEM

A. Two Classes of Cells: Nerve tissue is composed primarily of neurons, which transmit electrochemical messages (impulses), and the supporting cells that surround them. It contains relatively little extracellular material.

1. Neurons Neurons are discussed briefly here and in detail in section II.

a. Function Neurons perform all the specialized functions attributed to nerve tissue. They are characterized by **irritability,** ie, rapid and dramatic response to weak stimuli. Neurons can (1) receive and integrate stimuli from many sources simultaneously, (2) translate stimuli into a change in membrane potential (a difference in electrical charge between the inner and outer surfaces of their plasma membranes), (3) propagate this potential difference (the electrical message) rapidly over long distances and along specific pathways, (4) translate the electrical message into specific neurotransmitters (the chemical message), and (5) deliver neurotransmitters to target cells.

b. Structure A neuron has (1) a cell body, also called the **soma** (''body'') or **perikaryon** (''around the nucleus''), consisting of the nucleus and its surrounding cytoplasm and plasma membrane; (2) a variable number of cytoplasmic processes called dendrites that collect incoming messages and carry them toward the soma; and (3) a single cytoplasmic process called an axon that transmits messages to the target cells. The axons of most neurons have a whitish **myelin sheath** produced by supporting cells and interrupted by gaps called **nodes of Ranvier.** The segments of axon between the gaps are called **internodes.**

2. Supporting cells Supporting cells, also called **neuroglia** ("nerve glue") or **glial cells,** vary greatly in structure according to their functions. These include structural and nutritional support of neurons, electrical insulation, and enhancement (by means of myelin sheaths) of the speed of impulse conduction along axons (VII.B). Some authors reserve the terms neuroglia and glial cells for supporting cells of the central nervous system (brain and spinal cord). Supporting cells are discussed in detail in section III.

B. Impulse Conduction: Within a neuron, signals (impulses) are propagated as a wave of depolarization along the plasma membrane of the dendrites, soma, and axon. Depolarization is accomplished through the membrane, allowing ions (eg, Na^+, K^+) to enter or exit the cell. In an unmyelinated axon, depolarization is continuous along its plasma membrane (axolemma). In myelinated axons, depolarization occurs only at the nodes of Ranvier. The insulating effect of the myelin prevents depolarization between nodes. Thus the impulse jumps from node to node, a phenomenon called **saltatory conduction.** Myelinated axons therefore carry impulses faster than do unmyelinated axons of the same diameter.

C. Synapses: Signals pass via specialized connections termed synapses from a neuron to its target cell. The target may be another neuron or a cell in the end organ (eg, gland or muscle) it supplies. At **chemical synapses,** the signal is transmitted by exocytosis of **neurotransmitters,** chemical substances such as acetylcholine that cross the narrow gap (synaptic cleft) between the cells to initiate depolarization of the target cell. Chemical synapses are discussed in section IV. At **electrical synapses,** which are much less common, the signal is transmitted by ions flowing through a gap-junctionlike junctional complex.

D. Subsystems of the Nervous System: The nervous system is highly integrated but divisible into 2 overlapping pairs of subsystems:

1. Central and Peripheral Nervous Systems These 2 subsystems are defined mainly by location.

a. The **central nervous system (CNS)** includes the brain and spinal cord. In the CNS, collections of neuron cell bodies (with their dendrites and the proximal portions of their axons) constitute the **gray matter;** collections of mostly myelinated axons are called **white matter.** Localized groups of neuron cell bodies in the gray matter are termed **nuclei.**

b. The **peripheral nervous system (PNS)** includes all other nerve tissue. In the PNS, collections of neuron cell bodies are called **ganglia** and collections of mostly myelinated axons are called **peripheral nerves,** or simply **nerves**. The term **nerve fiber** refers to a single axon in a peripheral nerve (along with its myelin sheath if it is myelinated).

2. Autonomic and Somatic Nervous Systems These 2 subsystems are defined according to function but have distinctive anatomic features as well. Each has CNS and PNS components.

a. The **autonomic nervous system (ANS)** controls involuntary visceral functions (eg, glandular secretion, smooth muscle contraction) and has both motor and sensory pathways. Each motor pathway consists of 2 neurons that synapse (connect) in a peripheral autonomic ganglion (V.B). The cell body of the first neuron, called the **preganglionic motor neuron,** is in the CNS; the cell body of the second neuron, called the **postganglionic motor neuron,** is in the peripheral ganglion. Visceral sensory pathways, while crucial to autonomic function, are unfortunately excluded by some authors from the autonomic nervous system. The **sensory neurons** of the ANS have cell bodies in craniospinal ganglia (V.A) and processes extending to the periphery. The ANS is subdivided into the sympathetic and parasympathetic systems. When they innervate the same end organ, sympathetic and parasympathetic nerves usually have opposing effects.

(1) The motor pathways of the **sympathetic system** (the thoracolumbar outflow) have preganglionic neurons with cell bodies in the intermediolateral cell column of spinal cord segments T1–L3. The postganglionic neurons have cell bodies located mainly in the sympathetic chain ganglia (close to the spinal column). The sympathetic nervous system is therefore characterized by short preganglionic and long postganglionic nerve fibers. The neurotransmitter of the preganglionic fibers is **acetylcholine;** that of the postganglionic fibers is either **epinephrine** (adrenalin) or **norepinephrine** (noradrenalin). The sensory component consists of sensory neurons with cell bodies in the dorsal root ganglia and long dendrites that reach the periphery.

(2) The motor pathways of the **parasympathetic system** (the craniosacral outflow) are classified in 2 divisions. The **cranial division** has preganglionic neurons with cell bodies in nuclei of the medulla and midbrain. Axons of these neurons leave the CNS through cranial nerves III, VII, IX, and X. The **sacral division** has preganglionic cell bodies in the intermediate gray matter of the sacral spinal cord segments and postganglionic cell bodies in intramural and other ganglia close to their site of action. The parasympathetic nervous system is therefore characterized by long preganglionic and short postganglionic fibers. The neurotransmitter of both the pre- and the postganglionic fibers is acetylcholine. The sensory neuron cell bodies are located in sacral dorsal root ganglia and cranial ganglia.

b. The **somatic nervous system** includes all nerve tissue except the autonomic nervous system. It controls somatosensory perception (eg, touch, heat, cold) and somatomotor (voluntary) functions (eg, skeletal muscle contraction). Acetylcholine is the most common somatic neurotransmitter.

E. Development of Nerve Tissue: All neurons and supporting cells derive from embryonic ectoderm. Cells of the midline dorsal ectoderm of the early embryo are induced by the underlying notochord to form a thickened **neural plate.** The lateral border of the neural plate thickens and the center invaginates, forming a troughlike **neural groove.** As the groove deepens, the lateral borders contact each other to close the groove and form the **neural tube.** The cells lining the tube transform into a mitotically active pseudostratified columnar epithelium (neuroepithelium) and eventually form the layers that give rise to the entire central nervous system. As the neural groove is closing, cells at its lateral borders proliferate to form 2 columnar masses that come to lie dorsal to the neural tube and form the **neural crest.** Neural crest cells migrate away from the neural tube and form much of the peripheral nervous system, including the sensory neurons of the craniospinal ganglia, the postganglionic neurons of the autonomic nervous system, the Schwann cells of the peripheral nerves, and the satellite cells of the ganglia. Neural crest cells also form the meninges (see below) and most of the mesenchyme of the head and neck. Neural crest derivatives covered in other chapters include the odontoblasts of the developing teeth (see Chapter 15), the melanocytes of the epidermis and hair follicles (see Chapter 18), and the chromaffin cells and ganglion cells of the adrenal medulla (see Chapter 21).

F. Aging and Repair: Neurons are incapable of further mitosis once they mature and are often used as examples of terminally differentiated cells. Neurons of the elderly may contain abundant lipofuscin pigment. Their inability to divide makes repair of injured nerve tissue more difficult than for other tissues. Neuron cell bodies lost through injury or surgery cannot be replaced, but if an axon is severed or crushed and the cell body remains intact, regeneration of the injured axon is possible. Supporting cells can divide if stimulated by injury.

G. Meninges: The brain and spinal cord are separated from the bony compartments in which they lie (skull and vertebral canal) by 3 layers of specialized connective tissue termed the **meninges.** The outer layer, or **dura mater,** is dense connective tissue bound tightly to the periosteum of the surrounding bone. The middle layer, or **arachnoid,** has 2 components:

(1) a layer of loose connective tissue in direct contact with the dura mater, and (2) many connective tissue strands, or trabeculae, that attach the arachnoid layer to the underlying pia mater. The spaces between the arachnoid trabeculae are filled with the **cerebrospinal fluid.** Avascular projections of the arachnoid into sinuses in the dura are called arachnoid villi. The innermost layer, or **pia mater,** is a thin, richly vascularized layer of loose connective tissue that is firmly attached to the surface of the brain or spinal cord but separated from the neurons and their processes by neuroglial cell processes. Ramified, cuboidal epithelium-covered projections of the pia mater in the brain's ventricles are collectively termed the **choroid plexus;** they produce the cerebrospinal fluid by selective ultrafiltration of blood plasma.

H. Blood-Brain Barrier: Nerve tissue of the central nervous system receives oxygen and nutrients from capillaries in the pia mater. These capillaries are relatively impermeable, because (1) their endothelial cells lack fenestrations and are joined at the borders by tight junctions, and (2) they are partially surrounded by the cytoplasmic processes of neuroglia called astrocytes (III.A.1.a). These features contribute to a structural and functional **blood-brain barrier** that protects CNS neurons from many extraneous influences and prevents certain antibiotics and chemotherapeutic agents from reaching the CNS.

II. NEURONS

A. Cell Body: The cell body (soma, perikaryon) is the synthetic and trophic center of the neuron. It can receive signals from axons of other neurons through synaptic contacts on its plasma membrane and transmit them to its own axon.

1. Nucleus Neuron nuclei are usually large, centrally located, and euchromatic. Each has a prominent nucleolus and heterochromatin around the inner surface of the nuclear envelope.

2. Cytoplasm The cytoplasm of the perikaryon contains many organelles, including mitochondria, lysosomes, and centrioles. The numerous free ribosomes, polyribosomes, and RER-associated ribosomes appear as clumps of basophilic material, collectively called **Nissl bodies,** in light microscopic preparations. The Golgi complex is well developed and is the site for packaging of neurotransmitters into neurosecretory or synaptic vesicles. In some neurons, neurosecretory products are glycosylated in the Golgi complex prior to packaging. **Neurotubules** (microtubules) and bundles of **neurofilaments** (intermediate filaments) are distributed throughout the perikaryon and extend into the axon and dendrites. Some neurons (eg, in the substantia nigra of the midbrain) contain **melanin** in their perikarya.

B. Dendrites: Dendrites, extensions of the perikaryon specialized to increase the surface available for incoming signals, become thinner farther from the soma through successive branching. They are often covered over much of their surface with synaptic contacts; some have numerous sharp projections, termed **dendritic spines** or **gemmules,** that act as synaptic sites. Dendrites lack Golgi complexes but may contain small numbers of the other organelles found in the perikaryon.

C. Axon: Each neuron has one axon, a complex cell process that carries impulses away from the soma. An axon is divisible into several regions:

1. The **axon hillock** is the part of the perikaryon that leads directly into the axonal process. It differs from the rest of the perikaryon in that it contains no Nissl bodies. While the entire axon is usually not visible in sectioned material, its origin is distinguishable from that of the dendrites by the absence of Nissl-related basophilia.

2. The **initial segment** is the part of a myelinated axon between the apex of the axon hillock and the beginning of the myelin sheath. It is characterized by a thin layer of electron-dense material beneath the plasma membrane termed the **dense undercoating** and contains neurotubule and neurofilament bundles originating in the axon hillock.

3. The **axon proper** is the main trunk of the axon, excluding the initial segment. Axons tend to have a constant diameter along their entire length. The larger the diameter of the axon, the more likely it is to be myelinated and the faster its rate of impulse conduction. Some axons have branches, termed **collaterals,** which may contact other neurons or even return to the cell body of origin to modulate their own subsequent depolarization. The **axoplasm** (cytoplasm) contains few organelles but usually has some mitochondria and parallel bundles of neurotubules and neurofilaments. It has very limited metabolic activity, but it conveys metabolic products to and from the axon terminals (VII.A). Signal transmission (VII.B) relies heavily on the asymmetric distribution of ionic charges (potential difference) on either side of the **axolemma,** or axonal plasma membrane.

4. **Terminal arborization** Many axons undergo branching, or arborization, near their terminations. The degree of terminal branching depends upon the size and function of the axon.

5. **Boutons** Each terminal branch of an axon ends in a bulbous enlargement called a **terminal end-bulb** or **terminal bouton** (terminal boutons or boutons terminaux). Swellings in the wall of an axon before its termination are termed **boutons en passage.** Each bouton typically contains abundant mitochondria and neurosecretory vesicles. A specialized region of its plasma membrane, the **presynaptic membrane,** forms part of a synapse (IV).

D. Classification of Neurons:

1. By the configuration of their cell processes

a. **Multipolar neurons,** the most abundant type, have a least 2 and usually more dendrites. *Examples:* **motor neurons** with cell bodies in the ventral horn of the spinal cord gray matter, **pyramidal cells** of the cerebral cortex, and **Purkinje cells** of the cerebellar cortex. The dendrites of most multipolar neurons radiate in many directions, but those of Purkinje cells usually have a fanlike configuration, extending from the soma in a single plane.

b. **Bipolar neurons** have a single dendrite, which arises from the pole of the soma opposite the axon. These sensory neurons are found only in the retina, the olfactory mucosa, and the cochlear (spiral) and vestibular ganglia of the inner ear.

c. **Pseudounipolar neurons** begin in the embryo as bipolar cells whose axon and dendrite later fuse to form a single T-shaped process. These generally sensory neurons are found in dorsal root ganglia and in most cranial ganglia. In adults, both branches of the T are structurally and functionally similar to axons. Nerve impulses are carried only by the processes, bypassing the soma at the branch-point of the T.

d. **Unipolar neurons** have a single short axon and no dendrites. The photoreceptor cells of the retina (rods and cones; see Chapter 24) are the best examples.

2. By cell size

a. **Golgi type I** neurons have a long axon and a large soma (eg, motor neurons of the spinal cord, pyramidal cells of the cerebral cortex).

b. In **Golgi type II** neurons, the short axon undergoes extensive terminal arborization close to the small soma (eg, interneurons of the spinal cord).

3. By function

a. **Motor neurons** carry nerve impulses to peripheral end organs and induce or inhibit muscular contraction, glandular secretion, or both. Both the somatic and the autonomic nervous systems have motor components.

b. **Sensory neurons** receive impulses generated by the stimulation of peripheral sensory cells and organs and carry them toward the central nervous system.

c. Interneurons have short processes and mediate interactions between (1) a sensory and a motor neuron, as in reflex actions (eg, knee jerk); (2) one motor neuron and another, as in the concerted action of different muscle groups, and (3) 2 sensory neurons. Reflex actions mediated by interneurons may be automatic but not necessarily autonomic.

4. By neurotransmitters released Neurons may be named according to the neurotransmitters they release; eg, **cholinergic neurons** release acetylcholine, **GABAergic** neurons release gamma aminobutyric acid (GABA). Sympathetic and parasympathetic subdivisions of the ANS are distinguished mainly by the neurotransmitters their postganglionic fibers release: Sympathetic postganglionic neurons are **noradrenergic** or **adrenergic** (release noradrenalin or adrenalin), while parasympathetic postganglionic neurons are cholinergic (release acetylcholine). Other neurotransmitters include dopamine, serotonin, glycine, and perhaps several other biogenic amines (eg, histamine).

III. SUPPORTING CELLS.

Supporting cells provide neurons with both functional and structural support and play a passive role in generating and transmitting nerve impulses. Positioned between the blood and the neurons, they establish compartments and monitor the passage of materials from one compartment to another. It is difficult to maintain neurons in tissue culture without supporting cells.

A. Supporting Cells of the CNS:

In the CNS, there are about 10 neuroglial, or glial, cells per neuron. Glial cells are generally smaller than neurons. Their cytoplasmic processes, although abundant and extensive, are difficult to distinguish without special stains, so histologic identification is usually based on nuclear morphology. There are 4 major types of CNS neuroglial cells: oligodendroglia, astrocytes, microglia, and ependymal cells. The first 2 types are called macroglia.

1. Macroglia

a. Astrocytes are the largest glial cells. Their nuclei, also the largest, are irregular, spheric and pale-staining and have a prominent nucleolus. Astrocytes have long, branching cytoplasmic processes, many of which have expanded pedicles at their tips. These pedicles are termed **vascular end-feet,** because they often surround capillaries of the pia matter, where they are important components of the blood-brain barrier (I.H). There are 2 types of astrocytes:

(1) Protoplasmic astrocytes, also called **mossy cells,** are most numerous in gray matter. They have abundant granular cytoplasm and thicker, shorter, more highly branched processes than fibrous astrocytes.

(2) Fibrous astrocytes are most common in white matter. Special silver stains show their cytoplasm to be filled with a fibrillar material believed to be precipitated intermediate filaments. They have long, highly attenuated processes, less branched than those of protoplasmic astrocytes.

b. Oligodendroglia, or **oligodendrocytes,** are the most numerous glial cell type. Their spheric nuclei are intermediate in size and staining intensity between the nuclei of astrocytes and those of microglia (see below). Like the Schwann cells of PNS, they form myelin and occur in the long rows required to myelinate an entire axon. Unlike a Schwann cell, an oligodendrocyte has several cell processes and may provide myelin for segments of several axons.

2. Microglia, the smallest and least numerous of the glia, are found in both gray and white matter. Their nuclei are small and elongate (often bean-shaped), and their chromatin is so condensed that they often appear black in H&E-stained sections. Their processes are shorter than those of astrocytes and are covered with thorny branches. Microglial cells possibly derive from mesenchyme, or they may be **glioblasts** (immature oligodendrocytes) of neuroepithelial origin. Some microglia may be components of the mononuclear phagocyte system and have phagocytic capabilities. However, when neural injury is unaccompanied by vascular injury, phagocytic cells in the area of the injured neurons appear to derive solely from macroglia.

3. Ependymal cells are derived from ciliated neuroepithelial cells of the internal lining of the neural tube. In adults, they retain their epithelial nature and some cilia and line the remnants of the neural tube (ventricles of the brain and central canal of the spinal cord). Superficially, the lining resembles a simple columnar epithelium, but ependymal cells have basal cell processes that extend deep into the gray matter. The ependymal lining is continuous with the cuboidal epithelium of the choroid plexuses.

B. Supporting Cells of the PNS:

1. Schwann cells are the supporting cells of the peripheral nerves. A single Schwann cell may envelop segments of several unmyelinated axons or provide a segment of a single myelinated axon with its myelin sheath. A myelinated axon segment is surrounded by multiple layers of a Schwann cell process with most of its cytoplasm squeezed out; the remaining multilayered Schwann cell plasma membrane, called **myelin,** is composed mainly of a phospholipid complex. The gaps between the myelin-sheath segments formed by individual Schwann cells are the **nodes of Ranvier.** Schwann cell nuclei often appear ovoid or flattened and lie at the periphery of the axon they support. They are usually less heterochromatic than the nuclei of the fibrocytes found scattered among the axons of a peripheral nerve.

2. Satellite cells are specialized Schwann cells found in the dorsal root ganglia and autonomic ganglia of the PNS, where they form a one-cell-thick covering over the cell bodies of the neurons (ganglion cells). Their nuclei are spherical with a mottled chromatin pattern; in sectioned tissue, the nuclei typically appear as a "string of pearls" surrounding the much larger ganglion cell bodies.

IV. SYNAPSES (Chemical).

Artificially stimulated axons can propagate a wave of depolarization in either direction, but the signal can travel in only one direction across a synapse, which thus functions as a unidirectional valve. Synapses are named according to the structures they connect, eg, axodendritic, axosomatic, axoaxonic, and dendrodendritic synapses. Each synapse has 3 major structural components:

A. Presynaptic Membrane:

This is the portion of the terminal bouton membrane closest to the target cell. It consists of an electron-dense thickening into which are inserted many short intermediate filaments, making it resemble a hemidesmosome. Upon stimulation, neurosecretory vesicles in the bouton fuse with the presynaptic membrane and release their neurotransmitters into the synaptic cleft (see below). The vesicle membrane added to the presynaptic membrane is removed and recycled by invagination and budding of the bouton membrane lateral to the synaptic cleft.

B. Synaptic Cleft:

The synaptic cleft, or **synaptic gap,** is a fluid-filled space, generally about 20 nm in diameter, between the pre- and postsynaptic membranes. It is shielded from the rest of the extracellular space by supporting cell processes and a basal-laminalike structure that binds the pre- and postsynaptic membranes together. Some synaptic clefts are traversed by dense filaments that form structural links between the membranes and perhaps guide neurotransmitters across the gap.

C. Postsynaptic Membrane:

This is a thickening of a portion of the plasma membrane of the next neuron or target cell (eg, muscle). It is structurally similar to the presynaptic membrane but also contains highly selective receptors for neurotransmitters. When enough receptors are occupied by neurotransmitter molecules, hydrophilic channels are opened, resulting in depolarization of the postsynaptic membrane (VII.B.2.a).

D. Removal of Excess Neurotransmitter:

Acetylcholine remaining in the cleft after stimulation of the postsynaptic neuron (or other end organ) is degraded by acetylcholinesterase in the cleft. The degradation products are endocytosed by coated pits (see Chapter 3) in the membrane of the end bulb, peripheral to the presynaptic thickening. Other neurotransmitters are disposed of by other mechanisms. Removal of excess transmitter prevents continuous firing of the postsynaptic neuron in response to a single presynaptic stimulus.

V. GANGLIA.

Peripheral collections of neuron cell bodies, called ganglia, may be divided into 2 major types:

A. Craniospinal Ganglia: These include (1) the **ganglia of the cranial nerves,** and (2) the **dorsal root** (or **spinal) ganglia** associated with the spinal cord. They are predominantly sensory in function and, except for the spiral ganglion of the auditory system, contain mostly pseudounipolar neurons. Because impulses pass from the peripheral process of such a cell directly to the central process, bypassing the cell body, there are no synapses in these ganglia. Craniospinal ganglia can be distinguished in histologic section because their satellite cells are more numerous than those of autonomic ganglia, have more spheric nuclei, and completely surround the soma of each ganglion cell. Also, the ganglion cell bodies in craniospinal ganglia are concentrated peripherally around the core of abundant cell processes. Ganglion cell bodies in autonomic ganglia are more randomly distributed. The smaller nuclei lying at the center of craniospinal ganglia belong mainly to Schwann cells.

B. Autonomic Ganglia: These are predominantly visceromotor in function, controlling the contraction of smooth muscle and the secretory activity of certain glands. They contain mostly multipolar neurons and have synapses. Their satellite cells are less numerous than those of the craniospinal ganglia, have more ovoid nuclei, and form a discontinuous sheath around the multipolar ganglion cell bodies. The location of autonomic ganglia depends upon their function. **Sympathetic ganglia** are found closer to the CNS and occur primarily in the sympathetic chain. **Parasympathetic ganglia** usually occur farther from the CNS, often as part of the organs they supply (eg, the submucosal and myenteric plexuses in the walls of the digestive tract).

VI. PERIPHERAL NERVES.

Peripheral nerves contain myelinated and unmyelinated axons, Schwann cells, and fibroblasts. They contain no neuron cell bodies; nuclei seen in sections of peripheral nerves belong to Schwann cells or fibrocytes (fibroblasts). Schwann cell nuclei are generally larger and lighter-staining than fibrocyte nuclei.

A. Coverings: Each peripheral nerve is surrounded by a layer of dense connective tissue, the **epineurium.** Branches of this covering penetrate the nerve and separate the fibers into bundles called **fascicles.** The connective tissue sheath surrounding each fascicle is termed the **perineurium.** Fine slips of reticular connective tissue from the perineurium penetrate the fascicles to surround each nerve fiber, forming the **endoneurium.** Branches of the blood vessels in the epineurium penetrate the nerve along with the connective tissue, providing Schwann cells and axons with their vascular supply.

B. Types of Nerve Fibers: **Type A** fibers are myelinated, large-diameter axons with long internodes and rapid impulse conduction. **Type B** fibers are medium-diameter, myelinated axons with shorter internodes and a medium rate of impulse conduction. **Type C** fibers are small-diameter, unmyelinated axons with slow impulse conduction.

VII. HISTOPHYSIOLOGY OF NERVE TISSUE

A. Axonal Transport: Movement of metabolic products through the axoplasm is called axonal transport, or axoplasmic transport, and can be as fast as 400 mm/d. The movement of newly synthesized products and synaptic vesicles toward the terminal arborization is termed **anterograde** or **orthograde** axoplasmic transport, while the return of worn materials to the perikaryon for degradation or reutilization is termed **retrograde** axoplasmic transport. Both transport phenomena appear to involve neurotubules and neurofilaments.

B. Signal Generation and Transmission: The basic function of nerve tissue is the generation and transmission of signals in the form of nerve impulses, or **action potentials,** from one part of the body to another. The anatomic arrangement of neurons in chains and circuits allows integration of simple on-off signals into complex information. The microscopic structure of nerve tissue (eg, the diameter of axons and the presence or absence of myelin) exploits physicochemical phenomena to regulate the rate and sequence of signal transmission.

1. The resting membrane potential The K^+ concentration is 20 times higher inside neurons than outside, while the Na^+ concentration is 10 times higher outside than inside. Because the plasma membrane is much more permeable to K^+ than to other ions, K^+ ions tend to diffuse into the extracellular fluid until the accumulated positive charge outside the cell inhibits further K^+ movement across the membrane. In this state of equilibrium, the inside of the cell is negatively charged relative to the outside; this potential difference or voltage across the membrane is termed the **resting membrane potential.** The cell interior is at -40 to -100 millivolts (mV) relative to the exterior, which is considered to be at ground potential (0 V). Energy-requiring pumps in the plasma membrane help maintain the resting potential, thus keeping the neuron in a state of readiness to receive and transmit signals. The best known pump is Na^+/K^+-ATPase, which can exchange internal sodium for escaped potassium when adenosine triphosphate (ATP) is available.

2. The action potential

a. Firing and propagation of the action potential Binding of excitatory neurotransmitters (eg, acetylcholine) to receptors in the postsynaptic membrane allows positive ions to enter the cell, gradually reducing the potential difference across the membrane. When this membrane depolarization reaches a critical level (eg, when the potential difference is reduced from -90 mV to -70 mV), the **threshold** is reached, opening the voltage-gated Na^+ channels (integral membrane proteins that function as Na^+ ion channels and open or close in response to changes in voltage across membrane). Na^+ ions flow into the cell and reverse the membrane potential (ie, the interior becomes positive with respect to the exterior) in one region of the plasma membrane. Incoming Na^+ ions diffuse to adjacent sites within the cell, where they cause threshold depolarization and the opening of Na^+ channels; thus, a wave of depolarization spreads along the surface of the neuron. Spread of the wave of depolarization along the membrane surface is termed **propagation** of the action potential. Events leading to and including propagation of the action potential are referred to as the **firing** of the action potential. The firing of an action potential is an "all-or-none" event and will not occur unless the threshold is reached.

b. The refractory period Reversal of the membrane potential at threshold causes voltage-gated K^+ channels to open and K^+ ions to flow out of the cell, returning the membrane to its resting potential (repolarization). The membrane may achieve an even greater potential difference, or **hyperpolarization,** before stabilizing at normal resting levels. The refractory period is the 1- to 2-ms interval between the firing of an action potential and restoration of the resting potential during which an impulse cannot be generated. Na^+/K^+-ATPase helps restore the normal balance of Na^+ and K^+ inside and outside the cell during the refractory period.

c. Direction of signal transmission When the action potential is set off by neurotransmitters crossing the synapse, the sequence of depolarization is usually dendrites, cell body, axon, synapse, next neuron (or end organ). This is termed **orthodromic spread,** in which the impulse travels along the axon away from the cell body. Two factors normally prevent **antidromic spread** toward the cell body: (1) the portion of the axon directly behind the newly depolarized region is usually refractory, and (2) the signal cannot be propagated in a reverse direction across a synapse. When an action potential is generated artificially, by electrical stimulation of the axon, both orthodromic and antidromic spread occur, but the antidromic spread has no effect on other neurons because the signal is unable to cross a synapse.

d. Saltatory conduction Depolarization of myelinated axons can occur only at the nodes of Ranvier, where insulation is reduced and Na^+ and K^+ channels are concentrated. The action potential must therefore jump from node to node along the axon, a phenomenon called saltatory conduction. The result is a more rapid conduction of the impulse, less dramatic changes in ion concentrations, and a lower energy requirement for recovery of the resting membrane potential than in continuous conduction by unmyelinated neurons. A myelinated axon conducts impulses more rapidly than an unmyelinated one of the same diameter.

3. Blocking signal transmission Cold, heat, and pressure on a nerve fiber can block impulse conduction. Local anesthetics allow more complete and reversible impulse blocking by disturbing the resting potential. Certain poisons block ionic channels and prevent propagation of the action potential.

VIII. RESPONSE OF NERVE TISSUE TO INJURY

A. Damage to the Cell Body: Because mature neurons cannot divide, dead neuron cell bodies cannot be replaced. Neurons not connected with other functioning neurons or end organs are useless, and mechanisms have evolved to dispose of them. Thus, if a neuron makes synaptic contact with only one other neuron and the latter is destroyed, the former undergoes autolysis, a process termed **transneuronal degeneration.** However, most neurons have multiple connections.

B. Damage to the Axon: Axon regeneration can occur if the axon is injured or severed far enough from the soma to avoid cell death. Response to such injuries involves partial degeneration followed by regeneration.

1. Degeneration A crushed or severed axon degenerates both distal and proximal to the injury.

a. Primary, ascendant, or retrograde degeneration Proximal to the site of injury, degeneration of the axon and sheath is similar to that described below but incomplete. This process proceeds for about one or 2 internodes before the injured axon is sealed off. The cell body also undergoes degenerative changes in response to injury. The perikaryon enlarges; **chromatolysis,** or dispersion of Nissl substance, occurs; and the nucleus moves to an eccentric position. Degeneration and cell-body changes take about 2 weeks.

b. Secondary, Wallerian, or descendent degeneration Distal to the site of injury, both the axon and myelin sheath undergo complete degeneration because the connection between the distal segment and the cell body is severed. During this distal degeneration, which usually takes 2–3 days, nearby Schwann cells proliferate, phagocytose the degenerated tissue, and invade the remaining endoneurial sheath, or **endoneurial channel.**

2. Regeneration Regeneration of the injured axon begins in the third week after an injury. As the perikaryon gears up for increased protein synthesis, the Nissl bodies reappear. The proximal stump of the axon gives rise to a profusion of smaller processes termed **neurites;** one of these encounters and grows into the endoneurial channel, and the others degenerate. The neurite in the channel grows 3–4 mm/d distally, guided and then myelinated by the Schwann cells. Growth is maintained by orthograde axoplasmic transport of material synthesized in the perikaryon. When the growing tip of the neurite (regenerating axon) reaches its termination, it establishes a connection with its end organ or another neuron in the chain. If the cut ends of a severed nerve are matched according to size and arrangement of fascicles and sutured together by their epineural sheaths within 3–4 weeks after injury, sensory and motor innervation can often be restored.

Study-Focusing Questions*

1. List the basic functions of nerve tissue (160).
2. Compare the CNS and the PNS in terms of:
   a. Their major structural components (organs) (160)
   b. The term used for collections of nerve cell bodies (160)
   c. The term used for collections of nerve cell fibers (160)
   d. The types of supporting cells (neuroglia) present (168, 172, 187)
   e. The cell type responsible for myelination (171, 172, 173)
3. Beginning with the formation of the neural plate, list the basic steps in the development of the nervous system (160).
4. List the cell types derived from the embryonic neural crest (160).
5. Compare multipolar, bipolar, and pseudounipolar neurons (162) in terms of their:
   a. Number of axons
   b. Number of dendrites
   c. Usual function (sensory, motor, or both)
   d. Location in the body
   e. Relative abundance
6. How do pseudounipolar neurons form their single cell process (162)?
7. Compare neuronal cell bodies, axons, and dendrites in terms of:
   a. Their content of Nissl bodies (162, 164), Golgi complexes (162, 164), and mitochondria (162, 164)
   b. The number of synaptic contacts on their plasma membranes (162, 164, 166)
8. Compare axons (164–166) and dendrites (164) in terms of:
   a. The number per neuron
   b. Their average length
   c. The presence of surface projections
   d. Their primary function
   e. Their content of Nissl bodies (rough endoplasmic reticulum and ribosomes)
   f. The arrangement of their microtubules where the cell process originates from the perikaryon
   g. Their degree of branching
   h. The variation in their diameters as a function of distance from the perikaryon
   i. Their content of synaptic vesicles
9. Make a schematic drawing of a terminal bouton and the associated synapse (166) and label the following:
   a. Synaptic vesicles
   b. Mitochondria
   c. Presynaptic membrane
   d. Synaptic cleft
   e. Postsynaptic membrane
10. Compare protoplasmic astrocytes (170) and fibrous astrocytes (170) in terms of their location and the length and diameter of their cell processes.
11. Compare astrocytes (169–170), oligodendrocytes (170–171), and microglia (171) in terms of:
   a. The shape, size, and staining intensity of their nuclei
   b. The number of their cell processes
   c. Their ability to form myelin
   d. Their relationship to the mononuclear phagocyte system
12. Describe ependymal cells (171–172) in terms of their:
   a. Embryonic origin
   b. Location
   c. Similarities to epithelial cells (especially with regard to their arrangement and the specializations of their apical and lateral surfaces)

*The page references in this section refer to *Basic Histology,* 6th ed., Junqueira L, Carneiro J, Kelley R (editors), Appleton & Lange, 1989. **HR** (for Histology Review) is occasionally used instead of a page reference to indicate that the information referred to can be found in this book.

13. Compare neurons and neuroglia in terms of:
    a. The staining properties and visibility of their cytoplasm in routine H&E preparations (162, 168)
    b. The usual size of their nuclei (162, 168)
    c. Their numbers in the CNS (168)
    d. Their capability for proliferation in adults (168)
    e. Their embryonic origin (160)
    f. Their general function (160)
14. What part of a Schwann cell comprises the myelin sheath and what is myelin's predominant biochemical constituent (173)?
15. Compare myelinated and unmyelinated axons of the peripheral nervous system in terms of:
    a. Their impulse conduction velocity (172–173, 182)
    b. Their usual diameter (172)
    c. The number of axons ensheathed by a single Schwann cell (176)
    d. The presence of nodes of Ranvier (173, 176)
    e. Their means of propagating an action potential (181–182)
16. Compare large- and small-diameter axons (172, 182) in terms of their:
    a. Relative impulse conduction velocity
    b. Relative likelihood of being myelinated
17. Compare Schwann cells and oligodendrocytes in terms of:
    a. Their location (172)
    b. The number of axons each can myelinate (171, 172)
    c. The number of cells per internode of an individual axon (173)
    d. Their ability to ensheathe unmyelinated axons (171, 176)
18. Make a schematic drawing of a cross section of a nerve (177, 178, 179) and label the following:
    a. Epineurium
    b. Perineurium
    c. Endoneurium
    d. Schwann cell nuclei
    e. Myelin sheaths
    f. Axolemma
    g. Axoplasm
    h. Axons
19. List the basic features of the autonomic nervous system that distinguish it from the rest of the nervous system (176–177).
20. Compare the sympathetic nervous system and the parasympathetic nervous system (177–178) in terms of:
    a. The location of the cell bodies of their preganglionic neurons
    b. The location of the cell bodies of their postganglionic neurons
    c. The primary neurotransmitter released by the axons of their postganglionic neurons
    d. Their primary function (sensory or motor)
21. Compare the internal and external environments of a resting-state neuron (181) in terms of their:
    a. Potassium ion concentration
    b. Sodium ion concentration
    c. Charge differential (resting membrane potential) in millivolts
22. How does the neuron maintain the resting membrane potential (181)?
23. Beginning with an excitatory synaptic stimulus, list the sequence of events leading to the generation of an action potential (181).
24. After depolarization, how does a neuron reestablish its resting membrane potential (181)? Does this process require energy in the form of ATP? How long does it take?
25. Compare type A, type B, and type C nerve fibers (182) in terms of:
    a. The presence of myelin
    b. The diameter of their fibers
    c. The length of their internodes
    d. Their conduction velocity
26. Beginning with the spread of the action potential into a terminal bouton, list the sequence of events leading to depolarization of the postsynaptic membrane (182–183).

27. What happens to the neurotransmitter acetylcholine after it binds to its receptor in the postsynaptic membrane (183)?
28. Examine your answers to questions 23 through 26 and try to appreciate the cyclic nature of events occurring as a signal is relayed along a chain of several neurons.
29. List several neurotransmitters. Which one is known to be inhibitory (183)?
30. List the structures and substances moved by:
    a. Slow anterograde axoplasmic transport (183)
    b. Fast anterograde axoplasmic transport (183)
    c. Retrograde axoplasmic transport (183)
31. What happens to the following structures after a nerve is cut (184–187)?
    a. The distal stumps of the injured axons
    b. The myelin around the axons distal to the cut
    c. The Schwann cells distal to the cut
    d. The Nissl bodies of the perikaryons
    e. The volume of the perikaryons
    f. The position of the nuclei in the perikaryons
    g. The proximal stumps of the axons
32. If there is a large gap between the proximal and distal cut surfaces of a nerve, what may happen to the:
    a. Regenerating nerve fiber sprouts (neurites) growing from the proximal stump (186)
    b. Effector organ formerly innervated by the nerve (186)
33. Compare craniospinal and autonomic ganglia (187–189) in terms of:
    a. Their location
    b. Their primary function (sensory or motor)
    c. The class of neurons present
    d. The location of ganglion cell (neuronal) perikaryons
    e. The position of the nucleus in the ganglion cell body
    f. The completeness of the layer of satellite cells associated with the perikaryons
34. How do the ganglion cells of the spiral ganglion (of the acoustic nerve) differ from those in other craniospinal ganglia (187)?
35. How do intramural ganglia differ from other autonomic ganglia (188)?
36. Compare gray matter and white matter (189–190) in terms of:
    a. Their location in the spinal cord, the cerebrum, and the cerebellum
    b. Their predominant neuronal components (cell bodies, axons, dendrites)
    c. The amount of myelin present
    d. The predominant type of astrocyte (170)
    e. The abundance of synapses
37. Compare the dura mater, arachnoid, and pia mater (190–191) in terms of:
    a. Their location
    b. Their attachment to other structures (eg, periosteum, brain, spinal cord)
    c. Their tissue type
    d. The presence of blood vessels
38. Describe the blood-brain barrier in terms of its structural correlates and its function (191).
39. Describe the cerebrospinal fluid (192) in terms of its:
    a. Function(s)
    b. Composition
    c. Production site
    d. Circulation route
    e. Reabsorption site

Multiple-Choice Questions

For questions 9–1 through 9–7, select the single best answer.

9–1. Thorny spines (gemmules) that project from dendrites:
    A. Often have a larger diameter than the dendrites themselves

B. Contain numerous synaptic vesicles
C. Represent sites of synaptic contact with boutons terminaux
D. Are found at the nodes of Ranvier
E. Are also called neurites

9–2. Collections of neuron cell bodies (somata) in the central nervous system are called:
A. Ganglia
B. Nuclei
C. Nodes of Ranvier
D. Neuroglia
E. White matter

9–3. The part of the neuron that serves as its trophic center is the:
A. Terminal arborization
B. Dendrite
C. Axon
D. Cell body (soma)
E. Axon hillock

9–4. The blood vessels that serve the brain and spinal cord are most abundant in which layer?
A. Dura mater
B. Epineurium
C. Arachnoid mater
D. Perineurium
E. Pia mater

9–5. The structure shown in Fig 9–1 is:
A. Gray matter
B. White matter
C. A spinal ganglion
D. A peripheral nerve
E. Dura mater

9–6. All the following are true of synaptic vesicles *except* that they:
A. May be found in terminal boutons

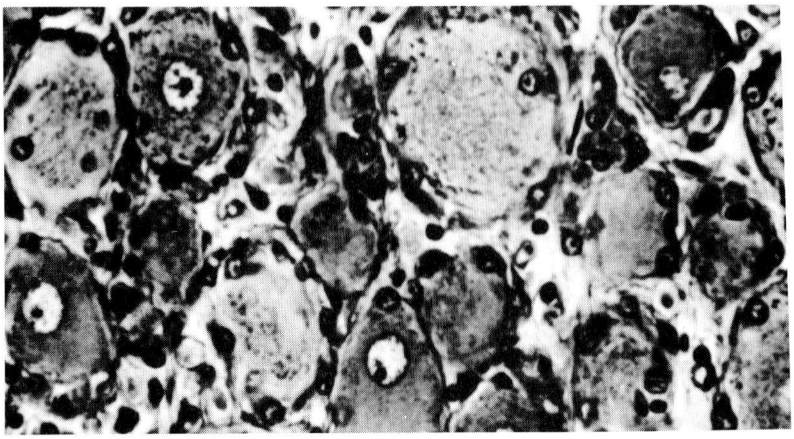

Figure 9–1.

B. May be found in the synaptic cleft
C. Contain neurotransmitters
D. Bud off from the Golgi complex
E. Are not found in dendrites near the postsynaptic membrane

9–7. The cells whose nuclei are labeled "n" in Fig 9–2 are:
A. Oligodendrocytes
B. Protoplasmic astrocytes
C. Pseudounipolar neurons
D. Multipolar neurons
E. Fibrous astrocytes

MATCHING (questions 9–8 through 9–28): Each choice may be used once, more than once, or not at all.

Questions 9–8 through 9–18:

A. Microglia
B. Oligodendrocytes
C. Protoplasmic astrocytes
D. Fibrous astrocytes
E. Schwann cells
F. Satellite cells
G. Ependymal cells
H. None of the above

9–8. Myelinate axons in the central nervous system
9–9. Myelinate axons in the peripheral nervous system
9–10. Found predominantly in white matter
9–11. Found predominantly in gray matter
9–12. May provide myelin for several axons
9–13. Provide myelin for only one axon
9–14. Surround the perikaryons of neurons in ganglia
9–15. Characterized by vascular end-feet

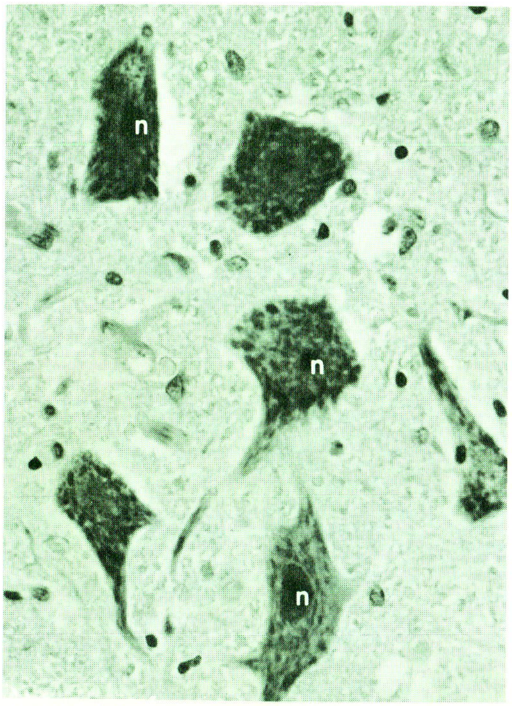

Figure 9–2.

9–16. Certain of these may be derived from monocytes
9–17. Most abundant glial cell type in the central nervous system
9–18. Derived from the neuroepithelium lining the embryonic neural tube

Questions 9–19 through 9–23:

A. Dura mater
B. Arachnoid
C. Pia mater
D. All of the above
E. None of the above

9–19. Tightly attached to periosteum of the skull and spinal column
9–20. Forms trabeculae between which the cerebrospinal fluid flows
9–21. Tightly attached to the surface of the brain and spinal cord
9–22. Covers the capillaries in the gray matter to form the blood-brain barrier
9–23. Composed primarily of dense collagenous connective tissue

Questions 9–24 through 9–28 use the letters in Fig 9–3.

9–24. Presynaptic membrane
9–25. Postsynaptic membrane
9–26. Synaptic vesicles
9–27. Synaptic cleft
9–28. Terminal bouton (end bulb)

For questions 9–29 through 9–68, either, both, or neither of the answers may be correct. Select

A if only A is correct
B if only B is correct
C if both A and B are correct
D if neither A nor B is correct

Questions 9–29 through 9–38:

A. Central nervous system
B. Peripheral nervous system
C. Both
D. Neither

9–29. Includes the brain and spinal cord
9–30. Includes the craniospinal ganglia

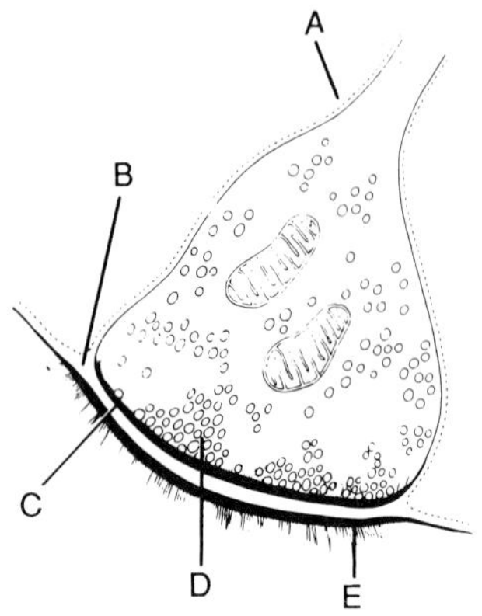

Figure 9–3.

9–31. Contains components of the autonomic nervous system
9–32. Composed of neurons and supporting cells
9–33. Includes gray matter and white matter
9–34. Covered by the meninges
9–35. Includes epineurium, perineurium, and endoneurium
9–36. Contains Schwann cells
9–37. Contains satellite cells
9–38. Contains ependymal cells

Questions 9–39 through 9–44:

A. Gray matter
B. White matter
C. Both
D. Neither

9–39. Astrocytes are mostly of the fibrous type
9–40. Contains oligodendrocytes
9–41. Outermost layer of the cerebrum (not including meninges)
9–42. Outermost layer of the spinal cord (not including meninges)
9–43. Contains neuron cell bodies
9–44. Contains mostly axons and neuroglial cells

Questions 9–45 through 9–54:

A. Axons
B. Dendrites
C. Both
D. Neither

9–45. May contain Nissl bodies
9–46. May contain Golgi complexes
9–47. Contain neurofilaments and neurotubules
9–48. Covered by thorny spines (gemmules)
9–49. Constant diameter along their entire length
9–50. One per neuron
9–51. May be myelinated
9–52. Number per neuron varies and may be used to classify neuron type
9–53. Contain synaptic vesicles
9–54. Typically exhibit boutons terminaux

Questions 9–55 through 9–61:

A. Sympathetic nervous system
B. Parasympathetic nervous system
C. Both
D. Neither

9–55. Concerned primarily with the motor control of involuntary functions
9–56. Primary postganglionic neurotransmitter is norepinephrine
9–57. Preganglionic neuron cell bodies found in the thoracic and lumbar segments of the spinal cord
9–58. Postganglionic neuron cell bodies found in ganglia
9–59. Long preganglionic axons and short postganglionic axons
9–60. Cell bodies of postganglionic neurons may be found in intramural ganglia
9–61. Preganglionic fibers of this system supply the adrenal medulla

Questions 9–62 through 9–68:

A. Myelinated axons
B. Unmyelinated axons

C. Both
D. Neither

9–62. May be covered by Schwann cells in the peripheral nervous system
9–63. May be covered by oligodendrocytes in the central nervous system
9–64. In general, have the largest diameter
9–65. Have the fastest conduction velocity, owing to saltatory conduction
9–66. Have nodes of Ranvier
9–67. Several may be associated with a single Schwann cell
9–68. Several may be associated with a single oligodendrocyte

For questions 9–69 through 9–75, one, more than one, or all of the answers may be correct. Select

A if only (1), (2), and (3) are correct
B if only (1) and (3) are correct
C if only (2) and (4) are correct
D if only (4) is correct
E if all answers are correct

9–69. Nissl bodies:
(1) Are composed of ribosomes and rough endoplasmic reticulum
(2) Undergo chromatolysis following injury to the axon
(3) Are important in protein synthesis
(4) Are found in the axon hillock

9–70. Mitochondria may be found in:
(1) The perikaryon
(2) Axons
(3) Dendrites
(4) Schwann cells

9–71. Following injury to an axon, the changes that occur in the proximal stump include:
(1) Complete degeneration of the entire myelin sheath back to the initial segment.
(2) Degeneration of the axon for a distance of a few internodes from the site of injury
(3) Chromatolysis
(4) Neurite outgrowth

9–72. Synapses:
(1) Permit transmission of a nerve impulse in only one direction
(2) In which gamma aminobutyric acid (GABA) serves as the neurotransmitter generally have an inhibitory rather than excitatory effect
(3) May occur between an axon and a neuron cell body
(4) Contain some basal lamina in the synaptic cleft

9–73. In the resting state:
(1) The K^+ concentration inside the neuron is greater than that outside the neuron
(2) The Na^+ concentration outside the neuron is greater than that inside the neuron
(3) The interior of the cell is negatively charged with respect to the exterior
(4) The Na^+/K^+-ATPase pump in the plasma membrane is inactive

9–74. Cell types derived from the neural crest include:
(1) Chromaffin cells of the adrenal medulla
(2) Schwann cells of the peripheral nerves
(3) Melanocytes of the skin
(4) Postganglionic neurons of the sympathetic ganglia

9–75. Cerebrospinal fluid:
(1) Is produced by the choroid plexus
(2) Flows through the subarachnoid space
(3) Is resorbed by the blood in the arachnoid villi
(4) Comes in direct contact with the apical surface of ependymal cells

Muscle Tissue 10

Objectives

This chapter should help the student to:

- Know the 3 major types of muscle tissue and compare them in terms of structure, function, and location in the body.
- Know the function(s) of muscle tissue and contemplate what measures would have to be taken to sustain life without it.
- Know the relationships between muscle fascicles, muscle fibers, myofibrils, and myofilaments.
- Explain the role of the T tubules and the sarcoplasmic reticulum in striated muscle function.
- Describe the mechanisms of skeletal muscle stimulation, contraction, and relaxation at the molecular, cellular, and tissue level.
- Recognize the type of muscle tissue present in a slide or photomicrograph of an organ and describe its probable function.

Synopsis

I. GENERAL FEATURES OF MUSCLE TISSUE

A. Terminology: Many special terms are applied to muscle. Most include the prefixes sarco- or myo-.

B. Specialization for Contraction: Muscle cells are structurally and functionally specialized for contraction, which requires 2 types of special protein filaments called myofilaments: thin filaments containing **actin** and thick filaments containing **myosin.**

C. Mesodermal Origin: Nearly all muscle cells arise from mesoderm. Mesenchymal cells differentiate into muscle cells through a process involving accumulation of myofilaments in the cytoplasm and development of special membranous channels and compartments. ***Exception:*** Smooth muscles of the iris arise from ectoderm.

D. Cell Shape: Muscle cells are typically longer than they are wide, sometimes reaching lengths of 4 cm. Muscle cells are therefore often called **muscle fibers,** or **myofibers**.

E. Organization: Muscle tissues are composed of groups of muscle cells organized by connective tissue elements. Their arrangement allows the groups to act together or separately, generating mechanical forces of varying strength. Named muscles of the body (eg, biceps brachii) are organs made up of highly organized muscle tissue (II.G).

F. Types of Muscle Tissue: The main muscle tissue types are **smooth muscle** and the 2 types of **striated muscle,** skeletal and cardiac. Smooth muscle (IV) is found mainly in the walls of hollow organs (eg, intestines and blood vessels); its contraction is slow, often in waves, and under involuntary control. In histologic section, it lacks the banding pattern, or striation, seen in the other type 2 types. **Skeletal muscle** (II) is found mainly in association with bones, which act as pulleys and levers to multiply the force of its quick, strong, voluntary contractions. **Cardiac muscle** (III) is found exclusively in the walls of the heart; its contractions are quick, strong, rhythmic, and involuntary. Characteristics of the different muscle types are summarized in Table 10–1.

II. SKELETAL MUSCLE

A. Histogenesis: Skeletal muscle arises from mesenchyme of mesodermal origin. The mesenchymal cells retract their long cytoplasmic processes and assume a shortened spindle shape to become **myoblasts;** these fuse to form multinucleated **myotubes.** Myotubes elongate by incorporating additional myoblasts while myofilaments accumulate in their cytoplasm. Eventually, the accumulated myofilaments organize into myofibrils (II.B.1.c) and displace the nuclei and other cytoplasmic components peripherally.

B. Skeletal Muscle Cells: Mature skeletal muscle fibers are elongated, unbranched, cylindrical, multinucleated cells. The flattened, peripheral nuclei lie just under the **sarcolemma** (muscle cell plasma membrane); most of the organelles and **sacroplasm** (muscle cell cytoplasm) are near the poles of the nuclei. The sarcoplasm contains many mitochondria, glycogen granules, and an oxygen-binding protein called **myoglobin,** and it accumulates lipofuscin pigment with age. Mature skeletal muscle fibers cannot divide.

1. Myofilaments In skeletal muscle fibers, these are of 2 major types.

a. Thin filaments Thin (actin) filaments have several components.

(1) Filamentous actin (F-actin) is a polymeric chain of **globular actin (G-actin)** monomers. Each thin filament contains a pair of F-actin strands wound around each other in a double helix.

(2) Tropomyosin is a long, thin, double helical polypeptide that wraps around the actin double helix and lies in the grooves on its surface. Each tropomyosin molecule spans 7 G-actin monomers.

Table 10–1. Distinguishing Characteristics of Muscle Types.

Features	Skeletal Muscle (Striated)	Cardiac Muscle (Striated)	Smooth Muscle (Unstriated)
Cells	Thick, long, unbranched, cylindric	Branched, cylindric	Small, spindle-shaped
Nuclei	Many, peripheral	One or 2, central	One, central
Filament ratio	Six thin/one thick	Six thin/one thick	Twelve thin/one thick
Sarcoplasmic reticulum and myofibrils	Highly organized sarcoplasmic reticulum surrounds myofibrils	Less organized sarcoplasmic reticulum; no distinct myofibrils	Poorly organized sarcoplasmic reticulum; no distinct myofibrils
T tubules	At A-I band junctions; form triads	At Z lines; form dyads	None
Motor end-plates	Present	Absent	Absent
Motor control	Voluntary	Involuntary	Involuntary
Other	Prominent fascicles	Intercalated disks at cell-to-cell junctions	Abundant caveolae
	Thick perimysium and epimysium		Cells overlap

(3) Troponin is a complex of 3 globular proteins. **TnT** (troponin T) attaches each complex to a specific site on each tropomyosin molecule, **TnC** binds calcium ions, and **TnI** inhibits the interaction between the thin and thick filaments.

b. Thick filaments A myosin molecule is a long golf club-shaped polypeptide. A thick (myosin) filament is a bundle of myosin molecules with their shafts pointing toward and overlapping in the bundle's middle and their heads projecting from the bundle's ends. This arrangement leaves a headless region in the center of each filament corresponding to the H band (II.B.1.d). Treating myosin molecules with papain (a proteolytic enzyme) cleaves them, at a point near the head, into 2 pieces. The piece containing the bulk of the thin shaft is termed **light meromysin;** the head and associated section of the shaft comprise **heavy meromyosin.** The head portion of heavy meromysin has an ATP-binding site and an actin-binding site, both necessary for contraction.

c. Organization of the myofilaments The banding pattern of skeletal muscle (II.B.1.d) reflects the grouping of its myofilaments into parallel bundles of thick and thin filaments called **myofibrils.** Each muscle fiber may contain several myofibrils, the number depending on its size.

(1) Appearance of the myofibrils in cross section Viewed with an electron microscope, cross sections of myofibrils reveal patterns of large and small dots corresponding to the thick and thin filaments, respectively. Sections containing both filament types have 6 thin filaments in hexagonal array around each thick filament. Each thick filament shares 2 of its surrounding thin filaments with each adjacent thick filament to form a repeating crystalline pattern.

(2) Appearance of the myofibrils in longitudinal section At both light and electron microscopic levels, each myofibril exhibits repeating, linearly arranged, functional subunits called **sarcomeres,** which have bands (striations) running perpendicular to the long axis of the myofibril. The sarcomeres of each myofibril lie in register with those in adjacent myofibrils so that their bands appear continuous. The sarcomere is separated from its neighbors at each end by a dense **Z line,** or **Z disk.** A major protein of the Z disk, **alpha actinin,** anchors one end of the thin filaments and helps maintain proper spatial distribution. The thin filaments extend to the middle of the sarcomere. The center of each sarcomere is marked by the **M line,** which holds the thick filaments in place. The thick filament bundles lie at the center of each sarcomere, are bisected by the M line, and overlap the free ends of the thin filaments. The pattern of overlapping between the thick and thin filaments is responsible for the banding pattern and differs depending on the myofibrils' state of contraction.

d. The bands With the light microscope, skeletal muscle exhibits alternating light- and dark-staining bands running perpendicular to the long axis of the muscle fibers.

(1) I bands The light-staining bands contain only thin filaments. They are known as **I bands** (isotropic) because they do not rotate polarized light. Each I band is bisected by a Z line. Thus each sarcomere has 2 half I bands, one at each end.

(2) A bands One dark-staining band lies in the middle of each sarcomere and shows the position of the thick filament bundles. This is known as an **A band** (anisotropic) because it is birefringent (rotates polarized light). At the EM level, each A band has a lighter-staining central region termed the **H band,** which is bisected by an M line. The H band lies between the free ends of the thin filaments and contains only the shafts of myosin molecules. The darker peripheral portions of the A bands are regions of overlap between the thick and thin filaments and contain the heads of the myosin molecules. The interaction between the myosin heads of the thick filaments and the free ends of the thin filaments causes muscle contraction.

2. Sarcoplasmic reticulum This is the smooth endoplasmic reticulum of striated muscle cells, specialized to sequester calcium ions. In skeletal muscle, it consists of an anastomosing complex of membrane-limited tubules and cisternae that ensheathe each myofibril. At each **A-I band junction,** a tubular invagination of the sarcolemma termed a **transverse tubule,** or **T tubule,** penetrates the muscle fiber and comes to lie close to the surface of the myofibrils. On each side of the T tubule lies an expansion of the sarcoplasmic reticulum termed a **terminal cisterna.** A complex of 2 terminal cisternae and an intervening T tubule constitutes a **triad.** Triads have an important role in initiating muscle contraction (II.D).

3. Types of skeletal muscle fibers Three types of skeletal muscle fibers differ in myoglobin content, number of mitochondria, and speed of contraction. In humans, most skeletal muscles are composed of a mixture of these fiber types.

a. Red fibers contain the most myoglobin and the greatest number of mitochondria and are capable of sustained contraction. Their contraction in response to nervous stimulation is slow and steady, resulting in their designation as **slow fibers.** They predominate in postural muscles and in the limbs.

b. White fibers contain the least myoglobin and the fewest mitochondria. They react quickly, with brief, forceful contractions, but cannot sustain contraction for long periods. They are thus also termed **fast fibers.** They predominate in the extraocular muscles.

c. Intermediate fibers have structural and functional characteristics intermediate between those of red and white fibers but are considered a subclass of the latter. They are found dispersed among the red and white fibers in muscles where either type predominates.

C. Motor End-Plates: A motor end-plate, or **myoneural junction,** is a collection of specialized synapses between the terminal boutons of a motor neuron and the sarcolemma of a skeletal muscle fiber. It transmits nerve impulses to muscle cells, initiating contraction. Each myoneural junction has 3 major components:

1. The **presynaptic (neural) component** consists of the terminal bouton. Although extensions of Schwann cell cytoplasm cover the bouton, the myelin sheath ends before reaching it. The bouton contains many mitochondria, as well as synaptic vesicles filled with acetylcholine. The portion of the bouton's plasma membrane directly facing the muscle fiber is termed the **presynaptic membrane.**

2. The **synaptic cleft** lies between the presynaptic membrane and the opposing postsynaptic membrane and contains a continuation of the muscle fiber's **basal lamina.** It also contains acetylcholinesterase, which breaks down the neurotransmitter so that when neural stimulation ends, contraction ends. The **primary synaptic cleft** lies directly beneath the presynaptic membrane and communicates directly with a series of **secondary synaptic clefts** created by infoldings of the postsynaptic membrane.

3. The **postsynaptic (muscular) component** includes the sarcolemma (postsynaptic membrane) and the sarcoplasm directly under the synapse. The postsynaptic membrane contains receptors for acetylcholine and is thrown into numerous **junctional folds.** The sarcoplasm beneath the folds contains nuclei, mitochondria, ribosomes, and glycogen granules.

D. The Mechanism of Contraction: According to the **sliding filament hypothesis,** skeletal muscle contraction is initiated by and includes the following chain of events:

1. The nerve impulse is carried along the motor neuron's axon and causes

2. depolarization of the presynaptic membrane (Na^+ influx), which causes

3. fusion of the synaptic vesicles with the presynaptic membrane and exocytosis of acetylcholine into the synaptic cleft.

4. Acetylcholine crosses the synaptic cleft and binds to receptors in the postsynaptic membrane, causing

5. depolarization of the sarcolemma (influx of Na^+), causing

6. depolarization of the T tubules (sarcolemmal invaginations), causing

7. depolarization of the terminal cisternae, causing

8. depolarization of the rest of the sarcoplasmic reticulum, causing

9. release of sequestered Ca^{2+} from the sarcoplasmic reticulum into the sarcoplasm surrounding the myofibrils.

10. Ca^{2+} binds to the TnCs of the troponin complexes, causing

11. a conformational change of each troponin complex, causing

12. the TnIs of the troponin complexes to move away from the myosin-head binding sites on the actin filaments, allowing the

13. myosin heads to bind to actin, causing

14. activation of the ATPase in the myosin heads, causing

15. the production of energy and ADP from ATP (II.F) and movement of the myosin heads, which

16. pull the actin filaments toward the center of the sarcomere, resulting in

17. simultaneous shortening of the sarcomeres by shortening of the I bands (A bands do not narrow), resulting in

18. shortening of the myofibrils, resulting in

19. shortening of the entire muscle fiber.

E. Relaxation: When neural stimulation ends, all the membranes repolarize, allowing the sarcoplasmic reticulum to sequester CA^{2+} from the sarcoplasm by active transport. This removes Ca^{2+} from the TnC and returns the TnI to a position in which it inhibits binding of the myosin head to the actin filament.

F. Energy Production: Muscles use glucose (from stored glycogen and from the blood) and fatty acids (from the blood) to form the ATP and phosphocreatine that provide chemical energy for contraction. When ATP is not available, actin-myosin binding becomes stabilized, accounting for **rigor mortis,** the muscular rigidity that occurs shortly after death.

G. Organization of the Skeletal Muscles: Named muscles are bundles of muscle **fascicles** surrounded by a sheath of dense connective tissue termed the **epimysium.** Each fascicle is a bundle of muscle fibers surrounded by a dense connective tissue sheath called the **perimysium,** which consists of septumlike inward extensions of epimysium. Each muscle fiber is a bundle of myofibrils surrounded by a delicate connective tissue sheath termed the **endomysium,** which consists of a basal lamina and a loose meshwork of reticular fibers. Each myofibril is a bundle of myofilaments surrounded by an investment of sarcoplasmic reticulum, with a triad at both A-I junctions of each sarcomere. The connective tissue investments are continuous with one another. They bind together subunits that function together and separate subunits that function independently.

H. Muscle-Tendon Junctions: The attachment of a muscle to a tendon must be secure to prevent the muscle from tearing away during contraction. The tendon's collagen fibers blend with the epimysium and penetrate the muscle along with the perimysium. Near the junction with the tendon, the ends of the muscle cells taper and exhibit many infoldings of their sarcolemmas. Collagen and reticular fibers enter the infoldings, penetrate the basal lamina, and attach directly to the sarcolemma's outer surface. The attachment of actin filaments to the sarcolemma's inner surface helps stabilize the association between the collagen fibers and the muscle cell.

I. Pattern of Innervation: Each motor neuron has a single axon that may terminate on a single muscle fiber or undergo terminal branching (arborization) and terminate on multiple muscle fibers. A motor neuron and all the muscle fibers it innervates (one to > 100) is termed a **motor unit.** Muscles responsible for delicate movements (eg, extraocular muscles) are composed of many small motor units; those responsible for coarser movements (eg, gluteus maximus) are composed of a few large motor units.

III. CARDIAC MUSCLE

A. Histogenesis: Cardiac muscle arises as parallel chains of elongated splanchnic mesenchymal cells in the walls of the embryonic heart tube. Cells within each chain develop specialized junctional complexes between them and often branch and bind to cells in nearby chains. As development continues, the cells accumulate myofilaments in their sarcoplasm. The branched network of myoblasts forms interwoven bundles of muscle fibers, but cardiac myoblasts do not fuse.

B. Cardiac Muscle Cells: Cardiac muscle fibers are elongated, branched cells with one or 2 elongated, central nuclei. The sarcoplasm near the nuclear poles contains many mitochondria and glycogen granules and some lipofuscin pigment. Mitochondria lie in chains between the myofilaments. The arrangement of myofilaments yields a pattern of striations identical to that of skeletal muscle.

1. Sarcoplasmic reticulum and T tubule system The sarcoplasmic reticulum in cardiac muscle fibers is less organized than that of skeletal muscle and does not subdivide myofilaments into discrete myofibrillar bundles. Cardiac T tubules are located at the Z line instead of the A-I junction. In most cells, cardiac T tubules are associated with a single expanded cisterna of the sarcoplasmic reticulum; thus, cardiac muscle contains **dyads** instead of triads.

2. Intercalated disks These unique histologic features of cardiac muscle appear as dark transverse lines between the muscle fibers and represent specialized junctional complexes. With the electron microscope, intercalated disks can be seen to have 3 major components arranged in a stepwise fashion.

a. The **fascia adherens,** similar to a zonula adherens (see Chapter 4), is a half Z line found in the vertical (transverse) portion of the step. Its alpha actinin anchors the thin filaments of the terminal sarcomeres.

b. The **macula adherens (desmosome;** see Chapter 4) is the second component of transverse portion of the junction. It prevents detachment of the cardiac muscle fibers from one another during contraction.

c. The **gap junctions** (see Chapter 4) of intercalated disks comprise the horizontal (lateral) portion of the step. They provide electrotonic coupling between adjacent cardiac muscle fibers and pass the stimulus for contraction from cell to cell.

3. Types of cardiac muscle fibers

a. Atrial cardiac muscle fibers are small and have fewer T tubules than ventricular cells. They contain many small membrane-limited granules that contain a precursor of **atrial natriuretic factor,** a hormone secreted in response to increased blood volume that opposes the action of aldosterone (see Chapters 19 and 21) and acts on the kidneys to cause sodium and water loss.

b. Ventricular cardiac muscle fibers are larger cells with more T tubules and no granules.

C. Organization of Cardiac Muscle: Because of the abundant capillaries in the endomysium of each fiber, cardiac muscle fibers appear more loosely arranged in histologic section than those of skeletal muscle. The whorled arrangement of cardiac muscle fibers in the wall of the heart accounts for the ability of the myocardium to "wring out" blood in the heart chambers (see Chapter 11).

D. Mechanism of Contraction: While the arrangement of the sarcoplasmic reticulum and T tubule complex of cardiac muscle fibers differs from that of skeletal muscle, the composition and arrangement of myofilaments are almost identical. Thus, at the cellular level, skeletal and cardiac muscle contraction are essentially the same.

E. Initiation of Cardiac Muscle Contraction: Unlike skeletal muscle fibers, which rarely contract without direct motor innervation, cardiac muscle fibers contract spontaneously with an intrinsic rhythm. The heart receives autonomic innervation that cannot initiate contraction but can speed up or slow down the intrinsic beat. The initiating stimulus for contraction is normally provided by a collection of specialized cardiac muscle cells called the sinoatrial node; it is delivered by other specialized fibers, called Purkinje fibers, to the other cardiac muscle cells. The stimulus is passed between adjacent cells through the gap junctions of the intercalated disks. The gap junctions establish an ionic continuity among cardiac muscle fibers that allows them to work together as a functional syncytium. For more details, see Chapter 11.

IV. SMOOTH MUSCLE

A. Histogenesis: Most smooth muscle cells differentiate from mesenchymal cells of mesodermal origin in the walls of developing hollow organs of cardiovascular, digestive, urinary, and reproductive systems. During differentiation, the cells elongate and accumulate myofilaments. Smooth muscles of the iris arise from ectoderm.

B. Smooth Muscle Cells: Mature smooth muscle fibers are elongated, spindle-shaped cells with a single central ovoid nucleus. The sarcoplasm at the nuclear poles contains abundant mitochondria, some rough endoplasmic reticulum, and a large Golgi complex. Each fiber produces its own basal lamina, consisting of proteoglycan-rich material and type III collagen fibers.

1. Myofilaments

a. Thin filaments The actin filaments of smooth muscle are like those of skeletal and cardiac muscle. They are always present in the cytoplasm and are anchored in **dense bodies** associated with the plasma membrane.

b. Thick filaments The myosin filaments of smooth muscle are less stable than those in striated muscle cells; they are not always present in the cytoplasm but seem to form in response to a contractile stimulus (IV.D). Unlike the thick filaments in striated muscle cells (II.B.1.b), those in smooth muscle have heads along most of their length and bare areas at the ends of the filaments.

c. Organization of the myofilaments The filaments run mostly parallel to the long axis of smooth muscle fibers, but they overlap much more than those of striated muscle, accounting for the absence of cross striations. The greater overlap of thick and thin filaments results from the unique organization of the thick filaments (see above) and permits greater contraction. The ratio of thin to thick filaments in smooth muscle is about 12:1, and the arrangement of the filaments is less regular and crystalline than in striated muscle (II.B.1.c).

2. Sarcoplasmic reticulum Smooth muscle cells contain a poorly organized sarcoplasmic reticulum that participates in the sequestration and release of Ca^{2+} but does not divide the myofilaments into myofibrillar bundles. They contain abundant surface-associated membrane-limited vesicles termed **caveolae** that appear to aid in Ca^{2+} uptake and release. The small size and slow contraction of these fibers make an elaborate stimulus-conducting system unnecessary; these fibers have no T tubules and no dyads or triads.

3. **Types of smooth muscle fibers** While all smooth muscle cells exhibit similar morphology in histologic section, they can be classified according to developmental, biochemical, and functional differences.

a. **Visceral smooth muscle** derives from splanchnopleural mesenchyme and is found in the walls of the hollow thoracic, abdominal, and pelvic organs of the respiratory, digestive, urinary, and reproductive systems. In addition to thick myosin and thin actin filaments, its cells contain networks of 10-nm intermediate filaments composed of **desmin.** Because of their poor nerve supply, the cells transmit contractile stimuli to one another through their abundant gap junctions, acting as a functional syncytium. Contraction is slow and in waves. Visceral smooth muscle is classed as **unitary smooth muscle.**

b. **Vascular smooth muscle** differentiates in situ from mesenchyme around developing blood vessels. Its cells have intermediate (10-nm) filaments that are composed of **vimentin** as well as desmin. It has the same functional features as visceral smooth muscle and is also classed as unitary smooth muscle, although its waves of contraction are not sustained and are limited to a localized area.

c. **Smooth muscle of the iris,** ie, of the sphincter and dilator pupillae muscles, differs from other smooth muscle. Its cells are derived from ectoderm and have a rich nerve supply. It is classed as **multiunit smooth muscle** because the cells can contract individually; it is capable of precise and graded contractions.

C. Organization of Smooth Muscle: Unlike striated-muscle fibers, which abut end-to-end, smooth muscle fibers overlap to varying degrees and attach to one another by fusing their endomysial sheaths. The sheaths are interrupted by many gap junctions, which transmit the ionic currents that initiate contraction. Smooth muscle fibers form fascicles that vary in size but are usually smaller than those in striated muscle. The fascicles, each surrounded by a meager perimysium, are often organized in layers separated by the thicker epimysial connective tissue. Fibers in adjacent layers often lie perpendicular to one another.

D. Mechanism of Contraction: The mechanism of smooth muscle contraction appears to be a modification of the sliding filament mechanism. At the beginning of the contraction, the myosin filaments appear, and the actin filaments are pulled toward and between them. Continued contraction involves the formation of more myosin filaments and further sliding of the actin filaments. The sliding of the actin filaments pulls the attached dense bodies closer together, shortening the cell. Unlike striated muscle fibers, individual smooth muscle fibers may undergo partial peristaltic, or wavelike, contractions. During relaxation, and myosin filaments decrease in number. They are believed to disintegrate into soluble cytoplasmic components.

E. Initiation of Smooth Muscle Contraction: Like cardiac muscle fibers, smooth muscle fibers are capable of spontaneous contraction that may be modified by autonomic innervation. Motor end-plates are not present. Neurotransmitters diffuse from terminal expansions of the nerve endings between smooth muscle cells to the sarcolemma. Both sympathetic (adrenergic) and parasympathetic (cholinergic) endings are present and exert antagonistic (reciprocal) effects. In some organs, contractile activity is enhanced by cholinergic nerves and decreased by adrenergic nerves, while in others the opposite occurs.

V. RESPONSE OF MUSCLE TO INJURY. The response of muscle to injury depends on the muscle type. The wound-closure mechanism always involves the proliferation of fibroblasts in the perimyseal and epimyseal connective tissue and the synthesis of connective tissue matrix materials.

A. Skeletal Muscle: Small, mononucleated **satellite cells** are scattered in adult skeletal muscles within the basal lamina of the mature fibers. While mature skeletal muscle fibers are incapable of mitosis, the normally quiescent satellite cells can be stimulated to divide following muscle injury, differentiate into myoblasts, and fuse to form new skeletal muscle fibers.

B. Cardiac Muscle: Cardiac muscle has little regenerative ability beyond early childhood. Lesions of the adult heart are repaired entirely by replacement with noncontractile connective tissue scars.

C. Smooth Muscle: Smooth muscle contains a population of relatively undifferentiated mononucleated smooth muscle precursors that proliferate and differentiate into new smooth muscle fibers in response to injury. The same mechanism appears to be involved in the addition of new muscle to the myometrium as the uterus enlarges during pregnancy to accommodate the growing fetus.

Study-Focusing Questions*

1. Compare skeletal, cardiac, and smooth muscle in terms of:
   - **a.** The size and shape of their muscle cells (eg, cylindric, spindle-shaped, branched, unbranched) (194)
   - **b.** The orientation of their adjacent cells (eg, abutting end-to-end, overlapping) (194, 195, 207, 211, 212)
   - **c.** The presence of striations (194)
   - **d.** The ratio of thick to thin filaments and their arrangement (197, 198, 207)
   - **e.** The presence of distinct myofibrils (196, 210, 211)
   - **f.** The composition and arrangement of intracellular membrane systems (eg, triads, dyads, caveolae) (202, 205, 208, 211)
   - **g.** The position of their T tubules in relation to the banding pattern (201–202, 207, 211)
   - **h.** The characteristic number of nuclei in each type of muscle cell (194, 207, 210)
   - **i.** The position of the nuclei in each type of muscle cell (194, 195, 207, 210)
   - **j.** Their type of motor control (voluntary or involuntary) (194)
   - **k.** The presence of motor end-plates (myoneural junctions) (203, 212)
   - **l.** The presence of intercalated disks (207)
   - **m.** The prominence of their perimysium, epimysium, and fascicles (195, 206–207, 210)
   - **n.** The abundance of their capillaries (196, 207)
2. Compare named muscles (195, 198), muscle fascicles (195, 198), muscle fibers (195, 198), and myofibrils (196, 198, 205) of skeletal muscle in terms of:
   - **a.** Their largest structural subunits
   - **b.** The named structure that ensheathes each
3. Sketch a longitudinal section of 2 resting sarcomeres attached end-to-end and label the following (198):

*The page references in this section refer to *Basic Histology,* 6th ed., Junqueira L, Carneiro J, Kelley R (editors), Appleton & Lange, 1989. **HR** (for Histology Review) is occasionally used instead of a page reference to indicate that the information referred to can be found in this book.

  a. Thin filaments
  b. Thick filaments
  c. A band
  d. I band
  e. Z line
  f. H band
  g. M line
4. Which of the bands or lines in question 3 contain the following?
  a. Thin filaments only (197, 198)
  b. Thick filaments only (197, 198)
  c. Both thick and thin filaments (197, 198)
  d. α-Actinin (199)
  e. No actin (197, 198)
  f. No myosin (197, 198)
5. Sketch the arrangement of myofilaments (198) in a cross section of a sarcomere cut through:
  a. The H band lateral to the M line
  b. The A band lateral to the H band
  c. The I band
6. Sketch a longitudinal section through 2 adjacent sarcomeres during contraction (200, 201, 202). Which bands or lines shrink (as compared to your drawing for question 3)?
7. How are the thin filaments attached to the Z lines in skeletal muscle (199) and to dense bodies in smooth muscle (213)?
8. Compare thick filaments and thin filaments in terms of:
  a. Their proteins (197–200)
  b. The names and arrangement of their subunits or components (197–200)
9. Compare troponin and tropomyosin (199, 200–201) in terms of their:
  a. Structure
  b. Association with thin filaments
  c. Function during contraction
10. Sketch a myoneural junction (motor end-plate) and label the following (202):
  a. Terminal bouton
  b. Synaptic (acetylcholine) vesicles
  c. Presynaptic membrane
  d. Postsynaptic membrane
  e. Junctional folds
  f. Primary synaptic cleft
  g. Secondary synaptic clefts
  h. Basal lamina
11. How does the localized membrane depolarization caused by the binding of acetylcholine to the postsynaptic membrane of the myoneural junction spread throughout the muscle fiber (201–202)?
12. Beginning with an impulse traveling down the axon of a motor neuron, list the events of skeletal muscle fiber stimulation, contraction, and relaxation (200–204).
13. Compare red and white skeletal muscle fibers (204–206) in terms of:
  a. Their myoglobin content
  b. Their cytochrome content
  c. The rate of their contractions
  d. Their main source of energy
  e. Their capacity for sustained activity
  f. The body sites where they may be found
14. List the components of an intercalated disk and describe the structure and function of each (207, 209).
15. Compare atrial and ventricular cardiac muscle cells (208–210) in terms of:
  a. The number of their T tubules
  b. Their cell size
  c. The number of their small cytoplasmic granules
16. Compare vascular and nonvascular smooth muscle in terms of the type(s) of intermediate filaments they contain (212).

Multiple-Choice Questions

For questions 10–1 through 10–6, select the single best answer.

10–1. Intercalated disks:
- **A.** Are found only in smooth muscle
- **B.** Are autonomic myoneural junctions
- **C.** Consist of desmosomes, fascia adherens, and gap junctions
- **D.** Are located at the M line
- **E.** Are the middle components of the triads

10–2. The troponin complex includes a globular protein that inhibits the binding of myosin to actin. What is the name of this protein?
- **A.** TnC
- **B.** TnA
- **C.** TnM
- **D.** TnT
- **E.** TnI

10–3. The filamentous protein that winds around F-actin and lies in grooves in its surface is called:
- **A.** Tropomyosin
- **B.** Desmin
- **C.** Troponin
- **D.** Myoglobin
- **E.** Myosin

10–4. Motor units:
- **A.** Are found only in cardiac muscle
- **B.** Are largest in muscles responsible for delicate movements
- **C.** Consist of a muscle fiber and all the nerves that supply it
- **D.** Consist of a motor neuron and all the muscle fibers it supplies
- **E.** Are the same as myoneural junctions

10–5. The order of membrane depolarization in skeletal muscle fibers after acetylcholine crosses the synaptic cleft is:
- **A.** T tubule, terminal cisternae, sarcoplasmic reticulum, sarcolemma
- **B.** Sarcoplasmic reticulum, T tubule, presynaptic membrane, sarcolemma
- **C.** Terminal cisternae, sarcolemma, sarcoplasmic reticulum, caveolae
- **D.** Sarcolemma, T tubule, terminal cisternae, sarcoplasmic reticulum
- **E.** Sarcolemma, sarcoplasmic reticulum, T tubule, terminal cisternae

10–6. The diagram in Fig 10–1 represents a cross section through which portion of a sarcomere?
- **A.** A band
- **B.** I band
- **C.** H band
- **D.** M line
- **E.** Z line

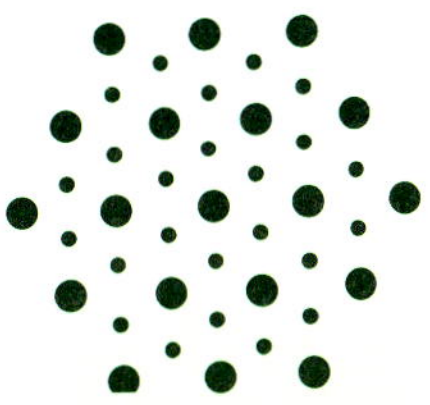

Figure 10–1.

MATCHING (questions 10–7 through 10–40): Each choice may be used once, more than once, or not at all.

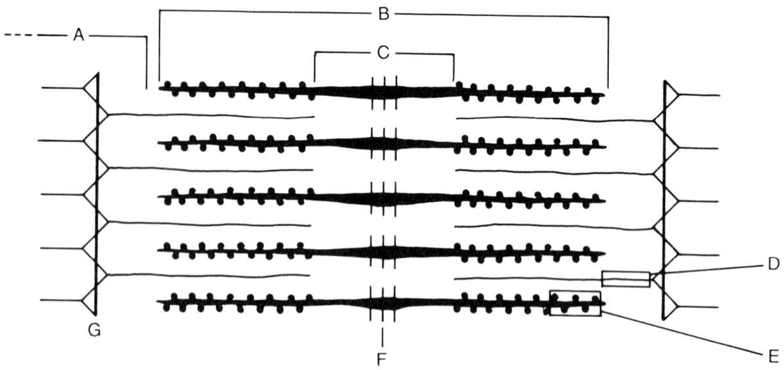

Figure 10-2.

10–7. A band
10–8. H band
10–9. M line
10–10. I band
10–11. Z line
10–12. Actin-containing filament
10–13. Myosin-containing filament
10–14. Shrinks during contraction

Questions 10–15 through 10–20:

A. Epimysium
B. Perimysium
C. Endomysium
D. Sarcoplasmic reticulum
E. None of the above

10–15. Surrounds individual myofilaments
10–16. Surrounds whole named muscles
10–17. Surrounds individual myofibrils
10–18. Surrounds individual fascicles
10–19. Surrounds individual muscle fibers
10–20. Includes the basal lamina

Questions 10–21 through 10–40:

A. Skeletal muscle
B. Cardiac muscle
C. Smooth muscle
D. A and B only
E. B and C only
F. A, B, and C

10–21. Contain(s) sarcoplasmic reticulum
10–22. Contain(s) abundant caveolae
10–23. Contain(s) intercalated disks
10–24. Contain(s) thin (actin) filaments
10–25. Contain(s) tropomyosin
10–26. Exhibit(s) motor end-plates
10–27. Contain(s) sarcomeres
10–28. Centrally located nuclei
10–29. Contain(s) thick (myosin) filaments

10-30. Cells are often branched
10-31. Contain(s) dyads
10-32. Cells are striated
10-33. Cells are multinucleated
10-34. Endomysium surrounds cells
10-35. Cells lack T tubules
10-36. T tubules lie across Z lines
10-37. Thin filaments attach to dense bodies
10-38. Each thick filament is surrounded by 6 thin filaments
10-39. Thick to thin filament ratio is about 1:12
10-40. Has distinct myofibrils

For questions 10-41 through 10-62, either, both, or neither of the answers may be correct. Select

A if only A is correct
B if only B is correct
C if both A and B are correct
D if neither A nor B is correct

Questions 10-41 through 10-55:

A. Thick filaments
B. Thin filaments
C. Both
D. Neither

10-41. Contain myosin
10-42. Contain actin
10-43. Contain tropomyosin
10-44. Contain troponin
10-45. Contain heavy meromyosin
10-46. Contain light meromyosin
10-47. Contain ATPase
10-48. Contain desmin
10-49. Contain vimentin
10-50. Globular heads project from filament
10-51. Found in the I band
10-52. Found in the A band
10-53. Found in the H band
10-54. Anchored in Z lines
10-55. Anchored in M lines

Questions 10-56 through 10-62:

A. Red fibers
B. White fibers
C. Both
D. Neither

10-56. Type of smooth muscle fibers
10-57. Type of skeletal muscle fibers
10-58. Predominate in postural muscles
10-59. Predominate in extrinsic ocular muscles
10-60. React quickly with brief, forceful contractions (fast fibers)
10-61. React slowly and are capable of sustained contraction (slow fibers)
10-62. Contain more glycogen and myoglobin

For questions 10–63 through 10–67, one, more than one, or all of the answers may be correct. Select

A if only (1), (2), and (3) are correct
B if only (1) and (3) are correct
C if only (2) and (4) are correct
D if only (4) is correct
E if all answers are correct

10–63. The sarcoplasmic reticulum of skeletal muscle:
- **(1)** Is a specialized form of smooth endoplasmic reticulum
- **(2)** Expands into terminal cisternae near the A-I band junction
- **(3)** Can actively transport calcium ions across its membranes
- **(4)** Is an invagination of the sarcolemma

10–64. Myosin molecules:
- **(1)** Can be divided into light and heavy meromyosin by the proteolytic enzyme papain
- **(2)** Have a head portion that exhibits ATPase activity
- **(3)** Have a head portion that includes an actin-binding site
- **(4)** Shorten during contraction

10–65. The synaptic cleft of a myoneural junction:
- **(1)** Contains a narrow continuation of the basal lamina
- **(2)** Contains acetylcholinesterase
- **(3)** Is divisible into a single primary and numerous secondary clefts
- **(4)** Contains myelin

10–66. T tubules:
- **(1)** Are invaginations of the sarcolemma
- **(2)** Sequester calcium during relaxation
- **(3)** Carry the depolarization into the interior of the muscle fiber
- **(4)** Are found overlying the A-I junction in cardiac muscle cells

10–67. Smooth muscle fibers of the iris:
- **(1)** Are of ectodermal origin
- **(2)** Are unitary smooth muscles
- **(3)** Receive a rich nerve supply
- **(4)** Are incapable of precise and graded contractions

INTEGRATIVE MULTIPLE-CHOICE QUESTIONS: BASIC TISSUE TYPES

For questions BT–1 thorugh BT–6, select the single best answer.

BT–1. The tissue shown in the photomicrograph in Fig BT–1 is:
- **A.** Nerve tissue
- **B.** Bone
- **C.** Mesenchyme
- **D.** Mucous connective tissue
- **E.** Stratified squamous epithelium

BT–2. The tissue shown in the photomicrograph in Fig BT–2 is:
- **A.** Smooth muscle
- **B.** Skeletal muscle
- **C.** Cardiac muscle
- **D.** Dense regular connective tissue
- **E.** Nerve tissue

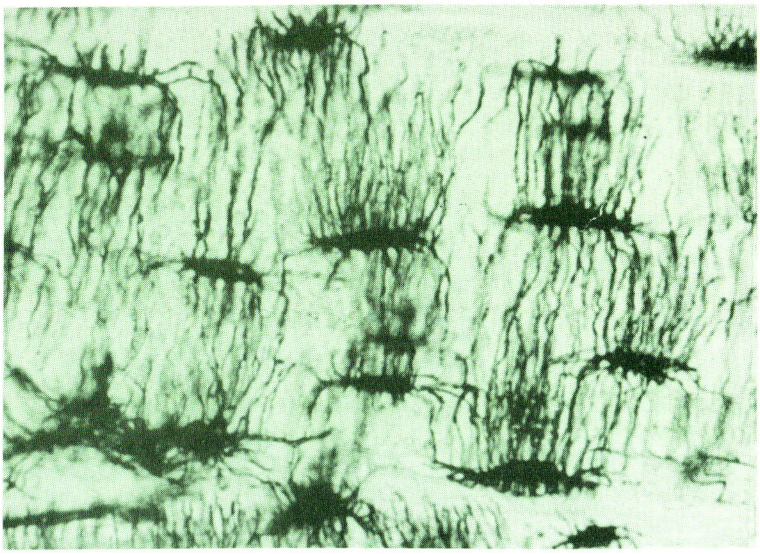

Figure BT–1.

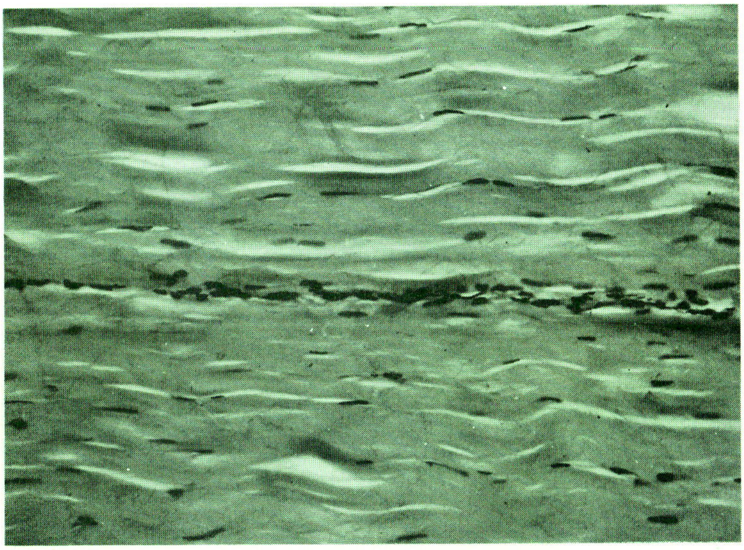

Figure BT–2.

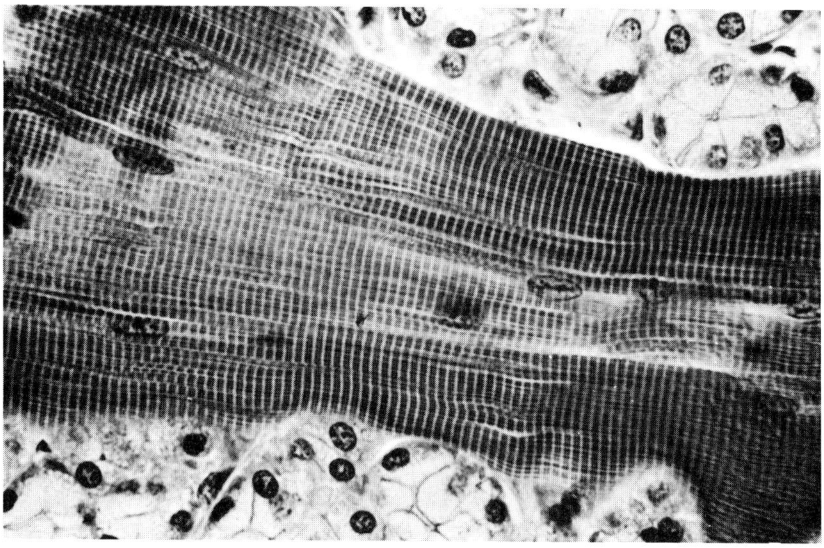

Figure BT-3.

BT-3. The 2 predominant tissue types in the photomicrograph in Fig BT-3 are:
- **A.** Cardiac muscle and nerve tissue
- **B.** Smooth muscle and dense regular connective tissue
- **C.** Skeletal muscle and glandular epithelium
- **D.** Cardiac muscle and smooth muscle
- **E.** Dense regular connective tissue and transitional epithelium

BT-4. The type of epithelium shown in the photomicrograph in Fig BT-4 is:
- **A.** Stratified squamous
- **B.** Pseudostratified columnar
- **C.** Stratified cuboidal
- **D.** Simple cuboidal
- **E.** Transitional

BT-5. The 2 predominant tissue types in the photomicrograph in Fig BT-5 are:
- **A.** Stratified squamous epithelium and dense irregular connective tissue
- **B.** Smooth muscle and dense irregular connective tissue
- **C.** Cardiac muscle and dense irregular connective tissue
- **D.** Dense regular connective tissue and nerve tissue
- **E.** Transitional epithelium and dense irregular connective tissue

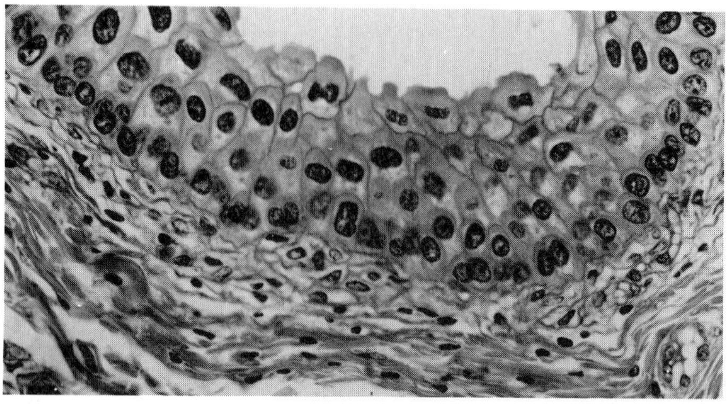

Figure BT-4.

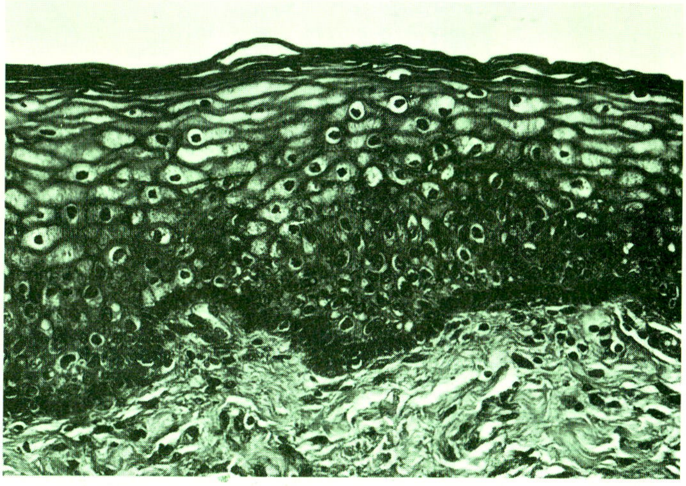

Figure BT-5.

BT-6. The cell type least likely to contain more than one nucleus is:
- **A.** Skeletal muscle fiber
- **B.** Osteoclast
- **C.** Domelike surface cells of transitional epithelium
- **D.** Cardiac muscle fiber
- **E.** Smooth muscle fiber

MATCHING (questions BT-7 through BT-24): Each choice may be used once, more than once, or not at all.

Questions BT-7 through BT-19:

- **A.** Epithelial tissues
- **B.** Connective tissues
- **C.** Nerve tissues
- **D.** Muscle tissues
- **E.** All of the above

BT-7. Derived from all 3 embryonic germ layers (ectoderm, mesoderm, and endoderm)
BT-8. Contain the widest variety of cell types
BT-9. Derived primarily from ectoderm
BT-10. Secretion is not a major function of its cells
BT-11. Some types derived from endoderm
BT-12. Basal cells are polarized and their basal surface rests on a basal lamina
BT-13. Contain cells capable of ameboid movement
BT-14. Cover body surfaces and line hollow organs
BT-15. Extracellular matrix predominates
BT-16. Cells have specializations on their apical surfaces including cilia, stereocilia, and microvilli
BT-17. Contain the longest cells in the body
BT-18. Cells contain desmin
BT-19. Cell renewal and replacement occurs continuously through mitosis

For questions BT–20 through BT–24, either, both, or neither of the answers may be correct. Select

A if only A is correct
B if only B is correct
C if both A and B are correct
D if neither A nor B is correct

Questions BT–20 through BT–24:

A. Nerve tissue
B. Muscle tissue
C. Both
D. Neither

BT–20. Fully differentiated cells incapable of mitosis
BT–21. Cells may accumulate a large amount of lipofuscin pigment with increasing age
BT–22. May be divided into fascicles by connective tissue
BT–23. Includes component(s) of motor units
BT–24. Cells may have receptors for acetylcholine in their plasma membranes

For questions BT–25 and BT–26, one, more than one, or all of the answers may be correct. Select

A if only (1), (2), and (3) are correct
B if only (1) and (3) are correct
C if only (2) and (4) are correct
D if only (4) is correct
E if all the answers are correct

BT–25. Tissues characterized by an abundant supply of capillaries include:
(1) Adipose tissue
(2) Stratified squamous epithelium
(3) Cardiac muscle
(4) Hyaline cartilage

BT–26. Cells whose functional activity may be altered according to the amount and type of innervation they receive include:
(1) Neurons
(2) Multilocular adipocytes
(3) Skeletal muscle fibers
(4) Certain glandular epithelial cells

Part III: Organs & Organ Systems

Circulatory System 11

Objectives

This chapter should help the student to:

- Name the types and subtypes of components of the circulatory system and know the major function of each.
- Name the 3 layers of tissue (tunics) that make up the walls of all circulatory system components, and know the type of tissue found in each tunic.
- Compare and contrast the components of the circulatory system in terms of size and wall structure.
- Relate the structure of the walls of each component of the circulatory system to its major functions.
- Describe the impulse generating and conducting system of the heart in terms of the structure, function, and location of its components and how the impulse is conveyed through them to the cardiac muscle fibers.
- Recognize the types of vessels present in a slide or photomicrograph of a cross section, longitudinal section, or oblique section of an organ, and be able to identify the tunics, valves, cell and tissue types, and other named structural components.
- Distinguish between cardiac muscle fibers and Purkinje fibers and identify the endocradium, myocardium, and epicardium in a slide or photomicrograph of the heart.
- Predict the functional consequences of a structural defect in one of the tunics of any component of the circulatory system.

Synopsis

I. GENERAL FEATURES OF THE CIRCULATORY SYSTEM

A. General Function: The circulatory system is responsible for the transport and homeostatic distribution of oxygen, nutrients, wastes, body fluids and solutes, body heat, and immune system components.

B. The 2 Subsystems:

1. The cardiovascular system This system is comparable to a closed system of plumbing, through which the **blood** circulates with the aid of an inline pump. It includes 4 types of components:

a. The **heart,** which serves as the muscular pump;

b. Arteries, which carry blood away from the heart toward the tissues;

c. Veins, which carry blood from the tissues toward the heart;

d. Capillaries, which intervene between the arteries and the veins, allowing exchange of nutrients, oxygen, and waste products between the blood and other tissues.

2. The lymphatic vascular system This system comprises an additional set of vessels, in which **lymph** moves in only one direction (toward the junction of the lymph vessels with the jugular and subclavian veins). This system lacks a separate pump. It includes 3 types of vessels:

a. Lymphatic capillaries, which are blind-ending, endothelial tubes that collect lymph (excess tissue fluid, cellular debris, and extravasated lymphocytes) from the intercellular spaces.

b. Lymphatic vessels, which collect lymph from lymphatic capillaries.

c. Lymphatic ducts, which collect lymph from the lyphatic vessels and empty it into the large veins in the neck.

C. Walls of the Blood and Lymphatic Vessels: Components of the circulatory system are described in terms of their wall structure. The walls are constructed on a general plan of 3 concentric layers, or **tunics,** that differ slightly in thickness and composition from one component to the next. The borders between the tunics of lymphatic vessels are less distinct than in blood vessels. Local weakening of vessel walls due to embryonic defects, disease, or lesions may lead to the development of a thin-walled outpocketing, or **aneurysm,** that may rupture and cause a hemorrhage.

1. The **tunica intima,** the innermost layer, borders directly on the lumen. The intima of the arteries and veins and that of the heart (the endocardium) are essentially identical. It consists of the **endothelium** (a simple squamous epithelium that borders the lumen and is underlain by a thin basal lamina) and the **subendothelial layer** of connective tissue. Capillaries are often composed solely of the endothelium. In arteries, the intima is separated from the tunica media by a fenestrated layer of elastin called the **internal elastic lamina.**

2. The **tunica media** is the middle layer. In blood vessels, it consists mainly of circumferentially arranged **vascular smooth muscle** fibers. Arteries generally have a thicker media, containing more muscle and elastic fibers, than that of veins or lymphatic vessels. Large arteries often exhibit an **external elastic lamina** between the media and the tunica adventitia. The media of the heart (the myocardium) is several times thicker than that of the largest artery (the aorta) and is composed of cardiac muscle.

3. The **tunica adventitia,** the outermost layer, consists chiefly of type I collagen and elastic fibers that anchor the vessel in the surrounding tissues. In veins, the adventitia is the thickest layer; in large veins it may contain longitudinal bundles of smooth muscle. In large vessels of each type, the adventitia contains small blood vessels **(vasa vasorum)** that supply oxygen and nutrients to cells in the vessel wall too far from the lumen to be nourished by simple diffusion. The outer layer of the heart (epicardium) is not an adventitia, but rather a **serosa,** composed of connective tissue covered on its outer surface by a **mesothelium.** The smooth surface helps reduce friction between the beating heart and surrounding structures.

D. Arteries: Arteries generally have a thicker tunica media than veins. The media is best exemplified in medium-sized (muscular) arteries. Large arteries (elastic arteries) contain more elastin in their media and adventitia than any other vessels. Arteries are also distinguished by refractile eosinophilic internal and external elastic laminae. In most tissues and organs, arteries are accompanied by veins. In cross sections through paired vessels, the arteries appear rounder than the veins, with thicker walls, and smaller lumens. For more detail, see II.A.

E. Veins: In cross sections, veins often present a collapsed appearance. They have thinner walls than arteries and are more likely to contain erythrocytes in their lumen. They are characterized by a thicker adventitia, which in larger veins may contain longitudinal smooth muscle. Veins contain valves that help maintain unidirectional blood flow. For more detail, see II.C.

F. Lymphatic Vessels and Ducts: These have walls that resemble those of veins. The beaded appearance of lymphatic ducts and vessels reflects the presence of numerous valves that control the direction of lymph flow. The adventitia is thin and lacks smooth muscle. The media contains both longitudinal and circular smooth muscle, but longitudinal fibers predominate.

G. Blood Capillaries: These are the smallest vascular channels in the body, with an average diameter of 7–9 μm. Their walls consist of a single layer of simple squamous epithelial (endothelial) cells rolled into a tube covered on the outer surface by a thin basal lamina. The cells attach to one another at their borders by junctional complexes, including tight (occluding) junctions and gap junctions. Some blood capillaries have fenestrations (pores) in their endothelial linings. For more detail, see II.B.

H. Lymphatic Capillaries: These differ from blood capillaries in that they have a larger diameter (up to 100 μm) and a thinner basal lamina. They lack fenestrations and have fewer tight junctions (zonulae occludentes) than blood capillaries.

I. The Heart: The heart has 4 **chambers:** 2 atria, which collect returning blood, and 2 ventricles, which eject blood from the heart. The **walls of the heart** have 3 layers. The internal layer (endocardium) has same basic structure as the intima of the vessels. The middle layer (myocardium) contains the specialized cardiac muscle fibers and is greatly thickened in relation to the corresponding media of the vessels. The walls of the ventricles are much thicker than those of the atria, owing to the presence of a thicker myocardium, and contract more forcefully. The external layer (epicardium) is not an adventitia but a serous covering. The **fibrous skeleton** of the heart to which the muscles of the myocardium attach, is composed of dense connective tissue. Together with the orientation of the muscle fibers, the fibrous skeleton directs the force of myocardial contraction so that the heart "wrings out" the blood in its chambers. Cardiac valves (flaps suspended from the fibrous skeleton) control the direction of blood flow. The heart is described in detail in section III. The **impulse generating and conducting system** of the heart is composed of specialized cardiac muscle cells. The system includes 2 nodes, the **sinoatrial (SA) node** (or pacemaker), and the **atrioventricular (AV) node.** It also includes the **atrioventricular bundle of His,** the **right and left bundle branches,** and the **Purkinje fibers.** Cardiac muscle fibers pass impulses from cell to cell by electrotonic coupling through the gap junctions of their intercalated disks.

II. BLOOD VESSELS

A. Arteries:

1. Types of arteries Arteries are classified according to size.

a. Elastic arteries Elastic arteries, or **large arteries,** are the largest diameter arteries in the body and are often considered organs. The best example is the aorta. Elastic arteries are also termed **conducting arteries,** since they conduct blood away from the heart. They are important in maintaining a constant pressure in the arterial system. When the left ventricle of the heart contracts (**systole**), blood is expelled into the aorta under high hydrostatic pressure, causing the elastic arteries to stretch. During relaxation of the ventricle (**diastole**), the ventricular pressure drops and the elastic walls of the large arteries recoil (contract), converting the force that caused them to expand back into hydrostatic pressure.

(1) Intima The tunica intima of elastic arteries is thicker than that of muscular arteries. The endothelium rests on a thin basal lamina, which is often so hard to distinguish that the endothelial cells seem to rest directly on a thickened layer of subendothelial connective tissue. A porous internal elastic lamina may be present between the intima and the media, but is difficult to distinguish because of the abundance of elastin in the media.

(2) Media The tunica media of elastic arteries contains abundant elastin, which appears as concentrically arranged, fenestrated membranes that increase in number with increasing age. Several layers of circumferentially arranged smooth muscle fibers are found between the elastic membranes. The muscle cells are interwoven with reticular fibers (type III collagen) and immersed in chondroitin sulfate-containing ground substance.

(3) Adventitia The tunica adventitia of elastic arteries is thin relative to the diameter of the vessel. It contains elastic and type I collagen fibers and an external elastic lamina that may be difficult to distinguish.

b. Muscular arteries Muscular arteries, or **medium-sized arteries,** also called **distributing arteries,** vary in diameter. They are common in many tissues and organs as major distributing branches of elastic arteries. Examples include the named arteries of the limbs (eg, brachial) and of the abdominal cavity (eg, the superior mesenteric).

(1) Intima The tunica intima of muscular arteries contains typical endothelium and subendothelial connective tissue. The prominent internal elastic lamina appears as a wavy, refractile line between the intima and the media.

(2) Media The tunica media of muscular arteries is relatively thick, containing up to 40 layers of smooth muscle fibers interspersed with variable amounts of collagen and elastic fibers as well as proteoglycans. The larger the artery, the greater the amount of elastin in the media.

(3) Adventitia The tunica adventitia of muscular arteries is relatively thin, and contains mostly collagen fibers.

c. Arterioles These are small arterial vessels, 0.5 mm or less in diameter.

(1) Intima The tunica intima of arterioles includes a typical endothelium. The endothelial cells of all vessels larger than capillaries contain rod-shaped **Weibel-Palade granules** that store components of von Willebrand's factor (factor VIII). The intima of arterioles often lacks the subendothelial connective tissue and the internal elastic lamina.

(2) Media The tunica media of arterioles has 1–5 layers of smooth muscle oriented circumferentially around the vascular lumen.

(3) Adventitia The tunica adventitia of arterioles is very thin and composed of collagen fibers.

d. Metarterioles These are small branches of arterioles. Their endothelium is surrounded by an incomplete single layer of smooth muscle cells. Constriction of these vessels helps regulate the amount of blood that reaches the capillaries, but it cannot completely halt the flow of blood to them.

2. Precapillary sphincters These are rings of smooth muscle fibers surrounding the metarterioles where capillaries originate. They can halt blood flow in the capillaries completely.

B. Capillaries:

1. Capillary beds The basic plan of the arterial tree is that a small number of large diameter arteries branch to feed a successively larger number of smaller diameter vessels. Capillaries are the smallest diameter vessels in this chain, and so the most numerous. They commonly occur as components of a profusion of anastomosing (interconnecting) channels referred to as a **capillary bed.**

2. Cells of capillaries

a. Endothelial cells, the chief structural component of capillaries, are simple squamous epithelial cells of mesenchymal origin joined by intercellular junctions (including zonula occludens) to form an epithelial tube. The nucleus causes the central part of each cell to bulge into the capillary lumen, but the cell thins toward its periphery to as little as 0.2 μm thick. There are abundant pinocytotic vesicles throughout the cytoplasm and small amounts of major organelles and filaments near the nucleus. Key functions carried out by endothelial cells include:

(1) Conversion of angiotensin I to angiotensin II. **Angiotensin** helps to regulate blood pressure by causing arterial smooth muscle contraction (see Chapter 19).

(2) Inactivation of a variety of bioactive compounds, including bradykinin, serotonin, prostaglandins, norepinephrine, and thrombin, which helps regulate their effects.

(3) Breakdown of lipoproteins (lypolysis) to yield triglycerides and cholesterol (substrates for energy metabolism, hormone synthesis and cell membrane assembly).

(4) Prevention of **thrombus** (clot) formation. Endothelial cells release prostacyclin, a powerful inhibitor of platelet aggregation. Damage to these cells may induce local clotting by decreasing prostacyclin release and uncovering the basal lamina, whose collagen stimulates thrombogenesis.

(5) Participation in capillary transport (see II.B.3).

b. Pericytes, or **advential cells,** are small mesenchymal cells found scattered along capillaries. Their long cytoplasmic processes allow them to cling to the outside of capillaries. Each pericyte is surrounded by its own basal lamina. They may or may not be contractile. Their mesenchymal nature allows pericytes to differentiate into a variety of cell types.

(3) Types of capillaries Capillaries are classified by wall structure.

a. Continuous capillaries have a smooth endothelial lining in which the endothelial cells are tightly attached to one another by junctional complexes and not interrupted by pores. Structures containing continuous capillaries include muscles, the brain, and peripheral nerves.

b. Fenestrated capillaries have endothelial cells perforated by pores (**fenestrae**). There are 2 types, one in which the pores are unobstructed, and another in which they are covered by thin **diaphragms** that limit the size of macromolecules that can pass through. Fenestrated capillaries are found in tissues where a rapid exchange of materials between tissues and the blood is required for tissue function. Organs containing fenestrated capillaries include the kidney, intestines, and certain endocrine glands.

c. Sinusoidal capillaries have 6 distinctive characteristics:

(1) They have unusually wide lumens (30–40 μm in diameter).

(2) They follow a tortuous path through the tissues they supply.

(3) They have distinct gaps between their endothelial cells, often large enough to allow entire cells to pass into and out of the sinusoidal lumen.

(4) They have an unusual abundance of fenestrations in their endothelial lining.

(5) They often have reticuloendothelial cells with well-developed phagocytic capabilities interspersed between their endothelial cells.

(6) They are surrounded by a discontinuous basal lamina.

4. Transport across capillary walls Capillaries are termed **exchange vessels,** because capillary beds serve as major sites for the exchange of oxygen, nutrients, and many other substances between the blood and other tissues. Most mechanisms of transcapillary transport are not well understood, but morphologic bases exist for at least 4 types:

a. Fenestrae penetrate completely through the endothelial cells lining capillaries. Some have diaphragms, the composition of which is poorly understood.

b. Intercellular clefts are spaces between neighboring endothelial cells through which particles and even some cells may pass. These are especially numerous in sinusoidal capillaries.

c. Pinocytosis is the process whereby small amounts of plasma or tissue fluid are endocytosed by the endothelial cells. This mechanism is followed by transport of membrane-bound **pinocytotic vesicles** across the endothelial cytoplasm in either direction.

d. Diapedesis is the process whereby some leukocytes pass from the blood into the tissues. The process may involve opening of the junctions between endothelial cells by means of locally released substances, eg, histamine, which is involved in inflammation and increases vascular permeability.

C. Veins:

1. Types of veins Veins are classified by size.

a. Large veins Examples of large veins are the superior and inferior vena cava.

(1) Intima The tunica intima of large veins is well developed and includes a thick layer of subendothelial connective tissue. Extensions of the intima protrude into the lumens of large veins in the form of valves (II.C.2).

(2) Media The tunica media of large veins contains several layers of smooth muscle fibers and abundant reticular and collagen fibers but sparse elastin.

(3) Adventitia The tunica adventitia of large veins is their best-developed layer. It commonly contains abundant collagen and longitudinal bundles of smooth muscle; the latter help strengthen the vessel wall to prevent excessive distention.

b. Small and medium-sized veins These are similar to large veins, but they have smaller diameters, thinner walls, fewer valves, and little if any muscle in the adventitia.

c. Venules These exhibit a still smaller version of general vein morphology, but they have no valves. **Postcapillary venules** are the vessels into which blood passes upon leaving the capillary beds.

2. Valves Valves, extensions of the intima into the lumen of a vein, are composed of a fibroelastic connective tissue core covered on both sides by a layer of endothelium. Since blood pressure is greatly diminished in veins, valves are needed to assure blood flow back to the heart and to help prevent blood from pooling. Pooling can lead to clot formation and obstruct blood flow.

D. Portal Vessels: Portal vessels convey blood directly from one capillary bed to another, or to a sinusoidal bed, without first returning to the heart. ***Examples:*** the hepatic portal vein between the intestines and the liver, the **hypophyseal portal veins** in the pituitary gland, and the **efferent arterioles** of the renal cortex.

E. Carotid and Aortic Bodies: These unencapsulated chemoreceptors consist of clumps and cords of epithelioid cells in close association with abundant fenestrated and sinusoidal capillaries. They receive a rich supply of unmyelinated nerve endings. **Carotid bodies** lie at the bifurcation of the common carotid artery. The **left aortic body** lies in the aorta's wall, medial to the origin of the subclavian artery. The **right aortic body** lies in the angle between the common carotid and subclavian arteries. Changes in oxygen and CO_2 levels in the blood or in blood pH generate nerve impulses that are carried to the brain by the glossopharyngeal nerve. In the brain, they elicit the physiologic response appropriate to maintaining homeostasis.

F. Carotid Sinus: This unencapsulated mechanoreceptor is found at the bifurcation of the common carotid artery, near the origin of the internal carotid. It consists of a dilation of the arterial lumen (sinus) and a thinned surrounding muscle layer, whose outer portion contains many large nerve endings. The sinus acts as a **baroreceptor,** responding to increased blood pressure by generating impulses that are carried by the glossopharyngeal nerve to the brain. Here the nerve impulses cause peripheral vasodilation and reflexive slowing of the heart.

G. Arteriovenous Anastomoses: These are direct connections between arteries and veins. The passage of blood is regulated by the contraction of smooth muscle in the walls of intervening vessels. When anastomoses are open, more blood passes directly from the arterial circulation to the venous circulation, bypassing the capillary bed. More complex anastomoses between arterioles and venules, termed **glomera,** occur mainly in the fingerpads, nail beds, and ears. The arterioles of glomera lack an internal elastic lamina and have more smooth muscle in their media. This muscle, upon contraction, can cause complete or partial closure of the vessels. Arteriovenous anastomoses allow efficient management of blood distribution during stress, heavy exertion, and temperature changes. They are also important in regulating blood pressure and other physiologic processes such as erection and menstruation.

H. Vasa Vasorum: The vasa vasorum (''vessels of the vessels'') form a capillary network for distribution of arterial blood in the walls of large vessels (eg, the aorta and venae cava). Oxygen, nutrients, and wastes cannot reach all cells in these thick vessel walls by simple diffusion from the lumen.

I. Innervation of Blood Vessels: The walls of all blood vessels except capillaries and some venules contain a rich supply of nerve fibers.

1. Unmyelinated vasomotor fibers (sympathetic fibers) arise in the sympathetic ganglia, ramify in the adventitia, and terminate in small knoblike endings in the media. They stimulate smooth muscle contraction. Arteries usually contain more of these fibers. Small **intra-adventitial ganglia** are found in the walls of the aorta and in certain other large arteries.

2. Myelinated fibers occur in bundles in the adventitia. Their unmyelinated (free) nerve endings appear to be sensory. Many terminate in the adventitia; some extend to the intima.

III. THE HEART

A. Chambers:

1. The **atria,** located at the base (top) of the heart, are smaller and thinner walled than the ventricles. The right atrium receives venous blood from the superior and inferior venae cava and contracts to force it into the right ventricle. The left atrium receives oxygenated blood from the pulmonary veins and contracts to force that blood into the left ventricle.

2. The **ventricles** are larger chambers located in the body and apex of the heart. They have thick, muscular walls that generate forceful contractions. The right ventricle receives blood from the right atrium and contracts to force it through the pulmonary arteries to the lungs. The left ventricle receives blood from the left atrium and contracts to force it into the aorta for distribution to the rest of the body.

B. Tunics:

1. The **endocardium** is homologous to the intima and has 3 major components:

a. The innermost layer is an endothelium, which is underlain by a thin, continuous basal lamina.

b. Beneath the endothelium lies a layer of subendothelial connective tissue with elastic fibers and some smooth muscle cells.

c. The **subendocardium** is a layer of loose connective tissue containing small blood vessels, nerves, and, in the ventricles, branches of the impulse-conducting system (bundle branches and Purkinje fibers).

2. The **myocardium** is homologous to the media and is composed mainly of cardiac muscle fibers. It contains the impulse conducting system and parts of the cardiac skeleton. Each cardiac muscle fiber is surrounded by an endomysium, and each small bundle of fibers (fascicle) is surrounded by perimysium.

a. Atrial cardiac muscle In the atrial myocardium, muscle is arranged in overlapping networks, giving the inner surface of the atria the appearance of parallel and crossing bundles of muscle (musculi pectinati). Cells in the outer layers of the atrial myocardium form a complex spiral (helical) pattern around the chamber, resembling the arrangement in the ventricles. Numerous collagen and elastic fibers are interspersed among the muscle cells. Atrial cardiac muscle cells differ from ventricular muscle cells in that the atrial cells (1) are somewhat smaller, (2) have many granules containing atrial natriuretic factor, (3) have a less extensive T tubule system, (4) have more abundant gap junctions, (5) conduct impulses at a faster rate, and (6) contract more rhythmically.

b. Ventricular cardiac muscle In the ventricular myocardium, muscle is arranged in complex layers of muscle fibers wound helically around the ventricular cavity. This arrangement aids in "wringing out" the heart during ventricular contraction, increasing the percentage of blood in the cavity that is expelled during each contraction. The superficial muscle layers surround both ventricles, whereas the deeper muscle layers surround each ventricle individually and contribute to the interventricular septum. There appear to be differences in metabolic activity between the cells of the inner and outer layers of the ventricular myocardium. Elastic connective tissue is less abundant in ventricular than in atrial myocardium.

3. The **epicardium,** or visceral pericardium, is the outermost coat of the heart. It is a **serosa** composed of:

a. A layer of mesothelial cells, which forms the outer layer and provides a smooth surface that reduces the friction between the heart and the surrounding structures generated during contraction;

b. A thin basal lamina beneath the mesothelium; and

c. A layer of subepicardial connective tissue, composed of areolar tissue, that binds the epicardium to the myocardium.

C. Cardiac Skeleton: The dense fibrous connective tissue scaffolding into which the cardiac muscle fibers insert and from which the cores of the cardiac valves extend is usually termed the cardiac skeleton, or **fibrous skeleton.** Portions of the skeleton may become calcified during certain disease processes and aging. The cardiac skeleton has 3 major groups of components.

1. The **annuli fibrosae** are rings of dense fibrous connective tissue that surround and reinforce the valve openings in the atrioventricular canals and at the origins of the aorta and pulmonary artery. The reinforcing cores of the valves are rooted in these rings.

2. The **trigona fibrosae** are 2 triangular masses of dense connective tissue, occasionally containing some islands of cartilage, that lie between the 2 groups of annuli fibrosae.

3. The **septum membranaceum** is a dense fibrous plate that forms the superior portion of the interventricular septum.

D. Cardiac Valves: The cardiac valves are folds of endocardium that enclose and are strengthened by a platelike core of dense connective tissue. The cores are anchored in and continuous with the annular rings of the cardiac skeleton. The cardiac valves include:

1. The **tricuspid valve,** located between the right atrium and right ventricle. This valve has 3 **cusps** (flaps), and the free edge of each cusp is anchored to **papillary muscles** in the floor of each ventricle by a number of fibrous cords called **chordae tendinae.**

2. The **bicuspid valve,** or **mitral valve,** located between the left atrium and left ventricle. This valve has 2 cusps, each anchored by chordae tendinae to papillary muscles in the ventricle floor.

3. The **semilunar valves,** each composed of 3 semilunar cusps. These valves are not attached by chordae tendinae. Each cusp has a characteristic thickening (nodule) at the center of its free edge. There are 2 semilunar valves.

a. The **aortic valve** is located between the left ventricle and the aorta.

b. The **pulmonary valve** is located between the right ventricle and the pulmonary artery.

E. The Impulse Generating and Conducting System: The heart's impulse generating and conducting system is composed of unusual cardiac muscle cells specialized for the initiation and conduction of electrochemical impulses. Due to the special distribution of these cells, the impulses they carry coordinate the contraction of the myocardium around the heart's chambers.

1. The **sinoatrial node (SA node),** or **pacemaker node,** is a small cell mass in the median wall of the right atrium, near the opening of the superior vena cava. All cardiac muscle cells beat (contract) automatically; the cells with the fastest intrinsic rhythm generate impulses that cause the surrounding cells to contract at a faster rate. Since the cells of the SA node have the fastest intrinsic rhythm, they serve as the pacemaker for the rest of the heart. Autonomic nerve fibers and ganglia are located close to the SA node and, while they do not directly dictate heart rhythm, they can increase or decrease the heart rate. Impulses generated in the SA node travel rather slowly through ordinary atrial cardiac muscle cells to the atrioventricular node. This slow conduction allows the atria to complete their contraction before ventricles begin theirs.

2. The **atrioventricular node (AV node)** is a collection of cells located on the right side of the interatrial septum. As the impulse leaves the AV node, it passes directly and rapidly along the atrioventricular bundle.

3. The **atrioventricular bundle (AV bundle),** or **bundle of His,** is a bundle of specialized cardiac muscle fibers, approximately 15 mm long and 2–3 mm wide, that passes from the interatrial wall into the interventricular septum. At its termination, it gives off a smaller bundle (bundle branch) to each ventricle.

4. The **right and left bundle branches** travel a short distance before branching further to form the Purkinje fibers.

5. **Purkinje fibers,** cardiac muscle cells specialized for conduction of electrochemical impulses, contain sparse myofilaments that are concentrated at the cytoplasmic periphery. These cells are generally larger than those in the bundle branches and, like typical cardiac muscle cells, may have one or 2 central nuclei. The impulses are transmitted through gap junctions between the Purkinje fibers and the cardiac muscle cells they contact.

6. **Cardiac muscle cells** can propagate the impulses they receive from Purkinje fibers and pass them on to their neighbors. Thus, the cardiac musculature functions effectively as a syncytium, allowing its constituent cells to contract in a synchronous, coordinated manner.

F. Blood Supply to the Heart: The **coronary arteries** arise near the origin of the aorta and supply oxygen-rich blood to the myocardium. Blockage of a coronary vessel or its branches due to a thrombus or to **atherosclerosis** (fatty deposits in the media and intima) may rob the tissue normally supplied by the blocked vessel of oxygen and nutrients and lead to localized tissue necrosis, called an **infarct.** Organs with high energy and oxygen demands, like the heart and brain, are particularly susceptible to infarcts. The density of capillaries in cardiac muscle is even greater than in skeletal muscle and is a diagnostic feature of cardiac muscle in histologic section. Most of the venous blood returns, through the **coronary sinus,** to the superior vena cava as it enters the heart. However, some venous blood passes directly from myocardial capillary beds into the ventricles through tiny venules (Thebesian veins).

G. Lymphatics of the Heart: The myocardium contains abundant lymphatic capillaries. These begin as blind-ending tubes in the myocardium (near the endocardium) and drain into larger vessels in the epicardial connective tissue.

H. Innervation of the Heart: Many myelinated and unmyelinated motor fibers (both sympathetic and parasympathetic) enter the base (top) of the heart and ramify, forming plexuses and innervating several ganglia. While there are no myoneural junctions in the heart, the autonomic nervous system can adjust the heart rate to meet changing demands by various organs and tissues. Generally sympathetic stimulation increases and parasympathetic stimulation decreases heart rate.

IV. ROUTE OF THE BLOOD: The route taken by the blood through the cardiovascular system may be summarized as follows. Venous blood returns to the heart via the **superior and inferior venae cava.** It enters the right atrium, which contracts and forces blood through the tricuspid valve into the right ventricle. Contraction of the right ventricle forces blood through the pulmonary (semilunar) valve into the pulmonary artery, through which it reaches the capillaries surrounding the alveoli in the lungs. Here, the blood picks up oxygen and releases carbon dioxide and other volatile wastes. Newly oxygenated blood is collected in the pulmonary veins and carried to the left atrium, which contracts to force it through the bicuspid (mitral) valve and into the left ventricle. The left ventricle then contracts, forcing blood through the aortic (semilunar) valve and into the **aorta** (a large elastic artery) for distribution to the body. The aorta gives off numerous branches (distributing arteries) through which blood passes to arteries of successivelv smaller diameters (muscular arteries, arterioles) until it reaches the capillary beds, where it releases its oxygen and nutrients to the tissues and picks up carbon dioxide and other metabolic byproducts. Some fluid also escapes from the capillaries into intercellular tissue spaces; part of this excess tissue fluid returns to the capillary lumen before the blood leaves the tissue. The blood in the capillary beds enters the venules and then veins of increasing diameters (medium-sized veins, large veins, finally returning to heart throught the largest veins, the superior and inferior vena cava.

V. ROUTE OF THE LYMPH: The route taken by the lymph is unidirectional. Excess tissue fluid not returned to the blood capillaries (see above) is collected by blind-ending lymphatic capillaries in the region of the blood capillary beds and carried through lymphatic vessels to lymphatic ducts. There is one major lymphatic duct for each side of the body, the **thoracic duct** on the left and the **right lymphatic duct** on the right. The lymphatic ducts return lymph to the blood by emptying into the venous system at the junction of the jugular and subclavian veins in the neck. The lymphatic system is discussed further in Chapter 14.

Study-Focusing Questions*

1. List the general functions of the circulatory system (214).
2. Name the 2 vascular systems that comprise the circulatory system (214).

*The page references in this section refer to *Basic Histology,* 6th ed., Junqueira L, Carneiro J, Kelley R (editors), Appleton & Lange, 1989. **HR** (for Histology Review) is occasionally used instead of a page reference to indicate that the information referred to can be found in this book.

3. Name the 4 types of components that comprise the blood vascular system (214).
4. Name the 3 types of components that comprise the lymphatic vascular system (214, 227).
5. Name the 2 points of functional contact between the blood vascular system and the lymphatic vascular system. That is, how does fluid from the blood vascular system enter the lymphatic vascular system, and how does fluid from the lymphatic vascular system enter the blood vascular system (214, 227)?
6. Name the 3 layers (tunics) that comprise blood vessel walls (214).
7. Name the basic tissue types characteristically found in each of the 3 layers named in the answer to question 6 (214).
8. Which of the layers named in the answer to question 6 are absent in blood capillaries (215–217)?
9. Name the 4 major types of blood capillaries (217) and compare them in terms of:
   a. Their diameter
   b. The presence of fenestrae, diaphragms, a continuous basal lamina, and phagocytic cells in and around the capillary wall
10. Describe 3 ways in which the exchange of substances (proteins, fluid, salts, etc) may occur across capillary walls between blood and tissue fluid (219–220).
11. List some of the structural features of blood capillaries in the brain that may account for the phenomenon of the blood-brain barrier (217, 220).
12. Describe the effects of the metabolic activities of capillary endothelial cells (220) on the following substances:
   a. Angiotensin I
   b. Bradykinin
   c. Serotonin
   d. Prostaglandins
   e. Norepinephrine
   f. Thrombin
   g. Lipoproteins
13. Discuss the role of capillary endothelial cells in inhibiting thrombus formation (220).
14. List the 3 classes of arteries according to diameter (220–222) and compare them in terms of:
   a. Their abundance in the body
   b. The composition of their tunica intima
   c. The composition of their tunica media
   d. The composition of their tunica adventitia
   e. Their function
15. Describe carotid bodies (223) in terms of:
   a. Their location
   b. The class of receptors to which they belong
   c. The changes in blood chemistry to which they are sensitive
   d. The types of cells they contain
   e. The type of capillaries that provide their vascular supply
16. List 4 important physiologic phenomena in which arteriovenous anastomoses participate (224).
17. List the 3 classes of veins according to their diameter (224–225) and compare them in terms of:
   a. Their abundance in the body
   b. The composition of their tunica intima
   c. The composition of their tunica media
   d. The composition of their tunica adventitia
   e. Their function
18. Compare arteries and veins (224) in terms of the:
   a. Composition of their tunica intima (214, 220–222, 224–225)
   b. Presence of valves (225)
   c. Presence of an internal elastic lamina (214)
   d. Composition of their tunica media (214, 220–222, 224–225)
   e. Thickness of their tunica media (214, 220–222, 224–225)
   f. Abundance of elastic fibers in their walls (221, 224–225)
   g. Composition of their tunica adventitia, especially the presence of smooth muscle (214, 225)

h. Thickness of their tunica adventitia (224)
i. Overall thickness of the walls of arteries and veins with comparable diameters (220, 224)
j. Presence of vasa vasorum in larger vessels (214–215)

19. Describe the innervation of blood vessels (215).
20. Name the 3 tunics of the heart (225). To which blood vessel tunic does each correspond (225)?
21. Name the basic tissue types characteristically found in each of the 3 tunics named in the answer to question 20 (225). Which tunic is thickest in the heart (225)?
22. Name the components of the fibrous skeleton of the heart (225–226).
23. Compare the structure of the valves in the heart with that of those found in veins (225, 226).
24. List, in order, the components of the impulse generating and conducting system of the heart through which an electrical stimulus must pass to cause contraction of the ventricular myocardium (226–227). ***Hint:*** Include the cardia muscle cells themselves.
25. Compare Purkinje cells (fibers) and typical cardiac muscle cells (fibers) in terms of:
    a. Their diameter (226–227)
    b. Their conduction velocity (226)
    c. The number and location of their nuclei (226–227)
    d. The amount and location of their myofilaments (227)
    e. The presence of intercalated discs (227)
26. If you were looking at a cross section of the heart, would you find the Purkinje fibers closer to the epicardium or the endocardium (226)?
27. How does the neural control of cardiac muscle differ from that of skeletal muscle (227)?
28. Compare the effects of sympathetic and parasympathetic innervation on heart rate (227).
29. Compare the structure of lymphatic capillaries with that of blood capillaries in terms of the:
    a. Type of epithelial lining (215, 227)
    b. Presence of fenestrations (217, 227)
    c. Presence of zonulae occludentes (216, 227)
    d. Thickness of the basal lamina (216, 227)
30. In what aspects are larger lymphatic vessels similar to veins (227)?
31. Name the 2 largest lymphatic vessels in the body (227).

Multiple-Choice Questions

For questions 11–1 through 11–9, select the single best answer.

11–1. Characteristics of sinusoidal capillaries include all of the following *except:*
- **A.** They have unusually wide lumens
- **B.** They have abundant fenestrations
- **C.** They usually follow a tortuous (twisting) course
- **D.** They usually have a continuous basal lamina
- **E.** They often have phagocytic cells inserted between the endothelial cells of their lining

11–2. The thickest layer in the walls of veins is the:
- **A.** Tunica media
- **B.** Tunica adventitia
- **C.** Subendothelial connective tissue
- **D.** Tunica intima
- **E.** Internal elastic lamina

11–3. The epicardium:
- **A.** Is lined by endothelium
- **B.** Lacks connective tissue
- **C.** Is also called the parietal pericardium
- **D.** Contains large lymphatic capillaries
- **E.** Contains no adipose tissue

11-4. Which of the structures indicated in the photomicrograph in Fig 11-1 are the Purkinje cells (fibers)?

11-5. Pericytes:
- **A.** Are specialized cardiac muscle cells
- **B.** Cling to the outside of capillaries
- **C.** Are specialized smooth muscle cells
- **D.** Are terminally differentiated
- **E.** Are multinucleated

11-6. Metabolic functions of endothelial cells include all of the following *except:*
- **A.** Activation of angiotensin I (to angiotensin II)
- **B.** Activation of bradykinin
- **C.** Lipolysis of triglycerides
- **D.** Inactivation of serotonin
- **E.** Production of an inhibitor of platelet aggregation (prostacyclin)

11-7. The cell whose nucleus is labeled "N" in the photomicrograph in Fig 11-2 is a(n):
- **A.** Pericyte
- **B.** Smooth muscle cell
- **C.** Endothelial cell
- **D.** Fibroblast
- **E.** Mesothelial cell

11-8. The structures indicated by the single arrows in the photomicrograph in Fig 11-3 are:
- **A.** Junctional complexes
- **B.** Micropinocytotic vesicles
- **C.** Coated pits
- **D.** Fenestrations closed by diaphragms
- **E.** None of the above

11-9. The photomicrograph in Fig 11-4 shows a cross section of a portion of the wall of what type of vessel?
- **A.** Aorta
- **B.** Muscular artery
- **C.** Medium-sized vein
- **D.** Vena cava
- **E.** Arteriole

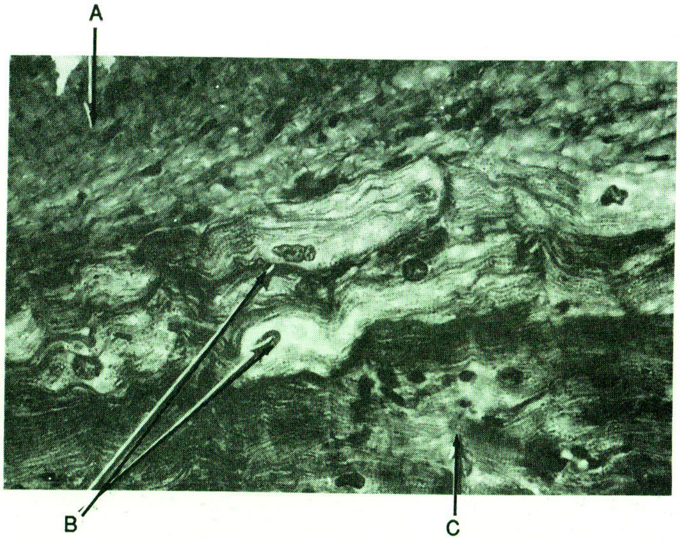

Figure 11-1.

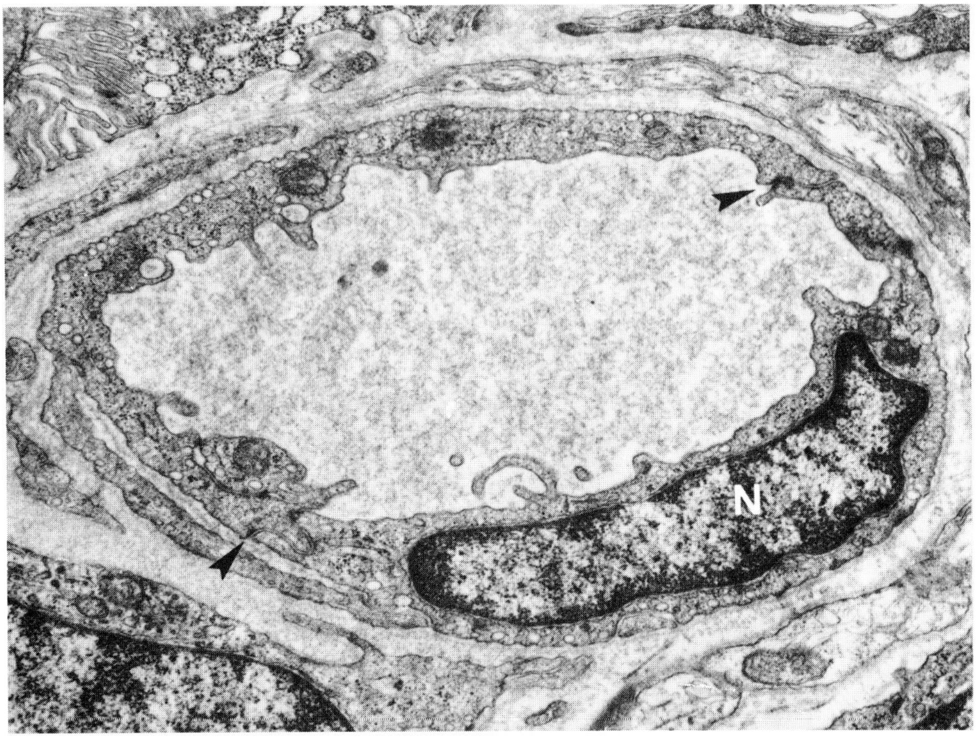

Figure 11-2.

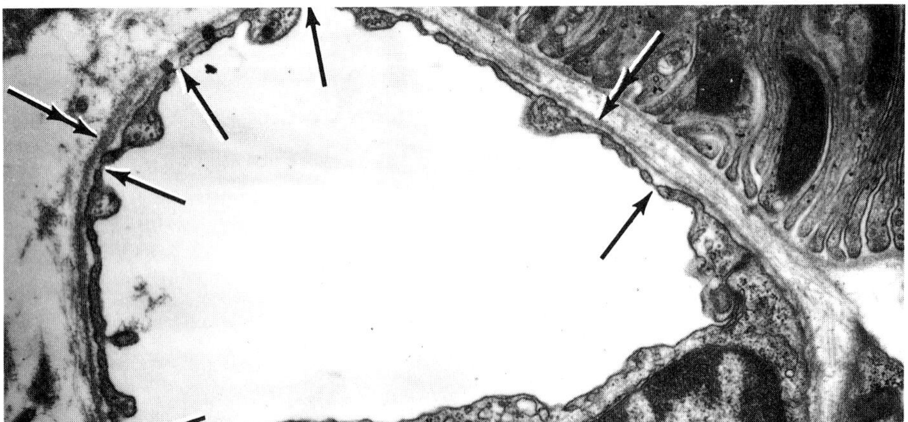

Figure 11-3.

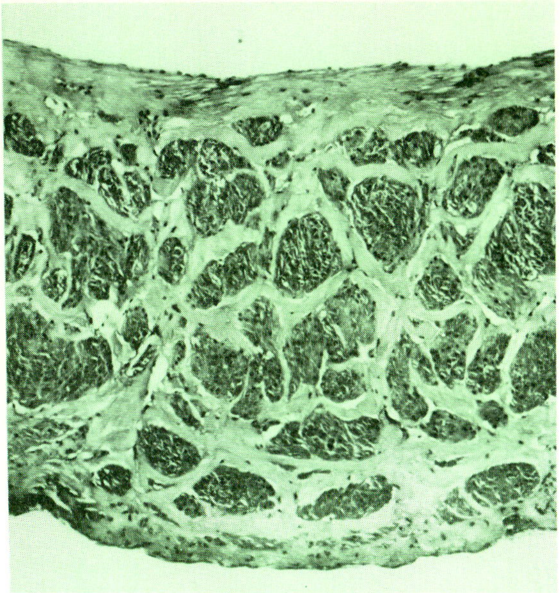

Figure 11-4.

MATCHING (questions 11-10 through 11-22): Each choice may be used once, more than once, or not at all.
Questions 11-10 through 11-16: From the following choices, indicate, in order, the structures through which an inpulse must be propagated so that the atria and ventricles contract in proper succession. Begin with the pacemaker (question 11-10).

A. Atrioventricular bundle of His
B. Sinoatrial (SA) node
C. Ventricular cardiac muscle
D. Atrioventricular (AV) node
E. Purkinje cells (fibers)
F. Right and left bundle branches
G. Atrial cardiac muscle

11-10. First step (pacemaker)
11-11. Second step
11-12. Third step
11-13. Fourth step
11-14. Fifth step
11-15. Sixth step
11-16. Seventh step

Questions 11-17 through 11-22 use the letters in Fig 11-5.

11-17. Sinoatrial node
11-18. Atrioventricular bundle of His
11-19. Pacemaker
11-20. Right bundle branch
11-21. Purkinje fiber system
11-22. Atrioventricular node

For questions 11-23 through 11-47, either, both, or neither of the answers may be correct. Select

A if only A is correct
B if only B is correct
C if both A and B are correct
D if neither A nor B is correct

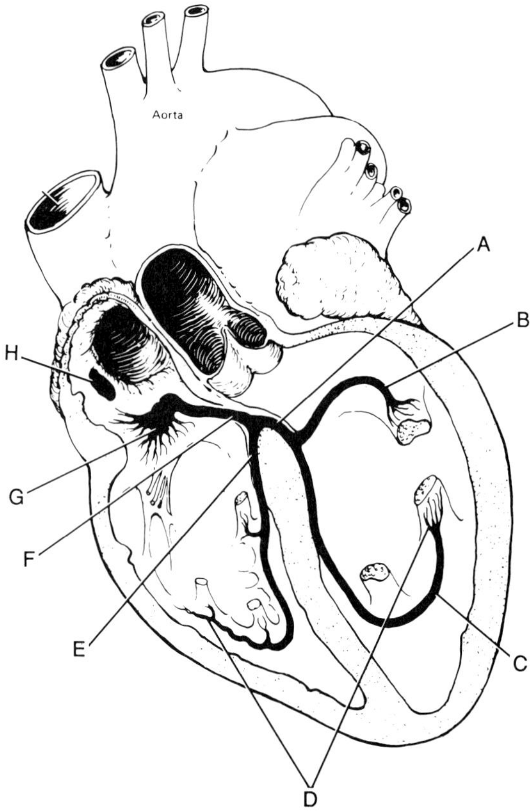

Figure 11-5.

Questions 11–23 through 11–33:

A. Arteries
B. Veins
C. Both
D. Neither

11–23. Large vessels may contain vasa vasorum
11–24. May contain valves
11–25. Exhibit a thicker tunica media
11–26. Adventitia is best-developed tunic
11–27. Medium-sized vessels contain a definitive internal elastic lamina
11–28. May contain longitudinal smooth muscle in the tunica adventitia
11–29. Generally have a more collapsed appearance in tissue sections
11–30. Classified by size
11–31. Receive an autonomic nerve supply
11–32. Most similar to lymphatic vessels
11–33. Have the largest amount of elastin in their tunica media

Questions 11–34 through 11–40:

A. Atria
B. Ventricles
C. Both
D. Neither

11–34. Thickest myocardium
11–35. Located at the base of the heart
11–36. Walls are composed of three layers
11–37. Right side receives blood from pulmonary veins
11–38. Cells in the myocardium contain abundant granules
11–39. Right side contains sinoatrial (pacemaker) node
11–40. Contain Purkinje fibers

Questions 11–41 through 11–47:

A. Lymphatic capillaries
B. Blood capillaries
C. Both
D. Neither

11–41. Contain erythrocytes
11–42. Contain lymphocytes
11–43. Blind-ending tubes
11–44. May have fenestrations in their walls
11–45. Contain valves
11–46. Have the thinner basal lamina
11–47. Characteristically exhibit occluding junctions between their lining endothelial cells

For questions 11–48 through 11–55, one, more than one, or all of the answers may be correct. Select

A if only (1), (2), and (3) are correct
B if only (1) and (3) are correct
C if only (2) and (4) are correct
D is only (4) is correct
E if all answers are correct

11–48. Fenestrated capillaries:
(1) Are found in the kidney
(2) Are important in the transport of macromolecules between blood and tissues
(3) Have a continuous basal lamina
(4) May have thin diaphragms covering their pores

11–49. The tunica intima:
(1) Has a layer of dense connective tissue
(2) Is avascular
(3) Is separated from the tunica media of arteries by the external elastic lamina
(4) Has a layer of simple squamous epithelium

11–50. Purkinje fibers:
(1) Are specialized cardiac muscle cells
(2) Are densely packed with myofilaments
(3) Communicate with typical cardiac muscle cells through gap junctions
(4) Are most commonly found directly beneath the ventricular epicardium

11–51. Basic tissue types found in large vessels include:
(1) Muscle
(2) Connective tissue
(3) Epithelium
(4) Nerve

11–52. Physiologic functions in which arteriovenous anastomoses play an important part include:
(1) Menstruation
(2) Thermoregulation
(3) Erection
(4) Regulation of blood pressure

11–53. Exchange of cells and other substances across capillary walls occurs through:
- **(1)** Fenestrae
- **(2)** Intercellular clefts
- **(3)** Pinocytotic vesicles
- **(4)** Diapedesis

11–54. Characteristics of the blood-brain barrier include:
- **(1)** Continuous (nonfenestrated) capillaries
- **(2)** The relative paucity of micropinocytotic vesicles in the capillary endothelial cells
- **(3)** Extremely tight occluding junctions between the capillary endothelial cells
- **(4)** Some intravenous drugs (eg, some antibiotics) that readily cross capillary walls elsewhere in the body are unable to cross the walls of capillaries in the brain

11–55. Lymphatic vessels:
- **(1)** Have walls resembling those of veins
- **(2)** Contain valves
- **(3)** Have indistinct borders between their tunics
- **(4)** Contain longitudinal smooth muscle fibers in their tunica media

12 Blood Cells

Objectives

This chapter should help the student to:

- Know the name, structure, and function of each of the formed elements normally found in blood.
- Know, in percentages, how much each of the formed elements contributes to the cell number (as determined by a differential cell count) and to blood volume (as determined by hematocrit measurement).
- Know the percentage of normal blood volume contributed by plasma.
- Know the composition of plasma and distinguish between plasma and serum.
- Describe in sequence the events of clot formation, including the roles of the platelets and various plasma proteins.
- Identify the various formed elements present in a slide or photomicrograph of a blood smear.

Synopsis

I. GENERAL FEATURES OF THE BLOOD

A. Two Divisions: Blood is divisible into 2 parts, the formed elements (III), which include the blood cells and platelets, and the plasma, or liquid phase (II), in which the formed elements are suspended and in which a variety of important proteins, hormones, and other substances are dissolved.

B. Two Basic Cell Types: There are 2 basic types of blood cells, the erythrocytes, or red blood cells (III.A) and the leukocytes, or white blood cells (III.B).

C. Clotting: Outside the blood vessels, blood undergoes a complex reaction called clot formation or coagulation (IV), which plays an important role in repairing damaged vessels and preventing blood loss.

D. Hematocrit: When anticoagulants (heparin, citrate, etc) are added, blood samples can be separated in a centrifuge into 3 major fractions. The erythrocytes constitute the densest fraction and end up at the bottom of the tube. The term **hematocrit** refers to the percentage of packed erythrocytes per unit volume of blood. In adults, normal hematocrit values vary from 35 to 50% and are sex-dependent. Leukocytes are less dense and less numerous (about 1% of blood volume) and form a thin white or grayish layer over the erythrocytes called the **buffy coat.** On the upper surface of the buffy coat is a thin layer of platelets. The least dense layer is the clear layer of plasma, which constitutes 42–47% of the blood and overlies the buffy coat.

E. Differential Cell Count: Blood is also studied by spreading a drop on a slide to produce a single layer of cells **(blood smear).** The cells are stained, differentiated by type, and counted to reveal any disease-related changes in their relative numbers. The smears are usually stained with modifications of dye mixtures containing eosin and methylene blue, ie, Romanovsky-type mixtures.

F. Staining Properties: All of the descriptions of the staining properties of blood cells in this chapter refer to their appearance after staining with Romanovsky-type mixtures (eg, Wright's stain or Giemsa stains). Blood cells and their components exhibit 4 major staining properties that allow the cell types to be distinguished:

1. Basophilia is an affinity for methylene blue. Basophilic structures stain purple to black.

2. Azurophilia is an affinity for the oxidation products of methylene blue called azures. Azurophilic structures stain red-blue.

3. Eosinophilia, or **acidophilia,** is an affinity for eosin. Eosinophilic structures stain yellow-pink to orange.

4. Neutrophilia is an affinity for a complex of dyes (originally thought to be neutral) in the mixture. Neutrophilic structures stain salmon pink to lilac.

II. COMPOSITION OF PLASMA

A. Water: Plasma contains 90% water by volume.

B. Solutes: Plasma contains 10% solutes by volume. These solutes include plasma proteins and other organic compounds as well as inorganic salts.

1. Plasma proteins Plasma contains a rich variety of soluble proteins, 7% by volume. Important examples include:

a. Albumin This is the most abundant plasma protein (3.5–5 g/dL of blood) and is mainly responsible for maintaining the osmotic pressure of blood. Substances that are partly or completely water-insoluble (eg, lipids) are transported in the plasma in association with albumin.

b. Globulins Alpha, beta, and gamma globulins are globular proteins dissolved in the plasma. The gamma globulins include the antibodies, or **immunoglobulins,** synthesized by plasma cells.

c. Fibrinogen This protein is converted by blood-borne enzymes into **fibrin** during clot formation. Fibrinogen is synthesized and secreted by the liver.

2. Other organic compounds Other organic molecules in plasma, 2.1% by volume, include nutrients such as amino acids and glucose, vitamins, and a variety of regulatory peptides, steroid hormones, and lipids.

3. Inorganic salts Inorganic salts in plasma, 0.9% by volume, include blood electrolytes such as sodium, potassium, and calcium salts.

III. THE FORMED ELEMENTS

A. Erythrocytes: Erythrocytes are also called **red blood cells,** or **RBCs.** Because of their presence in most tissues and organs, erythrocytes are useful to histologists and pathologists in estimating the size of other tissue and organ components (through estimates of multiples or fractions of RBC diameter).

1. Normal structure and function Red blood cells are structurally and functionally specialized to transport oxygen from the lungs to other tissues. Their cytoplasm contains the oxygen-binding protein hemoglobin. Their small diameter (7–8 μm) and biconcave shape (in humans) help to maximize their surface-to-volume ratio, facilitating oxygen exchange. Mature RBCs lack nuclei and cytoplasmic organelles, which they lose during differentiation. Because they lack mitochondria, the energy needed to maintain the hemoglobin in a functional state must be derived from anaerobic glycolysis. Because they lack ribosomes, the glycolytic enzymes and other important proteins cannot be renewed. Mature erythrocytes therefore have a limited lifespan (120 days) in the circulation before they are removed by macrophages in the spleen and bone marrow.

2. Abnormalities

a. Anisocytosis This term refers to the presence of a high percentage of RBCs with unusually great variations in size. Those larger than 9 μm in diameter are termed macrocytes and those smaller than 6 μm are termed microcytes.

b. Nuclear fragments In some disease states, nuclear fragments, or **Howell-Jolly bodies,** remain in otherwise mature RBCs. When these form circular filaments they are termed **Cabot rings.**

c. Reticulocytes Some RBCs recently released from the bone marrow contain a small amount of residual rough endoplasmic reticulum and ribosomes that can be precipitated into blue, netlike structures with the vital dye brilliant cresyl blue. When such cells, termed reticulocytes, constitute more than about 1% of the circulating RBCs, they indicate an increased demand for oxygen-carrying capacity (eg, from loss of RBCs due to hemorrhage or anemia, or to recent ascent to a higher altitude).

3. Hemoglobin Each hemoglobin molecule consists of 4 polypeptide subunits, each of which includes an iron-containing **heme** group. Hemoglobin can reversibly bind to oxygen, forming **oxyhemoglobin,** and to carbon dioxide, forming **carbaminohemoglobin.** However, hemoglobin binds irreversibly to carbon monoxide, forming **carboxyhemoglobin,** which reduces the oxygen-carrying capacity of the blood.

Hemoglobin (Hb) exists in a variety of forms, distinguishable on the basis of the amino acid sequence of their subunits. In humans, only 3 forms are considered normal in postnatal life: **HbA1** constitutes 97%, **HbA2** 2%, and **HbF** 1% of the hemoglobin of healthy adults. HbF comprises around 80% of the hemoglobin of newborns, however; this figure gradually decreases until it reaches normal adult levels at about 8 months of age. **HbS** is an abnormal form of HbA that is found in patients with **sickle cell anemia;** it differs by a single amino acid substitution in the beta chain (valine in HbS, glutamine in HbA). Unlike HbA, HbS becomes insoluble at low oxygen tensions and crystallizes into inflexible rods that deform the RBCs, giving them the characteristic sickle shape. When the rigid sickled cells pass through narrow capillaries, they cannot flexibly adapt to the passageway as normal RBCs do. They may become trapped, obstructing blood flow through the capillary, or rupture, decreasing the number of RBCs available for oxygen transport (anemia).

4. Plasmalemma and stroma When placed in a hypotonic solution, RBCs swell and release their hemoglobin into the surrounding solution, a process termed **hemolysis;** they leave behind an empty shell, or **red cell ghost,** composed of the plasmalemma and the stroma. The stroma is composed of proteins such as **spectrin** that are associated with the inner surface of the plasmalemma; it maintains the RBC's biconcave shape. The external surface of the plasmalemma is covered by a carbohydrate-rich glycocalyx, which contains genetically determined antigens that allow **blood types** (including A, B, O, and Rh groups) to be distinguished. The major integral membrane glycoprotein of RBCs is **glycophorin.**

B. Leukocytes: Leukocytes, or white blood cells, are nucleated and are larger and less numerous than erythrocytes. Leukocytes can be divided into 2 main groups, granulocytes and agranulocytes, according to their content of cytoplasmic granules. Each of these groups can then be further divided on the basis of size, nuclear morphology, ratio of nuclear to cytoplasmic volume, and staining properties. Two classes of cytoplasmic granules occur in leukocytes, specific and azurophilic granules. **Specific granules** are found only in granulocytes; their staining properties (neutrophilic, eosinophilic, or basophilic) distinguish the 3 granulocyte types. **Azurophilic granules** are found in both agranulocytes (III.B.1) and granulocytes (III.B.2). Unlike the RBCs, all leukocytes can leave the capillaries by squeezing between endothelial cells, a process termed **diapedesis,** and enter the surrounding connective tissue in response to infection or inflammation. The types and levels of activity expressed by extravascular leukocytes depends upon the specific cell type (see Chapter 5 for futher discussion).

1. Agranulocytes have unsegmented nuclei and are described as **mononuclear leukocytes.** They lack specific granules, but may contain azurophilic granules.

a. Lymphocytes constitute a diverse class of cells; they have similar morphologic characteristics but a variety of highly specific functions. They normally account for 20–25% of the white blood cells in adult blood, with a considerable range of normal variation (20–45%). Lymphocytes are also found outside the blood vessels, grouped in lymphatic organs (see Chapter 14) or dispersed in connective tissues. They respond to invasion of the body by foreign substances and organisms and assist in their inactivation. Unlike other leukocytes, lymphocytes never become phagocytic. The 2 major functional classes of lymphocytes are T cells and B cells (see below). Lymphocytes in the blood are predominantly (about 80%) T cells.

(1) Size Lymphocytes vary from 6 to 18 μm in diameter. Most of those found in blood are **small lymphocytes** in the 7- to 8-μm range, making them the smallest leukocytes, comparable in size to erythrocytes. A small number of **medium-sized** and **large lymphocytes** are also found in the circulation and probably represent lymphocytes activated by an antigen.

(2) Nucleus Lymphocyte nuclei are spheric and often flattened on one side. In small lymphocytes, the nucleus is densely heterochromatic, staining purplish-blue to black, and nearly fills the cell. In large lymphocytes, the nucleus is larger and less dense and stains reddish-purple.

(3) Cytoplasm Lymphocyte cytoplasm exhibits a pale basophilia and occasionally contains a few purplish azurophilic granules but lacks specific granules. In the smaller cells, the cytoplasm forms a thin rim around the nucleus; in the larger cells, it is more abundant. It contains many free ribosomes, few mitochondria, sparse endoplasmic reticulum, and a small Golgi complex.

(4) Memory cells and effector cells When stimulated by an antigen, lymphocytes undergo **blast transformation,** a process of enlargement and sequential mitotic divisions. Some of the daughter cells, called memory cells, return to an inactive state but retain the capacity to respond more quickly to the next encounter with the same antigen. Other daughter cells, called effector cells, become activated to carry out an immune response to the antigen. Effector cells may be derived from either B lymphocytes (B cells) or T lymphocytes (T cells). While circulating B and T cells are morphologically indistinguishable, they carry different cell-surface components (antigens recognized by other species) and can be identified by special procedures.

(a) B lymphocytes differentiate into **plasma cells** (see Chapter 5), which secrete specific antigen-binding molecules (antibodies or immunoglobulins) that circulate in the blood and lymph and serve as a major component of **humoral immunity.**

(b) T lymphocyte derivatives serve as the major cells of the **cellular immune response.** They produce a variety of factors, termed **lymphokines** (eg, interferon) that influence the activities of macrophages and of other leukocytes involved in an immune response. There are several types:

(i) Cytotoxic (killer) cells secrete substances that kill other cells and in some cases kill by direct contact; they play the major role in graft rejection.

(ii) Helper T cells enhance the activity of some B cells and other T cells.

(iii) Suppressor T cells inhibit the activity of some B cells and other T cells.

(5) Null cells are circulating cells that morphologically resemble lymphocytes but that exhibit neither B cell nor T cell surface antigens. They may represent circulating stem cells of lymphocytes or other blood cell types (see Chapter 13).

(6) The primary (central) lymphoid organs include the **thymus,** where lymphocyte precursors are programmed to become T cells and, in birds, the **bursa of Fabricius,** where lymphocyte precursors are programmed to become B cells. Humans have no bursa; our B cells appear to be programmed in the bone marrow.

b. Monocytes are often confused with large lymphocytes, but they are larger and constitute only 3–8% of the white blood cells in healthy adults. Monocytes are found only in the blood, but they remain in circulation for less than a week before migrating through capillary walls to enter other tissues or to become incorporated in the lining of sinuses. Once outside the bloodstream, they become phagocytic and apparently do not recirculate. The **mononuclear phagocyte system** (portions of which were formerly referred to as the reticuloendothelial system) consists of monocyte-derived phagocytic cells distributed throughout the body. Examples include the Kupffer cells of the liver and some of the macrophages of connective tissues.

(1) Size Monocytes in the blood of healthy adults have a diameter of 12–15 μm, but when they attach to surfaces they flatten and spread out, often reaching 20 μm in diameter.

(2) Nucleus Monocyte nuclei may be ovoid, but are usually kidney- or horseshoe-shaped and eccentrically placed; unlike lymphocyte nuclei, they are rarely spheric. The chromatin is less condensed than that of lymphocyte nuclei, has a "smudgy" appearance, and stains reddish-purple. There may be 2–3 nucleoli, but these are often difficult to distinguish.

(3) Cytoplasm The faint blue-gray cytoplasm of monocytes is more abundant than that of lymphocytes and contains many small azurophilic granules but no specific granules. It also contains many small mitochondria, a well-developed Golgi apparatus, and sparse rough endoplasmic reticulum and polyribosomes.

2. Granulocytes have segmented nuclei and are described as **polymorphonuclear leukocytes (PMNLs).** Depending on the cell type, the mature nucleus may have from 2 to 7 lobes connected by thin strands of nucleoplasm. Granulocyte types are most easily distinguished by their size and staining properties, and by the appearance (as seen with an electron microscope) of the abundant specific granules in their cytoplasm. These granules are all membrane-limited and bud off the Golgi complex. In addition to a small Golgi complex, each granulocyte contains a few mitochondria and free ribosomes and sparse endoplasmic reticulum.

a. Neutrophils are the most abundant leukocytes in the blood. They usually constitute 60–70% of the white blood cells in healthy adults, with a limited range of normal variation (50–75%). They are also found outside the bloodstream, especially in loose connective tissue. Neutrophils are the first line of cellular defense against the invasion of bacteria. Once they leave the bloodstream, they spread out, develop ameboid motility, and become active phagocytes. Unlike lymphocytes, neutrophils are all terminally differentiated cells and so are incapable of mitosis.

(1) Size Neutrophils in the blood are approximately 12 μm in diameter, while those in the tissues spread to a diameter of up to 20 μm.

(2) Nucleus Neutrophil nuclei contain highly condensed chromatin both in the lobes and in the attenuated chromatin bridges between them. Most have 3 lobes; however, lobe number increases from a single horseshoe-shaped nucleus in immature neutrophils, called **band neutrophils,** to more than 5 lobes in aging ones. The nuclei of certain diseased neutrophils, called **hypersegmented** neutrophils, also have more than 5 lobes. In females, a small heterochromatic body often extends from one of the nuclear lobes. This represents the inactive X chromosome, or **Barr body,** and is referred to as a **drumstick** because of its characteristic shape.

(3) Cytoplasm Neutrophil cytoplasm is abundant and filled with specific granules. The neutrophilic granules, with a diameter of 0.3–0.8 μm, are near the limit of resolution of the light microscope. They stain salmon pink with typical blood stains. The less numerous azurophilic granules are larger and stain a reddish-purple. The specific granules contain alkaline phosphatase and bactericidal cationic proteins called **phagocytins.** Azurophilic granules contain lysosomal enzymes and peroxidase. Neutrophils also contain more glycogen granules than other leukocytes.

b. Eosinophils constitute only 1–4% of the circulating leukocytes in healthy adults. They may leave the bloodstream by diapedesis, spread out, and move about in the connective tissues. They are capable of only limited phagocytosis, showing a preference for antigen-antibody complexes. The number of circulating eosinophils typically increases during allergic reactions and in response to parasitic infections, and rapidly decreases in response to treatment with exogenous corticosteroids.

(1) Size Eosinophils are usually slightly smaller than typical neutrophils, measuring about 9 μm in diameter in the blood and up to 14 μm in loose connective tissue.

(2) Nucleus Eosinophil nuclei contain condensed chromatin and usually have 2 lobes connected by a thin chromatin bridge. The nuclei are often partially obscured by the numerous specific granules in the cytoplasm.

(3) Cytoplasm The most characteristic structural feature of eosinophils is the presence of numerous large (0.5–1.5 μm in diameter), brightly eosinophilic granules (specific granules) in their cytoplasm. These granules are specialized lysosomes that lack lysozyme but contain acid phosphatase, cathepsin, and ribonuclease. In electron micrographs, each specific granule has an oblong shape and an elongated, centrally located, electron-dense crystalloid, or **internum,** lying parallel to its long axis. Between the granule membrane and the internum lies the electron-lucent **matrix,** or **externum.**

c. Basophils are the least numerous of the circulating leukocytes, constituting from 0 to 1% of the white blood cells of healthy adults. Like other white blood cells, basophils may leave the circulation, but they are capable of only very limited ameboid movement and phagocytosis in the tissues. Extravascular basophils are most often found at sites of inflammation and may be the major cell type at sites of **cutaneous basophil hypersensitivity.** Despite structural and functional similarities between basophils and mast cells (see Chapter 5), these cells are not the same and are distinguishable on the basis of ultrastructure.

(1) Size Basophils vary in diameter from 10 to 12 μm but are usually slightly smaller than neutrophils.

(2) Nucleus Basophil nuclei contain highly condensed chromatin and usually consist of 3 lobes twisted into an S shape. They are often obscured by the large, dark-staining cytoplasmic granules.

(3) Cytoplasm The specific granules of basophils are their most characteristic feature. These granules have irregular shapes and vary in size; the largest are the size of the specific granules of eosinophils, the smallest nearly as small as those of neutrophils. The granules stain metachromatically and appear reddish-violet to nearly black in stained blood smears. The specific granules of basophils (like those of the mast cells of connective tissue) contain heparin and histamine, which may be released by exocytosis in response to certain types of antigenic stimuli. The granules may contain inclusions, but they appear more homogeneously electron-dense than do those of eosinophils.

C. Platelets: Platelets, or **thrombocytes,** the smallest formed elements in the blood, are disklike cell fragments that vary in diameter from 2 to 5 μm. In humans, they lack nuclei and originate by budding from large cells in the bone marrow called **megakaryocytes** (see Chapter 13). They range in number from 150,000 to 300,000 per mm^3 (μL) of blood and have a lifespan of about 8 days. In blood smears they appear in clumps. Each platelet has a peripheral **hyalomere** region that stains a faint blue and a dense central **granulomere** that contains a few mitochondria and glycogen granules and a variety of purple granules. **Dense bodies,** or **delta granules,** are 250–300 nm in diameter and contain calcium ions, pyrophosphate, ADP, and ATP; they take up and store serotonin. **Alpha granules** are 300–500 nm in diameter and contain fibrinogen, platelet-derived growth factor, and other platelet-specific proteins. **Lambda granules** (platelet lysosomes) are 175–200 nm in diameter and contain only lysosomal enzymes. The hyalomere contains a **marginal bundle** of microtubules that helps to maintain the platelet's discoid shape. The glycocalyx is unusually rich in glycosaminoglycans and is associated with adhesion, the major functional characteristic of platelets. Platelets have an important physical role in plugging wounds, and they contribute to the cascade of molecular interactions among the various clotting factors dissolved in the plasma (see below).

IV. CLOT FORMATION

A. The Clot and Serum: Clotted blood consists of 2 parts: (1) the clot, or **thrombus,** which includes the formed elements and some of the proteins previously dissolved in the plasma, and (2) the serum, a clear yellow liquid that is similar to plasma except that it lacks fibrinogen and contains more serotonin.

B. Clotting Factors: Clotting involves a cascade of molecular interactions among several plasma proteins and ions (clotting facors I–XIII). The cascade can be initiated by 2 converging pathways, each of which results in the conversion of fibrinogen to fibrin by the enzyme **thrombin.** In the **intrinsic pathway,** initiation of the cascade occurs when factor XII is activated by contact with collagen underlying the endothelium (indicating damage to the endothelial lining of a vessel). In the **extrinsic pathway,** cells in a damaged vessel wall or the surrounding tissue release an ill-defined clot-promoting substance termed **thromboplastin** (factor III), which combines with blood calcium and factor VII to activate factor X, a plasma protein. Factor X is a point of convergence of the 2 pathways and, in its activated form, promotes the conversion of **prothrombin** (factor II) to thrombin. Both factor X and prothrombin are synthesized by the liver and require vitamin K as a cofactor in their synthesis. Thrombin enzymatically converts plasma fibrinogen (factor I, released into plasma by platelets and by the liver) into fibrin; this explains the lower concentration of fibrinogen in serum than in plasma. Other factors act as promoters and accelerators of the clotting process or help stabilize the fibrin once it has formed. An inherited abnormality in factor VIII (whose precise role in the clotting process is uncertain) results in the clotting disorder known as **hemophilia.**

C. The Role of Platelets:

1. **Primary aggregation** Platelets in the damaged region attach to collagen revealed by the discontinuity in the vessel wall, forming a **platelet plug.**

2. **Secondary aggregation** Platelets in the plug release the contents of their alpha and delta granules. This release of **serotonin** explains the higher concentration of serotonin in serum than in plasma. Serotonin, a vasoconstrictor, restricts blood flow to the damaged area by causing contraction of vascular smooth muscle.

3. **Blood coagulation** Platelets release fibrinogen in addition to that normally found in the plasma. The fibrinogen is converted by the clotting factor cascade into fibrin, which forms a dense fibrous mat to which more platelets and other blood cells attach, plugging the opening in the blood vessel wall.

D. Clot Retraction: The clot (thrombus) initially bulges into the vessel lumen, but later it contracts and condenses through the interactions of **thrombosthenin** (a contractile protein released by the platelets) and platelet actin, myosin, and ATP.

E. Clot Removal: As the vessel wall heals and the protection afforded by the clot is no longer needed, the clot is removed by the enzyme **plasmin.** Plasmin is formed by the action of **plasminogen activators** (released by endothelial cells) on the plasma proenzyme **plasminogen** (synthesized by the liver). Enzymes released by the lambda granules (lysosomes) of the platelets also aid in clot digestion.

Study-Focusing Questions*

1. Give the approximate total blood volume of adult humans (229).
2. Name the 2 major parts of blood (229).
3. Name the 3 classes of formed elements in blood (229).
4. Compare serum and plasma in terms of:
   a. The procedures involved in isolating them from whole blood (229)
   b. Their content of fibrinogen and serotonin (229)
5. Give the normal hematocrit values (229) for:
   a. Newborns
   b. Children (up to age 10)
   c. Adult females
   d. Adult males
6. As judged from the buffy coat obtained in measuring the hematocrit, what percentage of blood volume is composed of leukocytes (229)?
7. List the general functions of blood and name the blood components primarily responsible for each (229).
8. Describe the composition of plasma (229) in terms of:
   a. Its percentage of water
   b. Its percentage of plasma proteins
   c. Its percentage of inorganic salts
   d. The other types of substances present
9. List several types of plasma proteins (229).
10. To which class of plasma proteins do the circulating antibodies (immunoglobulins) secreted by the plasma cells belong (229)?
11. Name 2 or more examples of Romanovsky-type blood staining mixtures (230).
12. What is the normal diameter of a human erythrocyte (230)?
13. What is the functional significance of the biconcave shape of normal erythrocytes (231)?
14. Compare the erythrocytes of patients afflicted with sickle cell anemia with normal erythrocytes in terms of:
    a. Their amino acid composition (232)
    b. The type of hemoglobin (Hb) they contain (232)
    c. The effect of low oxygen tension on the solubility of their hemoglobin (232–233)
    d. The effect of low oxygen tension on cell shape and flexibility (232–233)
15. What biochemical components of the erythrocyte plasma membrane determine the blood group (ie, MN, ABO) to which an individual belongs (231)?
16. What happens to erythrocytes when they are placed in a:
    a. Hypotonic solution (232)
    b. Hypertonic solution (232)

*The page references in this section refer to *Basic Histology,* 6th ed., Junqueira L, Carneiro J, Kelley R (editors), Appleton & Lange, 1989. **HR** (for Histology Review) is occasionally used instead of a page reference to indicate that the information referred to can be found in this book.

17. Describe hemoglobin (232–233) in terms of:
  a. Its primary function
  b. The number of subunits per molecule
  c. The number of hemes per molecule
  d. The type of metal ion normally associated with the heme
  e. The types normally found in blood postnatally
  f. The predominant type found in adults
  g. The predominant type found in the fetus
18. Describe mature erythrocytes (233) in terms of:
  a. The organelles they contain
  b. Their capacity for protein synthesis
  c. Their source of energy (primary substrate and types of energy metabolism)
  d. Their site of production
  e. Their length of survival in the circulation
  f. Their site(s) of removal from the circulation
19. List the 5 types of leukocytes found in the blood (233).
20. Which of the types listed in the answer to question 19 are:
  a. Granulocytes (233)
  b. Agranulocytes (233)
21. Compare granulocytes and agranulocytes in terms of:
  a. Their content of specific granules (233)
  b. Their content of azurophilic granules (233, 235)
  c. The shape of their nuclei (233)
22. Leukocytes are considered a normal cellular component of what type of tissue besides blood (233)?
23. What are the structural and functional differences between leukocytes found in blood and those found in the tissue named in the answer to question 22 (233)?
24. What is the normal range of the leukocyte count (number of leukocytes per microliter of blood) and the predominant type or class of leukocyte present in humans at the following ages (233)?
  a. Birth
  b. 4 days
  c. 4 years
  d. 12 years
  e. 15 years
  f. During adulthood
25. What percentage of the leukocytes in normal adult blood is made up by each of the following cell types (233)?
  a. Neutrophils
  b. Lymphocytes
  c. Monocytes
  d. Eosinophils
  e. Basophils
26. Compare the 3 types of granulocytes in terms of:
  a. The staining properties of their specific granules (235, 236, 237–238)
  b. The contents of their specific granules (236)
  c. The size of their specific granules (235, 236, 237)
  d. The average number of nuclear lobes in a mature cell (234, 236, 237)
  e. The diameter of a mature cell (234, 236, 237)
  f. Their function (236, 237, 238)
27. Compare the 2 types of agranulocytes most commonly found in the blood in terms of:
  a. The amount of their cytoplasm (234, 239, 240)
  b. The staining properties of their cytoplasm (239, 240)
  c. The shape of their nuclei (239, 240)
  d. The staining properties of their nuclei (239, 241)
  e. The visibility of their nucleoli with Romanovsky-type stains (234, 239)
  f. Their cell diameter (239, 240)
  g. Their basic function (240, 241)
  h. Their ability to leave and reenter the circulation (241, 273)
28. Name the 2 types of granules found in neutrophils (235) and compare them in terms of their size (235) and contents (236).

29. Neutrophils constitute the first line of cellular defense against invading microorganisms such as bacteria. Describe the sequence of events whereby neutrophils:
    a. Leave the circulatory system and migrate to a site of infection (233, 236)
    b. Attack and kill invading organisms (236)
30. Sketch a specific granule of an eosinophil as it appears in a transmission electron micrograph (238) and label the following:
    a. Unit membrane
    b. Internum
    c. Externum (matrix)
31. List the effects of the following on the number of circulating eosinophils (237):
    a. Parasitic infection
    b. Allergic reaction
    c. Increased corticosteroid production
32. Name the connective tissue cell type most similar to basophils in terms of its staining properties, the content of its granules, and its function (238).
33. Of the 3 sizes of lymphocytes found in the blood, which is the most common (239)?
34. Compare large and small lymphocytes (239–240) in terms of the:
    a. Amount of their cytoplasm
    b. Number of polysomes in their cytoplasm
    c. Amount of heterochromatin in their nuclei
    d. Visibility of their nucleoli
    e. Number of their mitochondria
    f. Size of their Golgi complexes
35. On the basis of function, name the 2 fundamental classes of lymphocytes found in the blood (239–240) and compare them in terms of the:
    a. Type of immunity (humoral or cell-mediated) with which each is primarily associated
    b. Primary or central lymphoid organs in which each type develops in humans
    c. Predominant type found circulating in the blood
36. Name 3 functionally distinguishable types of T lymphocytes (T cells) found in the blood and generally describe the function of each (240).
37. During the rejection of a transplanted heart, which of the T cells named in the answer to question 36 are directly responsible for killing the cardiac muscle cells in the transplant (240, 269)?
38. Are the T cell types named in the answer to question 36 memory cells or effector cells (240, 261–262)?
39. Name the effector cell type into which B lymphocytes differentiate upon antigenic stimulation (240).
40. List the advantages of forming memory cells after the first encounter with an antigen for subsequent encounters with the same antigen (240).
41. What is the name for the diffuse system of cells derived from blood monocytes and found distributed in several tissues and organs? What functional capacity do these monocyte derivatives have in common (241)?
42. Make a schematic drawing of a platelet (243) and label the following:
    a. Hyalomere
    b. Granulomere
    c. Granules
    d. Marginal bundle of microtubules
43. List the contents of the following components of the granulomere (243):
    a. Delta granules (dense bodies)
    b. Alpha granules
    c. Lambda granules
44. Name the component of the endothelial basal lamina and subendothelial connective tissue to which platelets attach during primary aggregation if a gap in the endothelial lining appears (243).
45. The binding of platelets to a damaged vessel wall causes the release of the contents of alpha and delta granules from the attached platelets. What is the effect of the release of these substances on:
    a. Unattached platelets in the blood (243)
    b. The cascade of interactions involved in the formation of fibrin (243)
46. List the components of a blood clot (thrombus) (243). How does this differ from a platelet plug (243)?

47. Once a clot forms, what process helps prevent the clot from completely or partly occluding the vessel lumen until damage to the wall is repaired (243)?

48. The inactive proenzyme plasminogen is synthesized and added to the blood plasma by the liver. State:
   a. How it is converted to its active form (243)
   b. The name and function of its active form (243)
   c. The cells in which the substances that activate plasminogen are synthesized (243)

Multiple-Choice Questions

For questions 12–1 through 12–8, select the single best answer.

12–1. The term that refers to the percentage of packed erythrocytes per unit volume of blood is:
   A. Differential count
   B. Hemoglobin
   C. Hematocrit
   D. Hematopoiesis

12–2. The lifespan of an erythrocyte in the circulation is approximately:
   A. 20 days
   B. 1 year
   C. 5 weeks
   D. 4 months
   E. 8 days

12–3. The predominant form of hemoglobin in humans at birth is:
   A. HbA1
   B. HbA2
   C. HbB
   D. HbS
   E. HbF

12–4. The darker-staining central region of human platelets:
   A. Contains the marginal bundle of microtubules
   B. Contains the platelet nucleus
   C. Is termed the granulomere
   D. Is termed the hyalomere

12–5. The component of plasma responsible for maintaining the osmotic pressure of blood is:
   A. Plasmin
   B. Albumin
   C. Fibrinogen
   D. Gamma globulin
   E. Plasminogen activator

12–6. The biochemical constituent of the erythrocyte cell surface primarily responsible for determining blood type (eg, A, B, AB, O) is:
   A. Carbohydrate
   B. Protein
   C. Lipid
   D. Nucleic acid

12–7. The cell type shown in the electron micrograph in Fig 12–1 is a(n):
   A. Monocyte
   B. Erythrocyte
   C. Basophil
   D. Eosinophil
   E. Lymphocyte

12–8. The cell type shown in the electron micrograph in Fig 12–2 is a(n):
   A. Basophil
   B. Eosinophil

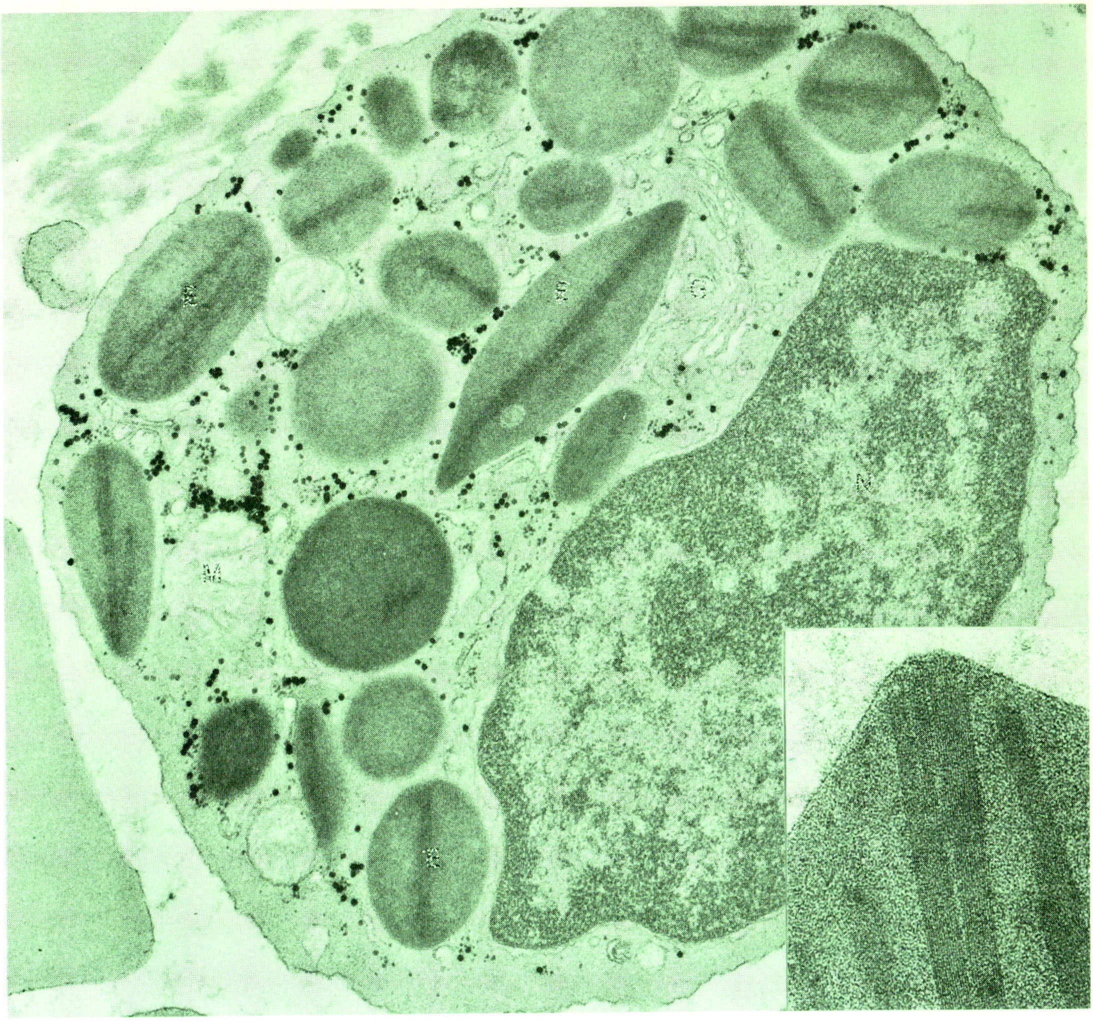

Figure 12-1.

C. Platelet
D. Erythrocyte
E. Neutrophil

MATCHING (questions 12-9 through 12-25): Each choice may be used once, more than once, or not at all. Each question may have more than one correct answer.

A. Lymphocytes
B. Monocytes
C. Eosinophils
D. Basophils
E. Neutrophils
F. All of the above

12-9. Agranulocytes
12-10. Granulocytes
12-11. Mononuclear leukocytes
12-12. Leukocytes
12-13. Least numerous of circulating leukocytes
12-14. Specific granules contain an elongated, electron-dense internum

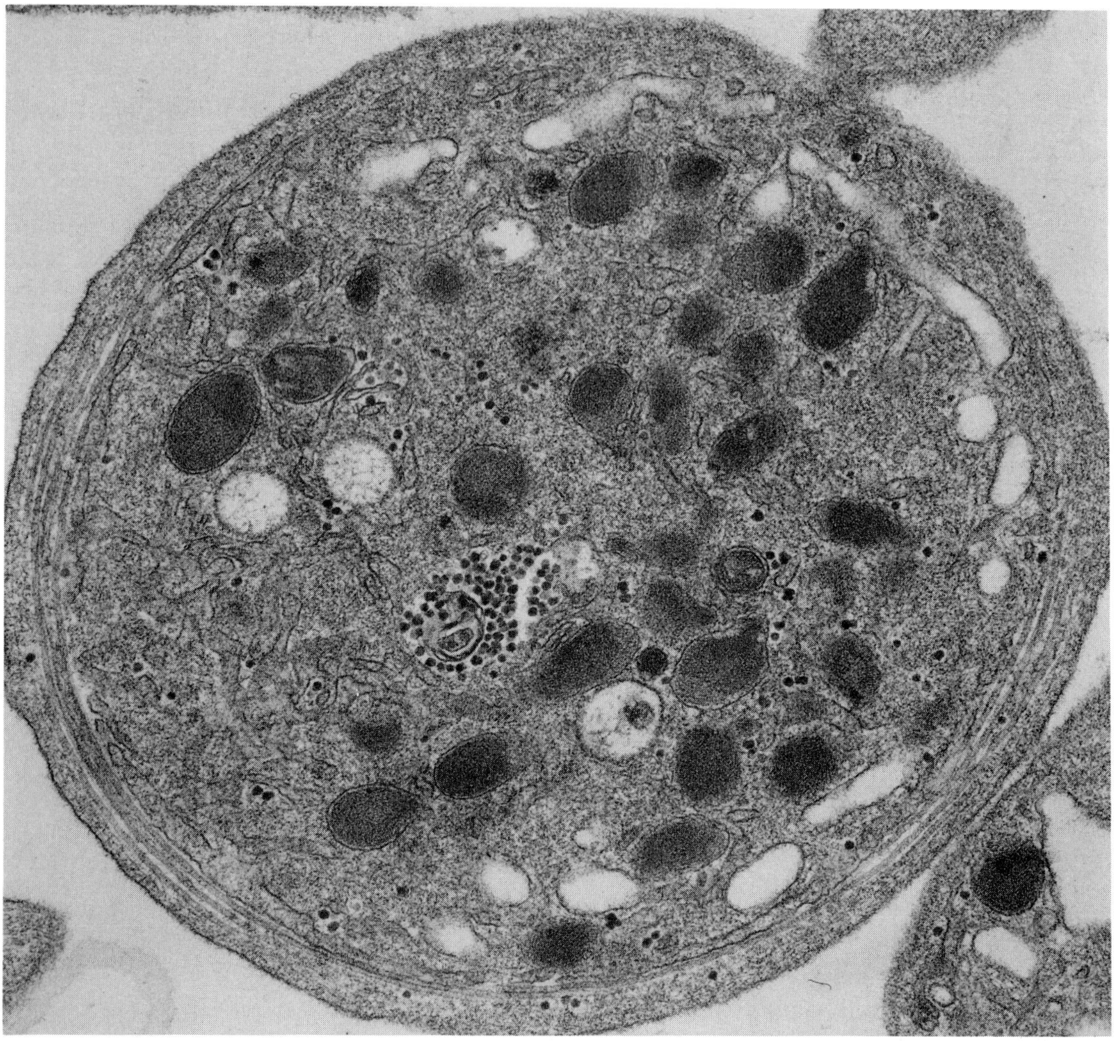

Figure 12-2.

12-15. First line of cellular defense against bacterial invasion
12-16. Found in the buffy coat in a hematocrit tube
12-17. Do not become phagocytic
12-18. Granulocyte type that increases in number in circulation during allergic reactions
12-19. Graft rejection cells
12-20. Precursor cells of the mononuclear phagocyte system
12-21. Most numerous of the circulating leukocytes
12-22. Specific granules contain heparin and histamine
12-23. Granules contain phagocytins
12-24. Capable of diapedesis
12-25. May be found in loose connective tissue

For questions 12-26 through 12-29, either, both, or neither of the answers may be correct. Select

A if only A is correct
B if only B is correct
C if both A and B are correct
D if neither A nor B is correct

Questions 12–26 through 12–29:

A. Plasma
B. Serum
C. Both
D. Neither

12–26. Contains fibrinogen
12–27. Contains albumin
12–28. Contains a higher concentration of serotonin
12–29. Contains immunoglobulins

For questions 12–30 through 12–34, one, more than one, or all of the answers may be correct. Select

A if only (1), (2), and (3) are correct
B if only (1) and (3) are correct
C if only (2) and (4) are correct
D if only (4) is correct
E if all answers are correct

12–30. Which of the following hematocrit values would be considered *abnormal* for an adult human?
(1) 45
(2) 67
(3) 39
(4) 26

12–31. Forms of hemoglobin that may be considered normal in adults include:
(1) HbA1
(2) HbF
(3) HbA2
(4) HbS

12–32. Azurophilic granules may:
(1) Be found in lymphocytes
(2) Be found in neutrophils
(3) Be found in monocytes
(4) Contain lysosomal enzymes

12–33. When the oxygen tension in the blood of patients with sickle cell anemia decreases, as it does at high altitudes, which of the following changes occur?
(1) The hemoglobin in their red blood cells (HbS) crystallizes
(2) Their erythrocytes become less flexible and may become trapped in narrow capillaries
(3) Many erythrocytes lose their normal biconcave shape
(4) Sickled erythrocytes may rupture

12–34. Null cells:
(1) May be circulating hematopoietic stem cells
(2) Are inactive B lymphocytes
(3) Are neither T nor B lymphocytes
(4) Are inactive T lymphocytes

13 Hematopoiesis

Objectives

This chapter should help the student to:

- Describe the structural and functional characteristics of a stem cell.
- Describe in general terms the relationships, similarities, and differences between mature circulating blood cells and hematopoietic stem cells.
- Know the difference between the monophyletic and polyphyletic theories of hematopoiesis.
- Know the general structural characteristics of hematopoietic tissues and describe the changes that occur in bone marrow composition with age.
- Describe the sequence of events in the life of each formed element of blood, from stem cell to death, and know where each event occurs.
- Describe the hormonal control of erythropoiesis.
- Name the 3 overlapping phases of intrauterine hematopoiesis, the sites in the body where each occurs, and any differences in the erythrocytes produced during each phase.
- Recognize the various precursors of mature erythrocytes and granulocytes in photographs or slides of bone marrow. For each cell type, be able to name the cell type of the stage immediately preceding and following.

Synopsis

I. GENERAL FEATURES OF HEMATOPOIESIS. **Hematopoiesis** is the term applied to blood cell production. It includes both the proliferation and the differentiation of hematopoietic stem cells and may be subdivided according to the cell type being formed into erythropoiesis, leukopoiesis, granulopoiesis, agranulopoiesis, lymphopoiesis, and thrombopoiesis (platelet formation).

A. Hematopoietic Stem Cells: These are undifferentiated mesodermal derivatives able to divide repeatedly and differentiate into mature blood cells. The nature and structure of the earliest blood cell precursors is still debatable. There is evidence for a **pluripotent stem cell** type (formerly called a **hemacytoblast**) that can form all blood cell types. Currently, hematopoietic stem cells are called **colony-forming units (CFUs),** because they form colonies of recognizable blood cell types in culture. Pluripotent CFUs were first demonstrated in spleen cell cultures and are called CFU-S. Some CFU-S cells may circulate in a form resembling lymphocytes. The progeny of a dividing CFU-S remain pluripotent or differentiate into one of several **unipotential stem cell** types, which retain their ability to divide but produce only one mature blood cell type each (eg, CFU-E cells form erythrocytes).

B. Theories of Hematopoiesis: The **monophyletic theory** suggests that a pluripotent stem cell (CFU-S) can form all mature blood cell types. The several **polyphyletic theories** suggest that each mature blood cell type is derived from a distinct stem cell.

C. Hematopoietic Tissues: These tissues are collections of CFUs and their progeny at various stages of maturation, suspended in a reticular connective tissue stroma. Active hematopoiesis shifts its location in overlapping stages during development (II.A): It occurs first in the extraembryonic mesoderm of the yolk sac, then in the fetal liver, spleen, and thymus, and finally in the bone marrow and lymphoid tissue.

D. Bone Marrow (III.A): Bone marrow, also called medullary tissue, is the primary hematopoietic tissue from the fifth month of fetal development on. The marrow of all bones begins as active hematopoietic tissue or **red marrow.** During growth, development, and aging, portions of the active red marrow are replaced by adipocytes to form **yellow marrow**. Yellow marrow can be reactivated to red marrow by an increased demand for blood cells (as occurs in chronic hypoxia and hemorrhage). Yellow marrow does not produce blood cells, however, so it is not mentioned in the discussions of hematopoietic tissue in this chapter. Red marrow has a limited distribution in adults. It contains alternating masses of reticular connective tissue **stroma** and the **hematopoietic cords** which contain the CFUs and their progeny. Red marrow also has a rich supply of vascular sinusoids whose walls are interrupted by openings through which maturing blood cells enter the circulation.

E. Blood Cell Lifespan: Blood cells have a limited lifespan in the circulation, owing to the recognition and removal of worn and damaged erythrocytes by macrophages and to the migration of many leukocytes into the surrounding tissues. To keep a constant amount of each blood cell type in circulation, hematopoiesis must occur continuously. If it does not, the result is a decrease in the number of circulating formed elements or **anemia.**

F. Regulation of Hematopoiesis: Regulation involves specific colony-stimulating factors (CSFs) such as erythropoietin, leukopoietin, and thrombopoietin. These hormones act at various steps in hematopoiesis to enhance proliferation and differentiation of CFUs, but except for erythropoietin (VII.A), their nature and actions are not clear.

II. DEVELOPMENT OF HEMATOPOIETIC TISSUES

A. Sites of Intrauterine Hematopoiesis:

1. Primordial (prehepatic) phase During the third week of embryonic development, cell clusters termed **blood islands** form in the extraembryonic mesoderm of the yolk sac, and cells at the periphery of each cluster form the endothelium of the primitive blood vessels. By a process called **megaloblastic erythropoiesis,** cells at the center form the first blood cells, called **primitive erythroblasts.** These differ from erythrocytes of later stages in that they are larger, contain a unique type of hemoglobin, and retain their nuclei. Leukocytes and platelets do not appear until the next phase.

2. Hepatosplenothymic phase: During the second month of development, hematopoiesis shifts to the liver, spleen, and thymus. Hematopoietic stem cells invade these organs and begin producing a wider variety of blood cell types.

a. The liver produces granulocytes, platelets, and red blood cells that may be nucleated (**definitive erythroblasts**) or enucleate (erythrocytes). Hematopoiesis in the liver declines during the fifth month, but continues at low levels until a few weeks after birth.

b. The spleen produces mainly erythrocytes and small numbers of granulocytes and platelets. Just before birth, lymphopoiesis becomes an important splenic function.

c. The thymus produces lymphocytes almost exclusively. Lymphocytes produced in the thymus become T cells and have a variety of specialized functions (Chapters 12, 14).

3. Medullolymphatic (definitive) phase During the third month of development, hematopoiesis begins to shift to the bone marrow and lymphoid tissue, where it remains throughout adulthood.

a. Medullary tissue Medullary tissue (bone marrow) first becomes a functional hematopoietic tissue in the diaphysis of the clavicle, between the second and third months of embryonic development. As other bones ossify, their marrow becomes active. By the fifth month, bone marrow is the primary hematopoietic tissue, producing platelets and all types of blood cells.

b. Lymphatic tissue Additional lymphocytes are formed in the developing lymphoid tissues and organs (eg, thymus, lymph nodes, spleen). Before birth, the lymph nodes may also produce red blood cells.

B. Sites of Postnatal Hematopoiesis: Beginning in infancy, hematopoiesis is restricted to the bone marrow (medullary or myeloid tissue) and the lymphoid tissues.

C. Extramedullary Hematopoiesis in Disease: In adults, the occurrence of erythropoiesis, granulopoiesis, and thrombopoiesis in sites other than the bone marrow is considered abnormal. When bone marrow is unable to meet the continuous demand for new blood cells, the liver, spleen, or lymph nodes may reassume some of their embryonic hematopoietic responsibilities.

III. GENERAL STRUCTURE OF MATURE HEMATOPOIETIC TISSUE.

Mature hematopoietic tissues share a basic architecture supported by a 3-dimensional scaffolding of reticular cells and fibers (stroma) permeated by many sinusoids. The meshwork between the sinusoids contains developing blood cells; as these complete their differentiation, they enter the circulation through openings in the sinusoid walls.

A. Bone Marrow: All bone marrow begins as red marrow, also called **active,** or **hematogenous** marrow. During growth, the blood cells of this active hematopoietic tissue are gradually depleted and replaced by adipocytes. In adults, red marrow is restricted to the skull, vertebrae, ribs, sternum, ilia, and the proximal epiphyses of some long bones. The fatty, nonhematopoietic replacement tissue found in other bony cavities is termed **yellow marrow.** Red bone marrow is composed of interdigitating masses of stroma and hematopoietic cords.

1. Stroma Stroma consists of adipocytes (up to 75% of red marrow), macrophages, and reticular connective tissue composed of **adventitial cells** (reticular cells) and the reticular fibers (type III collagen) they produce. Adventitial cells are highly branched, poorly differentiated mesenchymal derivatives resembling fibroblasts. Their processes separate the developing blood cells from the endothelium of the bone marrow sinusoids.

2. Hematopoietic cords These fill the interstices of the stroma and are crowded with overlapping blood cells of all types and at all stages of differentiation. Abundant sinusoids penetrate the cords and have openings in their walls through which maturing blood cells and platelets enter the circulation. In histologic section, the dense packing of the cells makes the tissue appear disorganized and identification of individual cell types difficult. In some sections, clusters of developing erythrocytes can be seen surrounding macrophages engaged in transferring iron to the maturing cells. Such groupings are called **erythroblastic islands.**

3. Bone marrow smears Differentiating blood cells are most commonly studied in smears. Hematopoiesis is a continuous process, and bone marrow smears contain many cells at stages of differentiation between those given specific names. Students should concentrate on representative examples of the named stages and not attempt to identify every cell in a given smear.

4. Bone marrow functions In addition to being the primary site for hematopoiesis, bone marrow helps destroy old red blood cells. Macrophages in the bone marrow, spleen, and liver break down hemoglobin to form (1) **globin,** which is quickly hydrolyzed; (2) **porphyrin rings,** which are coverted to **bilirubin;** and (3) **iron,** which is complexed with and transported by the plasma protein **transferrin** to the bone marrow for reuse by developing erythrocytes. Iron is stored in bone marrow macrophages as **ferritin** (iron complexed with the protein **apoferritin**) and **hemosiderin.** The latter represents iron (free or complexed with apoferritin) bound to lysosomal enzymes, carbohydrates, and lipids; it is located in cytoplasmic vacuoles termed **siderosomes.** Macrophages transfer iron to developing red blood cells in erythroblastic islands.

B. Lymphoid Tissues and Organs: The thymus, spleen, lymph nodes, and lymphatic aggregations such as the tonsils and Peyer's patches contribute to postnatal hematopoiesis primarily by providing sites for the proliferation, programming, and differentiation of lymphocytes. These organs and tissues are described in Chapter 14.

IV. ERYTHROPOIESIS

A. General: In healthy adults, erythropoiesis (red blood cell formation) occurs exclusively in the bone marrow. Erythrocytes are derived from CFU-Es, which are in turn derived from CFU-Ss. The differentiation of erythrocytes from stem cells is commonly described by naming cell types at specific stages in the process according to their histologic characteristics (IV.B). Cellular changes that occur during erythroid differentiation include (1) decrease in cell size, (2) condensation of nuclear chromatin, (3) decrease in nuclear diameter, (4) accumulation of hemoglobin in the cytoplasm (increased acidophilia), (5) decline in the number of ribosomes in the cytoplasm (decreased basophilia), and (6) ejection of the nucleus.

B. Stages of Erythroid Differentiation: Erythrocyte maturation is commonly divided into 6 stages. Cells at these stages are identified by examining their overall diameter, the size and chromatin pattern of their nuclei, and the staining properties of their cytoplasm. Cells in transition between these stages are commonly found in bone marrow smears. Cell division occurs throughout the early stages, but once cells reach the normoblast stage they generally lose their ability to divide. The following discussion starts with the least mature cells; the sixth stage is the mature erythrocyte, described in Chapter 12.

1. Proerythroblasts are large (14–17 μm in diameter) and contain a large, centrally located, pale-staining nucleus with 1 or 2 large nucleoli. The small amount of cytoplasm (about 20% of cell volume) contains polyribosomes actively involved in hemoglobin synthesis. The resulting cytoplasmic basophilia allows these cells to be distinguished from myeloblasts, with which they are most easily confused. Proerythroblasts are capable of multiple mitoses and may be considered unipotential stem cells.

2. Basophilic erythroblasts are slightly smaller than proerythroblasts, with a diameter of 13–16 μm. They have slightly smaller nuclei with a clock face chromatin pattern. Their nucleoli are difficult to distinguish. The cytoplasm is more intensely basophilic, typically staining a deep royal blue. A prominent, clear, juxtanuclear cytocenter is often visible. Basophilic erythroblasts continue hemoglobin synthesis at a high rate and are capable of mitosis.

3. Polychromatophilic erythroblasts are smaller yet (12–15 μm in diameter), with significant amounts of hemoglobin beginning to accumulate in their cytoplasm. The conflicting staining affinities of the polyribosomes (basophilic) and hemoglobin (acidophilic) give the cytoplasm a grayish appearance. The nucleus is smaller than in less mature cells, with more condensed chromatin that forms a checkerboard pattern. These cells retain the ability to synthesize hemoglobin and to undergo mitosis.

4. Normoblasts (orthochromatophilic erythroblasts) are easily identified because of their small size (8–10 μm in diameter), acidophilic cytoplasm with only traces of basophilia; and small, eccentrically placed nuclei with chromatin so condensed that it appears black. Although early normoblasts may be capable of mitosis, erythroid cells lose their ability to divide during this stage, which ends with the extrusion of the **pyknotic** (degenerated, dead) nucleus.

5. Reticulocytes are difficult to distinguish from mature erythrocytes with standard stains, but when stained with the supravital dye cresyl blue, **residual polyribosomes** form a blue-staining, netlike precipitate in the cytoplasm. Reticulocytes complete their maturation to become erythrocytes (Chapter 12) during their first 24–48 hours in the circulation. This process involves ejection or enzymatic digestion (by ubiquitin) of their remaining organelles and assumption of the biconcave shape.

V. LEUKOPOIESIS.

Leukopoiesis (white blood cell formation) encompasses both granulopoiesis and agranulopoiesis. Leukopoietic CFUs that have been identified include: CFU-GM (forms both granulocytes and macrophages), CFU-G (forms all granulocyte types), CFU-M (forms macrophages), CFU-Eo (forms only eosinophils). All these CFUs with limited capabilities are derived from the pluripotential CFU-S.

A. Granulopoiesis:

1. General–Granulopoiesis occurs in the bone marrow of healthy adults. The three types of granulocytes—neutrophils, basophils, and eosinophils—may all derive from a single precursor (CFU-G). The structural changes occurring in the cells include (1) decrease in cell size, (2) condensation of nuclear chromatin, (3) changes in nuclear shape (flattening → indentation → lobulation: a progression resembling the gradual deflation of a balloon) and (4) accumulation of cytoplasmic granules.

2. Stages of granulocyte differentiation Granulocyte maturation is commonly divided into 6 stages. Cells at these stages are identified by examining their overall diameter; the size, shape, and chromatin pattern in their nuclei; and the type and number of specific granules in their cytoplasm. The specific granules, with their characteristic staining properties, first appear at the myelocyte stage; from this point, the cells are named according to the mature granulocyte type they will form (eg, neutrophilic myelocyte). In the granulocyte series, cell division ceases at the metamyelocyte stage. The following discussion starts with the least mature cells; the sixth stage is the mature granulocyte, discussed in Chapter 12.

a. Myeloblasts, the earliest recognizable granulocyte precursors, are 10–15 μm in diameter. They are difficult to distinguish from other stem cells, because they are morphologically undifferentiated. Each has a large, spherical, euchromatic nucleus with up to 3 smudgy nucleoli. Their cytoplasm is more basophilic than that of their CFU precursors, but less basophilic than that of proerythroblasts, with which they are most often confused.

b. Promyelocytes may be slightly larger than myeloblasts, and their chromatin is slightly more condensed. Their otherwise spheric nuclei are often flattened on one side and may contain nucleoli. Their cytoplasm is more basophilic than that of myeloblasts and contains azurophilic granules that differ from the specific granules (Chapter 12) that appear during the next stage. Since azurophilic granules are synthesized mainly during this stage, their relative number decreases as the cells divide and mature.

c. Myelocytes are large (16–24 μm in diameter). This is the first stage at which sufficient numbers of specific granules accumulate in the cytoplasm to allow one to distinguish the 3 immature granulocyte types—**neutrophilic myelocytes, eosinophilic myelocytes,** and **basophilic myelocytes.** Myelocyte nuclei are kidney-shaped, with more highly condensed chromatin than at previous stages. Like their precursors, myelocytes can divide.

d. Metamyelocytes The 3 types of metamyelocyte—**neutrophilic metamyelocytes, eosinophilic metamyelocytes,** and **basophilic metamyelocytes**—are smaller and more densely packed with specific granules than their respective myelocyte precursors. By this stage the nucleus is deeply indented, often resembling a mask, and its chromatin is more condensed. During this stage, the capacity for mitosis is lost.

e. Band cells The 3 band cell types—**neutrophilic band, eosinophilic band,** and **basophilic band**—have horseshoe-shaped nuclei. Like the reticulocytes of the erythroid series, these nearly mature cells circulate in relatively small numbers (3–5% of the circulating leukocytes), but may appear in larger numbers when granulopoiesis is hyperstimulated. During final maturation, the nuclei undergo further chromatin condensation and lobulation. Mature granulocytes, ie, neutrophils, eosinophils, and basophils are also found in the bone marrow.

B. Agranulopoiesis: Agranulocytes (monocytes and lymphocytes), like the other blood cell types, are derived from CFU-Ss. The morphologic changes these cells undergo during maturation include a decrease in overall cell diameter, a decrease in nuclear diameter, and an increase in nuclear heterochromatin content. However, the morphologic characteristics of agranulocytes at immature stages are much less distinct than those of erythrocytes and granulocytes.

1. Monocytopoiesis The CFU-derivatives that give rise to monocytes are called **monoblasts** and are difficult to identify in bone marrow smears. A product of the monoblast, the **promonocyte,** is only slightly easier to identify and serves as the immediate precursor of monocytes. Promonocytes are larger (10–20 μm in diameter) than monocytes and have pale-staining nuclei and basophilic cytoplasm. The similarity between monocyte precursors and other stem cells in the bone marrow makes definitive identification difficult.

2. Lymphopoiesis In adults, lymphopoiesis occurs mainly in lymphoid tissues and organs and to a lesser extent in bone marrow. Prior to division, the precursor, or **lymphoblast,** is usually much larger than the typical circulating lymphocyte. However, many circulating lymphocytes can respond to antigenic stimulation by blasting (enlarging to assume the typical lymphoblast morphology), indicating that they are dormant stem cells. Some of these cells, called **null cells,** are neither T nor B cells and may represent a circulating form of the CFU-Ss.

VI. THROMBOPOIESIS.

Platelet (thrombocyte) production is carried out in the bone marrow by unusually large cells called **megakaryocytes.** Immature megakaryocytes, called **megakaryoblasts,** are derived from CFU-Megs, which in turn are derived from CFU-Ss. Megakaryoblasts undergo a series of successive incomplete mitoses involving repeated DNA replications without cellular or nuclear division. The result of this process, called **endomitosis,** is a single large megakaryocyte with a large, **polyploid** (up to 64n) nucleus. Maturation involves lobulation of the nucleus and development of an elaborate **demarcation membrane system** that subdivides the peripheral cytoplasm, outlining cytoplasmic fragments destined to become platelets. As the demarcation membranes fuse to form the plasma membranes of the platelets, ribbonlike groups of platelets are shed from the megakaryocyte periphery into the marrow sinusoids to enter the circulation.

VII. COMPARTMENTS AND THE LIFE CYCLE OF BLOOD CELL TYPES

A. Erythrocytes: The total population of mature and developing red blood cells constitutes a widely dispersed but functionally discrete organ called the **erythron,** divisible into 2 compartments. The **circulating compartment** includes all the mature erythrocytes in the circulation (about 2.5×10^{13}). The **medullary compartment** (erythropoietic pool) includes the parts of the bone marrow where erythropoiesis is occurring. Erythrocytes usually leave the bone marrow to enter the circulation as reticulocytes and undergo final maturation within 24–48 hours. Mature erythrocytes circulate for about 120 days before being retired by macrophages (primarily in the spleen, but also in the bone marrow and liver). The iron in the hemoglobin is conserved and eventually returned to the marrow by transferrin. The iron-free portion of hemoglobin is converted by the liver into the bile pigment **bilirubin.** Red cell replacement is controlled by the hormone **erythropoietin,** which stimulates erythrocyte precursors in the bone marrow to proliferate and differentiate. Erythropoietin is produced by unknown cells in the kidney cortex in response to low oxygen tension in the blood. Other factors affecting erythrocyte production and function include iron, intrinsic factor, vitamin B_{12}, and folic acid.

B. Granulocytes: Neutrophils and other granulocytes have life cycles best described in terms of the 4 compartments they occupy. They are continually produced in the bone marrow, and since their numbers remain relatively constant, they must also be continually destroyed. Granulocytes constantly move from the marrow to the circulation to the tissues, where many of them die.

1. The **medullary formation compartment** in the bone marrow includes the stem cells and is the site of granulopoiesis. Cells spend about 7 days in this compartment.

2. The **medullary reserve compartment** in the bone marrow includes newly formed granulocytes that have yet to enter the circulation. Neutrophils remain here for another 4 days.

3. The **circulating compartment** includes mature granulocytes circulating in the blood. The number of cells in the circulating compartment remains relatively constant, even though most granulocytes circulate only for a few hours. When the cell number in this compartment decreases as a result of margination or removal of the cells from the blood (eg, by leukopheresis), granulocyte production in the bone marrow is stimulated to replace the missing cells by an unknown mechanism. This stimulation of bone marrow activity appears to be mediated by an unidentified CSF called **leukopoietin.**

4. The marginating compartment includes cells that have entered the circulation but have attached to the walls of blood vessels, become confined by vasoconstriction in certain capillary beds, or passed through intercellular junctions between endothelial cells to move out of the blood vessels and into the connective tissues, a process called **diapedesis.** Once in the tissues, granulocytes rarely reenter the circulation. However, exchanges between the rest of the marginating compartment and the circulating compartment are normal and occur continuously. The total time spent in the circulating and marginating compartments is about 6 to 7 hours.

C. Lymphocytes: Precursors of both B cells and T cells are produced in the bone marrow. Those destined to become T cells migrate to the thymus, where they are programmed to assume the specialized functions of this lymphocyte class before reentering the circulation and moving to the spleen or lymph nodes for final maturation. Mature T cells return to the circulation and have a lifespan measured in years in humans. Precursors destined to become B cells never enter the thymus but are programmed as B cells in the bone marrow, then distributed to the spleen, lymph nodes, and other lymphatic aggregations to be programmed to respond to specific antigens. B cells have a lifespan of at least 6 weeks in humans. Upon antigenic stimulation they proliferate and differentiate into plasma cells. Lymphopoiesis and lymphocyte function are discussed further in Chapter 14.

D. Monocytes: Monocytes are formed in the bone marrow and remain in circulation for about 2 days before leaving the bloodstream by passing between the endothelial cells in the walls of capillaries and venules. They enter the connective tissues to differentiate into **macrophages** and other mature components of the mononuclear phagocyte system, including the Kupffer cells in the liver and osteoclasts in bone.

E. Platelets: Platelets are formed in the bone marrow, probably in response to increased blood levels of one or more CSFs, tentatively termed **thrombopoietin.** Platelets have a lifespan of about 10 days in the circulation. Other than their involvement in clot formation and the eventual removal of clots by sloughing or phagocytosis, the ultimate fate of platelets is unknown.

Study-Focusing Questions*

1. Describe pluripotent hematopoietic stem cells (245) in terms of:
   a. The 2 names for these cells in scientific nomenclature
   b. Their embryonic germ layer of origin

*The page references in this section refer to *Basic Histology,* 6th ed., Junqueira L, Carneiro J, Kelley R (editors), Appleton & Lange, 1989. **HR** (for Histology Review) is occasionally used instead of a page reference to indicate that the information referred to can be found in this book.

   c. The degree of their differentiation (maturity)
   d. Their ability to produce a variety of cell types
   e. The frequency of their cell divisions
   f. The average percentage of their daughter cells that undergo differentiation (0%, 50%, 100%)
2. Name the 2 types of bone marrow and compare them in terms of:
   a. Their hematopoietic activity (245)
   b. The relative number of adipocytes (245)
   c. The predominant form (in terms of total amount) in infants (245)
   d. The predominant form (in terms of total amount) in adults (246)
   e. The sites in the body where they are found in adults (246)
3. List the structural components of active bone marrow other than the developing blood cells in terms of the:
   a. Cell types present (246)
   b. Type of capillaries present (246)
   c. Type of connective tissue present, including predominant collagen type (118, 246)
4. List the functions of active bone marrow other than hematopoiesis (246–247).
5. List 3 organs that contain macrophages actively involved in the destruction of old red blood cells (246).
6. Name 3 byproducts of the breakdown of hemoglobin and describe the fate of each (246–247).
7. What are the effects of hypoxia and hemorrhage on yellow bone marrow (247)?
8. During the differentiation and maturation of erythrocytic cells, what general changes (increase, decrease, or no change) are observed in the following:
   a. Cell volume and diameter (247)
   b. Nuclear volume and diameter (247)
   c. Amount of heterochromatin in the nucleus (247)
   d. Size and visibility of the nucleoli (247)
   e. Number of polyribosomes in the cytoplasm (247)
   f. Cytoplasmic basophilia (247)
   g. Amount of hemoglobin in the cytoplasm (247)
   h. Cytoplasmic acidophilia (247)
   i. Number of mitochondria in the cytoplasm (247)
9. Beginning with the first recognizable cell type in the erythroid series, list, in order, the names of the 6 stages in the differentiation of erythrocytes (247–249).

   (1)

   (2)

   (3)

   (4)

   (5)

   (6)

10. Return to your list of stages in question 9 and indicate at which stage(s) or between which stages the following events occur:
  a. Cells divide (249)
  b. Intense RNA synthesis takes place (247)
  c. Cytoplasmic basophilia reaches its peak (247)
  d. Hemoglobin synthesis accelerates (247)
  e. First patches of cytoplasmic acidophilia appear and cytoplasm acquires a grayish tinge (248)
  f. Hemoglobin synthesis peaks and begins to decline (249)
  g. Capacity for mitosis is lost (249)
  h. Nucleus is extruded (249)
  i. Protein (hemoglobin) synthesis ceases (249)
  j. Cells leave hematopoietic cords and enter sinusoids (249)
  k. Cell lacks nucleus but retains some ribonucleoprotein that can be precipitated and stained with cresyl blue (249)
  l. Remaining organelles are broken down by nonlysosomal enzymes (233)
  m. Cells are mature (249, 230–233)

11. Describe each of the 6 cell types listed in question 9 (247–249, 230) in terms of their:
  a. Cell diameter
  b. Nuclear morphology (diameter, chromatin pattern, visibility of nucleoli)
  c. Cytoplasmic staining properties

12. Describe 2 ways in which erythrocyte precursors receive iron for complexing with hemoglobin molecules.

13. Describe the erythron (249) in terms of:
  a. Its general functions
  b. Its 2 functional compartments
  c. The approximate number of erythrocytes in the circulation at any time in adults
  d. The average life span of a circulating erythrocyte
  e. The approximate number of erythrocytes produced and destroyed each day

14. Describe the hormone erythropoietin (249–250) in terms of:
  a. Its biochemical composition
  b. Its site(s) of synthesis
  c. The effect of hypoxia on its rate of synthesis and concentration in the blood
  d. Its effect on the rate of mitosis of erythroid progenitor cells
  e. Its effect on the rate of erythroid precursor differentiation
  f. Its effect on the rate of RNA synthesis in erythroid precursor cells
  g. Its effect on the transit time from the medullary to the circulating compartment of the erythron
  h. Its effect on the number of reticulocytes in the circulation

15. List some dietary factors (eg, vitamins and minerals) that are essential to erythropoiesis (250).

16. What is the effect of increased circulating levels of the following hormones on hematocrit values (increase, decrease, no effect):
  a. Thyroxine (250)
  b. Testosterone (250)
  c. Cortisol (250)
  d. Estrogen (250)
  e. Growth hormone (250)

17. Beginning with the first recognizable cell type in the granulocytic series, list, in order, the names of the 6 stages in the differentiation of granulocytes (250–253).
  (1)

  (2)

(3)

(4)

(5)

(6)

18. Return to your list of stages in question 17 and indicate at which stage(s) or between which stages the following events occur:
- **a.** Cells divide (253)
- **b.** Azurophilic granules are formed (253)
- **c.** Azurophilic granules first appear (253)
- **d.** Specific granules appear (253)
- **e.** Neutrophilic, eosinophilic, and basophilic precursors first become distinguishable from one another (253)
- **f.** Capacity for mitosis is lost (253)
- **g.** Cells are mature
- **h.** Cells leave hematopoietic cords and enter sinusoids (253)

19. Describe each of the 6 cells types listed in question 17 in terms of:
- **a.** Their cell diameter (252–253)
- **b.** Their nuclear morphology (shape, chromatin pattern, visibility of nucleoli) (252–253)
- **c.** Their cytoplasmic staining properties (252–253)
- **d.** The types of granules present in each (252–253)

20. Compare azurophilic granules and specific granules in terms of their:
- **a.** Diameter (235, 252–253)
- **b.** Contents (236)
- **c.** Staining properties (235, 252–253)
- **d.** Order of appearance (252)
- **e.** Changing abundance (increase or decrease) in the cytoplasm of granulocytic precursor cells as differentiation and maturation proceed (253)

21. List, in order, the hematologic compartments through which a neutrophil passes from its differentiation to the time it undergoes diapedesis to enter the connective tissue. Indicate the approximate amount of time the cells spend in each compartment and its location (253–255).

22. Compare the neutrophilia (255) that results from exercise (intense muscular activity) and that which results from bacterial infection in terms of the:
- **a.** Source of the neutrophils added to the circulation
- **b.** Duration of neutrophilia

23. A decrease in the number of neutrophils in which compartment serves as a potent stimulus of neutrophilopoiesis (255)

24. Name the sites in the body where the following occur:
- **a.** Lymphoblasts divide to form prolymphocytes (255)
- **b.** Prolymphocytes or their derivatives are programmed to become T lymphocytes (255)
- **c.** Prolymphocytes or their derivatives are programmed to become B lymphocytes (255)

25. List 4 stages in life cycle of monocytes leading to the formation of macrophages and name the sites in the body where cells at each stage may be found (256).

26. Name the cell type that produces platelets (256) and describe it in terms of:
    a. The name of the cell type from which it is derived (256–257)
    b. Its size (257)
    c. The staining properties of its cytoplasm (257)
    d. The shape of its nucleus (257)
    e. The amount of DNA it contains as compared to most other cells (257)
27. How are platelets formed (257)?
28. List, in order, the 3 overlapping stages of intrauterine hematopoiesis and name the sites in the body where hematopoiesis occurs in each stage (257–259).
29. Compare primitive erythroblasts, definitive erythroblasts, and erythrocytes in terms of their size, site of production, and the presence of a nucleus (258).
30. During which of the stages listed in the answer to question 31 are leukocytes first produced (258)?
31. In adults whose bone marrow has become injured, diseased, or destroyed, which organs can help to compensate for the loss by resuming hematopoietic functions (259)?

Multiple-Choice Questions

For questions 13–1 through 13–8, select the single best answer.

13–1. The most widely held theory of hematopoiesis, in which all cell types are believed to be derived from a single pluripotential stem cell, is termed:
- **A.** The polyphyletic theory
- **B.** The medullolymphatic theory
- **C.** The monophyletic theory
- **D.** The monopoietic theory

13–2. The correct order of the phases of intrauterine hematopoiesis is:
- **A.** Hepatosplenothymic, medullolymphatic, primordial
- **B.** Primordial, medullolymphatic, hepatosplenothymic
- **C.** Hepatosplenothymic, primordial, medullolymphatic
- **D.** Primordial, hepatosplenothymic, medullolymphatic

13–3. The component of bone marrow that generally increases in abundance as hematopoietic activity declines is:
- **A.** Hematopoietic cords
- **B.** Sinusoids
- **C.** Adipocytes
- **D.** Stem cells
- **E.** Erythroblastic islands

13–4. In adults, red bone marrow may be found in all of the following *except:*
- **A.** The sternum
- **B.** The vertebrae
- **C.** The tibia
- **D.** The diploe of the skull
- **E.** The ribs

13–5. Which cell type has a nucleus with a checkerboard pattern and grayish-staining cytoplasm due to the presence of roughly equal amounts of basophilic and acidophilic components?
- **A.** Polychromatophilic erythroblast
- **B.** Normoblast (orthochromatophilic erythroblast)
- **C.** Basophilic erythroblast
- **D.** Proerythroblast
- **E.** Reticulocyte

13–6. The dark precipitate formed in reticulocytes upon staining with the vital dye cresyl blue consists mainly of residual:
- **A.** Golgi complexes
- **B.** Nucleoli
- **C.** Smooth endoplasmic reticulum

D. Polyribosomes
E. Nuclear fragments

13–7. An immature neutrophil with a deeply indented, or mask-shaped, nucleus is called a:
A. Neutrophilic myelocyte
B. Neutrophilic metamyelocyte
C. Neutrophilic band
D. Mature neutrophil
E. Promyelocyte

13–8. The cell type depicted in Fig 13–1 is a:
A. Promyelocyte
B. Mature (segmented) neutrophil
C. Band neutrophil
D. Megakaryocyte
E. Hypersegmented neutrophil

MATCHING (questions 13–9 through 13–24): Each choice may be used once, more than once, or not at all.

Questions 13–9 through 13–13:

A. Proerythroblast
B. Reticulocyte
C. Erythrocyte
D. Basophilic erythroblast
E. Polychromatophilic erythroblast
F. Orthochromatophilic erythroblast

13–9. Stage at which cells usually leave bone marrow
13–10. First cell type in series incapable of mitosis
13–11. Also called a normoblast
13–12. Contains a pyknotic nucleus
13–13. Cell type in which nucleoli are most easily visualized

Questions 13–14 through 13–20:

A. Myeloblast
B. Promyelocyte

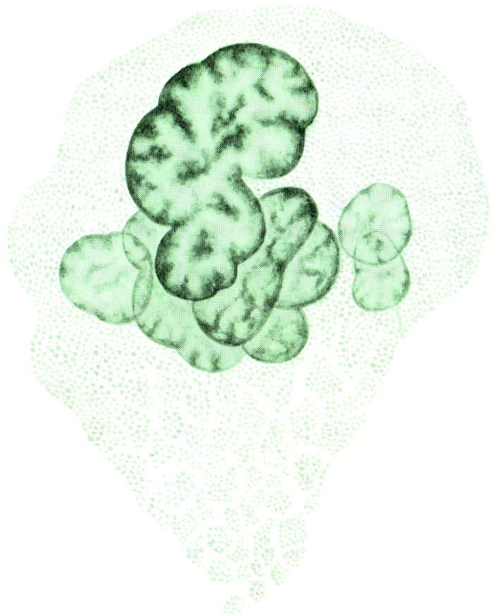

Figure 13–1.

C. Myelocyte
D. Metamyelocyte
E. Band form
F. Mature form

13–14. Earliest stage at which specific granulocyte types can be differentiated from one another
13–15. Earliest recognizable stage of granulopoiesis
13–16. Stage at which azurophilic granules first accumulate
13–17. Stage at which specific granules first accumulate
13–18. Smallest cell type listed
13–19. First cell type in series incapable of mitosis
13–20. Appearance of large numbers of this cell type in the blood is termed a "shift to the left" and may be indicative of a bacterial infection

Questions 13–21 through 13–24:

A. Hemoglobin
B. Transferrin
C. Erythropoietin
D. Bilirubin
E. None of the above

13–21. Waste product of erythrocyte destruction
13–22. Carries iron from the site of erythrocyte destruction to bone marrow for reuse
13–23. Breaks down to yield iron, globin, and a porphyrin ring
13–24. Hormone whose synthesis is stimulated during hypoxia

For questions 13–25 through 13–31, either, both, or neither of the answers may be correct. Select

A if only A is correct
B if only B is correct
C if both A and B are correct
D if neither A nor B is correct

A. Erythrocyte maturation
B. Granulocyte maturation
C. Both
D. Neither

13–25. Overall cell diameter generally decreases
13–26. Overall nuclear size decreases
13–27. Cytoplasmic content of hemoglobin increases
13–28. Nuclear euchromatin content generally increases
13–29. Nucleus is expelled
13–30. Cells eventually lose their capacity for mitosis
13–31. Nucleus becomes increasingly lobulated

For questions 13–32 through 13–37, one, more than one, or all of the answers may be correct. Select

A if only (1), (2), and (3) are correct
B if only (1) and (3) are correct
C if only (2) and (4) are correct
D if only (4) is correct
E if all answers are correct

13–32. In patients whose bone marrow is unable to produce an adequate number of erythrocytes due to disease, which of the following organs may reassume some of their embryonic erythropoietic activity?

(1) Liver
(2) Thymus
(3) Spleen
(4) Kidneys

13–33. Megakaryocytes:
(1) Are multinuclear
(2) Are polyploid
(3) Secrete thrombopoietin
(4) Produce platelets

13–34. Erythrocytes:
(1) Enter the circulation only after becoming fully mature
(2) Undergo mitosis in the circulation in response to erythropoietin
(3) Secrete hemosiderin
(4) Are removed from circulation by macrophages in the spleen and bone marrow after circulating for about 120 days

13–35. General trends that occur during the differentiation of erythroid cells include:
(1) A decrease in cellular diameter
(2) A decrease in nuclear diameter
(3) An increase in the amount of hemoglobin in the cytoplasm
(4) An increase in the number of ribosomes in the cytoplasm

13–36. Once granulocytes have entered the marginating compartment they may:
(1) Enter the connective tissues by passing through capillary walls
(2) Undergo mitosis
(3) Reenter the circulating compartment
(4) Differentiate into tissue macrophages

13–37. Monocytes:
(1) Are derived from precursor cells in the bone marrow that are virtually indistinguishable from early granulocyte precursors
(2) Usually remain in the circulation for several weeks
(3) Contain azurophilic granules that are primary lysosomes
(4) Undergo no further maturation once they leave the bone marrow

Lymphoid System 14

Objectives

This chapter should help the student to:

- Know the functions of the lymphoid system.
- Know the names, locations, and functions of the cells, tissues, and organs of the lymphoid system and be able to identify them, as well as the named structural elements of the organs, on a slide or in a photomicrograph.
- Know the distinguishing features of the lymphoid organs.
- Know the difference between central and peripheral lymphoid organs.
- Know the differences between cell-mediated and humoral immunity.
- Know the structural characteristics of antigens and antibodies.
- Describe the steps in the differentiation of lymphocytes from stem cells to T or B memory and effector cells.
- Know the 5 classes of immunoglobulin and their distinguishing features.
- Describe the steps in lymphocyte activation by antigens.

- Describe the steps in the disposal of antigens by cell-mediated and humoral mechanisms.
- Describe the path taken by lymph as it flows through the lymph nodes.
- Describe the path taken by blood as it flows through the spleen according to the open and closed theories of splenic circulation.

Synopsis

I. GENERAL FEATURES OF THE LYMPHOID SYSTEM

A. Components of the System: The lymphoid system's major functional components, **lymphocytes,** consist principally of 2 widely distributed types, T and B lymphocytes, which circulate in the blood and lymph and are scattered in loose connective tissue. Lymphocytes also occur in clusters called **lymphatic** (or **lymphoid) aggregates.** These can be large and encapsulated, forming lymphoid organs, such as the thymus, spleen, and lymph nodes. They also form smaller, partly encapsulated organs, such as the tonsils. Smaller unencapsulated aggregates often occur in the walls of the respiratory, digestive, and urinary tracts. In addition to lymphocytes, lymphoid tissues typically include a reticular connective tissue stroma in whose meshwork lymphocytes, macrophages, and a variety of antigen-presenting cells are suspended.

B. Classification of Lymphoid Tissues and Organs: These are classed as either central (primary) or peripheral (secondary). In **peripheral lymphoid organs** (lymph nodes, spleen, tonsils, Peyer's patches, other unencapsulated lymphoid aggregates), lymphocyte production is antigen-dependent and provides committed **immunocompetent cells** that respond to specific antigens. In **central lymphoid organs** (thymus, bone marrow, bursa of Fabricius [in birds]), lymphocyte production is antigen-independent and provides a supply of uncommitted T lymphocyte (thymus) or B lymphocyte (bone marrow, bursa) precursors that later move to peripheral organs and tissues. Mounting effective immune responses to new antigens requires ongoing production of uncommitted lymphocytes by the central lymphoid organs.

C. Lymphoid Nodules (Follicles): These are found in all lymphoid aggregates except the thymus. During the production of lymphocytes, the nodules have a dark-staining periphery, or **mantle zone,** that contains tightly packed small lymphocytes. Their lighter-staining cores, or **germinal centers,** contain numerous **immunoblasts (lymphoblasts),** ie, lymphocytes stimulated by antigens to enlarge and proliferate. The lighter staining reflects the increased cytoplasm and decreased nuclear heterochromatin that accompany lymphocyte activation.

D. General Functions of Lymphoid Tissues: All lymphoid tissues and organs produce lymphocytes. Lymph nodes also filter lymph and add antibodies to it, while the spleen filters blood, adds antibodies to it, and removes and destroys old red blood cells. Unencapsulated lymphoid aggregates filter tissue fluid and add antibodies to it. Although the thymus has no significant filtration or antibody-secreting functions, it serves as a site for the proliferation and programming of T lymphocyte precursors. The thymus is also responsible for the secretion of hormones (eg, thymosin, thymopoietin) that promote the development and maintenance of the lymphoid tissues in general and T cells in particular. The functions of the lymphoid system are all directed toward a single objective: antigen disposal. This involves 2 major mechanisms:

1. Cellular (cell-mediated) immunity Activated T lymphocytes differentiate into specialized cell types, some of which contact and kill intruding cells, while others release **lymphokines,** substances that enhance other aspects of the immune response.

2. Humoral immunity Activated B lymphocytes differentiate into plasma cells that secrete the antigen-binding **immunoglobulins (antibodies)** that circulate in the blood and lymph.

E. Immunoglobulins: There are 5 major classes of circulating antibodies, or immunoglobulins (Ig's): IgM, IgA, IgD, IgG, and IgE (easily recalled with the mnemonic MADGE). All are secreted by plasma cells, but each class has distinguishing features (described in detail in II.B). Each Ig binds with great specificity to its antigen to inactivate toxic substances and to mark (**opsonize**) them for removal by macrophages, neutrophils, or eosinophils.

F. Lymphocyte Programming and Activation: This multistep process can be described as follows:

1. Lymphocyte precursors are programmed in the bone marrow or thymus as B or T lymphocytes, respectively;

2. They next move to peripheral organs where each cell is programmed—committed—to respond to a specific antigen. The response is enhanced by concentrating antigens on the surfaces of special **antigen-presenting cells** or the delivery of processed antigens to lymphocytes by macrophages rather than by random lymphocyte-antibody collisions;

3. Contact with an antigen (activation) stimulates lymphocytes to enlarge and form lymphoblasts (blast transformation) that then proliferate (clonal expansion);

4. The products of this division then differentiate into 2 basic cell types: **effector cells,** which begin immediately to dispose of the appropriate antigen (primary immune response), and **memory cells,** which are held in reserve for the next encounter with the antigen (secondary immune response). T lymphocyte derivatives form 3 types of effector cells (helper, suppressor, and cytotoxic T cells), which enter the circulation and search the body for their antigens, providing cellular immunity. B lymphocyte derivatives form only one effector cell type, plasma cells. While these cells usually remain in the tissue or organ where they differentiated, they secrete immunoglobulins into the body fluids, providing humoral immunity; and

5. When the antigen is again encountered, memory cells undergo the same process—blast transformation, clonal expansion, and differentiation—as in the primary response, but more rapidly and effectively than before. This is the secondary response.

G. Antigens: These foreign (nonself) substances are able to elicit an immune response (cellular, humoral, or both). They can be entire cells (eg, bacteria, tumor cells) or large molecules (eg, proteins, polysaccharides, nucleoproteins). Their **antigenicity** is determined by several factors: Larger and more complex (eg, branched or folded) molecules are more potent antigens than are smaller, simpler molecules; proteins are more antigenic than carbohydrates; and lipids are nonantigenic unless complexed with a more potent antigen. An antigen's site of entry into the body can also affect its antigenicity. The specific part of an antigen that elicits the immune response (and to which antibodies bind) is called an **antigenic determinant,** or **epitope,** which can consist of a monosaccharide or as few as 4–6 amino acids. Thus, a bacterium can have many antigenic determinants and elicit many cellular and humoral immune responses.

II. IMMUNOGLOBULINS.

These antibodies (Ig's) are proteins secreted by plasma cells into the body fluids (blood, lymph, tissue fluid, saliva, tears, milk, mucus) in response to stimulation by antigens. They bind with high affinity to the antigenic determinants that stimulated their production and make up most of the gamma globulins of blood plasma.

A. Structure of Immunoglobulins: Students should be familiar with the Y shaped structure common to all Ig's and with the positions of their components.

1. Heavy and light chains Each IgG consists of 2 heavy chains (MW 50,000 each) and 2 light chains (MW 23,000 each). The heavy chains are adjacent and parallel to each other; they are connected by disulfide bonds near the branch point of the Y (hinge region). The smaller light chains are also parallel; they lie lateral to the heavy chains and are located in the arms of the Y. Each is attached to its adjacent heavy chain by a disulfide bond near the hinge region.

2. Constant and variable domains Each chain (whether heavy or light) includes both a region of constant structure that varies little from one IgG to another and a region of variable structure that determines the binding specificity of the antibody. The variable domains are at the distal ends of the arms, while the constant regions are in the stem and proximal portions of the arms.

3. Fc and Fab regions The proteolytic enzyme papain cleaves the Ig into 3 fragments at its hinge region. There is one Fc (fragment crystallizable; stem) region that includes a part of the constant domain and binds to the cell surface of macrophages and mast cells. There are also 2 Fab (fragments, antigen-binding; arms) regions that include the entire light chain and variable portions of both light and heavy chains. These fragments retain the antigen-binding specificity of the original Ig.

4. Carboxy and amino termini The carboxy termini of the heavy chains are found at the base of the stem; the carboxy terminus for the light chains is found toward the hinge region of the arms. The amino termini for both light and heavy chains are at the free ends of the arms.

5. Antigen-binding region The amino terminal region of the variable portion at the end of each arm of the Y constitutes the specific antigen-binding region of each Ig molecule.

6. Disulfide bonds While interchain disulfide bonds link heavy chains to each other and light to heavy chains in the hinge region, intrachain disulfide bonds also occur at various sites along both light and heavy chains.

B. Characteristics of Immunoglobulins: Human immunoglobulins are divided into 5 major groups:

1. IgG The most abundant type in blood, constituting 75% of serum Ig, IgG occurs primarily as a monomer. It is produced more slowly than IgM and is slightly less effective in complement activation, but it shows greater antigen-binding specificity. It constitutes most of the secondary humoral immune response and can remain active in blood for many weeks (6 times as long as IgM). IgG is the only immunoglobulin that crosses the placenta to confer passive immunity on the fetus; it is also found in human milk.

2. IgA The secretory antibody, this is the main Ig in body secretions (saliva, tears, mucus, colostrum, semen, vaginal fluid), but constitutes only 0.2% of serum Ig. Secretory IgA comprises 2 IgA monomers that are linked by a polypeptide called **protein J** and combined with another protein, the **secretory,** or **transport, component.** The IgA monomers and protein J are plasma cell products, the transport component is produced by mucosal epithelial cells.

3. IgM This Ig constitutes only 10% of the serum Ig, but it is the major immunoglobulin in the primary immune response. Secreted soon after a new antigenic challenge, IgM is less antigen-specific than IgG. It is found, along with IgD, on the surface of B lymphocytes. When antigen binds to these surface antibodies, B cells differentiate into plasma cells. IgM is effective in complement activation (11.C.2); it usually occurs as a pentamer.

4. IgE Normally occurring as a monomer, IgE is present in very small amounts in serum. Its Fc portion binds with high avidity to cell surface receptors on mast cells and basophils, leaving its antigen-binding sites extending away from the cell surface. The binding of antigens to IgE cross-links the receptors and stimulates the release of such substances as histamine, heparin, leukotrienes (including slow-reacting substance of anaphylaxis [SRS-A]) and eosinophil chemotactic factor of anaphylaxis (ECF-A) from the cytoplasmic granules. Antigens that bind to IgE or stimulate its production are termed **allergens,** and IgE thus plays a major role in **allergic reactions.** Elevated levels of IgE are also found in the blood of patients infested with parasites.

5. IgD This is the least understood of the immunoglobulins. Its concentration in plasma is low—only 0.2% of serum Ig. It is found on the surface of B lymphocytes along with IgM, IgD is thought by some to function as an embryonic or fetal type of Ig.

C. General Mechanisms of Immunoglobulin Action

1. Opsonization Foreign cells and molecules that have been bound by antibodies are more easily recognized as intruders by the antigen-disposing cells (macrophages, cytotoxic T cells, neutrophils, eosinophils). Antibody-labeled intruders are thus opsonized (marked for phagocytosis or destruction). IgG, IgM, and certain components of the complement system act as **opsonins.**

2. Complement activation The complement system is a complex group of plasma enzymes that catalyze a cascade of enzymatic interactions when activated (both IgG and IgM can initiate the interactions). Biologic effects of complement activation include (1) increased blood flow to the affected area (inflammation); (2) **chemotaxis** of the inflammatory cells (eosinophils, basophils, neutrophils, cytotoxic T cells); (3) opsonization; and (4) lysis of the invading cells (ie, components of the system act together to puncture the invading cell's plasma membrane).

3. Formation of antigen-antibody complexes Antigenic molecules in body fluids precipitate out when antibodies bind to them. In the process, the antigens may be inactivated; ie, their toxicity is decreased or eliminated. These antigen-antibody complexes are then phagocytosed by macrophages, neutrophils, or eosinophils.

III. CELLS OF THE LYMPHOID SYSTEM

A. Lymphocytes: These are the principal cells of the lymphoid system. Although their ability to recognize and respond to foreign (nonself) cells and substances is the basis for initiating an immune response, lymphocytes are not phagocytic. The 2 functional classes of lymphocytes (B and T lymphocytes) differ in cell-surface composition and in their response to antigenic challenges, but they are indistinguishable with standard histologic stains. (The appearance of lymphocytes in connective tissue and in the blood is described in Chapters 5 and 12 respectively, and the origin of lymphocyte precursors in bone marrow is described in Chapter 13.) Bone marrow-derived precursors enter the circulation and then populate other lymphoid organs. Those in the thymus become T lymphocytes. Although the precise B lymphocyte-programming site (called the bursa equivalent or bursa analogue in humans) is unclear, evidence favors specific microenvironments in bone marrow.

1. B lymphocytes (B cells) These cells, which are primarily responsible for humoral immunity (I.D.2), carry IgM and IgD on their membranes as receptors for specific antigens. When antigens bind to these antibodies, B lymphocytes undergo blast transformation and clonal expansion (I.F). Most of the resulting daughter cells differentiate into **plasma cells** (III.C), while others become memory cells that react to the same antigen in subsequent encounters. B cells require assistance from helper T cells to respond to many antigens; these antigens are called **T-dependent (thymus-dependent) antigens.**

2. T lymphocytes (T cells) Primarily responsible for cell-mediated immunity (I.D.1), T cells carry antibodylike antigen receptors (but not Ig's) on their surfaces. When antigens bind to these receptors, T lymphocytes undergo blast transformation and proliferation and produce both effector and memory cells (I.F); they may require the aid of macrophages for an optimal response. There are 3 major types of T lymphocyte effector cells: (1) **Helper T cells** aid B lymphocytes in mounting a humoral immune response to T-dependent antigens; (2) **suppressor T cells** moderate helper cell activity, thereby helping to regulate humoral immune responses; (3) cytotoxic (killer) T cells recognize, surround, adhere to, and kill—by cell lysis—invading bacteria, virus-infected cells, and tumor cells. Antigen-stimulated T cells and macrophages also release lymphokines, the proteins (eg, blastogenic factor, migration-inhibiting factor, proliferation-inhibiting factor) that control B and T cell proliferation and macrophage activity. T lymphocyte precursors programmed in the thymus enter the circulation and populate T-dependent regions of the lymph nodes (paracortical area) and spleen (periarterial lymphatic sheaths). T lymphocyte effector cells reenter the circulation more readily than do B lymphocyte effector cells (plasma cells).

B. Macrophages: These are commonly monocyte derivatives, ie, components of the mononuclear phagocyte system (the morphologic characteristics of these large, often migratory phagocytic cells are described in Chapter 5). They participate in both cellular and humoral immunity, phagocytosing antigens and enhancing their antigenicity by developing a number of antigenic determinants from a single antigen. They also phagocytose antigen-antibody complexes. Macrophages interact with T lymphocytes primarily through direct cell contact. The T cells thus activated differentiate into T lymphocyte effector cells (for cellular immunity). Activated helper T cells cooperate with B cells to stimulate their differentiation into immunoglobulin-secreting plasma cells (for humoral immunity). Macrophages are found lining sinuses, distributed among the lymphocytes of lymphoid organs and tissues and dispersed in loose connective tissues.

C. Plasma Cells: These differentiated B lymphocyte effector cells secrete the Ig's primarily responsible for humoral immunity. (Their morphologic characteristics, including a ''clock face'' nucleus and the abundant rough endoplasmic reticulum (RER) typical of protein-secreting cells, are described in Chapter 5.) Plasma cells, found in all lymphoid tissues and organs except the thymus, occur in higher concentrations in the medullary cords of lymph nodes, the red-pulp cords in the spleen, and the lamina propria underlying mucosal and glandular epithelia. Each plasma cell secretes only one class of antibody that will bind to a single antigenic determinant.

D. Reticular Cells: Usually stellate, these cells have long cell processes that form a meshwork within which lymphocytes, plasma cells, and other tissue components are suspended. Lymphoid organs contain 2 major types of reticular cells:

1. Reticular cells of the lymph nodes, spleen, tonsils, and bone marrow are of mesodermal origin. Each has a central nucleus with a prominent nucleolus and pale, sparse cytoplasm that contains RER, a Golgi complex, free ribosomes, lysosomes, and glycogen granules. They produce a network of reticular fibers (see Chapter 5) upon which they are suspended and which they partially surround with their long filopodia. Other functions ascribed to these cells and their derivatives include: (1) Phagocytosing antigenic organisms, inert foreign matter, dead cells, and cell debris; (2) trapping antigens on their surfaces and subsequently stimulating adjacent B lymphocytes (causing them to differentiate into plasma cells); and (3) acting as hematopoietic (lymphoid and myeloid) stem cells.

2. Reticular cells of the thymus (epithelial-reticular cells) are of endodermal origin (the lining of the third pharyngeal pouch). Like the mesoderm-derived reticular cells, these cells may assume a stellate shape, but they differ in that they do not secrete reticular fibers. They form their reticular meshwork by attaching to one another at the tips of their long cell processes with **desmosomes.** The cells have large, pale, oval nuclei with prominent nucleoli; the cytoplasm contains a Golgi complex, RER, and ribosomes. They also contain small (0.1 μm) dense granules thought to be secretory granules that contain thymic hormones (eg, serum thymic factor, thymic humoral factor, thymopoietin, thymosin). In the thymic medulla, these cells assume many shapes; some become flattened to form tight concentric bodies called **Hassall's corpuscles.** In the cortex, they contribute to the formation of the **blood-thymus barrier** (VI.A.2.b).

E. Antigen-Presenting Cells: These cells bind antigen-antibody complexes on their surfaces for long periods of time without phagocytosing them. In this way, they collect and concentrate antigens for presentation to and stimulation of lymphocytes. Many of these cells derive from reticular cells. Antigen-presenting cells appear in the lymph nodes as **follicular**

dendritic cells of the cortex and **dendritic cells** of the paracortical zone; in the spleen, they are the dendritic cells of the marginal zone; in the skin (see Chapter 18), they are **Langerhans' cells;** and in the liver (see Chapter 16), they are **Kupffer's cells.** While macrophages (III.B) also have important antigen-presenting functions, their first task is usually the phagocytosis of the antigenic material.

IV. LYMPHOID NODULES.

These spheric collections of lymphocytes constitute the primary functional subunits of all encapsulated and unencapsulated lymphoid aggregates except the thymus. While B lymphocytes predominate, smaller numbers of helper T cells may also be present. Lymphoid nodules are commonly divided into 2 classes:

A. Primary Nodules:

Containing only small lymphocytes, primary lymphoid nodules are present prenatally and in the absence of antigens (eg, in animals housed in sterile surroundings). Primary nodules, which lack a germinal center, become secondary nodules on exposure to antigens.

B. Secondary Nodules:

These nodules, which appear after birth, are primary nodules that have been activated by exposure to antigens; their size and number are proportional to the amount of antigenic stimulation. They occur in the same sites as the primary nodules. Structurally, the nodule is characterized by a narrow, dark-staining peripheral halo of small lymphocytes surrounding a larger, lighter-staining **germinal center** that contains mainly lymphoblasts. The dark periphery often shows a **cap,** a localized crescent-shaped thickening. The size of the germinal center gradually decreases when antigenic stimuli are removed, and the nodules eventually assume a form more like that of a primary nodule. Although thin sections through a cap or periphery of an active secondary nodule may resemble primary nodules, the presence of primary nodules is doubtful if nearby nodules contain germinal centers.

V. UNENCAPSULATED LYMPHATIC AGGREGATES.

These aggregations consist of lymphoid nodules that occur singly or in small clusters. The classic example of these structures is **Peyer's patches,** clusters of lymphoid nodules that are found in the lamina propria of the small intestine (ileum; see Chapter 15). Nodule clusters also occur in the appendix, and there are scattered solitary nodules beneath the epithelium in the walls of the digestive, respiratory, urinary, and genital passageways. These occur especially at branch-points and the sites at which one organ joins another (eg, esophageal cardiac-stomach junction, recto-anal junction). While lacking the connective tissue capsule that surrounds lymphoid organs, nodules may be covered by a layer of flattened reticular cells.

VI. MAJOR LYMPHOID ORGANS (Thymus, Lymph Nodes, & Spleen)

A. Thymus:

Several features of this organ make it unique among lymphoid organs. It is the only discrete primary lymphoid organ in humans. It produces only T lymphocyte precursors. Unlike the secondary lymphoid tissues and organs, the thymus has neither lymphoid nodules nor plasma cells. Its reticular cells derive from endoderm, not mesoderm, and produce no reticular fibers. The thymus is the only organ that contains **Hassall's corpuscles.** The age-dependent structural atrophy of the thymus, **involution** (discussed below) is also unique among lymphoid organs.

1. Structural features The thymus is found in the mediastinum anterior to the large vessels emerging from the heart. Its 2 lobes are connected and covered by a thin loose-connective-tissue **capsule** that penetrates the parenchyma of each lobe as septa. These divide each lobe into several incomplete lobules. Each lobule has a peripheral dark-staining **cortex** adjacent to the capsule and septa, and a central light-staining **medulla.** The septa penetrate only to the cortico-medullary junction, so that the medulla of each lobule is continuous with that of adjacent lobules.

a. Cortex This is the dark-staining periphery of each lobule. While small lymphocytes predominate, large and medium-sized lymphocytes are also present. The dark color reflects the tight packing of lymphocyte nuclei, which are suspended in a meshwork of elongated epithelial reticular cell processes. The reticular cells, which are stellate and less numerous than in the medulla, form a boundary between the cortex and the connective tissue of the capsule and septa. They also ensheathe the cortical capillaries, the only blood vessels found in the cortex. The cortex is the site of active thymic lymphocyte production and the blood-thymus barrier.

b. Medulla Found at the core of each lobule, the medulla connects adjacent lobules. In effect, each lobe has a single medulla that extends into the core of each of the lobules. The medulla's light staining reflects the presence of more epithelial reticular cells and fewer lymphocytes than are found in the cortex. The medullary reticular cells assume many shapes and sizes; some have granules containing thymic hormones. The lymphocytes, which are more mature than in the cortex, enter the circulation from the medulla to populate the T-dependent areas of other lymphoid organs. The spheric **Hassall's corpuscles,** which range from 30 to 150 μm in diameter, are composed of concentric layers of flattened epithelial reticular cells. With age, cells in the core of the corpuscles may die and become calcified; the function of these structures is unknown.

2. Functional features

a. T lymphocyte production This is the primary function of the thymus, and T lymphocyte precursors populate the thymic cortex. The cortical environment influences these thymic lymphocytes, or **thymocytes,** to proliferate extensively and to acquire the ability to become T lymphocytes. For reasons that are not known, some cortical thymocytes die and are phagocytosed by local macrophages. As the survivors mature, they move toward the medulla, where they enter the circulation through postcapillary venules or efferent lymphatic vessels. They populate the thymus-dependent regions of secondary lymphoid organs, eg, the lymph nodes and spleen. Here, the thymocytes further differentiate into functional T lymphocytes. The vast majority of thymocytes are functionally inert and cannot respond to antigenic stimulation. Therefore, thymocytes—especially those in the thymic cortex—should be considered as distinct from, but precursors to, the T lymphocytes outside the thymus that carry out the cellular immune response.

b. Blood supply and blood-thymus barrier The arterial supply enters the thymus through the capsule, penetrating the organ through the septa. Branches of septal vessels extend along the border between the cortex and medulla, fedding capillaries that penetrate both the cortex and medulla. The cortical capillaries arch through the cortex and empty into **postcapillary venules** in the medulla, as do the medullary capillaries. The venous drainage of the organ follows the arterial route in reverse. The thymus contains continuous (nonfenestrated) capillaries surrounded by a thick basal lamina. In the cortex, processes of the capillary endothelial cells may penetrate the basal lamina and contact processes of the epithelial reticular cells that ensheathe the cortical capillaries. This 3-layered structure (nonfenestrated capillary endothelium, thick basal lamina, and reticular cell sheath) forms what is termed the blood-thymus barrier. This barrier, which occurs only in the cortex, separates proliferating thymocytes from the blood. Together with the disposition of the blood vessels (which directs the blood flow toward the medulla and away from the cortex), the barrier helps reduce the amount of antigenic material to which the thymocytes are exposed before they leave the thymus. This helps maintain a supply of stem cells for later programming during encounters with new antigens.

c. Hormone production Epithelial reticular cells of the thymic medulla have cytoplasmic granules thought to contain certain thymic hormones (eg, **thymopoietin, thymosin**). These humoral factors have a trophic effect on the entire lymphoid system and promote thymocyte proliferation and T cell differentiation.

d. Effects of exogenous hormones Adrenocorticosteroids and ACTH diminish thymocyte proliferation and reduce the thickness of the thymic cortex. Androgens and estrogens accelerate thymic involution; castration has the opposite effect. Growth hormone stimulates thymic growth in general.

e. Effects of thymectomy Destruction or removal of the thymus at birth results in complete failure of T lymphocyte production. It reduces the number of circulating lymphocytes, and T-dependent regions of the spleen and lymph nodes remain unpopulated. There is no cell-mediated immune response—and consequently, no delayed hypersensitivity or graft rejection. Neither is there any T-dependent humoral immune response, and the lack of thymic hormones causes general atrophy of other lymphoid organs. By 3–4 months after postnatal thymectomy, the animal becomes weaker; it loses weight and finally dies. Thymectomy in adults has less dramatic effects because many thymocytes have already left the thymus. Functional T lymphocytes are already distributed in the tissues and T-dependent regions of the secondary lymphoid organs. The number of circulating lymphocytes is reduced, however, and response to new and unusual antigens may be compromised. At any age, grafting thymic tissue into thymectomized animals reverses the effects of thymectomy. The graft is repopulated with thymocyte precursors from the host bone marrow, and thymic function is restored.

f. Histogenesis and involution The thymus arises from the ventral portion of the paired third pharyngeal pouch, whose endodermal lining gives rise to the epithelial reticular cells. After the sixth week of gestation, the thymic rudiments detach from the pharyngeal wall and migrate to the mediastinum, where they partially fuse to form the 2 lobes of the thymus. The thymus is populated by hematopoietic stem cells from the yolk sac, liver, and bone marrow during the primordial, hepatosplenothymic, and medullary phases of hematopoiesis, respectively; the stem cells divide and fill the thymic cortex with thymocytes. Although the thymus increases in size until puberty, it reaches its maximum size (relative to body weight) shortly after birth. At puberty, the process of involution begins. The cortex gradually thins as the rate of thymocyte proliferation slows and more cells leave the thymus. The relative area of the medulla increases, and the Hassall's corpuscles enlarge, sometimes becoming calcified. Even in adults, the thymus can produce large numbers of thymocytes when needed. In the elderly, much of the active thymic tissue is replaced by connective and adipose tissue.

B. Lymph Nodes: These are the smallest, but most numerous encapsulated lymphoid organs. Scattered in groups along lymphatic vessels, they act as inline filters of the lymph, removing antigens and cellular debris and adding immunoglobulins.

1. Structural features Lymph nodes are bean-shaped structures with both convex and concave surfaces. The parenchyma consists of a peripheral cortex, adjacent to the convex surface, and a central medulla lying near the depression (hilum) in the concave surface. The connective tissue capsule that covers the node's surface gives off **trabeculae** that penetrate between the cortical nodules and subdivide the cortex. Blood vessels enter and leave through the hilum.

a. Cortex In active lymph nodes, the cortex is dark-staining because of the presence of tightly packed lymphocytes. These are suspended in a reticular connective tissue network and arranged as a layer of typical secondary lymphoid nodules (containing primarily B lymphocytes) with germinal centers. The cortex also contains reticular cells, antigen-presenting follicular dendritic cells, macrophages, a few plasma cells, and some helper T cells.

b. Medulla Lighter staining than the cortex, the medulla is composed of cords of lymphoid tissue **(medullary cords)** separated by **medullary sinuses.** The lymphocytes are mainly small, less numerous than in the cortex, and concentrated in the cords. The cords are also rich in reticular cells and fibers and contain many plasma cells that have migrated from the cortex.

c. Paracortical zone This is the T-dependent region, lying between the cortical lymphoid nodules and the medulla. It contains mainly T-lymphocytes suspended in a reticular connective tissue network. B lymphocytes, plasma cells, macrophages, and antigen-presenting interdigitating dendritic cells may also be present. This zone is also characterized by the presence of many **high-endothelial postcapillary venules.** T lymphocytes leave the blood to enter the paracortical zone by passing between the cuboidal endothelial cells of these vessels.

d. Lymphatic vessels Lymphatic vessels associated with lymph nodes are of 2 types. Both contain valves to ensure a unidirectional flow of lymph through the node. **Afferent**

lymphatic vessels deliver lymph by penetrating the capsule at several points on the node's convex surface. **Efferent lymphatic vessels** carry filtered lymph away from the node, exiting through the hilum on the concave surface.

e. Sinuses The sinuses of the lymph nodes filter the lymph passing through them and direct its flow. Partly lined by reticular cells and many macrophages, they are not simply open spaces, but are traversed by a meshwork of reticular cells and fibers, macrophages, and follicular dendritic cells. The complex seiving action slows lymph flow to facilitate the removal of antigens. Lymph is delivered by the afferent vessels to the cuplike **subcapsular sinus** between the capsule and cortical parenchyma. From here it passes directly into the **peritrabecular sinuses** on either side of the trabeculae. It then flows through the anastomotic network of **medullary sinuses** that converge on the efferent lymphatic vessels exiting through the hilum.

2. Functional features

a. Filtration of lymph Cellular debris and antigens carried by incoming lymph are removed by the macrophages and follicular dendritic cells of the sinuses (similar cells are found in the cortical nodules and medullary cords). The lymphocytes carried by the lymph may flow through the nodes, contacting antigen-presenting cells and macrophages in the sinuses, they may instead leave the sinuses and enter the parenchyma. By the time the lymph reaches the efferent lymphatic vessels, more than 90% of the antigens and cellular debris have been removed. More than 99% of the lymph remains in the sinuses as it passes through the nodes.

b. Lymphopoiesis

(1) T lymphocytes Stimulated by antigens removed from the lymph, these cells undergo blast transformation and clonal expansion, then differentiate into effector and memory cells that recognize and respond to the specific antigen. T lymphocyte effector cells may leave the paracortical zone to seek and destroy the antigen, entering the sinuses and leaving the node through efferent vessels. The cells typically reenter the blood at the point where the lymphatic vascular system empties into the venous system.

(2) B lymphocytes Similarly stimulated, B lymphocytes typically move to the germinal centers of cortical nodules to undergo the blast transformation and clonal expansion that yield memory and effector (plasma) cells. Differentiated plasma cells migrate to the medullary cords (where they occur in large numbers). Memory B lymphocytes either return to the nodule's peripheral mantle zone or leave the node by migrating into the sinuses.

c. Immunoglobulin production Most plasma cells remain in the medullary cords, secreting immunoglobulins into the lymph as it passes through the medullary sinuses and exits through the efferent lymphatic vessels. These immunoglobulins reach the blood as the lymph empties into the venous system in the neck.

C. Spleen: The largest of the lymphoid organs, the spleen's functions include lymphopoiesis, immunoglobulin production, and filtering the blood for cellular debris and antigens. Because it serves as the immunologic filter of the blood, its blood supply and circulation are especially important. Unlike other lymphoid organs, the spleen lacks a definitive cortex and medulla. The parenchyma (splenic pulp) lacks true lobules; however, the dense connective tissue capsule gives rise to trabeculae that divide the splenic pulp into incomplete compartments.

1. Structural features

a. Splenic pulp This is composed of many erythrocytes, leukocytes, and macrophages, as well as a variety of blood vessels, all suspended within a supporting meshwork of reticular cells and fibers. Unstained slices of splenic pulp exhibit numerous whitish islands of lymphoid tissue (white pulp) embedded in a sea of dark red erythrocyte-rich tissue (red pulp).

(1) White pulp Consisting of the lymphoid tissue surrounding each of many **central arteries,** the white pulp has 2 major components. The sleeves of lymphoid tissue immediately surrounding each central artery are called **periarterial lymphatic sheaths (PALS).**

These contain mainly T lymphocytes and constitute the thymus-dependent zones of the spleen. Surrounding each PALS or appended to one of its sides is the second component, the **peripheral white pulp** (PWP). PWP contains mainly B lymphocytes and usually includes a typical secondary lymphoid nodule.

(2) Red pulp This makes up most of the spleen and also has 2 major components: the red pulp cords and the splenic sinusoids that lie between them.

(a) Red pulp cords (Billroth's cords) Irregular sheets of reticular connective tissue, these cords branch and anastomose to surround the sinuses. They vary in thickness according to the distention of the adjacent sinusoids. In addition to reticular cells and fibers, the cords contain many cell types, including all the formed elements of blood, dendritic cells, macrophages, plasma cells, and lymphocytes.

(b) Splenic sinusoids These differ from common capillaries; the lumen is wider and more irregular; there are 2–3 μm spaces between the lining endothelial cells and a sparse, discontinuous basal lamina that is composed largely of reticular fibers arranged in bands that run roughly perpendicular to the length of the vessel. The overall arrangement resembles a barrel, with the endothelial cells (elongated on the sinusoid's long axis) as the wooden staves and the bands of the basal lamina as the hoops. The slitlike spaces between the endothelial cells permit extensive exchange of fluids, solutes, and flexible cells between the sinusoids and cords. Macrophages in the cords extend their processes through the slits and phagocytose material in the sinusoid lumen.

(3) Marginal zone Forming the border between white and red pulp, this zone consists of a moatlike arrangement of blood sinuses and loose lymphoid tissue containing few lymphocytes. Blood-borne antigens delivered to the **marginal sinuses** are phagocytosed by the many macrophages and trapped by interdigitating dendritic cells in the zone. Its rich blood supply, cellular composition, and location next to the white pulp make the marginal zone important in concentrating blood-borne antigens for presentation to the spleen's lymphocytes.

b. Splenic circulation

(1) Arterial supply The spleen receives blood from the **splenic artery** (a branch of the celiac trunk of the aorta). Near the hilum, the splenic artery branches into a series of **trabecular arteries.** These enter the spleen through the trabeculae and branch to enter the parenchyma as the numerous central arteries around which the white pulp is organized. After passing through the white pulp, the arteries give rise to many **penicillar arterioles,** which in turn give rise to many capillaries and sheathed arterioles. Near their termination, the sheathed arterioles have localized wall thickenings that consist of macrophages. Many of the capillaries arising from the central artery loop back toward the white pulp to feed the marginal sinuses. Others, including those arising from the penicillar and sheathed arterioles, feed the sinusoids of the red pulp.

(2) Open and closed theories of splenic circulation The way in which blood in the splenic capillaries reaches the sinusoid lumens is not clear. The **closed theory** of circulation holds that the capillary walls are continuous with the walls of the sinusoids and the capillaries empty directly into the sinusoid lumens. The **open theory** holds that the capillaries end abruptly in the red pulp cords and that blood reaches the sinusoid lumens by percolating through the cords and passing through openings in the sinusoid walls. For humans, current evidence favors the open theory.

(3) Venous drainage From the sinusoids, blood flows into red pulp veins that converge on the trabeculae and empty into trabecular veins; these are unusual in that their walls lack a distinct tunica media. The trabecular veins exit the spleen through the hilum, emptying into the **splenic vein,** which joins the inferior mesenteric vein and empties into the hepatic portal vein just before it enters the liver.

2. Functional features

a. Filtration of blood The removal of antigenic material and cellular debris involves several aspects of splenic structure and function. Antigens carried by capillaries to the marginal sinuses are removed by macrophages and dendritic cells; they are concentrated and processed for presentation to lymphocytes in the white pulp. Other macrophages are found in red pulp cords and sinusoids and in the sheaths surrounding sheathed arterioles. Antigenic material in red pulp sinusoids can be removed by macrophage processes that extend into the lumen; in the cords, such materials are cleared by scattered macrophages and dendritic cells.

b. Lymphopoiesis Both B and T lymphocytes are activated in by the spleen. Lymphocyte-antigen interactions are more intense in the white pulp, particularly near the marginal zone, but they also occur in red pulp. T lymphocyte effector cells formed in the PALS migrate through the pulp cords to the sinusoids to enter the circulation. B lymphocytes stimulated in the marginal zone move to germinal centers of the PWP, where they divide. Plasma cells generated in this way leave the white pulp. They migrate and remain in red pulp cords, producing immunoglobulins that percolate into the sinusoids and leave the spleen in the venous blood.

c. Destruction of worn red blood cells This occurs in both the spleen and the bone marrow. Toward the end of their average 120-day lifespan, erythrocytes become less flexible; they can fragment before or during their passage through the spleen. Fragments trapped in red pulp cords are phagocytosed and digested by macrophages there. The hemoglobin is degraded into several components. The protein portion (globin) is hydrolysed to amino acids for reuse in protein synthesis. Iron released from the heme is transported, with transferrin, to the bone marrow for reuse in erythropoiesis. The heme's porphyrin ring is metabolized to bilirubin and carried by the hepatic portal vein to the liver to be processed and excreted in the bile.

d. Extramedullary hematopoiesis In pathologic conditions such as leukemia, where bone marrow function (medullary hematopoiesis) is compromised, the spleen may resume its embryonic erythropoietic or granulopoietic activity. In some cases, the liver and lymph nodes resume similar functions.

D. Tonsils: These incompletely encapsulated lymphoid aggregates contain many lymphoid nodules; they underlie the mucous membranes (epithelial lining) of the mouth and pharynx. Together with the diffuse subepithelial lymphoid tissue that connects them to form a ring, they guard the common entrance to the digestive and respiratory tracts. The 3 types of tonsils (named according to their locations) differ in number, epithelial covering, presence (or absence) and number of epithelial invaginations or **crypts,** and presence (or absence) of a definitive partial capsule.

1. Palatine tonsils These are 2 dense lymphoid aggregates found in the lateral walls of the oral pharynx, below the back of the soft palate. Each tonsil is covered by nonkeratinized stratified squamous epithelium and partly penetrated by 10–20 crypts. The tonsils are separated from underlying tissues by a partial capsule of dense connective tissue that acts as a barrier against the spread of tonsillar infections.

2. Pharyngeal tonsil A single small lymphoid aggregation at the back of the nasopharynx above the soft palate, this is covered by ciliated pseudostratified columnar epithelium. Its surface may be pleated, but it has no crypts. A thin partial capsule separates it from underlying structures.

3. Lingual tonsils The smallest and most numerous tonsils, these are located at the back of the tongue. Covered by partly keratinized stratified squamous epithelium, each tonsil has a single crypt but no definitive capsule.

Study-Focusing Questions*

1. Describe the general structure of lymphoid tissue in terms of the:
  - **a.** Type of connective tissue that makes up the stroma (118, 260)
  - **b.** Types of cells and fibers that make up the stroma (118, 260)

*The page references in this section refer to *Basic Histology,* 6th ed., Junqueira L, Carneiro J, Kelley R (editors), Appleton & Lange, 1989. **HR** (for Histology Review) is occasionally used instead of a page reference to indicate that the information referred to can be found in this book.

c. Types of cells suspended within the spaces of the stroma (260)
d. Organ in which the composition of the stroma differs from the others (260, 262)

2. Compare cellular and humoral immunity in terms of the:
   a. Type of lymphocyte (B or T) primarily associated with each (260)
   b. Need for direct lymphocyte contact in antigen disposal (260)
   c. Names of the effector cells involved in each type (261–262)
   d. Need for accessory cells (eg, macrophages) in an optimal response (108, 262)
3. Compare central and peripheral lymphoid organs (260) in terms of the:
   a. Names of the organs that fall into each group
   b. Antigen-dependence or antigen-independence of lymphocyte proliferation in these organs
4. Make a generalized schematic drawing of an IgG molecule and label the following:
   a. Light chains
   b. Heavy chains
   c. Fc portion
   d. Fab portion
   e. Constant regions
   f. Variable regions
   g. Cell-binding region
   h. Antigen-binding region
5. List the 5 types of immunoglobulins (Ig's) secreted by plasma cells and indicate the Ig for each of the following characteristics.
   a. Most abundant Ig in blood (261)
   b. Can cross the placenta (261)
   c. Secretory form consists of 2 Ig's, protein J, and a transport component (261)
   d. Predominant Ig in bodily secretions (eg, mucus, tears, saliva) (261)
   e. Usually exists as a pentamer (261)
   f. Most effective Ig in activating the complement system (261)
   g. Fc portion has a great affinity for the surface of mast cells and basophils (261)
   h. Primary mediator of allergic reactions (261)
   i. The Ig that is least well understood
   j. Two Ig's found on the surface of B lymphocytes (261)
6. Indicate the numerical order in which both T and B lymphocytes undergo the following processes after encountering their appropriate antigens.
   a. Differentiation into effector and memory cells
   b. Blast transformation (formation of immunoblasts)
   c. Clonal expansion (proliferation)
7. List the effector cells of the T lymphocyte lineage and describe the basic functions of each (261).
8. Name the effector cell of the B lymphocyte lineage and describe its basic function and its most abundant cytoplasmic organelle (110–112, 261).
9. In what ways do memory cells make the response to subsequent encounters with a particular antigen (secondary immune response) more effective than to the first encounter (primary immune response) (262)?
10. Describe the thymus in terms of:
    a. Its general functions (260)
    b. Its location in the body (262)
    c. Its classification as a central or peripheral, encapsulated or unencapsulated lymphoid organ (260, 262)
    d. Its embryonic germ layer(s) of origin (262)
    e. The embryonic pharyngeal pouch(es) from which it is derived (262)
    f. The source of the lymphocyte precursors that populate it before birth and after birth (255, 262)
    g. The type of reticular cells it contains and their embryonic germ layer of origin (262, 263)
    h. The presence or absence of lymphoid nodules (263)
11. List 4 cell types found in a postnatal thymus (263).
12. List 4 thymic hormones that may be secreted by the epithelial reticular cells (263). What is the general effect of these hormones on other lymphoid organs (263, 268)?
13. Compare the cortex and medulla of the thymus in terms of the:
    a. Packing density of lymphocytes (263–264)

   b. Number of reticular cells (264)
   c. Presence of Hassall's corpuscles (263, 264)
   d. Type of blood vessels present (263, 265)
   e. Location of the blood-thymus barrier (264)
   f. Site of T cell programming (264)
   g. Site where involution begins (265)

14. List, in order, the layers through which a substance in the blood would have to pass to cross the blood-thymus barrier (264).

15. What is the probable function of the blood-thymus barrier (264)?

16. What happens to the size and functional activity of the thymus, beginning at puberty and continuing into old age? What is this process called (265)?

17. Compare the thymus and other lymphoid organs in terms of:
   a. Their embryonic germ layer(s) of origin (262)
   b. The lymphocyte type(s) they produce (262, 266–268)
   c. The primary type of reticular cells present (261, 262–263)
   d. The presence of lymphoid nodules (263, 271, 274)
   e. Their filtering functions (266, 271, 273)

18. Compare normal animals with those that have undergone thymectomy at birth in terms of the:
   a. Number of lymphocytes found in their blood and lymph (268)
   b. Ability to mount a delayed hypersensitivity reaction (268)
   c. Ability to reject a foreign graft (269)
   d. Animals' length of survival (268)
   e. Ability to mount a cellular immune response (260)
   f. Ability to mount a humoral immune response (260)

19. Describe lymph nodes in terms of:
   a. Their general functions (271)
   b. Their location in the body (271)
   c. Their classification as central or peripheral (260) and encapsulated or unencapsulated (271) lymphoid organs
   d. Their embryonic germ layer(s) of origin
   e. The source(s) of the lymphocyte precursors that populate them (255, 262, 271)
   f. The type of reticular cells they contain and the cells' embryonic germ layer of origin (260, 261, 271)

20. Make a schematic drawing of a lymph node (270) and label the following:
   a. Capsule
   b. Hilum
   c. Afferent lymphatic vessels
   d. Trabeculae
   e. Subcapsular sinus
   f. Peritrabecular sinus
   g. Lymphoid nodules
   h. Germinal centers
   i. Paracortical zone
   j. Medullary cords
   k. Medullary sinuses
   l. Efferent lymphatic vessels
   m. Cortex
   n. Medulla
   o. Thymus-dependent region

21. Beginning with the afferent lymphatic vessels and ending with the efferent lymphatic vessels, trace the path of lymph through a lymph node (270, 273). What percentage of the lymph actually penetrates the nodules (273)?

22. Name the cells and structures commonly found in the lumens of a lymph node's sinuses (271).

23. How does the composition of the lymph change as it passes through a lymph node? What substances are removed or added? By which cell types (273)?

24. In what parts of a lymph node are the following cell types found? If a cell type is found throughout the node, indicate any sites where it occurs in higher proportions
   a. B lymphocyte (271–273)
   b. T lymphocyte (271)
   c. Immunoblast (271)

  d. Memory cell (271)
  e. Plasma cell (271–273)
  f. Follicular dendritic cell (271)
  g. Macrophage (271)
  h. Reticular cell (271)

25. What is the basic function of each cell type named in question 24 (271–273)?

26. Through which blood vessels in a lymph node can lymphocytes (primarily T lymphocytes) directly exit the blood stream? Where in the lymph node are these vessels found (273)?

27. Describe the spleen in terms of:
  a. Its general functions (273, 278)
  b. Its location in the body (**HR**)
  c. Its classification as a central or peripheral, encapsulated or unencapsulated lymphoid organ (260)
  d. Its embryonic germ layer(s) of origin (262)
  e. The source(s) of the lymphocyte precursors that populate it
  f. The type of reticular cells it contains and the cells' embryonic germ layer of origin (255, 260, 274)

28. Beginning with the splenic artery and ending with the splenic vein, name the vessels, sinuses, and any other structures through which blood travels as it passes through the spleen, according to both the open and closed theories of splenic circulation (274–277)

29. Compare the white and red pulp of the spleen in terms of the:
  a. Amount of each in the spleen (274)
  b. Predominant cell type present (277)
  c. Site of activated lymphocyte production (277)
  d. Site of red blood cell destruction by splenic macrophages (277–278, 279)
  e. Site of the highest concentrations of mature, active plasma cells (277)

30. Name the 2 major components of the white pulp (277) and compare them in terms of:
  a. Their location (276)
  b. The predominant type of lymphocyte each contains (277)
  c. The presence of a germinal center (274–277)

31. Describe the sequence of events in the life cycle of a B lymphocyte following its encounter with an appropriate antigen in the marginal zone of the white pulp (277).

32. Name the 2 major components of red pulp (277–278).

33. Compare the red pulp sinusoids with common capillaries (277–278) in terms of:
  a. Their luminal diameter
  b. The presence of openings between the lining endothelial cells
  c. The continuity and distribution of the endothelial basal lamina
  d. The shape of the endothelial cells

34. Describe collections of unencapsulated lymphoid tissue (280) in terms of:
  a. Their location in the body
  b. The predominant type of lymphocytes (T or B) they contain
  c. The presence of germinal centers
  d. The predominant type of immunoglobulin (Ig) secreted by plasma cells in or near these lymphoid arggregates

35. Name the 3 types of tonsils in the human mouth and pharynx (280–281) and compare them in terms of:
  a. Their location
  b. The number of each type
  c. The number of crypts per tonsil (for each type)
  d. The type of epithelium covering each type

Multiple-Choice Questions

For questions 14–1 through 14–4, select the single best answer.

14–1. All of the following statements are true of the epithelial reticular cells of the thymus *except:*

A. They are derived from embryonic endoderm
B. They are structural components of the blood-thymus barrier
C. They are structural components of Hassall's corpuscles
D. They attach to one another at the tips of their long cytoplasmic processes via desmosomes
E. They synthesize and secrete reticular fibers

14–2. One function carried out by all lymphoid tissues and organs is:
A. Filtering lymph
B. Filtering blood
C. Extramedullary erythropoiesis
D. Production of lymphocytes
E. Destruction of old erythrocytes

14–3. All of the following statements are true of the thymic cortex *except:*
A. It is the site of the blood-thymus barrier
B. The only blood vessels it contains are capillaries
C. It contains Hassall's corpuscles
D. It lacks reticular fibers
E. It is the site where thymic involution begins

14–4. Indicate the order in which lymph passes through the sinuses of lymph nodes:
A. Subcapsular → medullary → peritrabecular
B. Medullary → subcapsular → peritrabecular
C. Medullary → peritrabecular → subcapsular
D. Peritrabecular → subcapsular → medullary
E. Subcapsular → peritrabecular → medullary

MATCHING (questions 14–45 through 14–48): Each choice may be used once, more than once, or not at all. Questions 14–5 through 14–12 use the letters in Figure 14–1.

Questions 14–5 through 14–12:

14–5. Light chain
14–6. Heavy chain
14–7. Fc fragment
14–8. Fab fragment
14–9. Constant region

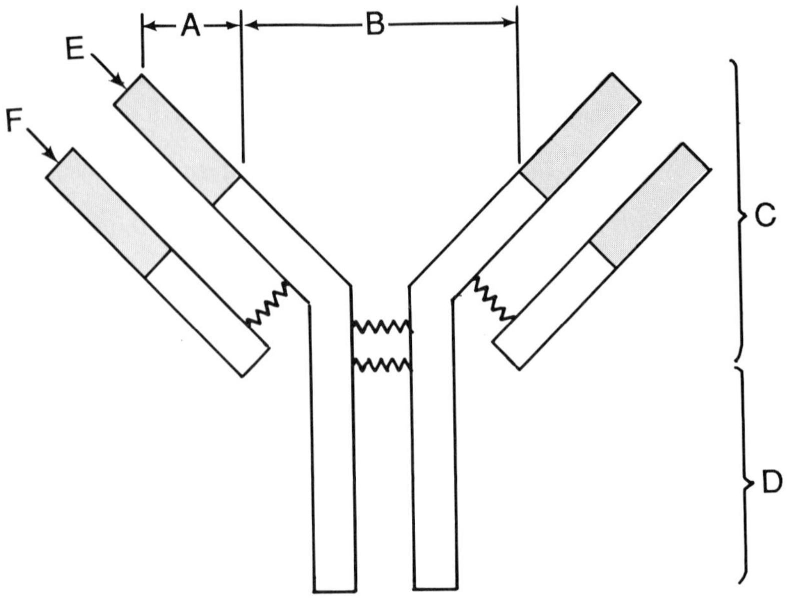

Figure 14–1.

14–10. Variable region
14–11. Cell-binding region
14–12. Antigen-binding region

Questions 14–13 through 14–17:

A. Lymphocytes
B. Macrophages
C. Reticular cells
D. Plasma cells
E. Dendritic cells

14–13. Nonphagocytic cells that bind antigen on their surfaces and present them to lymphocytes for recognition and stimulation
14–14. Derived from blood monocytes
14–15. Secrete immunoglobulins
14–16. Primary cellular component of the stroma of the lymph nodes and spleen
14–17. Contain the largest amount of rough endoplasmic reticulum of those listed

Questions 14–18 through 14–28:

A. IgA
B. IgM
C. IgG
D. IgD
E. IgE
F. All of the above

14–18. The most abundant immunoglobulin in serum
14–19. Secretory form consists of 2 Ig's, protein J, and a transport component
14–20. Antibody
14–21. May cross the placenta
14–22. Most effective Ig in activating the complement system
14–23. Predominant Ig in bodily secretions (eg, mucus, tears)
14–24. Usually occurs as a pentamer
14–25. Cell-binding region has a great affinity for the surface of mast cells and basophils
14–26. A major component of B lymphocyte surface
14–27. Primary mediator of allergic reactions
14–28. The Ig that is least well understood

Questions 14–29 through 14–33:

A. Palatine tonsils
B. Pharyngeal tonsils
C. Lingual tonsils
D. All of the above

14–29. Characteristically lack crypts
14–30. Contain(s) lymphoid nodules
14–31. Are paired structures
14–32. The most numerous type of tonsil
14–33. Covered by ciliated pseudostratified columnar epithelium

Questions 14–34 through 14–48:

A. Thymus
B. Spleen
C. Lymph nodes
D. All of the above
E. A and C only
F. B and C only

14–34. Exhibit(s) a cortex and a medulla
14–35. Contain(s) significant numbers of B lymphocytes
14–36. Contain(s) significant numbers of T lymphocytes
14–37. Primary immunologic filter of blood
14–38. Primary immunologic filter of lymph
14–39. Contain(s) lymphoid nodules
14–40. Encapsulated organ(s)
14–41. Central (primary) lymphoid organ(s)
14–42. Peripheral (secondary) lymphoid organ(s)
14–43. Capsule contains some smooth muscle
14–44. Contain(s) cords and sinuses
14–45. Contain(s) a subcapsular sinus
14–46. Contain(s) Hassall's corpuscles
14–47. Receive(s) afferent lymphatic vessels
14–48. Contain(s) periarterial lymphatic sheaths

For questions 14–49 through 14–54, either, both, or neither of the answers may be correct. Select

A if only A is correct
B is only B is correct
C if both A and B are correct
D if neither A nor B is correct

Questions 14–49 through 14–54:

A. T lymphocytes
B. B lymphocytes
C. Both
D. Neither

14–49. Respond to antigenic stimulation by blast transformation and proliferation
14–50. Primarily associated with humoral immunity
14–51. Primarily associated with cell-mediated (cellular) immunity
14–52. Form both memory and effector cells
14–53. Differentiate into plasma cells
14–54. Differentiate into cytotoxic (killer/graft rejection) cells

For questions 14–55 through 14–60, one, more than one, or all the answers may be correct. Select

A if only (1), (2), and (3) are correct
B if only (1) and (3) are correct
C if only (2) and (4) are correct
D if only (4) is correct
E if all answers are correct

14–55. Effector cell types derived from T lymphocytes include
(1) Helper cells
(2) Suppressor cells
(3) Cytotoxic cells
(4) Plasma cells
14–56. Central lymphoid organs
(1) Include the human thymus
(2) Include the bursa of Fabricius of birds

(3) Include human bone marrow
(4) Are capable of antigen-independent lymphopoiesis

14–57. Thymus-dependent regions of lymphoid organs include the
(1) Paracortical zone of lymph nodes
(2) Germinal centers of Peyer's patches
(3) Periarterial lymphatic sheaths in the spleen
(4) Crypts of the pharyngeal tonsils

14–58. Plasma cells
(1) Contain abundant rough endoplasmic reticulum in their cytoplasm
(2) Are located in the medullary cords of lymph nodes
(3) Derive from B lymphocytes
(4) Are located in the red pulp cords (Billroth's cords) in the spleen

14–59. B lymphocytes are the major type of lymphocytes found
(1) In Peyer's patches
(2) In the palatine tonsils
(3) In the peripheral white pulp of the spleen
(4) Circulating in the blood

14–60. Thymectomy at birth causes
(1) A decrease in the number of circulating lymphocytes
(2) The inability to mount a humoral response to T-dependent antigens
(3) Generalized atrophy of peripheral lymphoid organs
(4) The pool of B lymphocytes to be decreased by 75%

INTEGRATIVE MULTIPLE CHOICE QUESTIONS: CIRCULATORY, HEMATOPOIETIC AND LYMPHOID SYSTEMS

For the following questions, select the SINGLE BEST ANSWER.

CHL–1. All of the following are derived from embryonic mesoderm EXCEPT:
- **A.** Endothelial cells
- **B.** Erythrocytes
- **C.** Epithelial reticular cells
- **D.** Lymphocytes
- **E.** Vascular smooth muscle

CHL–2. The only cells capable of reentering the bloodstream after leaving the circulation are
- **A.** Neutrophils
- **B.** Monocytes
- **C.** Basophils
- **D.** T-lymphocytes
- **E.** Eosinophils

CHL–3. The process by which leukocytes leave the circulation by passing between endothelial cells to enter the surrounding connective tissue is termed:
- **A.** margination
- **B.** diapedesis
- **C.** leukopoiesis
- **D.** endocytosis
- **E.** none of the above

CHL–4. All of the following occur during a bacterial infection of loose connective tissue EXCEPT:
- **A.** increased diapedesis
- **B.** neutrophilia
- **C.** a "shift to the left"
- **D.** inhibition of the release of neutrophils from the medullary storage compartment
- **E.** increased numbers of band neutrophils enter the circulation

MATCHING (each choice may be used once, more than once, or not at all)
Questions CHL–5 through CHL–14

- **A.** Ubiquitin
- **B.** Thymosin
- **C.** Histamine
- **D.** Serotonin
- **E.** Albumin
- **F.** Immunoglobulin
- **G.** Phagocytins
- **H.** Atrial natriuretic factor
- **I.** Bilirubin
- **J.** Erythropoietin

CHL–5. Hormone secreted by epithelial reticular cells
CHL–6. Secreted by basophils
CHL–7. Secreted by the liver
CHL–8. By-product of the destruction of erythrocytes
CHL–9. Produced by the kidney
CHL–10. Found in the specific granules of neutrophils
CHL–11. Released by platelets during clot formation
CHL–12. Hormone secreted by the heart
CHL–13. Enzyme involved in the maturation of reticulocytes into erythrocytes
CHL–14. Secreted by plasma cells

For the following questions, EITHER, BOTH or NEITHER of the answers may be correct. Select

A if only A is correct
B if only B is correct
C if both A and B are correct
D if neither A nor B are correct

Questions CHL-15 through CHL-23

A. T-lymphocytes
B. B-lymphocytes
C. Both
D. Neither

CHL-15. Predominant lymphocyte type in blood vessels
CHL-16. Predominant lymphocyte type in lymphatic vessels
CHL-17. Predominant lymphocyte type in lymph nodes
CHL-18. Predominant lymphocyte type in Peyer's patches
CHL-19. Predominant lymphocyte type in the thymus
CHL-20. Produce memory cells upon antigenic stimulation
CHL-21. Produce effector cells that attack virus-infected cells (first line of cellular defense against viruses)
CHL-22. Produce effector cells that can secrete immunoglobulins that attach to the surface of bacteria
CHL-23. First line of cellular defense against bacteria

For the following questions, ONE, MORE THAN ONE, or ALL of the answers may be correct. Select

A if only (1), (2), and (3) are correct
B if only (1) and (3) are correct
C if only (2) and (4) are correct
D if only (4) is correct
E if all answers are correct

CHL-24. Cell types capable of undergoing further cell division after they leave the hematopoietic organ where they were formed include:
(1) Erythrocytes
(2) Neutrophils
(3) Eosinophils
(4) Lymphocytes

CHL-25. Organs capable of intrauterine erythropoiesis include:
(1) Bone marrow
(2) Liver
(3) Spleen
(4) Thymus

CHL-26. In diseased adults, extramedullary erythropoiesis may occur in the:
(1) Spleen
(2) Bone marrow
(3) Liver
(4) Thymus

CHL-27. Allergic reactions:
(1) are characterized by eosinophilia
(2) involve the binding of antigens to IgE
(3) involve the degranulation of mast cells
(4) are characterized by inflammation

Digestive Tract

15

Objectives

This chapter should help the student to:

- Name the parts of the digestive tract.
- Name the primary function of each part of the digestive tract.
- Describe the structure of the tongue.
- Describe the development of the teeth.
- Describe the layered structure of the teeth, the structures that hold them in place, and the composition of the gingiva.
- Name the 4 layers that form the walls of the tubular organs of the digestive tract and the tissue types found in each layer.
- Compare the tubular organs of the digestive tract in terms of the structure of each of their layers and relate any structural variations to differences in organ function.
- Know the distinguishing structural features of the various regions of each of the tubular organs of the digestive tract.
- Name the secretory product(s), distinguishing structural features, and (where appropriate) the staining properties for each type of secretory cell in the digestive tract mucosa.

Table 15-1. Distinguishing features of the walls of the digestive tract.

		Mucosa	
Organ	**Region**	**Epithelium**	**Lamina Propria**
Esophagus	Upper third	Nonkeratinized stratified squamous.	Mucous glands.
	Middle third		
	Lower third		Cardiac glands (mostly mucous).
Stomach	Cardia	Simple columnar.	
	Fundus and body		Gastric glands (fundic type with shallow pits).
	Pylorus		Gastric glands (pyloric type with deep pits).
Small Intestine	Duodenum	Simple columnar; striated border; goblet cells.	Crypts of Lieberkühn; lamina propria forming the core of villi; lymphoid nodules.
	Jejunum		
	Ileum		Peyer's Patches.
Colon & Rectum	Appendix	Simple columnar; shorter microvilli; abundant goblet cells.	Many lymphoid nodules.
	Cecum		No villi; few crypts.
	Ascending and descending colon		
	Transverse and sigmoid colon		
	Rectum	Rectal columns.	
Anal Canal	Anorectal area	Nonkeratinized stratified squamous.	Large venous plexus (hemorrhoidal plexus).
	Anocutaneous area	Keratinized stratified squamous.	No distinguishing features.
	Cutaneous area		Pilosebaceous follicles and apocrine sweat glands.

- List the features of the small intestine that promote nutrient absorption and trace the steps in this process.
- Identify the organ, region, cell types present, and type of section (ie, transverse or longitudinal) from a slide or photomicrograph of a section of any part of the digestive tract.

Synopsis

I. GENERAL FEATURES OF THE DIGESTIVE TRACT

A. Components of the Tract: The digestive tract is a series of organs forming a long muscular tube whose continuous lumen opens to the exterior at both ends. The organs include the oral cavity, oral pharynx (oropharynx), esophagus, stomach, small intestine (duodenum, jejunum, and ileum), large intestine (cecum and appendix; ascending, transverse, descending, and sigmoid colon), rectum, and anal canal.

B. General Structural Features: The walls of each organ consist of 4 concentric layers: the **mucosa, submucosa, muscularis externa,** and **serosa or adventitia.** (The fastest way to master digestive-tract histology is first to learn the general composition and location of each of these layers and then focus on the similarities of and differences between the organs; see Table 15–1).The structural features of these organs are more easily understood in terms of the contribution each makes to the functions detailed in I.C.

Table 15-1 (cont'd).

Muscularis Mucosa	Submucosa	Muscularis Externa	Adventitia/ Serosa
Thick.	Esophageal glands (mostly mucous, some serous).	Skeletal muscle.	Adventitia.
Thin.		Skeletal and smooth muscle.	
		Smooth muscle.	
Two layers with radial projections into the lamina propria.	No distinguishing features, no permanent folds.	Three layers of smooth muscle (inner oblique, middle circular, outer longitudinal).	Serosa.
Elevated by plicae circulares.	Brunner's glands.	2 layers of smooth muscle (inner circular, outer teniae coil.)	Adventitia and serosa.
	Circular folds formed by submucosa (plicae circulares).		Serosa.
Discontinuous.	Lymphoid nodules.	Very thin.	Serosa.
	No circular folds.	2 layers of smooth muscle (inner circular, outer teniae coil.)	Adventitia and serosa.
	Semicircular folds.		Serosa.
No distinguishing features		Circular folds formed by submucosa thickened inner circular layer of smooth muscle. Internal sphincter formed by thickened inner circular layer of smooth muscle. External sphincter formed by outer layer of skeletal muscle.	Adventitia.

1. Mucosa Bordering the lumen, the mucosa has 3 parts. The epithelium, or **mucous membrane,** is stratified squamous in the oral cavity, oral pharynx, esophagus, and anal canal; it is simple columnar in the stomach, intestines, and rectum. The **lamina propria** is a layer of loose connective tissue beneath the epithelium; it contains small blood and lymphatic vessels. The **muscularis mucosae** is a thin layer of smooth muscle bordering the submucosa.

2. Submucosa This connective tissue layer contains blood and lymphatic vessels, and the submucosal (Meissner's) plexus. Some organs are characterized by the presence of glands and lymphoid nodules in this layer.

3. Muscularis externa This consists of 2 layers of smooth muscle—an inner circular and an outer longitudinal—through most of the tract. Between these layers lies the **myenteric (Auerbach's) plexus.** Any muscle present surrounding the oral cavity is skeletal; in other sites such as the hard palate and gingiva muscle is absent, and the submucosa binds tightly to bone. In the upper third of the esophagus, this layer contains primarily skeletal muscle, which is replaced by smooth muscle in the lower portion. The stomach's muscularis externa has 3 layers: an outer longitudinal, a middle circular, and an inner oblique. The colon's outer longitudinal layer is gathered into 3 bands, the **teniae coli.** The smooth and skeletal muscle encircling the tract in the anal canal form involuntary and voluntary sphincters, respectively.

4. Serosa and adventitia The outer covering of the digestive tract differs in its various parts. The esophagus and rectum are surrounded by an adventitia of connective tissue like that surrounding blood vessels. **Intraperitoneal** organs (eg, stomach, jejunum, ileum, transverse and sigmoid colons) are suspended by mesenteries and covered by a serosa (visceral peritoneum) consisting of a thin layer of loose connective tissue that is covered by simple squamous epithelium (mesothelium). **Retroperitoneal** organs (eg, duodenum, ascending and descending colons) are bound to the abdominal wall by adventititia; they are covered on their free (anterior) surfaces by serosa.

C. General Functional Features: The main functions of the digestive tract are the absorption of nutrients and water and the excretion of wastes and toxins.

1. Digestion Enzymatic degradation of food is a prerequisite for absorption; enzymes act mainly at food particle surfaces. Teeth aid absorption by breaking up food to expose more surface area. Lip, cheek, and tongue muscles help position food between the teeth. Saliva dissolves water-soluble particles and contains enzymes that attack carbohydrates (see Chapter 16). Taste buds (see Chapter 24) check for contaminants and toxins. The tongue moves chewed food back into the **oral pharynx** and closes the epiglottis to protect the airway. Skeletal muscle in walls of the oral pharynx and the upper third of the **esophagus** aid the tongue in swallowing and move food down the esophagus to where smooth muscle takes over. In the esophagus, mucus is added to reduce friction, but the main role of this muscular tube is moving material from the oral cavity to the **stomach.** Glands in the stomach wall add acid (HCl), a protease (pepsin), and mucus to the mixture (now called chyme). Smooth muscles in the stomach wall mix and further pulverize the chyme and move it to the **small intestine** (duodenum) where pancreatic enzymes and bile are added. The enzymes hydrolyze nutrients to an absorbable form. The detergent action of bile disperses water-insoluble lipid into tiny droplets, increasing the surface area available to pancreatic lipases. The lining epithelial cells **(enterocytes)** of the small intestine have additional enzymes on their luminal surfaces to complete the hydrolysis of certain nutrients.

2. Absorption This primary function of the digestive tract occurs mainly in the intestines; the small intestines generally absorb nutrients and the large intestines absorb water. To maximize the absorptive surface, the small intestine's lining has multiple permanent folds including plicae circulares and villi. Intestines are lined by absorptive cells (enterocytes) whose apical microvilli further increase the absorptive surface. These cells absorb most nutrients from the lumen. They transfer amino acids and sugars to capillaries in the lamina propria, whose blood carries them to the liver for further processing. Enterocytes assemble chylomicrons from absorbed lipids and transfer them to lymphatic capillaries (sometimes called lacteals) in the lamina propria. From here lipids reach the blood through the lymphatic vascular system.

3. Excretion Metabolic wastes are excreted by the liver as bile and emptied into the duodenal lumen by the bile duct. Smooth muscles in the walls of the small intestine move undigested material and waste products to the large intestine (colon). Here, mucus is added and most of the water is extracted. This concentrates and solidifies the intestinal contents, forming feces. This material is further dehydrated and stored in the rectum and finally expelled through the anal canal.

4. Endocrine function Individual cells with the characteristics of the diffuse neuroendocrine system (DNES; see Chapter 4) are scattered among the epithelial cells lining the digestive tract's mucosal glands and crypts. (These enteroendocrine cells were at one time known as argentaffin, argyrophilic, and enterochromaffin cells because of their affinity for stains containing silver or chromium.) They secrete hormones and amines (eg, serotonin, secretin, gastrin, somatostatin, cholecystokinin, glucagon) that affect such local gastrointestinal functions as gut motility and the secretion of acid, digestive enzymes, and hormones by other types of cells.

5. Innervation Distributed along and in the walls of the tract are the myenteric (Auerbach's) and submucosal (Meissner's) autonomic plexuses. These include postsynaptic sympathetic fibers, pre- and postsynaptic parasympathetic fibers, parasympathetic ganglion cell bodies, and some visceral sensory fibers. After voluntary swallowing, these autonomic plexuses coordinate peristalsis—wavelike contractions of the muscularis externa that propel ingested material through the tract. They also control the independent activity of the muscularis mucosa, which maintains contact between the mucosa and the contents of the tract and helps empty mucosal glands. These plexuses also modulate the secretory activity of certain DNES-like cells. In general, sympathetic action inhibits gut motility and parasympathetic action has the opposite effect.

6. Blood supply The arterial supply to the abdominal parts of the tract arises from mesenteric branches of the abdominal aorta that branch further in the mesenteries to form a series of arcades. Small arteries penetrate the walls of the tract to feed capillaries in the lamina propria. Only the smaller veins accompany branches of the mesenteric arteries. The larger veins draining these organs diverge from the arterial path and empty either directly or through tributaries into the **hepatic portal vein,** which branches within the liver to feed the **hepatic sinusoids** (see Chapter 16). Amino acids, sugars, small fatty acids, and any toxins absorbed in the intestine thus travel directly to the liver to be metabolized, stored or detoxified before reaching the general circulation.

7. Protection The large size of the digestive tract's absorptive surface increases the risk of infection by foreign substances and organisms. The body is protected from invasion and infection by immunoreactive cells—including IgA-secreting plasma cells—in the lamina propria and submucosa. Other defenses include the lysozyme secreted by the Paneth cells, the digestive enzymes in the lumen, the layer of mucus covering the epithelium, and the tight junctions found between absorptive cells. Toxic substances that do reach the blood are carried directly to the liver for detoxification in the smooth endoplasmic reticulum of the hepatocytes.

II. ORAL CAVITY.

This upper end of the digestive tract is bounded anteriorly, by the teeth and lips; posteriorly, by the oral pharynx; laterally, by the teeth and cheeks; superiorly, by the hard and soft palate; and inferiorly, by the tongue and floor of the mouth.

A. Wall Structure:

1. Mucosa This nonkeratinized stratified squamous epithelium (mucous membrane) covers all internal surfaces of the oral cavity and pharynx except the teeth. The underlying lamina propia is a vascular connective tissue with papillae like those of the dermis (see Chapter 18). The papillae contain capillaries that nourish the epithelium. There is no muscularis mucosae.

2. Submucosa A somewhat more fibrous connective tissue than the lamina propria, the submucosa contains many blood vessels and small salivary glands.

3. Muscle and bone The oral cavity lacks a standard muscularis externa. Skeletal muscle underlies the submucosa in the lips, cheeks, tongue, floor of the mouth, oral pharynx, and the soft palate and its downward extension, the **uvula.** Bone underlies the thin submucosa of the hard palate and gingiva.

B. Lips: There is a transition from nonkeratinized mucous membrane to the keratinized stratified squamous epithelium of the epidermis on the lips. The thin keratinized layer covering the lip's vermillion border allows the reddish color of blood in vessels of the lamina propria to show through. Hair follicles and keratin help distinguish the outer lip surface from the inner in tissue sections.

C. Tongue: This structure is a mass of skeletal muscle covered by a mucosa, bound tightly to the muscle by the lamina propria, which penetrates between the bundles of muscle fibers. There is little or no submucosa.

1. Muscle The mass of muscle is arranged in bundles of many sizes; these are separated by connective tissue and cross each other in 3 planes. This arrangement gives the tongue the flexibility required for speech, for positioning food for chewing, and for swallowing.

2. Mucosa The mucosa of the tongue differs on the dorsal (upper) and ventral (lower) surfaces. The ventral surface has a thin nonkeratinized stratified squamous epithelium underlain by a lamina propria. The dorsal surface, however, is covered by a stratified squamous epithelium that is partly keratinized. The anterior two-thirds of the dorsal surface is separated from the posterior third by a V-shaped groove. Behind this groove, the epithelium invaginates to form the crypts of the lingual tonsils (see Chapter 14). Cryptless patches of lymphoid tissue in the lamina propria cause surface bulges in this region. The anterior two-thirds of the dorsal surface has many **papillae**—mucosal projections that extend from the surface. There are 4 types of lingual papillae:

a. Filiform papillae Sharp, often partly keratinized conical projections, these are the most numerous of the papillae; they lack taste buds.

b. Fungiform papillae These resemble mushrooms. They occur singly and are scattered among the filiform papillae. Each papilla has taste buds (see Chapter 24) on its expanded upper surface but not on its narrow stalk.

c. Foliate papillae Poorly developed in humans, these occur in rows that are separated by furrows into which serous glands drain. The furrow walls (sides of the papillae) harbor many taste buds.

d. Circumvallate papillae These are the largest and least numerous papillae, with only 7–12 occurring near the V-shaped groove at the back of the tongue. Each papilla is surrounded by a ringlike ridge of mucosa from which it is separated by a circular furrow. The walls of the furrow contain taste buds, often on both sides. As with the foliates, ducts from serous (von Ebner's) glands empty into the furrow and periodically wash chemical stimuli from the taste buds, allowing new tastes to be sensed. (Chapter 24 describes the taste bud cells.)

D. Teeth and Associated Structures:

1. Classification of teeth

a. Shape Humans have 4 types of teeth, each with a distinctive crown and root structure. The structure and location of each type allow it to perform specific functions.

(1) Incisors Located directly behind the lips, each has a single root and a chisel-shaped crown for cutting.

(2) Canines (cuspids) These lie lateral to the incisors. Each has a single root and a conical crown for grasping and tearing.

(3) Premolars (bicuspids) Lying posterolateral to the canines, each has 2 roots and a squat ovoid crown with a flattened upper surface for crushing. Their location near the front of the mouth allows the premolars to assist in grasping.

(4) Molars (tricuspids) These lie behind the premolars. Each has 3 roots and a rounded, boxlike crown with a flat upper surface for crushing and grinding. Their location near the angle of the jaw allows them to exert greater crushing force than do the premolars.

b. Permanent and deciduous teeth

(1) Permanent (adult) teeth Human adults (barring loss to decay, accident, or other causes) normally have 32 permanent teeth arranged in 2 arches (maxillary, or upper; mandibular, or lower). Each arch has 2 bilaterally symmetric quadrants. The 8 teeth in each quadrant define the adult "dental formula": 2 incisors, 1 canine, 2 premolars, and 3 molars.

(2) Deciduous (baby) teeth These develop first and are normally shed upon replacement by permanent teeth. The arrangement of the 20 deciduous teeth is like that of the permanent teeth, but there are no molars. The dental formula for the 5 deciduous teeth in each quadrant is 2 incisors, 1 canine, and 2 premolars.

2. Tooth structure In cross section, each tooth exhibits concentric tissue layers from core to periphery. Each tooth has the following named parts that lie above, at, or below the gum line:

a. Crown (corona) This is the part of the tooth that projects above the **gingiva** (gum) and is the only part covered by **enamel.**

b. Root (radix) This projects below the gum and into the bony socket (**alveolus**) in which the tooth is anchored. Depending on its type, a tooth can have 1–3 roots, which are covered by **cementum.** A small opening at the root's apex (**apical foramen**) allows vessels and nerves to enter the pulp cavity.

c. Neck (cervix) Lying at the crown-root junction at or just below the gum line, this is defined as the point where the enamel and cementum meet.

d. Pulp cavity Found at the core of the tooth, it lies mainly in the root, with a portion extending into the crown. It is filled with **pulp,** a loose connective tissue that contains many vessels and nerves, which enter through the apical foramen. Some nerve fibers lose their myelin after entering the cavity; they may extend for short distances into **dentinal tubules** (small canals). The only sensation transmitted by these sensory nerves in teeth is pain.

e. Dentin A relatively thick layer of bonelike calcified tissue, dentin surrounds the pulp cavity in both crown and root.

(1) Matrix composition Hydroxyapatite crystals (see Chapter 8) make up 70% of dentin's dry weight, placing it between bone and enamel in hardness. Organic components include type I collagen and glycosaminoglycans.

(2) Tissue organization The dentin and pulp cavity are separated by a single layer of columnar cells called **odontoblasts.** These have basal nuclei, a well-developed Golgi complex, rough endoplasmic reticulum (RER), and many ribosomes. A long, branched, tapered odontoblast process (**Tomes' fiber**) extends from each cell's apical (dentinal) surface and penetrates the dentin's width in a dentinal tubule. Transverse sections through the dentin have a honeycomblike appearance (dentin forms the comb; the Tomes' fibers and surrounding tissue fluid represent the honey).

(3) Histogenesis Dentin's organic matrix components, together termed **predentin,** are secreted by odontoblasts from their apical surfaces. As the predentin is deposited, the cells retreat, leaving in place a thin cell process that gradually elongates to form a Tomes' fiber while the dentin layer thickens. Mineralization begins when the cells release into the predentin membrane-limited **matrix vesicles** containing fine hydroxyapatite crystals. These crystals act as nucleation sites for further mineral deposition that occurs as the crystals themselves grow by accruing more mineral from the tissue fluid.

f. Enamel A thick layer of calcified material covering the dentin of the crown, enamel is not considered a true tissue when mature, because it lacks cells.

(1) Composition Mineral salts (mainly hydroxyapatite) make up 95% of enamel, making it the hardest substance in the body. Unlike bone and dentin, its inorganic components do not include collagen. They do, however, include 2 unique classes of proteins—**amelogenins** and **enamelins**—whose role in organizing the mineral components is not yet clear.

(2) Organization Enamel is arranged at tightly packed columns of hydroxyapatite. These **enamel rods (prisms)** are bound together by **interrod enamel.**

(3) Production During tooth formation, production of enamel is a function of tall columnar cells, **ameloblasts.** Each has a basal nucleus, a well-developed Golgi complex, RER, and a short apical cell process (**Tomes' process**). This process extends into the enamel matrix; it contains secretory vesicles filled with the glycoproteins that later constitute the organic portion of enamel. As the organic material is secreted from the ameloblast's apical surface, the cell recedes. Unlike the Tomes' fibers of the odontoblasts, Tomes' processes of the ameloblasts recede along with the cell, leaving behind a solid rod of organic preenamel. Calcification begins at the periphery of each rod and proceeds toward its core. Ameloblasts do not accompany the tooth during eruption; they degenerate. Once worn away or destroyed by bacteria (which cause dental caries), therefore, enamel cannot be replaced.

g. Cementum This bonelike tissue covering the dentin of the roots is thicker at the apex of the root than near the neck of the tooth. It contains **cementocytes** that, like osteocytes, lie in lacunae, communicate through canaliculi, and produce the surrounding matrix. Cementum is an active tissue that can undergo either enhanced production or resorption, depending upon the stresses to which it is subjected. It thus helps keep the roots in close contact with the walls of the alveoli.

3. Associated structures

a. Periodontal ligament A dense connective tissue sling surrounding the root, its fibers insert into both cementum and alveolar bone. This ligament serves as the periosteum of alveolar bone and binds the root to the walls of the socket (alveolus), suspending the tooth in the socket and permitting slight movement. It contains many pressure-sensitive nerve endings that warn against excess pressure and thus soften the impact of chewing. This action prevents the resorption of alveolar bone that would otherwise accompany direct transmission of pressure to the socket walls. Like immature tissues, it contains soluble collagen and glycosaminoglycans. Because its matrix components undergo rapid and continual turnover, it is particulary susceptible to nutritional deficiencies. Vitamin C or protein deficiencies may cause it to degenerate, resulting in the loosening or loss of teeth.

b. Alveolar bone This is simply the bone of the mandible and maxilla that lines the alveoli and to which the teeth are attached by the periodontal ligament. Even in adults it consists of primary (woven) bone (see Chapter 8).

c. Gingiva (gum) The oral mucosa covering the mandibular and maxillary arches in which the teeth are anchored, the gum is composed of nonkeratinized stratified squamous epithelium. There is an underlying lamina propria whose long papillae interdigitate with ridges of the overlying epithelium. The lamina propria is bound tightly to the epithelium by hemidesmosomes and to the periosteum of the underlying bone by interwoven collagen fibers. The gingival epithelium forms a cuff around the base of the crown, separated from the tooth by a narrow gingival crevice. At the base of this crevice, the gingiva forms a basal lamina-like thickening, the **cuticle,** that encircles the tooth and attaches to the enamel. This is called the **epithelial attachment of Gottlieb.**

4. Tooth development Beginning in humans during the sixth week of gestation, this involves a cascade of epithelio-mesenchymal interactions and proceeds through a series of morphologic stages. The process can be more easily understood by following the changes in epithelium and mesenchyme that occur during each stage and by focusing on the specific tooth components formed by each tissue.

a. Epithelium This is the oral epithelium. It derives from ectoderm and gives rise to the ameloblasts that form enamel.

b. Mesenchyme This is the ectomesenchyme that underlies the oral epithelium. It is an embryonic connective tissue derived from the neural crest and gives rise to odontoblasts and cementoblasts, which form dentin and cementum, respectively. It also forms the dental pulp. Mesenchyme surrounding the developing teeth forms alveolar bone.

c. Crown development This process is completed shortly before eruption.

(1) Dental lamina stage Localized bands of proliferating cells in the basal layer of the stratified oral epithelium, peripheral to the developing tongue, form 2 (one in each jaw) horseshoe-shaped epithelial ridges, or **dental laminae,** over the mesenchyme of the future mandibular and maxillary arches.

(2) Bud stage Stimulated by local collections of neural ectoderm-derived cells in the mesenchyme, proliferation increases in the base of each dental lamina at the 10 sites of future deciduous teeth. These **epithelial tooth buds** enlarge and bulge into the underlying mesenchyme.

(3) Early cap stage With continued proliferation, the deep bud surfaces invaginate and broaden to form solid caps over clumps of mesenchyme. In the cap's core, the cell density decreases as internal cells become stellate and the interstices accumulate tissue fluid. The peripheral cells, which contact the basal lamina, form a simple epithelial shell and continue to divide, increasing the cap's size. A stalk of dental lamina connects each cap to the oral epithelium. The mesenchyme under the cap proliferates and condenses, indenting the cap's base.

(4) Late cap stage Mesenchyme in the indentation grows, forming the **dental papilla** and further indenting the cap's base. The epithelial cells over the papilla (**inner enamel epithelium**) become columnar, while those that form the rest of the shell (**outer enamel epithelium**) remain low cuboidal. The stellate cells and fluid inside the shell make up the **stellate reticulum.** Between the stellate reticulum and inner enamel epithelium lies a layer of epithelial cells, the **stratum intermedium.** Together, the inner and outer enamel epithelia, stratum intermedium, and stellate reticulum constitute the **enamel organ.** The outer enamel epithelium is continuous with the narrowing dental lamina; this gives rise to another tooth bud that will later form a permanent tooth.

(5) Bell stage As the cap grows, the indentation deepens, the inner enamel epithelium expands around the enlarging papilla, and the developing tooth becomes bell-shaped. Mesenchyme cells near the inner enamel epithelium condense, differentiate into a layer of columnar **odontoblasts,** and begin forming predentin. Mesenchyme in the papilla's core forms the dental pulp. Columnar inner enamel epithelial cells differentiate into **ameloblasts** and begin producing enamel soon after the dentin begins to calcify. Once the enamel layer is complete, the ameloblasts shorten and become inactive. The ringlike junction of the inner and outer enamel epithelium at the rim of the bell is termed the **cervical loop.** Capillaries indent the outer enamel epithelium, and it loses its connection with the oral epithelium as the dental lamina degenerates.

(6) Epithelio-mesenchymal interactions during crown development A wave of interactions between the epithelial cap and papillary mesenchyme begins at the top of the crown and progresses toward the cervical loop. Briefly stated, neuroectodermal mesenchyme clusters produce epithelial tooth buds, inducing the proliferation and condensation of papillary mesenchyme. This, in turn, induces formation of the inner enamel epithelium, causing the papillary mesenchyme cells to become odontoblasts. The inner enamel epithelial cells are induced to become ameloblasts, which cause the odontoblasts to produce predentin. On calcification, this induces the ameloblasts to produce enamel.

d. Root development Once the crown is formed, the cervical loop grows rootward and encloses the dental papilla. The inner and outer enamel epithelia fuse around the root, forming **Hertwig's root sheath,** whose inner layer induces odontoblast differentiation in the adjacent papillary mesenchyme. Once the predentin surrounding the root becomes calcified, the root sheath degenerates. This brings surrounding mesenchymal cells into contact with the dentin and stimulates them to become cementoblasts. Cementum secreted by these cells onto the root surface traps the ends of fibers produced by nearby fibroblats (the fibroblasts also remodel these fibers to form the periodontal ligament).

e. Eruption As the root elongates, newly formed alveolar bone limits its downward growth, forcing the crown upward. Tissue between the crown tip and gingival surface degenerates, allowing the crown to erupt into the oral cavity. Ameloblasts covering the crown degenerate. No new enamel is formed after eruption.

f. Development of permanent teeth In the late cap stage, a secondary (permanent) tooth bud arises from the labial surface of each dental lamina stalk. Dental lamina tissue from each second premolar burrows backward, successively budding off 3 permanent molar buds. Permanent tooth buds remain dormant until activated after birth; they then undergo the same developmental steps as deciduous teeth. As each developing permanent tooth enlarges, it induces osteoclast-mediated resorption of the alveolar bone that separates the bony crypt in which it lies and the baby tooth's socket. Continued growth of the permanent tooth leads to resorption of the baby tooth's root until only the crown is left, held in place only by its epithelial attachment to the gingiva. Once this is lost, the permanent tooth erupts into the oral cavity.

III. PHARYNX.

A short, broad, muscular tube that lies behind the tongue and soft palate, the pharynx is shared by the respiratory and digestive tracts. Its superior portion, the **respiratory pharynx,** lies above the level of the soft palate; it communicates with the nasal cavity and is lined by respiratory epithelium. The inferior portion, the **oral pharynx (oropharynx),** lies below the level of the soft palate. It communicates with the oral cavity and is lined by nonkeratinized stratified squamous epithelium. Its walls, whose structure resembles that of the oral cavity, contain the palatine and pharyngeal tonsils (see Chapter 14), many small subepithelial mucous glands, and skeletal muscle arranged as circular pharyngeal constrictors and longitudinal pharyngeal muscles. The pharynx also communicates with both the esophagus and the larynx. During swallowing, the back of the tongue helps close the epiglottis (see Chapter 17) to direct food away from the larynx and into the esophagus.

IV. ESOPHAGUS.

This is a long, narrow, muscular tube that transports food from the pharynx to the stomach. Its mucosa includes nonkeratinized stratified squamous epithelium, a lamina propria that interdigitates with the scalloped basal border of the epithelium, and a muscularis mucosae. The mucus-secreting **esophageal glands** that characterize its submucosa help distinguish the esophagus from the vagina (see Chapter 23) in histologic sections. The muscularis externa of the esophagus is composed of skeletal muscle in the upper third, a mixture of skeletal and smooth muscle in the middle third, and smooth muscle in the lower third. The outer surface is covered by adventitia, except for the short serosa-covered segment in the abdominal cavity between diaphragm and stomach. Mucus-secreting esophageal cardiac glands are found in the lamina propria of the region near the stomach.

V. STOMACH.

This dilated portion of the digestive tract temporarily holds ingested food, adding mucus, acid, and the digestive enzyme **pepsin.** Muscular contractions of the stomach blend these components into a viscous mixture called **chyme.** The chyme is then divided into parcels for further digestion and absorption by the intestines.

A. General Structure:

The stomach wall has the same layers as the rest of the tract. The complex mucosa contains numerous **gastric glands,** a 2–3 layer muscularis mucosae that helps empty the glands, and an intervening lamina propria. When the stomach is empty and contracted, the mucosa and underlying submucosa are thrown into irregular, temporary folds called **rugae,** that flatten when it is full. The smooth muscle of the muscularis externa is arranged in 3 layers: outer longitudinal, middle circular, and inner oblique. The stomach has 4 major regions; **cardia, fundus, body,** and **pylorus.**

B. Gastric Mucosa:

1. General features The stomach lining is covered with simple columnar epithelium and perforated by numerous small holes called **foveolae gastricae.** The foveolae are the openings of epithelial invaginations, the **gastric pits,** which penetrate the lamina propria to varying depths. The pits serve as ducts for the branched tubular gastric glands. Each gland has 3 regions: an isthmus at the bottom of the pit, a straight neck that penetrates deeper into the lamina propria (perpendicular to the surface), and a coiled base that penetrates deeper still and ends blindly just above the muscularis mucosae.

2. Mucosal epithelial cell types

a. Surface mucous cells These form the simple columnar epithelium lining the stomach, the gastric pits, and much of the isthmus of each gastric gland. These cells secrete a neutral mucus that protects the stomach's surface from the acidity of the gastric fluid.

b. Undifferentiated cells Low columnar cells with basal ovoid nuclei, these are found scattered in the neck of the gastric gland. Some cells divide in the neck and move upward to replace pit and surface mucous cells. Others move deeper into the glands and differentiate into the other cell types listed below. Surface mucous cells turn over more rapidly than do the other cell types.

c. Mucous neck cells These cells occur singly or in clusters between the parietal cells in the neck of the gland. They differ from surface mucous cells in that they secrete an acidic mucus.

d. Parietal (oxyntic) cells These cells secrete HC1 and intrinsic factor.

(1) Structure and location Found mainly between mucous neck cells in the neck of the gland, they are present, but scarce, in the base. These cells are large, pale, and round to pyramidal in shape. They have one or 2 central nuclei and an acidophilic cytoplasm. The many mitochondria indicate that their secretory activity is energy-dependent. Each cell has a circular invagination of its apical plasma membrane that is visible only with the electron microscope. When stimulated to produce HCl, the many **tubulovesicles** in the apical cytoplasm fuse with the invaginated plasma membrane to form a deeper, more highly branched invagination termed the **intracellular canaliculus.**

(2) Function HCl production involves active transport of H^+ and Cl^- ions across canalicular membranes into the lumen. The Cl^- derives from blood-borne chloride. H^+ formation involves a 2-step process in which CO_2 is converted by **carbonic anhydrase** to carbonic acid. This dissociates into H^+ and bicarbonate. **Intrinsic factor** is a glycoprotein that is required for absorption of vitamin B_{12}. B_{12} deficiency leads to a disorder of erythropoiesis called **pernicious anemia.** Parietal cell secretion is stimulated by cholinergic nerve endings. Acid production is greatly enhaced by histamine and gastrin produced by enteroendocrine cells in the gastric glands (and elsewhere).

e. Chief (zymogenic) cells These secrete pepsinogen and some lipase.

(1) Structure and location These cells, which predominate in the base of gastric glands, are smaller than parietal cells. They are basophilic as a result of the ribosomes associated with their RER. They also contain membrane-limited pepsinogen-filled zymogen granules.

(2) Function The RER synthesizes pepsinogen and lipase, which are packaged in granules by the Golgi complex and stored in the cytoplasm for secretion. **Pepsinogen** is an inactive proenzyme or zymogen that is converted to the active protease **pepsin** when exposed to the acidic environment of the stomach lumen. Gastric **lipase** has only weak lipolytic activity.

f. Enteroendocrine cells In the stomach, these cells (I.C.4) occur mainly in the base of gastric glands. They produce various endocrine and paracrine amines (eg, histamine, serotonin) and peptide hormones (eg, gastrin). They are considered components of the diffuse neuroendocrine system (DNES).

C. Regional Differences:

1. Cardia A narrow collarlike region, the cardia surrounds the point of entry of the esophagus. Here, the lamina propria contains simple or branched tubular cardiac glands like those in the terminal part of the esophagus. The basal portions of these glands are often coiled, with wide lumens. Although they produce mainly mucus and lysozyme, some parietal cells may be present.

2. Fundus and body These are similar in structure and function. The body is the stomach's largest region, extending from the cardia to the pylorus. The fundus is a smaller, roughly hemispheric region that extends above the cardia. Gastric glands—termed **fundic glands** in both regions—are characterized by shallow pits and long glands. The pits extend about a third of the distance from the mucosal surface to the base of the glands. Fundic glands contain abundant **parietal** and **chief cells.** Parietal cells are concentrated in the neck and upper part of the base, while chief cells predominate in the lower portion. **Serotonin (5-hydroxytryptamine)-secreting cells** are typically found at the bases of these glands.

3. Pylorus This makes up the distal 4–5 cm of the stomach, leading to the small intestine. **Pyloric glands** are characterized by deep pits and short glands (mnemonic: P for both pylorus and pits). The pits extend one-half to two-thirds of the distance from the mucosal surface to the base of the glands. While all glandular cell types may be present, large pale-staining mucus-secreting cells with basal nuclei predominate (these are hard to distinguish from mucous neck cells in H&E-stained sections), and parietal cells are fewer in number. Chief cells are especially scarce in this region. Gastrin-secreting cells **(G cells)** are typical of the bases of these glands. At the pylorus-small intestine junction, a thickened band of the middle circular layer of the muscularis externa, the **pyloric sphincter,** controls the passage of chyme.

VI. SMALL INTESTINE.

The small intestine, which includes the **duodenum, jejunum, and ileum,** receives chyme from the stomach, bile from the liver, and digestive enzymes from the pancreas. Here, nutrients are hydrolyzed into an absorbable form; they are absorbed and transferred to blood and lymphatic capillaries. Undigested material is moved to the large intestine by peristalsis. The word *small* refers to diameter, not length: the small intestine is longer and narrower than the large intestine.

A. General Structure:

The walls of the small intestine have the same layers as do the rest of the tract (I.B). The 2-layered muscularis externa (I.B.3) exhibits archetypal organization, as does the submucosa (I.B.2), except in the duodenum, where distinctive submucosal (Brunner's) glands (discussed below) are present. A series of permanent folds, the **plicae circulares (valves of Kerckring),** composed of both submucosa and mucosa, extend into the lumen and increase the surface area about 3-fold. The main distinguishing features of the small intestine (as viewed through the microsope) reside in the composition and organization of the mucosa.

B. Mucosa of the Small Intestine:

This consists of simple columnar epithelium with goblet cells, underlain by a lamina propria and separated from the submucosa by a muscularis mucosae.

1. Villi The presence of these epithelium-covered fingerlike mucosal projections into the lumen is the most outstanding diagnostic feature of small intestine structure. The lamina propria core of each is composed of loose connective tissue (see Chapter 5) and contains a central, blind-ending lymphatic capillary (often called a lacteal), as well as blood capillaries. Smooth muscle fibers run lengthwise in the villus core; however, the muscularis mucosae per se does not extend into the villi. Rhythmic contractions (shortening) of the villi speed up during digestion and help propel the nutrients in blood and lymphatic capillaries to the general circulation. The villi increase the mucosal surface area about 10-fold and thus enhance absorption; their shape and abundance differ according to the region in which they lie.

2. Intestinal glands Also known as the **crypts of Lieberkühn,** these are simple tubular glands (often coiled) in the lamina propria below the bases of the villi. They are lined by absorptive, goblet, Paneth, enteroendocrine, and undifferentiated cells. Their secretions enter the lumen via small openings between the villi. Similar glands are seen in the large intestine, where they contain many more globlet cells.

3. Mucosal epithelial cell types

a. Enterocytes These **absorptive cells** are the predominant cell type covering the villi. They occur in smaller numbers in the crypts.

(1) Structure These tall columnar cells with basal nuclei have densely-packed glycocalyx-covered **microvilli** extending from their apical surfaces into the lumen. The approximately 3000 microvilli per cell give the cell-lumen border a striped appearance, this is known as a **striated border.** Absorptive cells attach laterally to neighboring cells by junctional complexes (see Chapter 4), including tight junctions near the lumen.

(2) Function While their structure is comparatively simple, these cells perform several complex and important functions.

(a) Digestion Disacharidases and dipeptidases may be found associated with the luminal surfaces of the microvilli. These enzymes complete the hydrolysis of nutrients that was begun by pancreatic enzymes in the lumen. The resulting monosaccharides and amino acids are more readily absorbed.

(b) Absorption Apical microvilli increase the absorptive surface area about 20-fold and thus enhance absorption. Amino acids and monosaccharides are actively transported across the apical plasma membrane, while the products of lipid hydrolysis (fatty acids and monoglycerides) cross passively. Various large molecules may enter through the pinocytotic vesicles **(caveolae)** that form at the bases of the microvilli.

(c) Lipid processing and chylomicron assembly Absorbed monoglycerides and long-chain fatty acids collect in the smooth endoplasmic reticulum, where they are resynthesized into triglycerides and then assembled into chylomicrons—small lipid spheres with a thin surface coat of protein. Chylomicrons are packed in vesicles by the Golgi complex and move to the lateral plasma membrane for exocytosis; from here, most enter the lymphatic capillaries.

(d) Transport of smaller nutrients Amino acids, monosaccharides, and short-chain fatty acids cross the cytoplasm and then the basolateral cell membrane to reach the lamina propria, where they enter blood and lymphatic capillaries.

b. Goblet cells These lie between the absorptive cells, with more in the surface epithelium than in the crypts. They gradually increase in number from the duodenum to the ileum. The acid glycoproteins they secrete onto the mucosal surface lubricate the digestive tract's walls, protecting them from pancreatic enzymes and impeding bacterial invasion (see Chapter 4 for a discussion of the cell structure).

c. M cells These membranous epithelial cells are flat cells overlying solitary lymphoid nodules and Peyer's patches (see Chapter 14) of the intestinal lamina propria. Their apical (luminal) surfaces have small folds rather than microvilli. The cells help initiate immune responses by endocytosing antigens from the lumen and passing them to lymphoid cells in the underlying nodules.

d. Paneth cells Lying in the bases of the crypts, these cells synthesize a protein-polysaccharide complex. In addition to RER and Golgi complexes, they contain many large acidophilic secretory granules that contain **lysozyme** an antibacterial enzyme that may play a role in controlling intestinal flora.

e. Enteroendocrine cells Most known types of enteroendocrine cells (I.C.4) are found in the crypts of the small intestine. Those that occur mainly in this area produce hormones and amines such as secretin, which increases pancreatic and biliary bicarbonate and water secretion, cholecystokinin, which increases pancreatic enzyme secretion and gall bladder contraction; gastric inhibitory peptide, which decreases gastric acid production; and motilin, which increases gut motility.

f. Undifferentiated cells Mucosal epithelial cells undergo continual turnover. Replacement occurs through the mitosis of undifferentiated (stem) cells located near the base of the crypts. Products of these divisions differentiate into all the cell types described above; by a mechanism that is still unclear, they move toward the crypt base to become Paneth cells or toward the tips of the villi, where they are finally sloughed off into the lumen.

C. Regional Differences:

1. Duodenum The major distinguishing feature of this C-shaped first part of the small intestine is the presence of **duodenal (Brunner's) glands** in the submucosa. The mucous cells of these glands produce an alkaline secretion (pH 8.1–9.3) that protects the duodenal lining from the acidity of the chyme and raises the luminal pH to the optimum level for pancreatic enzyme activity. Unlike the jejunum and ileum, the duodenum is mostly a retroperitoneal organ (I.B.4). It is also the point of entry for the usually common, but sometimes separate, bile and pancreatic ducts, which penetrate the full thickness of the duodenal wall. It typically exhibits fingerlike or leaflike villi and relatively few goblet cells. Since the arms of the C cradle the head of the pancreas in situ, small pieces of pancreatic tissue often accompany duodenal sections, providing another clue for identification.

2. Jejunum An intraperitoneal organ, the jejunum has long leaflike villi, many plicae circulares, and an intermediate number of goblet cells. The key to its identification, however, is that while it has villi (and is thus part of the small intestine), it contains neither Brunner's glands nor Peyer's patches.

3. Ileum This intraperitoneal organ has fewer villi, which are short and broad-tipped (clublike), and relatively abundant goblet cells. Its lamina propria typically contains many lymphoid nodule clusters (Peyer's patches; see Chapter 14). These may be large enough to produce a visible bulge on the luminal surface and extend into the submucosa.

VII. LARGE INTESTINE (COLON).

This includes the cecum; the ascending, transverse, descending, and sigmoid colons; and the rectum. It converts undigested material received from the small intestine into feces by removing water and adding mucus. The large intestine is shorter than the small intestine and has a wider lumen. Its walls have structural features that distinguish it from the small intestine at both gross and microscopic levels.

A. Mucosa:

The colon's lining has no folds, except in the rectum, where many vertical folds, called the **rectal columns (of Morgagni),** occur at the recto-anal junction. No villi are present. The epithelium is simple columnar with a great abundance of goblet cells. The interposed absorptive cells have irregular short microvilli. Water absorption by these cells is passive; it follows the active transport of sodium out of their basal surfaces. The mucosa has many deep crypts of Leiberkühn containing abundant goblet cells and few enteroendocrine cells. The lamina propria has more lymphoid cells and nodules than does that of the small intestine. Nodules may extend into the submucosa.

B. Submucosa:

This is generally unremarkable except in the lower rectum where it contains portions of the **hemorrhoidal plexus** of veins, which extends into the lamina propria. The absence of valves in the veins within and draining this plexus, added to the great abdominal and pelvic pressure changes they are subjected to during straining, etc, often causes these veins to become varicosed, resulting in the formation of hemorrhoids (known familiarly as piles).

C. Muscularis Externa:

This portion of the colon is unique in that the outer longitudinal layer of smooth muscle is gathered into 3 thick longitudinal bands called **teniae coli.** A thin layer of longitudinal smooth muscle often exists between the bands. The inner circular muscle layer resembles that of the small intestine.

D. Adventitia and Serosa:

The type of outer covering found on the various parts of the colon depends on whether they are intraperitoneal (cecum, transverse, sigmoid) or retroperitoneal (ascending, descending) (see I.B.4 and Table 15–1). The rectum passes vertically through the pelvis, surrounded entirely by adventitia. The colon's serosa is characterized by the presence of many teardrop-shaped adipose-filled outpocketings termed **appendices epiploicae.**

VIII. APPENDIX (Vermiform Appendix). This is a narrow fingerlike evagination of the inferior end of the cecum. Histologically, it resembles the colon except that it has a smaller lumen, fewer and shorter crypts, more lymphoid nodules, and no teniae coli.

IX. ANAL CANAL. In humans, this canal is about 4 cm long, connecting the rectum and the anal opening. The mucosa of the first 2 cm has typical colonic epithelium with very short crypts. This is replaced by stratified squamous epithelium, which continues to the anal opening. The lamina propria contains extensions of the hemorrhoidal plexus, and the submucosa under the stratified epithelium contains typical sebaceous glands and large circumanal apocrine sweat glands (see Chapter 18). The muscularis in this region has a thickened inner circular layer of smooth muscle that forms the involuntary internal anal sphincter. Distal to this, the canal is encircled by the voluntary external anal sphincter, composed of skeletal muscle from the pelvic diaphragm.

Study-Focusing Questions*

1. List the organs of the digestive tract in the order in which food traverses them (282). (Before answering, read question 2. You may want to construct a table.)
2. What happens to the food in each of the organs listed in the answer to question 1 (282)?
3. Describe the oral cavity in terms of:
   a. Its epithelial lining (284)
   b. The type of muscle found in its walls (284)
   c. The structural difference between the hard and soft palate (284)
4. Describe the tongue in terms of:
   a. The predominant tissue it contains (284)
   b. Its covering epithelium (284–285)
5. Name the 4 types of lingual papillae and compare them in terms of their:
   a. Characteristic shape
   b. Number and distribution of taste buds
   c. Abundance
6. Sketch the upper (dorsal) surface of the tongue and indicate the location of the various types of papillae and the lingual tonsils (284–285).
7. Describe the oral pharynx (285) in terms of:
   a. Its epithelial lining
   b. The type of muscle found in its walls
8. List the 4 types (by shape) of teeth found in humans (285).
9. Compare the number of permanent and deciduous teeth found in each quadrant (the "dental formula") (285).
10. Sketch a tooth and its surrounding structures in sagittal (midline longitudinal) section (286) and label the following:
    a. Gingiva
    b. Alveolar bone (288)
    c. Crown
    d. Neck
    e. Root
    f. Apical foramen
    g. Enamel
    h. Cementum
    i. Dentin
    j. Pulp

*The page references in this section refer to *Basic Histology,* 6th ed., Junqueira L, Carneiro J, Kelley R (editors), Appleton & Lange, 1989. **HR** (for Histology Review) is occasionally used instead of a page reference to indicate that the information referred to can be found in this book.

   - **k.** Periodontal ligament
   - **l.** Epithelial attachment (of Gottlieb) (288)

11. Compare dentin (285), enamel (285–286), and cementum (287) in terms of:
   - **a.** Their hardness
   - **b.** Their porosity
   - **c.** Their collagen content
   - **d.** The cell type responsible for the formation of each
   - **e.** Their ability to be replaced in adulthood

12. Describe the composition of tooth pulp (286) in terms of its:
   - **a.** Predominant tissue
   - **b.** Major cell types
   - **c.** Blood supply
   - **d.** Innervation

13. Compare ameloblasts, odontoblasts, and cementoblasts in terms of:
   - **a.** Their embryonic tissue of origin (288)
   - **b.** The layer of tooth structure formed by each (285–286, 287)
   - **c.** Their survival into adulthood (285–286, 289)

14. Describe the periodontal ligament in terms of:
   - **a.** Its composition (287)
   - **b.** Its location (286, 287)
   - **c.** The structures to which it attaches (286, 287)
   - **d.** Its functions (287)
   - **e.** The effects of dietary vitamin C and protein deficiency on it (288)

15. Name the 2 embryonic tissue types whose interactions result in tooth development (288).

16. Beginning with the formation of the dental laminae, list, in order, the named stages in crown development (288–289).

17. Describe the dental laminae (288) in terms of their:
   - **a.** Number
   - **b.** Location
   - **c.** Shape
   - **d.** Cell type (ie, which of the 2 cell types listed in your answer to question 15)

18. Sketch a developing tooth in the bell stage (289) and label the following:
   - **a.** Ameloblasts
   - **b.** Odontoblasts
   - **c.** Enamel organ
   - **d.** Inner enamel epithelium
   - **e.** Outer enamel epithelium
   - **f.** Stellate reticulum
   - **g.** Dental papilla
   - **h.** Cervical loop

19. Identify the origin of each component listed in question 18 as epithelial or mesenchymal (288–289).

20. Name the events or structures that induce the following during tooth development (288–289):
   - **a.** Initiation of tooth-bud formation
   - **b.** Proliferation and condensation of dental papillary mesenchyme
   - **c.** Formation of the inner enamel epithelium
   - **d.** Differentiation of odontoblasts
   - **e.** Differentiation of ameloblasts
   - **f.** Production of predentin
   - **g.** Production of enamel

21. By the time a deciduous tooth is shed prior to the eruption of the permanent tooth, only the crown remains. What happens to the root (**HR**)?

22. Sketch a cross section of a generalized tubular organ of the digestive tract showing the layered structure of its walls (282, 283), and indicate the location of the following:
   - **a.** Lumen
   - **b.** Mucosa
   - **c.** Submucosa
   - **d.** Muscularis externa

- **e.** Serosa
- **f.** Epithelium
- **g.** Lamina propria
- **h.** Muscularis mucosae
- **i.** Meissner's (submocosal) plexus
- **j.** Auerbach's (myenteric) plexus
- **k.** Mesothelium
- **l.** Attachment of the mesentery

23. Compare the esophageal wall in the portion nearest the pharynx with that nearest the stomach (290) in terms of the:
- **a.** Epithelium
- **b.** Location of mucus-secreting glands
- **c.** Tissue type of the muscularis externa
- **d.** Outer covering (serosa versus adventitia)

24. Sketch the outline of the stomach and show the boundaries of the 4 named regions: cardia, fundus, body, and pylorus (291).

25. Name the type of epithelium covering the stomach's luminal surface and lining the gastric pits (foveolae) (290).

26. Compare the gastric glands found in the mucosa of the 4 regions of the stomach (292–296) in terms of:
- **a.** Their major secretory products
- **b.** Their minor secretory products
- **c.** The depth of their gastric pits

27. Name the 4 types of secretory cells found in the gastric glands (292–295) and compare them in terms of their:
- **a.** Secretory product(s)
- **b.** Staining properties
- **c.** Distribution in the glands
- **d.** Characteristic cytoplasmic organelles

28. How does the stomach's muscularis externa differ from that of the other tubular organs of the digestive tract (297)?

29. Name, in order of digestion, the 3 segments of the small intestine (297).

30. Name the type of epithelium lining the small intestine (298).

31. List 3 features of the wall of the small intestine that increase the surface area exposed to the lumen and thus promote absorption of nutrients (297–298).

32. Name 5 important cell types found in the epithelium lining the intestinal lumen and the crypts of Lieberkühn (298–300) and compare them in terms of their:
- **a.** Primary function (and secretory products, if any)
- **b.** Distribution
- **c.** Distinguishing structural characteristics
- **d.** Special staining properties, if any

33. Compare the duodenum and ileum in terms of the:
- **a.** Shape and number of villi (297–298)
- **b.** Presence of submucosal glands (300)
- **c.** Presence of lymphoid tissue (302)
- **d.** Number of goblet cells (300)

34. Sketch a cross section of a portion of the small intestine wall (283, 301, 305); include and label the following:
- **a.** Mucosa
- **b.** Submucosa
- **c.** Muscularis externa
- **d.** Serosa
- **e.** Plicae circulares
- **f.** Villi(us)
- **g.** Crypt(s) of Lieberkühn
- **h.** Epithelium
- **i.** Absorptive cell(s)
- **j.** Goblet cell(s)
- **k.** Paneth cell(s)
- **l.** Lamina propria
- **m.** Blood capillaries

n. Lymphatic capillary (lacteal)
o. Muscularis mucosae
p. Meissner's (submucosal) plexus
q. Auerbach's (myenteric) plexus
r. Mesothelium

35. Compare the absorption of lipids, amino acids, and monosaccharides from the small intestine lumen (305–306) in terms of:
    a. The mechanism by which they enter the absorptive cells
    b. Any modifications carried out in the absorptive cell (eg, packaging)
    c. Their selective uptake by blood versus lymph
36. List the functions of the large intestine (306).
37. Indicate how the large intestine differs from the small intestine in terms of the:
    a. Plicae circulares and villi (306)
    b. Number of goblet cells (306)
    c. Amount of lymphoid tissue (309)
    d. Outer layer of the muscularis externa (309)
38. Describe how the appendix differs from most of the large intestine in terms of:
    a. Its overall diameter (309–310)
    b. The depth of the crypts (310)
    c. The abundance of lymphoid follicles (310)
    d. Its muscularis externa (310)
39. Compare the rugae of the stomach (290) and the circular folds (plicae circulares) of the small intestine (297) in terms of their permanence.
40. List the segments of the digestive tract that are covered:
    a. Primarily by serosa
    b. Primarily by adventitia
    c. By both
41. Describe the trends in wall structure from duodenum through the colon in terms of the increase or decrease in the:
    a. Number of goblet cells (300, 306)
    b. Number of enteroendocrine cells (300, 303)
    c. Amount of lymphoid tissue (297, 302, 309)
    d. Number of villi (**HR**)
    e. Number of circular folds (297, 300)

Multiple-Choice Questions

For the questions 15–1 through 15–8, select the single best answer.

15–1. The dental formula for adults (permanent teeth) is:
- A. 1 incisor, 1 canine, 3 premolars, 3 molars
- B. 2 incisors, 1 canine, 2 premolars, 3 molars
- C. 2 incisors, 2 canines, 2 premolars, 2 molars
- D. 2 incisors, 1 canine, 3 premolars, 2 molars
- E. 3 incisors, 1 canine, 2 premolars, 3 molars

15–2. A cascade of interactions between which 2 tissue types is primarily responsible for tooth formation?
- A. Epithelium and nerve
- B. Ectomesenchyme and epithelium
- C. Blood and ectomesenchyme
- D. Blood and nerve
- E. Nerve and ectomesenchyme

15–3. The ectomesenchyme located in the region of developing teeth is derived from:
- A. Oral endoderm
- B. Mesoderm
- C. Oral ectoderm
- D. Neural crest
- E. None of the above

15-4. The organ shown in the photomicrograph in Fig 15-1 is the:
- **A.** Lower esophagus
- **B.** Rectum
- **C.** Cardiac stomach
- **D.** Upper esophagus
- **E.** Colon

15-5. The organ shown in the photomicrograph in Fig 15-2 is:
- **A.** Duodenum
- **B.** Fundic stomach
- **C.** Colon
- **D.** Pyloric stomach
- **E.** Cardiac stomach

15-6. The cell type depicted in the diagram in Fig 15-3 is a:
- **A.** Paneth cell
- **B.** Gastric chief cell
- **C.** Parietal (oxyntic) cell
- **D.** Enteroendocrine cell
- **E.** Mucous neck cell

15-7. The organ shown in the photomicrograph in Fig 15-4 is the:
- **A.** Ileum
- **B.** Duodenum
- **C.** Jejunum
- **D.** Pyloric stomach
- **E.** Colon

15-8. The organ shown in the photomicrograph in Fig 15-5 is the:
- **A.** Pyloric stomach
- **B.** Fundic stomach
- **C.** Cardiac stomach
- **D.** Ileum
- **E.** Colon

MATCHING (questions 15-9 through 15-45): each choice may be used once, more than once, or not at all.

Questions 15-9 through 15-13:

- **A.** Filiform papillae
- **B.** Foliate papillae

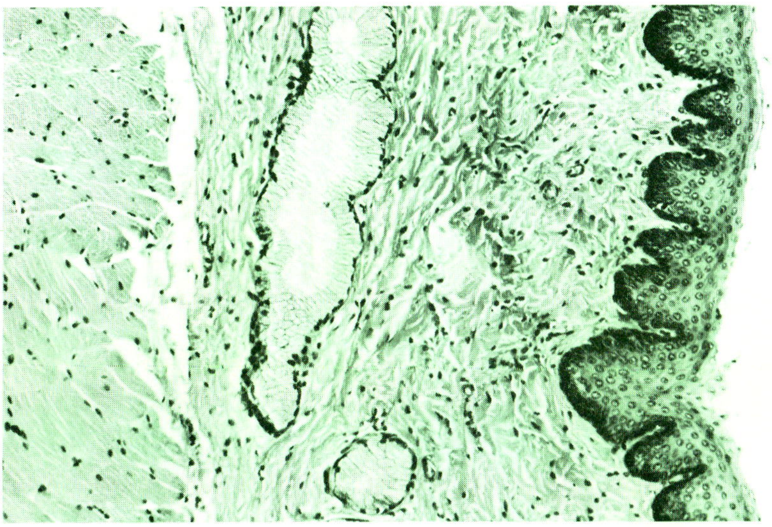

Figure 15-1.

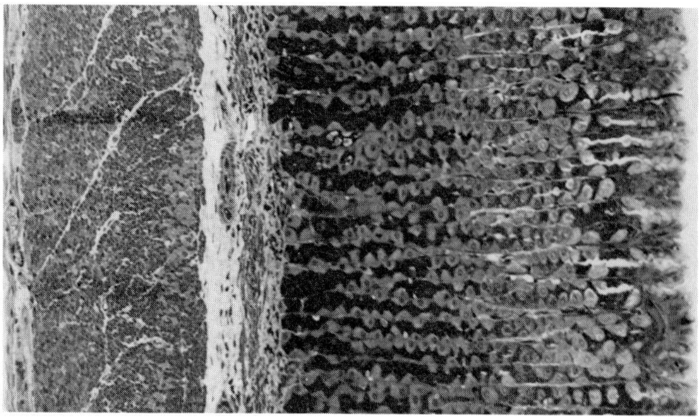

Figure 15-2.

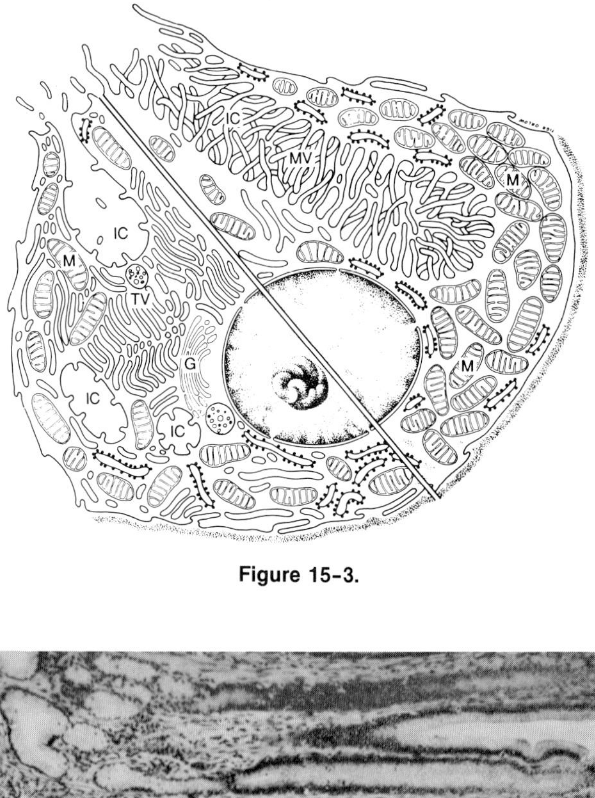

Figure 15-3.

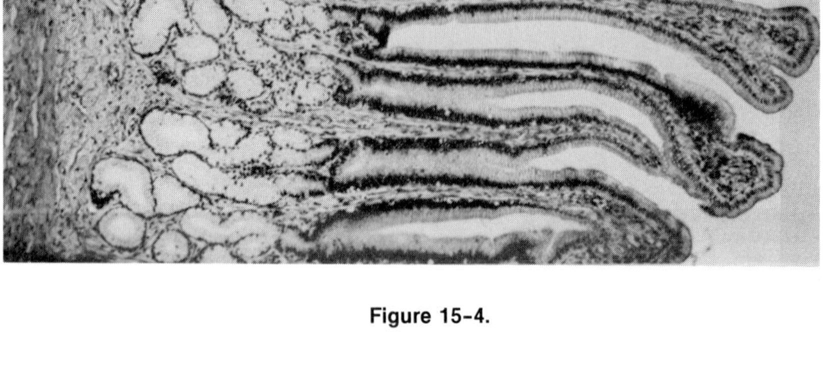

Figure 15-4.

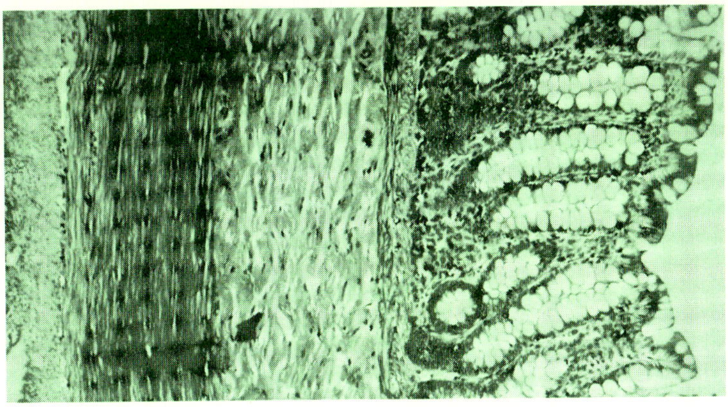

Figure 15-5.

C. Fungiform papillae
D. Circumvallate papillae

15-9. Are often partially keratinized
15-10. Have taste buds on upper surface of papillae
15-11. Are largest papillae
15-12. Lack taste buds
15-13. Ducts from glands open around the base

Questions 15-14 through 15-22 use the letters in Fig 15-6:

15-14. Dentin
15-15. Pulp
15-16. Enamel

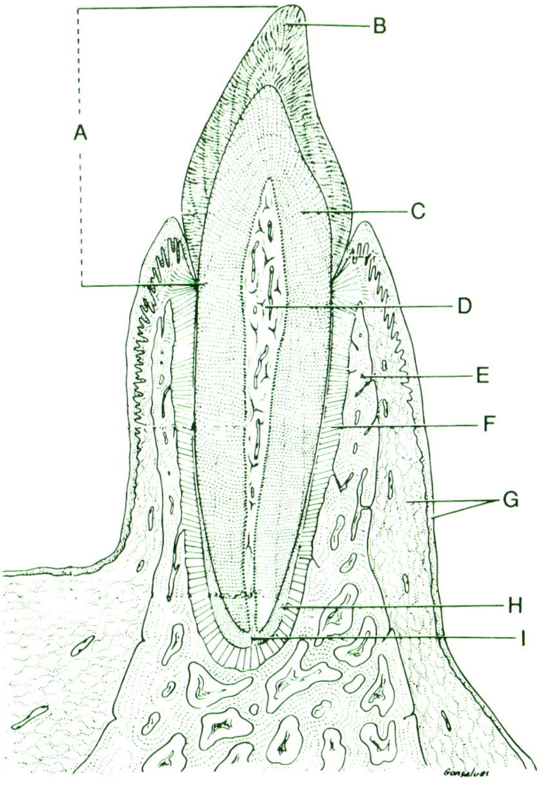

Figure 15-6.

15–17. Alveolar bone
15–18. Periodontal ligament (or membrane)
15–19. Crown of tooth
15–20. Gingiva
15–21. Cementum
15–22. Apical foramen

Questions 15–23 through 15–32 use the letters in Fig 15–7:

15–23. Cervical loop
15–24. Inner enamel epithelium
15–25. Outer enamel epithelium
15–26. Odontoblasts
15–27. Developing ameloblasts
15–28. Capillary
15–29. Basal lamina
15–30. Stellate reticulum
15–31. Together form enamel organ
15–32. Cells that produce dentin

Questions 15–33 through 15–45:

A. Parietal cells
B. Chief cells
C. Enteroendocrine cells
D. Paneth cells
E. Goblet cells
F. Enterocytes (absorptive cells)

15–33. Assemble chylomicrons
15–34. Secrete pepsinogen
15–35. Secrete gastrin
15–36. Secrete intrinsic factor
15–37. Secrete secretin
15–38. Secrete HCl
15–39. Predominate at the base of fundic glands
15–40. Secrete somatostatin
15–41. Secrete lysozyme
15–42. Secrete mucus

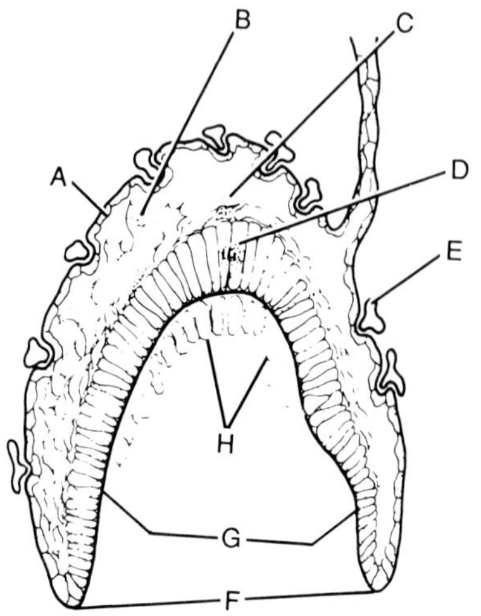

Figure 15-7.

15–43. Secrete cholecystokinin
15–44. Have intracellular canaliculi
15–45. Are basophilic cells in fundic glands

For questions 15–46 through 15–69, either, both, or neither of the answers may be correct. Select

A if only A is correct
B if only B is correct
C if both A and B are correct
D if neither A nor B are correct

Questions 15–46 through 15–53:

A. Ameloblasts
B. Odontoblasts
C. Both
D. Neither

15–46. Derived from ectoderm
15–47. Derived from ectomesenchyme
15–48. Produce dentin
15–49. Form Tomes' processes
15–50. Produce enamel
15–51. Produce cementum
15–52. Die soon after tooth erupts
15–53. Form Tomes' fibers

Questions 15–54 through 15–59:

A. Upper esophagus
B. Lower esophagus
C. Both
D. Neither

15–54. Nonkeratinized stratified squamous epithelium
15–55. Skeletal muscle in muscularis externa
15–56. Skeletal muscle in muscularis mucosae
15–57. Thickest muscularis mucosae
15–58. Mucous glands in submucosa
15–59. Mucous glands in lamina propria

Questions 15–60 through 15–69:

A. Small intestine
B. Large intestine
C. Both
D. Neither

15–60. Contain(s) more goblet cells per unit area
15–61. Has permanent circular folds (plicae circulares) in wall
15–62. Is more active in absorption of water
15–63. Is more active in absorption of nutrients
15–64. Exhibit(s) appendices epiploicae
15–65. Contain(s) villi
15–66. Contain(s) crypts of Lieberkühn
15–67. Contain(s) some enteroendocrine cells
15–68. Exhibit(s) teniae coli
15–69. Is lined by simple columnar epithelium

For questions 15-70 through 15-78, one, more than one, or all of the answers may be correct. Select

A if only (1), (2), and (3) are correct
B if only (1) and (3) are correct
C if only (2) and (4) are correct
D if only (4) is correct
E if all answers are correct

15-70. The periodontal membrane (ligament):
(1) Is composed primarily of elastic fibers
(2) Attaches directly to the dentin
(3) Attaches only to the crown of the tooth
(4) Attaches to the alveolar bone

15-71. Cells and structures derived from ectomesenchyme include:
(1) Odontoblasts
(2) Alveolar bone
(3) Dental pulp
(4) Ameloblasts

15-72. The mucosal glands of the fundus of the stomach:
(1) Are similar to those in the body of the stomach
(2) Have more parietal cells in their upper half than in their basal half
(3) Secrete more pepsinogen than do the pyloric glands
(4) Have deeper pits than those in the pyloric region

15-73. The wall of the stomach:
(1) Is thrown into temporary folds called rugae when empty
(2) Is covered on its inner surface by simple columnar epithelium
(3) Has 3 layers of smooth muscle in its muscularis externa
(4) Is covered on its outer surface by simple squamous epithelium

15-74. Structures that promote the absorption of nutrients by increasing the internal surface area of the small intestine include the:
(1) Villi
(2) Plicae circulares
(3) Microvilli
(4) Appendices epiploicae

15-75. A high rate of mitotic activity is normally found:
(1) In the neck region of the gastric glands
(2) In the germinal centers of Peyer's patch nodules
(3) In the crypts of Lieberkühn
(4) At the tips of the villi

15-76. Brunner's glands:
(1) Are a characteristic constituent of the wall of the duodenum
(2) Are found in the submucosal layer
(3) Empty their secretions into the crypts of Lieberkühn
(4) Produce a serous secretion rich in digestive enzymes

15-77. Absorptive cells (enterocytes) of the small intestine:
(1) Are covered on their apical surfaces by abundant microvilli
(2) Absorb lipids by passive diffusion
(3) Use absorbed lipids to resynthesize triglycerides
(4) Absorb amino acids and monosaccharides by passive diffusion

15-78. The appendix:
(1) Is a blind-ended evagination of the cecum
(2) Has abundant lymphoid nodules in its walls
(3) Has relatively shallow intestinal glands
(4) Has longitudinal smooth muscle collected into teniae coli

Glands Associated With the Digestive Tract 16

Objectives

This chapter should help the student to:

- Know the accessory glands attached, by their ducts, to the digestive tract.
- Name the primary exocrine secretory product(s) of each of these accessory glands and describe the role of each product in digestion.
- Compare the structure and function of the 3 major types of salivary glands.
- Compare the serous and mucous secretory cells of salivary glands.
- Compare the structures of the parotid gland and pancreas.
- Describe the liver's double blood supply.
- Describe the complex structure of a hepatocyte and relate its structure to its many functions.
- Describe the classic liver lobule, the portal lobule, and the hepatic acinus (of Rappaport).
- Describe the composition and production of bile.
- List several endocrine secretory products of the liver.
- List the functions of the gall bladder.
- Compare the wall of the gall bladder with that of the small intestine.
- Identify the gall bladder from a slide or photomicrograph and distinguish it from a similar section of small intestine.
- In a slide or photomicrograph of a section of a digestive gland, identify the type of gland; distinguish between adenomeres and ducts; identify the different types of ducts, cells, and other named substructures (eg, serous demilune, central vein, bile duct, sinusoid.

Synopsis

I. GENERAL FEATURES OF THE GLANDS ASSOCIATED WITH THE DIGESTIVE TRACT

A. Components of the System: The **salivary glands**—parotid, submandibular, and sublingual—**pancreas,** and **liver** are digestive glands situated outside the digestive tract. The main function of the **gall bladder,** also discussed in this chapter, is to store bile.

B. Embryonic Origin and Association With the Tract: Each component arises as an outpocketing of the embryonic gut tube and retains its connection with the lumen of the tract through a duct. The duct-lining cells and exocrine secretory cells are epithelial and of endodermal origin. The supporting connective tissue that forms the organ capsules and penetrates the glands to divide them into lobes and lobules derives from mesoderm.

C. Exocrine and Endocrine Functions: The presence of ducts indicates that these are exocrine glands; however, the pancreas and liver also have important endocrine functions.

D. Serous and Mucous Exocrine Secretory Cells: In general, the secretory cells of the liver, pancreas, and parotid gland are exclusively serous, while the submandibular and sublingual glands contain a mixture of serous and mucous cells (see Chapter 4).

E. Glandular Subunits: Exocrine glands are structurally and functionally subdivided by **septa,** plate-like invaginations of their connective tissue capsules. This arrangement applies mainly to the pancreas and salivary glands; the subdivision of the liver, which is more complex, is considered separately (IV.E).

1. Lobes The largest of the subunits, these are separated from one another by connective tissue septa.

2. Lobules These are subunits of the lobes and are separated by thin extensions of the septa.

3. Adenomeres The secretory subunits of lobules, adenomeres consist of all the secretory cells that release their products into a single intralobular duct.

4. Acini (or alveoli) These are smaller secretory subunits. Each acinus is a spheric collection of secretory cells surrounding the blind-ended termination of a single intercalated duct. An adenomere may include one or several acini.

F. Exocrine Ducts: Digestive gland ducts are classified by their location and identified by their location, size, and epithelial lining.

1. Intralobular ducts Several of these small ducts may be found within each lobule. They are generally lined by simple cuboidal epithelial cells with central or basal nuclei and surrounded by only a thin layer of connective tissue. They transport the secretory products from the adenomeres to the interlobular excretory ducts. There are also 2 special types of intralobular ducts.

a. Intercalated ducts These are the smallest ducts in a gland, with a narrow lumen that is continuous with the lumen of the acini. These ducts usually have a simple squamous or low cuboidal epithelial lining. They transport secretory products from the adenomeres to the larger intralobular ducts.

b. Striated ducts These differ from standard intralobular ducts mainly in the appearance of their lining epithelial cells. The nucleus is displaced toward the cell apex by extensive infoldings of the basal plasma membrane, giving the cell's base a radially striped (striated) appearance at high magnification. With the electron microscope, these infoldings can be seen to interdigitate with numerous mitochondria. This arrangement of the epithelial basal surface is characteristic of sites of energy-dependent ion transport activity, such as that performed by Na^+/K^+-ATPase (see Chapter 4). Striated ducts, which are typical of salivary glands, are seldom (if ever) found in the pancreas.

2. Interlobular ducts These ducts, located in the septa between the lobes and lobules, are larger than the intralobular ducts and are quickly distinguished by the greater amount of connective tissue surrounding them. Their lining is typically simple tall cuboidal to simple columnar to stratified columnar epithelium. Generally, the larger the duct, the taller the epithelial lining. These ducts include the large ducts within the glands and the still larger excretory ducts that exit the gland. They transport secretory products from the intralobular ducts to the lumen of the digestive tract.

II. SALIVARY GLANDS

A. General Structure and Function: Three major pairs of glands, the parotid, submandibular, and sublingual, surround the oral cavity. The lobules of each gland contain numerous adenomeres that empty their secretions (saliva) through a series of intercalated, striated, and interlobular ducts into the oral cavity. The saliva moistens the food, lubricates the digestive tract, and begins the enzymatic digestion of carbohydrates. The glands also excrete certain salts; they protect against bacterial invasion through the mouth by releasing **lysozyme** and **IgA** into the saliva.

B. Cell Types:

1. Serous and mucous cells These are the predominant secretory cells of salivary **adenomeres.** The key to identifying the 3 types of salivary glands in tissue sections lies in knowing the differences in the staining properties of the cells, their organization, and the proportion of each type found in each gland.

a. Serous cells These basophilic cells produce a protein-rich, watery secretion and usually form acinar (spheric) adenomeres.

b. Mucous cells More acidophilic than the serous cells, these may have a foamy appearance. They produce a thick glycosaminoglycan-rich secretion (mucus) and usually form tubular adenomeres.

2. Myoepithelial cells These contractile cells lie between the basal lamina and the epithelial cells of adenomeres and ducts. The cells surrounding the serous acini are often called **basket cells** because of their stellate shape and long cell processes that embrace the acinus. In the duct, the myoepithelial cells are spindle-shaped and lie parallel to its length. Both types contain abundant actin microfilaments and myosin, allowing them to help propel secretory products toward the oral cavity.

3. Other cells IgA-secreting plasma cells and other cells typically found in areolar tissue are scattered in the connective tissue surrounding the adenomeres.

C. Parotid Glands: These branched acinar glands contain secretory cells that are almost exclusively serous. The granules in these cells are PAS-positive (because of their polysaccharide content) and are rich in protein. The secretions of the parotids, which produce about 25% of the total salivary volume, contain amylase, maltase, sialomucin, and enzyme-resistant secretory IgA (see Chapter 14).

D. Submandibular (Submaxillary) Glands: These branched tubuloacinar glands contain both serous and mucous adenomeres (mostly serous). The serous acini are composed of small basophilic cells with PAS-positive cytoplasm and basal membrane infoldings. Their serous secretions contain sialomucin and have weak amylase activity. The mucous adenomeres may be capped by **serous demilunes** composed of several serous cells that secrete **lysozyme.** These glands produce about 70% of the salivary volume.

E. Sublingual Glands: These are also branched tubuloalveolar glands that contain both mucous and serous cells (mostly mucous). While only mucous adenomeres are present, many are capped by serous demilunes. These glands produce about 5% of the salivary volume.

F. Modulation of Salivary Composition by Duct Epithelium: The saliva produced by the secretory cells (**primary saliva**) is **isosmotic** with the blood; that reaching the oral cavity, however, is typically hypotonic and contains less sodium and more potassium than does blood. This is the result of the absorption of sodium and the addition of potassium and water by the cells lining the striated and excretory ducts. The ion-transporting cells lining the striated ducts, like those lining the distal tubules of the kidney (see Chapter 19), respond to aldosterone and help regulate the body's electrolyte balance.

G. Modulation of Salivary Volume by Autonomic Innervation: **Parasympathetic** stimulation (eg, sitting down to a meal) provokes high-volume secretion of watery saliva containing less than average amounts of organic material. **Sympathetic** stimulation (eg, fear and stress) yields low-volume viscous saliva, rich in organic material (sometimes known as cotton mouth).

III. PANCREAS

A. General Structure and Function: The pancreas is a compound acinar gland that resembles the parotid gland in its microscopic appearance. It differs in that is lacks striated ducts and contains islets of Langerhans. (These clusters of endocrine cells, discussed in Chapter 21, constitute the endocrine pancreas; only the exocrine pancreas will be considered here.) The lobules of the pancreas contain serous adenomeres that secrete a variety of digestive enzymes into a branched duct system that empties into the duodenum.

B. Cell Types:

1. Pancreatic acinar cells Each acinus consists of several pyramid-shaped enzyme-secreting cells whose apices border on a small lumen, and whose bases abut a basal lamina. The base of each cell is basophilic because of the ribosomes of the enzyme-synthesizing rough endoplasmic reticulum found here. Acinar cells synthesize a wide variety of enzymes that can hydrolyze proteins (proteases, such as trypsin, chymotrypsin, and elastase), lipids (lipases, such as triacylglycerol lipase and phospholipase A_2), carbohydrates (amylase), and nucleic acids (ribonuclease and deoxyribonuclease). Nascent enzymes are packaged and concentrated by the juxtanuclear Golgi complex and stored in the acidophilic apical region as membrane-bound **zymogen granules.** Here they await exocytosis in response to stimulation by **cholecystokinin,** which is produced by enteroendocrine cells in the small intestine, or parasympathetic stimulation via the vagus nerve. The enzymes in the granules are zymogens, which are inactive before their release. One such zymogen, trypsinogen, is enzymatically converted to the active protease trypsin in the small intestine by enterokinase, an enzyme that is secreted by enterocytes.

2. Centroacinar cells Unique to the exocrine pancreas, each centroacinar cell has a condensed nucleus and a clear cytoplasm. One or 2 can be found in the lumen of each acinus at the origin of the intercalated duct. These and other duct-lining cells produce a watery, bicarbonate-rich fluid in response to stimulation by **secretin,** an enteroendocrine product of the mucosa of the small intestine. This fluid helps adjust the acidic chyme to neutral pH and thus to optimize pancreatic enzyme activity.

IV. THE LIVER

A. General Structure: The liver is the body's largest gland. It is partly covered by a thin capsule **(Glisson's capsule)** and has a sparse, delicate, reticular connective tissue stroma accompanying the blood vessels as they penetrate the parenchyma. Its predominant cell type is the hepatocyte. These cells are arranged in one- or 2-cell-thick plates that are separated by the hepatic sinusoids. The liver has a dual blood supply, the portal vein and the hepatic artery; it also has 3 drainage systems, the hepatic veins, lymphatic vessels, and bile ducts.

B. General Functions: The liver has several important functions, most of which are carried out by hepatocytes. Its major role in digestion involves the enzymatic processing (metabolism) of nutrients absorbed by the intestines to provide the body with the chemical building blocks and fuel needed to support life. Some of the hepatocytes' enzymes assist in **detoxification** by modifying potentially dangerous chemicals and drugs and rendering them harmless. Hepatocytes synthesize many important proteins (eg, albumin, prothrombin, fibrinogen, lipoproteins) and secrete them into the blood, thus acting as an **endocrine gland.** They also synthesize bile from the wastes of erythrocyte destruction and secrete it into the biliary tract (IV.F.2), acting as an **exocrine gland.** The liver also serves as a storage site for glucose, fats, and vitamin A. Since the hepatocytes carry out most of the liver's functions, knowledge of their structure and functions (detailed in IV.D.1) is a prerequisite for understanding liver function.

C. Blood Supply: Because the liver's complex structure is organized around its many vessels and sinusoids, it is helpful to begin more detailed studies of liver structure by examining its unusual double blood supply.

1. Hepatic portal vein This large vein is formed by the junction of mesenteric and splenic veins. Mesenteric veins deliver oxygen-poor nutrient-rich blood from capillaries in the intestinal walls. The splenic vein delivers byproducts of red blood cell destruction from the splenic sinusoids (see Chapter 14). The hepatic portal vein, which supplies about 75% of the liver's total blood volume, enters through the **hilum** on the liver's inferior surface. It branches repeatedly to form the **portal venules** that penetrate the liver parenchyma and empty their blood into the hepatic sinusoids.

2. Hepatic artery This is a smaller vessel, a branch of the celiac artery, and enters the liver alongside the portal vein. It follows the latter's branching pattern and empties oxygen-rich blood into the same sinusoids. It supplies about 25% of the liver's blood volume.

3. Hepatic sinusoids Serving as the liver's blood capillaries, these lie between the radially oriented hepatocyte plates and receive blood from branches of both the portal vein and the hepatic artery. The mixed arterial and venous blood flows through the sinusoids and directly into the central veins. The sinusoid lumen is separated from the free surface of the hepatocyte plates by a discontinuous endothelial wall composed of typical endothelial cells and **Kupffer cells.** Between the endothelium and the hepatocytes is the narrow **space of Disse.** Blood plasma enters this space through openings between the endothelial cells that are too small to allow blood cells to pass. Blood-borne substances thus come in direct contact with the microvillus-covered free surface of the hepatocytes. In the space of Disse, hepatocytes absorb nutrients, oxygen, and toxins and release their endocrine secretory products. The spaces of Disse also serve as the liver's lymphatic capillaries, and the fluid in these spaces flows toward lymphatic vessels in the portal spaces, ie, in a direction opposite to the blood flow.

4. Central veins So named because each lies at the center of a classic liver lobule, these veins receive blood from the sinusoids and deliver it to larger **sublobular veins,** which merge to form even larger hepatic veins. They can be distinguished from other hepatic vessels by their position at the hub of the radially arranged hepatocyte plates and sinusoids and by the paucity of surrounding connective tissue.

5. Hepatic veins These collect oxygen- and nutrient-poor blood from the sublobular veins. They converge to form larger veins that exit the liver's upper surface and empty into the inferior vena cava.

D. Cell Types:

1. Hepatocytes These are the primary structural and functional subunits of the liver.

a. Hepatocyte structure and organization Hepatocytes can have one or 2 nuclei; they contain every type of membrane-bound organelle (see Chapter 3) as well as numerous glycogen granules and lipid droplets. Organized into one- or 2-cell-thick plates that are separated by the sinusoids; the polygonal hepatocytes are essentially cube-like, with 6 major surfaces. Four of these typically abut on similar surfaces of adjacent hepatocytes. The abutting hepatocyte plasma membranes are attached by desmosomes and are closely apposed, except where they form the walls of a **bile canaliculus.** These small, tubular, plasma membrane-bound gaps between adjacent hepatocytes receive bile (IV.F.1). They are sealed around their periphery with continuous occluding junctions to prevent the bile from leaking out between the hepatocytes and into the sinusoids. Short microvilli project into each canaliculus. Each of the other 2 free surfaces generally faces the sinusoids on either side of the plate and is covered with short microvilli that project into the space of Disse.

b. Hepatocyte function The metabolism of absorbed nutrients may involve their further degradation, the storage of any excess as glycogen granules or lipid droplets, or the use of one type of nutrient to synthesize another (eg, amino acids to make glucose). Unlike most endocrine glands, the liver's primary endocrine functions do not include hormone secretion, but instead involve the production of various processed nutrients (eg, glucose, lipoproteins) and the synthesis and secretion of plasma proteins (eg, albumin, fibrinogen). The liver's main exocrine function is the production and secretion of **bile.** Metabolic wastes, byproducts of red blood cell destruction, and toxic substances removed from the blood are enzymatically inactivated (detoxified) in the smooth endoplasmic reticulum and released into the bile canaliculi.

2. Kupffer cells Monocyte-derived members of the mononuclear phagocyte system, these are interspersed among the sinusoidal endothelial cells and on their luminal surfaces. They contain ovoid nuclei, many mitochondria, a well developed Golgi complex, scattered lysosomes, phagosomes, and rough endoplasmic reticulum. They are more easily distinguished from the endothelial cells in standard H&E preparations when they have phagocytosed colored particles (eg, india ink) prior to fixation.

3. Fat-storing cells These are stellate cells that are associated with the sinusoids, but which lie in the space of Disse. They accumulate fat and store vitamin A in the form of retinyl esters (eg, retinyl acetate, retinyl palmitate). Their precise function is unclear.

E. Liver Lobules: The relationship between hepatic structure and function can best be demonstrated through 3 models of liver subdivision: the classic lobule, the portal lobule, and the hepatic acinus (of Rappaport) as shown in Fig. 16–1.

1. Classic liver lobule This model is based on the direction of blood flow. In sections, the liver substructure exhibits a pattern of interlocking hexagons; each of these is a classic lobule. While lobules in pigs are defined by a sheath of connective tissue, there is less connective tissue in humans, and the lobule boundaries are less distinct. The boundaries of human lobules can often be discerned, however, by noting the positions of the portal triads at the lobule periphery, the central vein at its center, and the alternating hepatocyte plates and sinusoids that lie between them.

a. Portal triad One triad occupies a potential space (**portal space**) at each of the 6 corners of the lobule. Each triad contains 3 main elements surrounded by connective tissue: a **portal venule** (a branch of the portal vein), a **hepatic arteriole** (a branch of the

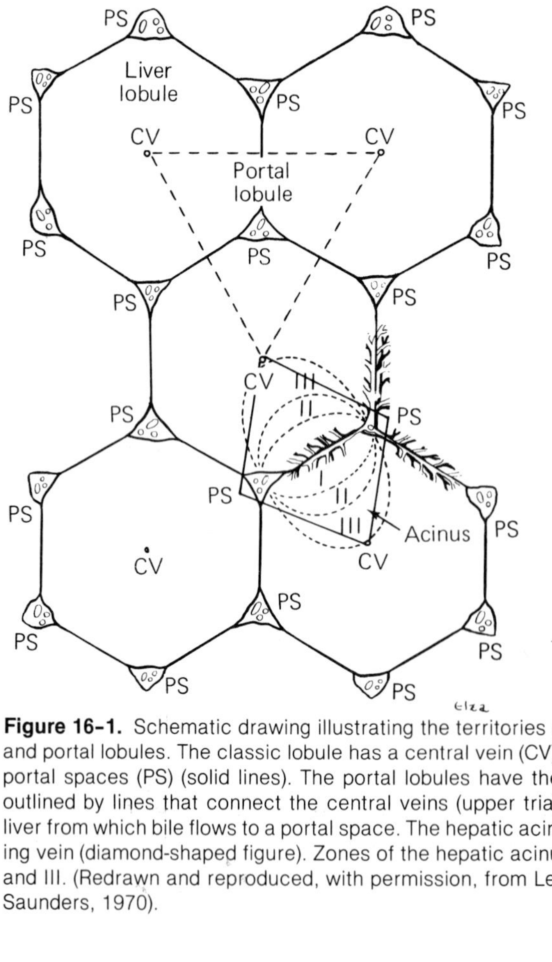

Figure 16–1. Schematic drawing illustrating the territories of the classic liver lobules, hepatic acini, and portal lobules. The classic lobule has a central vein (CV) and is outlined by lines that connect the portal spaces (PS) (solid lines). The portal lobules have their centers in the portal spaces and are outlined by lines that connect the central veins (upper triangle). They constitute the portion of the liver from which bile flows to a portal space. The hepatic acinus is the region irrigated by one distributing vein (diamond-shaped figure). Zones of the hepatic acinus are indicated by Roman numerals I, II, and III. (Redrawn and reproduced, with permission, from Leeson TS, Leeson CR: *Histology,* 2nd ed. Saunders, 1970).

hepatic artery), and a **bile ductule** (a tributary of the larger bile ducts). A lymphatic vessel may also be seen.

b. Central vein A single vein marks the center of each lobule. This vessel is easily distinguished from those in the portal triad by its larger opening and lack of a connective tissue investment.

c. Hepatocyte plates and hepatic sinusoids Many of these plates radiate from the central vein toward the lobule periphery (like the spokes of a wheel). The plates are separated by hepatic sinusoids, which receive blood from the vessels in the triads, converging on the lobule center to empty directly into the central vein.

2. Portal lobule This model is based mainly on the direction of bile flow, which is opposite to that of blood. From this perspective, the liver parenchyma is divided into interlocking triangles, each of which has a portal triad at the center and a central vein at each of its 3 corners. Bile, produced by the hepatocytes, enters the membrane-bound bile canaliculi between them, and flows within the hepatocyte plates toward the bile duct in the portal triad. Liver lymph in the spaces of Disse flows in the same direction as bile, toward lymphatic vessels in the triad.

3. Hepatic acinus (of Rappaport) This model is more abstract; it is based on changes in oxygen, nutrient, and toxin content as blood flows through the sinusoids and is acted on by hepatocytes. Each diamond-shaped acinus contains 2 central veins and 2 portal triads that define its 4 corners. The diamond is divided into 2 triangles by a line connecting the portal triads. Along this line run terminal branches of the portal and hepatic vessels that deliver blood to the sinusoids. Each triangle can be divided into 3 zones, according to their distance from the terminal distributing vessels. Zone I, for example, is closer to these vessels, while zone III is closer to the central vein. Blood in zone I sinusoids has higher oxygen, nutrient, and toxin concentrations than in the other zones. As the blood flows toward the central vein, these substances are gradually removed by hepatocytes. Zone I hepatocytes thus have a higher metabolic rate and larger glycogen and lipid stores. They are also more susceptible to damage by blood-borne toxins, and their energy stores are the first to be depleted during fasting. This model helps explain regional pathologic differences in patients with liver damage.

F. Biliary System: The synthesis and secretion of bile are the major exocrine functions of the liver.

1. Bile Consisting of bile acids, phospholipids, cholesterol, bilirubin, water, and electrolytes, bile's composition gives it detergent properties that aid in digesting dietary fat. About 90% of the bile comes from recycled substances that were added to the intestinal contents in the duodenum and then reabsorbed into the portal circulation by the epithelial lining of the distal part of the intestine. Hepatocytes merely reabsorb them from the sinusoids and transport them back to the bile canaliculi. About 10% of the bile is synthesized de novo in the hepatocyte's smooth endoplasmic reticulum.

a. Bile acids Cholic acid is synthesized from cholesterol and conjugated with glycine or taurine to form glycocholic and taurocholic acid, respectively.

b. Bilirubin This is a water-insoluble byproduct of the hemoglobin catabolism that accompanies the disposal of worn erythrocytes by cells of the mononuclear phagocyte system in the spleen, liver, and bone marrow. It is carried by the blood to the hepatocytes, which conjugate it with glucuronic acid to form **bilirubin glucuronide.** This now water-soluble substance is then secreted, with other bile components, into the bile canaliculi.

2. Biliary tract Bile in the canaliculi flows toward the portal triads (ie, opposite to the blood flow in the sinusoids). At the lobule periphery, the canaliculi empty into short, narrow **bile ductules** (also called **cholangioles** or **Hering's canals**), which are lined by cuboidal cells with clear cytoplasm. The ductules deliver the bile to **bile ducts** in the portal triads (in cross section, these small ducts resemble strings of beads). The bile ducts empty into successively larger ducts, ending in a single **hepatic duct** that joins the cystic duct from the gall bladder to form the **common bile duct (ductus choledochus).** This empties the bile into the duodenum. Where the common bile duct penetrates the duodenal wall, it is encircled by a thick layer of smooth muscle, the **sphincter of Oddi.** Although the liver produces bile continuously, the sphincter opens fully only when a particularly fatty meal enters the duodenum. When the sphincter is closed, bile backs up the common duct, through the cystic duct, and into the gall bladder.

V. GALL BLADDER. A small, blind-ending sac, the gall bladder is attached to the lower surface of the liver. Its function is to store and concentrate bile and to release stored bile in response to **cholecystokinin.** A hollow organ with layered walls, its microscopic structure resembles the digestive tract, but it lacks a definitive submucosa and therefore has only 3 of the 4 layers commonly present in the digestive tract wall.

A. Mucosa: This consists of simple columnar epithelium overlying a typical lamina propria. The epithelial cells secrete some mucus and they contain a sodium pump in their membranes to facilitate water absorption from stored bile. The numerous mucosal folds are branched, thus differing from intestinal villi. Near the **cystic duct,** the mucosa invaginates deeply into the lamina propria and often into the underlying muscularis. These invaginations form glands with large lumens whose continuity with the principal lumen of the organ may not be apparent in cross section. These large sinuses also help to distinguish gall bladder tissue from that of the intestines. The cells lining these sinuses contribute most of the mucus to the stored bile.

B. Muscularis: This is a layer of interwoven smooth muscle fibers underlying the lamina propria. These contract and empty the gall bladder in response to the release of cholecystokinin by enteroendocrine cells in the intestinal mucosa. This is triggered by the entry of dietary fat into the intestinal lumen.

C. Adventitia and Serosa: Like the retroperitoneal organs of the tract, the outer layer of the gall bladder consists of both an adventitia that attaches it to the liver and a typical serosa that covers its free (peritoneal) surface.

Study-Focusing Questions*

1. Compare serous cells with mucous cells (311) in terms of:
   a. Their secretory product
   b. Their shape
   c. Their staining properties
   d. The type of adenomeres they usually form (acinar or tubular)
2. Name the 3 types of paired salivary glands (311) and compare them in terms of:
   a. Their size (**HR**)
   b. Their contribution to salivary volume (314)
   c. The proportion of serous and mucous cells they contain (312, 314)
   d. The presence of serous demilunes (312, 314)
   e. The composition of their secretions (312, 314)
   f. The presence of striated ducts (311)
3. Describe the function of striated ducts (311).
4. Compare the viscosity of saliva produced in response to sympathetic versus parasympathetic stimulation (315).
5. Name the endocrine portion of the pancreas (315).
6. List 10 enzymes secreted by the exocrine pancreas (316).

*The page references in this section refer to *Basic Histology,* 6th ed., Junqueira L, Carneiro J, Kelley R (editors), Appleton & Lange, 1989. **HR** (for Histology Review) is occasionally used instead of a page reference to indicate that the information referred to can be found in this book.

7. Sketch a section through a pancreatic acinus (316) and label the following:
  a. Acinar cells
  b. Nucleus
  c. Rough endoplasmic reticulum
  d. Golgi complex
  e. Zymogen granules
  f. Basal lamina
  g. Lumen
  h. Centroacinar cell
  i. Intercalated duct

8. Describe 2 types of pancreatic exocrine secretions (316) in terms of:
  a. Their composition
  b. Their role in digestion
  c. The cells primarily responsible for their secretion
  d. The enteroendocrine hormone that stimulates their release

9. Into which segment of the digestive tract are the exocrine secretory products of the pancreas delivered (**HR**)?

10. Compare the exocrine pancreas with the parotid gland in terms of the:
  a. Predominant secretory cell type (serous or mucous) (312, 315–316)
  b. Presence of centroacinar cells (316)
  c. Presence of islets of Langerhans (315)
  d. Presence of striated intralobular ducts (316)

11. Name the 2 vessels that provide the liver's blood supply (320–321) and compare the blood they carry in terms of their:
  a. Origin (the vessels from which they arise)
  b. Contribution (%) to liver blood volume
  c. Oxygen content
  d. Nutrient content
  e. Bilirubin content

12. In which vessels in the liver does the dual blood supply first become mixed (321)?

13. Sketch a schematic diagram of a section through 3 adjacent classic liver lobules and include and label the following (317–324):
  a. Portal triads
  b. Branches of the hepatic artery
  c. Branches of the hepatic portal vein
  d. Bile ducts
  e. Central veins
  f. Hepatic sinusoids
  g. Space(s) of Disse
  h. Hepatocytes
  i. Endothelial cells
  j. Kupffer cells
  k. A portal lobule (outline)
  l. A hepatic acinus (outline)
  m. The direction of (show with arrows):
    (1) Blood flow (320)
    (2) Bile flow (325)
    (3) Lymph flow (320)

14. Name the 3 principal components of a portal triad (317). Which has the largest lumen (321)?

15. Name the 2 major cell types that border the hepatic sinusoids (324).

16. Name the 3 major cell types that border the space of Disse (324–325).

17. Name the cells that border on the bile canaliculi (324–325).

18. Name several proteins synthesized and secreted by hepatocytes (327–328). Are these endocrine or exocrine products?

19. Name the organelles or cellular inclusions of hepatocytes involved in the following hepatocyte functions:
  a. Protein synthesis and secretion (328)
  b. Drug detoxification and inactivation (330)
  c. Synthesis of bilirubin glucuronide (328–329)
  d. Synthesis of bile acids (328–329)

e. Storage of lipid (329–330)
f. Storage of glycogen (329–330)

20. Name the exocrine secretory product of the liver and describe its composition and function (328–339).
21. List in order the named structures through which bile flows after secretion by the hepatocytes (331) and name the segment of the digestive tract into which it is delivered (**HR**).
22. How is the flow of bile into the digestive tract regulated (331)?
23. List the functions of the gall bladder (333).
23. Compare the structure of the wall of the gall bladder with that of the small intestine in terms of the:
    a. Type of lining epithelium (331)
    b. Branching of mucosal folds (331)
    c. Presence of a submucosal layer (331)
    d. Orientation of muscle fibers in the muscularis (331)
24. Describe the process by which bile fills the gall bladder (**HR**).
25. Name the enteroendocrine hormone that stimulates the contraction of smooth muscle in the gall bladder wall, ejecting the bile into the duct system (333).

Multiple-Choice Questions

For questions 16–1 through 16–5, select the single best answer.

16–1. The gland type shown in the photomicrograph in Fig 16–2 is a:
A. Sublingual gland
B. Submandibular gland
C. Pancreas
D. Parotid gland
E. Liver

16–2. The gland type shown in the photomicrograph in Fig 16–3 is a:
A. Sublingual gland
B. Submandibular gland
C. Pancreas
D. Parotid gland
E. Liver

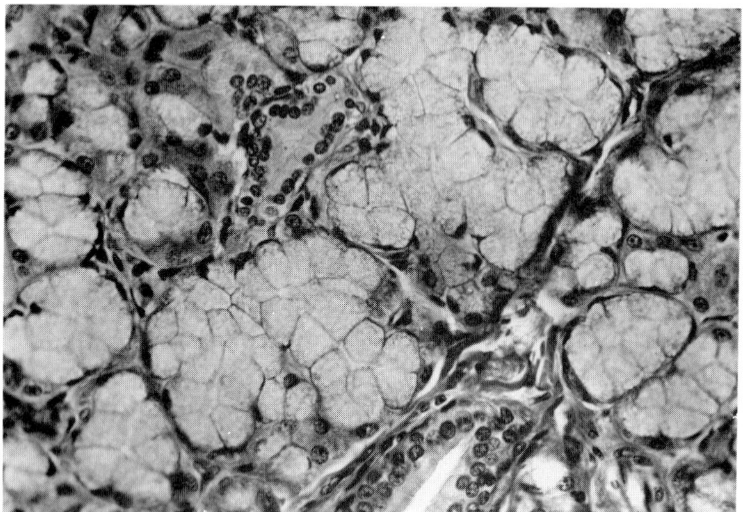

Figure 16–2.

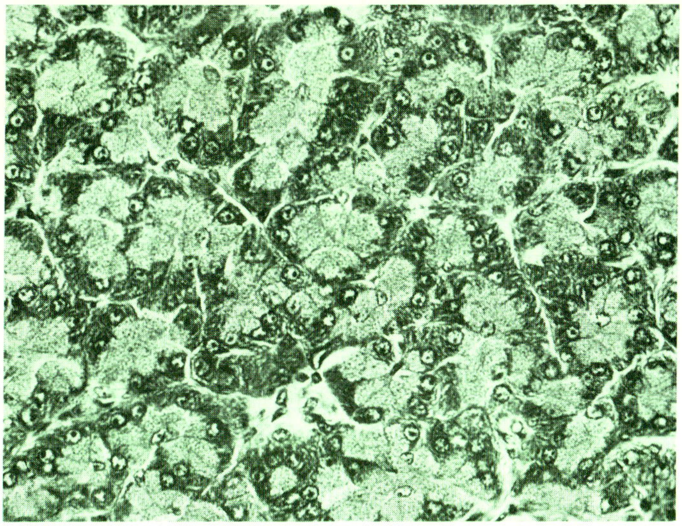

Figure 16-3.

16-3. The gland type shown in the photomicrograph in Fig 16-4 is a:
- **A.** Sublingual gland
- **B.** Submandibular gland
- **C.** Pancreas
- **D.** Parotid gland
- **E.** Liver

16-4. The gland type shown in the photomicrograph in Fig 16-5 is a:
- **A.** Sublingual gland
- **B.** Submandibular gland
- **C.** Pancreas
- **D.** Parotid gland
- **E.** Liver

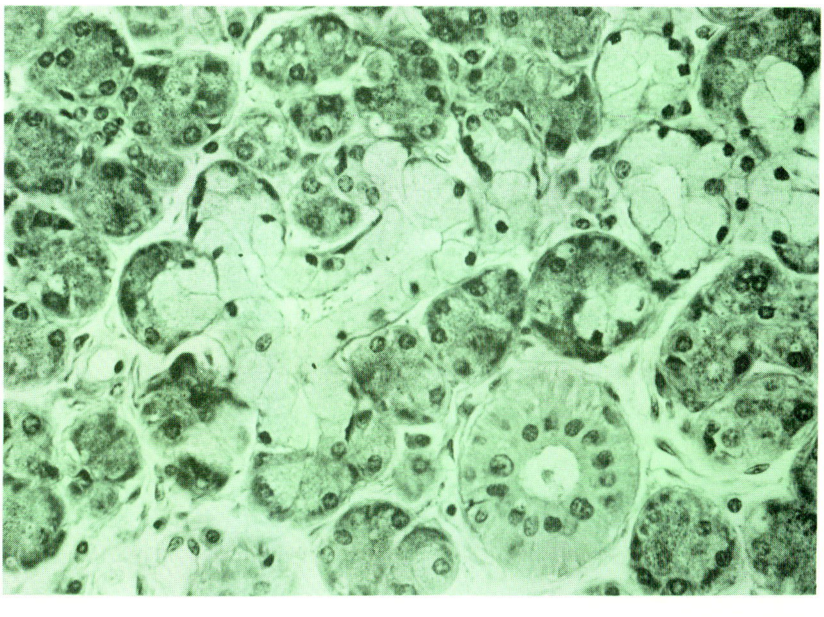

Figure 16-4.

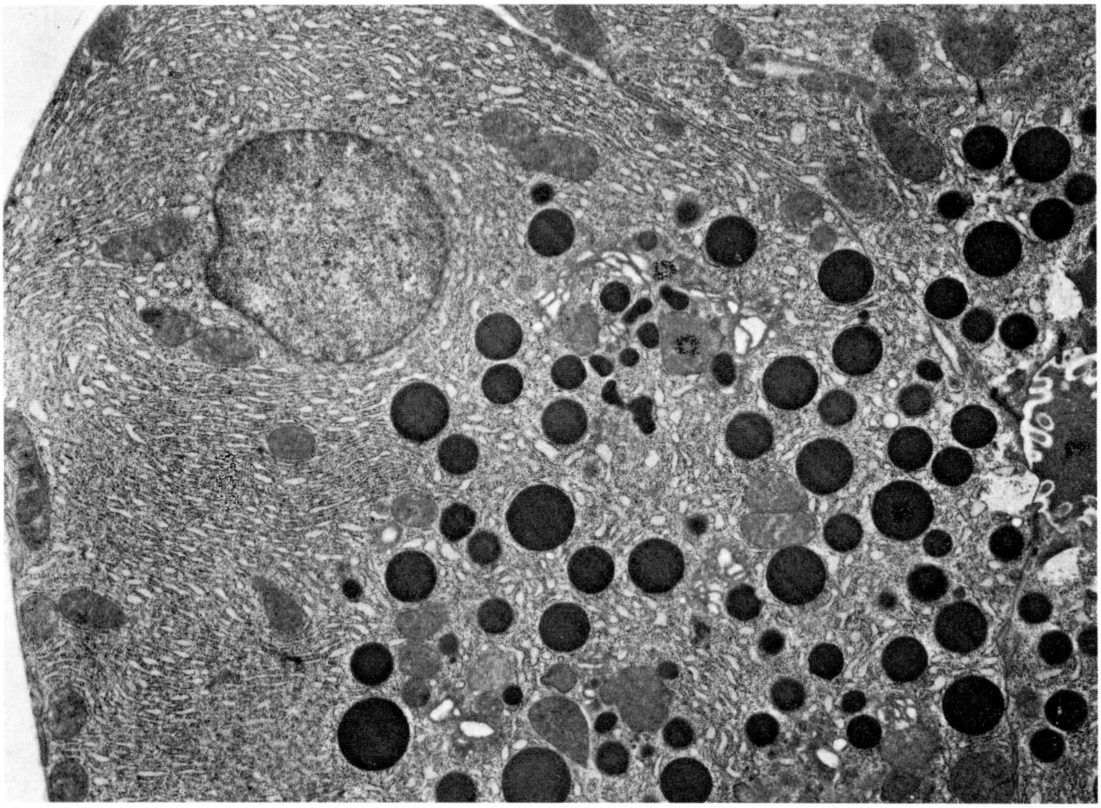

Figure 16-5.

16-5. The structure found at the center of a classic liver lobule is:
- A. Known as zone I
- B. A portal triad
- C. A central vein
- D. A branch of the hepatic portal vein
- E. A branch of the hepatic artery

MATCHING (questions 16-6 through 16-24): Each choice may be used once, more than once, or not at all.

Questions 16-6 through 16-13:

- A. Parotid gland
- B. Submandibular gland
- C. Sublingual gland
- D. All of the above
- E. B and C only
- F. None of the above

16-6. Contain(s) striated interlobular ducts
16-7. Contain(s) serous demilunes
16-8. Almost exclusively serous
16-9. Mostly mucous, no serous adenomeres
16-10. Contain(s) both serous and mucous adenomeres
16-11. Contribute(s) majority of the salivary volume
16-12. Largest gland
16-13. Exocrine gland(s)

Questions 16–14 through 16–24:

A. Hepatic sinusoids
B. Space of Disse
C. Bile canaliculus
D. All of the above
E. A and B only
F. B and C only

16–14. Bordered by hepatocytes
16–15. Bordered by endothelial cells
16–16. Bordered by Kupffer cells
16–17. Contain(s) red blood cells
16–18. Contain(s) plasma
16–19. Contain(s) reticular fibers
16–20. Fluid contents flow toward portal triads
16–21. Fluid contents flow toward central vein
16–22. Surrounded by space of Disse
16–23. Contents empty into a cholangiole (canal of Hering)
16–24. Lumen sealed by junctional complexes

For questions 16–25 through 16–53, either, both, or neither of the answers may be correct. Select

A if only A is correct
B if only B is correct
C if both A and B are correct
D if neither A nor B is correct

Questions 16–25 through 16–37:

A. Serous cells
B. Mucous cells
C. Both
D. Neither

16–25. Are relatively small and dark-staining
16–26. Are relatively large and pale-staining
16–27. Usually form acinar adenomeres
16–28. Usually form tubular adenomeres
16–29. Produce a viscous secretion rich in polysaccharides
16–30. Produce a watery secretion rich in protein
16–31. Are predominantly basophilic
16–32. Are predominantly acidophilic
16–33. Secrete lysozyme
16–34. Secrete IgA
16–35. Secrete amylase
16–36. Secrete mucinogen
16–37. Are found in all salivary glands

Questions 16–38 through 16–42:

A. Parotid gland
B. Pancreas
C. Both
D. Neither

16–38. Contain(s) predominantly serous cells
16–39. Contain(s) predominantly mucous cells
16–40. Contain(s) centroacinar cells

16–41. Contain(s) islets of Langerhans
16–42. Contain(s) striated interlobular ducts

Questions 16–43 through 16–48:

A. Hepatic portal vein
B. Hepatic artery
C. Both
D. Neither

16–43. Contains blood richest in nutrients
16–44. Contains blood richest in oxygen
16–45. Contains blood richest in bilirubin
16–46. Drains into hepatic sinusoids
16–47. Receives blood from central veins
16–48. Contributes majority of blood volume

Questions 16–49 through 16–53:

A. Secretin
B. Cholecystokinin
C. Both
D. Neither

16–49. Stimulates the contraction of smooth muscle in the gall bladder
16–40. Stimulates the release of zymogens by the pancreatic acinar cells
16–51. Stimulates the production of a watery, protein-poor, bicarbonate-rich secretion by pancreatic duct-lining cells
16–52. Produced by enteroendocrine cells in the intestinal mucosa
16–53. Produced by pancreatic acinar cells

For questions 16–54 through 16–62, one, more than one, or all of the answers may be correct. Select

A if only (1), (2), and (3) are correct
B if only (1) and (3) are correct
C if only (2) and (4) are correct
D if only (4) is correct
E if all answers are correct

16–54. Saliva contains:
(1) Amylase
(2) Secretory IgA
(3) Lysozyme
(4) Lactoferrin

16–55. Serous demilunes:
(1) Produce IgA
(2) Border directly on salivary intercalated ducts
(3) Produce mucinogen
(4) Produce lysozyme

16–56. The cells lining the striated ducts:
(1) Exhibit numerous infoldings of their basal plasma membranes
(2) Are characterized by basally located nuclei
(3) Contain numerous mitochondria
(4) Are characterized by their abundant, long, apical microvilli

16–57. Myoepithelial cells:
(1) Are usually found inside the acinar basal lamina
(2) Do not actually contract
(3) Contain actin and myosin in their cytoplasm
(4) Are found around bile canaliculi

16–58. Pancreatic zymogens are:
- **(1)** Synthesized on free polyribosomes
- **(2)** Packaged for secretion in the Golgi complex
- **(3)** Enzymatically inactive until they reach the duodenal lumen
- **(4)** Stored in the basal cytoplasm of pancreatic acinar cells

16–59. Within the connective tissue of a portal triad one may find a:
- **(1)** Branch of the hepatic artery
- **(2)** Bile duct
- **(3)** Branch of the hepatic portal vein
- **(4)** Lymphatic vessel

16–60. Kupffer cells:
- **(1)** Are phagocytic
- **(2)** Contain lysosomes
- **(3)** Are considered components of the mononuclear phagocyte system
- **(4)** Resemble endothelial cells in H&E-stained sections

16–61. Endocrine secretory products of the liver include:
- **(1)** Bilirubin glucuronide
- **(2)** Fibrinogen
- **(3)** Bile acids
- **(4)** Albumin

16–62. The gall bladder:
- **(1)** Concentrates bile
- **(2)** Secretes mucus
- **(3)** Lacks a definitive submucosa
- **(4)** Secretes bile

INTEGRATIVE MULTIPLE-CHOICE QUESTIONS: DIGESTIVE SYSTEM

For question DS–1 through DS–4, select the single best answer.

DS–1. The organ shown in the photomicrograph in Fig DS–1 is the:
- **A.** Gall bladder
- **B.** Duodenum
- **C.** Ileum
- **D.** Colon
- **E.** Stomach

DS–2. The organ shown in the photomicrograph in Fig DS–2 is the:
- **A.** Gall bladder
- **B.** Duodenum
- **C.** Ileum
- **D.** Colon
- **E.** Stomach

DS–3. The organ shown in the photomicrograph in Fig DS–3 is the:
- **A.** Gall bladder
- **B.** Duodenum
- **C.** Ileum
- **D.** Colon
- **E.** Stomach

DS–4. The organ shown in the photomicrograph in Fig DS–4 is the:
- **A.** Gall bladder
- **B.** Duodenum
- **C.** Ileum
- **D.** Colon
- **E.** Stomach

MATCHING (questions DS–5 through DS–26): Each choice may be used once, more than once, or not at all.

Questions DS–5 through DS–16:

- **A.** Ameloblast
- **B.** Parietal cell
- **C.** Centroacinar cell
- **D.** Odontoblast

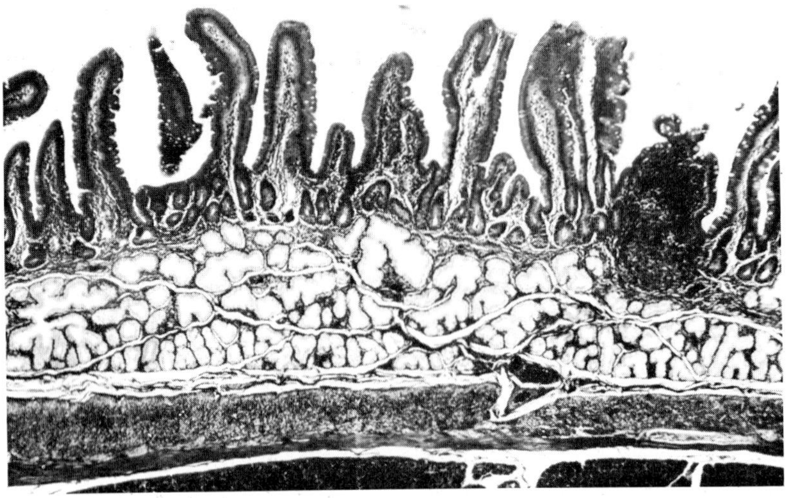

Figure DS–1.

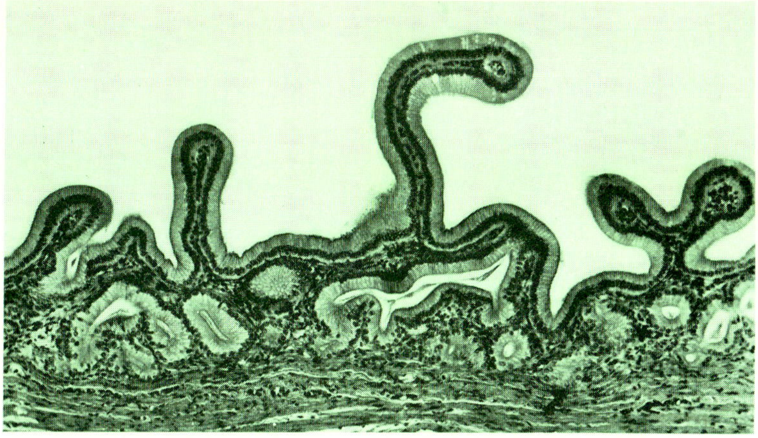

Figure DS-2.

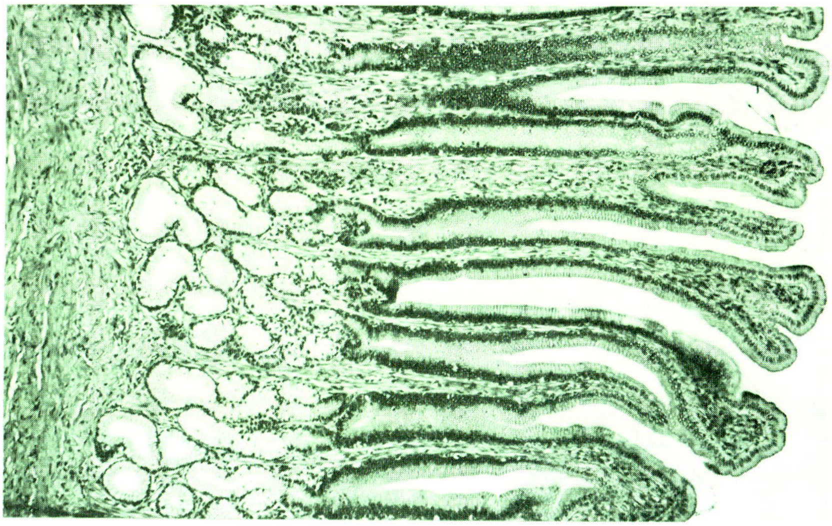

Figure DS-3.

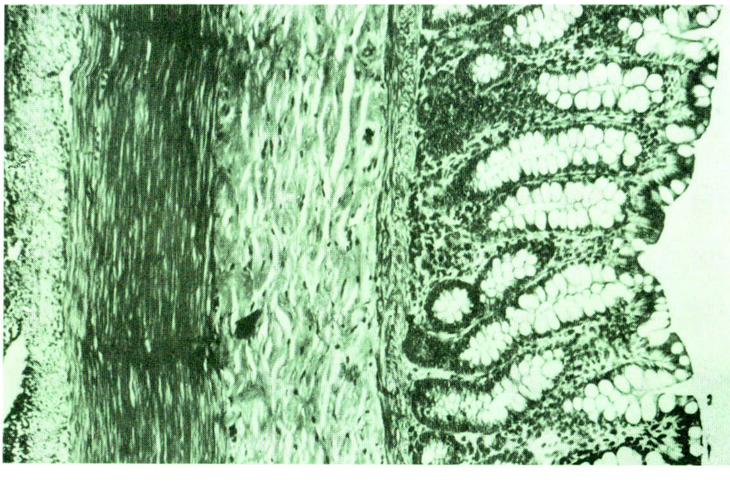

Figure DS-4.

E. Enteroendocrine cell
F. Gastric chief cell
G. Goblet cell
H. Hepatocyte
I. M cell
J. Paneth cell
K. Kupffer cell
L. Pancreatic acinar cell

DS–5. Is epithelial cell over Peyer's patch
DS–6. Secretes intrinsic factor
DS–7. Is duct-lining cell of pancreas
DS–8. Produces nonhormone endocrine secretions
DS–9. Lines bile canaliculi
DS–10. Is unicellular mucous gland
DS–11. Produces enamel
DS–12. Is phagocytic
DS–13. Produces dentin
DS–14. Produces mucus
DS–15. Secretes zymogens
DS–16. Secretes lysozyme

Questions DS–17 through DS–26:

A. Ectoderm (other than neural crest)
B. Neural crest
C. Mesoderm
D. Endoderm

DS–17. Source of hepatocytes
DS–18. Source of Kupffer cells
DS–19. Source of goblet cells
DS–20. Source of myenteric plexus
DS–21. Source of ameloblasts
DS–22. Source of hepatic endothelial cells
DS–23. Source of pancreatic acinar cells
DS–24. Source of epithelium covering lips
DS–25. Source of epithelium lining esophagus
DS–26. Source of intestinal absorptive cells

For questions DS–27 through DS–31, either, both or neither of the answers may be correct. Select

A if only A is correct
B if only B is correct
C if both A and B are correct
D if neither A nor B are correct

Questions DS–27 through DS–31:

A. Secretin
B. Cholecystokinin
C. Both
D. Neither

DS–27. Produced by enteroendocrine cells in the mucosa of the small intestine
DS–28. Stimulate(s) copious watery secretion by salivary glands
DS–29. Stimulate(s) contraction of the gall bladder muscularis
DS–30. Stimulate(s) secretion of watery, bicarbonate-rich fluid by cells lining pancreatic ducts
DS–31. Stimulate(s) secretion of zymogens by pancreatic acinar cells

For questions DS–32 through DS–37, one, more than one, or all of the answers may be correct. Select

A if only (1), (2), and (3) are correct
B if only (1) and (3) are correct
C if only (2) and (4) are correct
D if only (4) is correct
E if all answers are correct

DS–32. Contributors of mucus to the digestive tract lumen include:
(1) Brunner's glands
(2) Goblet cells
(3) Sublingual glands
(4) Gall bladder

DS–33. Contributors of enzymes to the digestive tract lumen include:
(1) Parotid glands
(2) Stomach
(3) Pancreas
(4) Liver

DS–34. Cell types of the digestive system that exhibit microvilli include:
(1) Intestinal absorptive cells
(2) Gall bladder epithelial cells
(3) Hepatocytes
(4) Cells lining striated ducts

DS–35. Organs that have both adventitial and serosal coverings include:
(1) Gall bladder
(2) Rectum
(3) Duodenum
(4) Transverse colon

DS–36. Organs that exhibit both endocrine and exocrine functions include:
(1) Pancreas
(2) Stomach
(3) Liver
(4) Salivary glands

DS–37. Parasympathetic stimulation provokes:
(1) Copious watery secretion by the salivary glands
(2) Meager viscous secretion by the salivary glands
(3) Increased secretion by the exocrine pancreas
(4) Secretion of bile by the gall bladder epithelium

Respiratory System 17

Objectives

This chapter should help the student to:

- Name the 3 divisions of the respiratory system and the components of each division.
- Compare the right and left lung.
- Name the important tissues and layers of the walls of the respiratory tract and describe the function of each.
- Compare the structure of the walls of the various components of the respiratory tract.

- Name 6 important cell types associated with the walls of the respiratory tract and describe the structure and function of each.
- Compare the terminal and respiratory bronchioles.
- Describe the structure of the interalveolar septum.
- Name the components of the blood-air barrier.
- Describe the blood supply to the lungs.
- Describe the lymphatic drainage of the lungs.
- Compare the responses of bronchial smooth muscle to sympathetic and parasympathetic stimulation.
- Describe the structure and function of the pleura.
- Identify the organ and the cell types present; distinguish between the various components of the respiratory tract from a slide or photomicrograph of a section of lung tissue.
- Identify the components of the blood-air barrier and differentiate between type I and type II alveolar cells in electron micrographs.

Synopsis

I. GENERAL FEATURES OF THE RESPIRATORY SYSTEM

A. Components and Basic Functions of the Respiratory System: The respiratory system consists basically of the lungs and airways (ie, pharynx, larynx, trachea, bronchi). Specialized for gaseous exchange between blood and air, including the uptake of oxygen and release of carbon dioxide, it is functionally divisible into 3 major parts: the conducting and respiratory portions and the ventilating mechanism.

1. Ventilating mechanism This mechanism, which creates pressure differences that move air into (inspiration) and out of (expiration) the lungs, includes the diaphragm, rib cage, intercostal muscles, abdominal muscles, and the elastic connective tissue in the lungs. Inspiration (inhalation) is active, involving muscle contraction. To inhale, the intercostal muscles lift the ribs while the diaphragm and abdominal muscles lower the floor of the thoracic cavity. This enlarges the cavity, creating a vacuum that draws air through the airways. The incoming air expands the airways, inflates the lungs, and stretches the elastic connective tissue. Expiration (exhalation) is more passive: Relaxing the muscles allows the elastic fibers to retract, contracting the lungs and forcing air out.

2. Conducting portion The walls of this system of tubes are specialized to carry air to and from the site of gas exchange without collapsing under the pressures created by the ventilating mechanism. This portion also conditions the air, warming, moistening, and cleaning it to enhance gas exchange. It includes the nasal cavity (II), nasopharynx (IV), larynx (V), trachea (VI), bronchi (VII), bronchioles (VII.D), and terminal bronchioles (VII.E).

3. Respiratory portion This portion is distinguished by alveoli (VIII), small, saccular structures whose thin walls enable the gas exchange between air and blood. Alveoli occur in clusters at the end of the bronchial tree. These clusters extend (like rooms from a hallway) (Fig 17–1) from the walls of respiratory bronchioles (VII.F), alveolar ducts (VII.G), and atria and alveolar sacs (VII.H).

B. Wall Structure: Like the digestive tract, the tubelike respiratory tract has layered walls whose lining epithelium derives from endoderm. The wall layers include an epithelium, a lamina propria that contains mucous glands as well as cartilages that prevent the tract from collapsing under pressure, smooth muscle that regulates the luminal diameter, and an adventitia that contains collagen and elastic fibers. Each of these layers undergoes gradual changes as the wall's overall thickness decreases from nasal cavity to alveoli (Table 17–1).

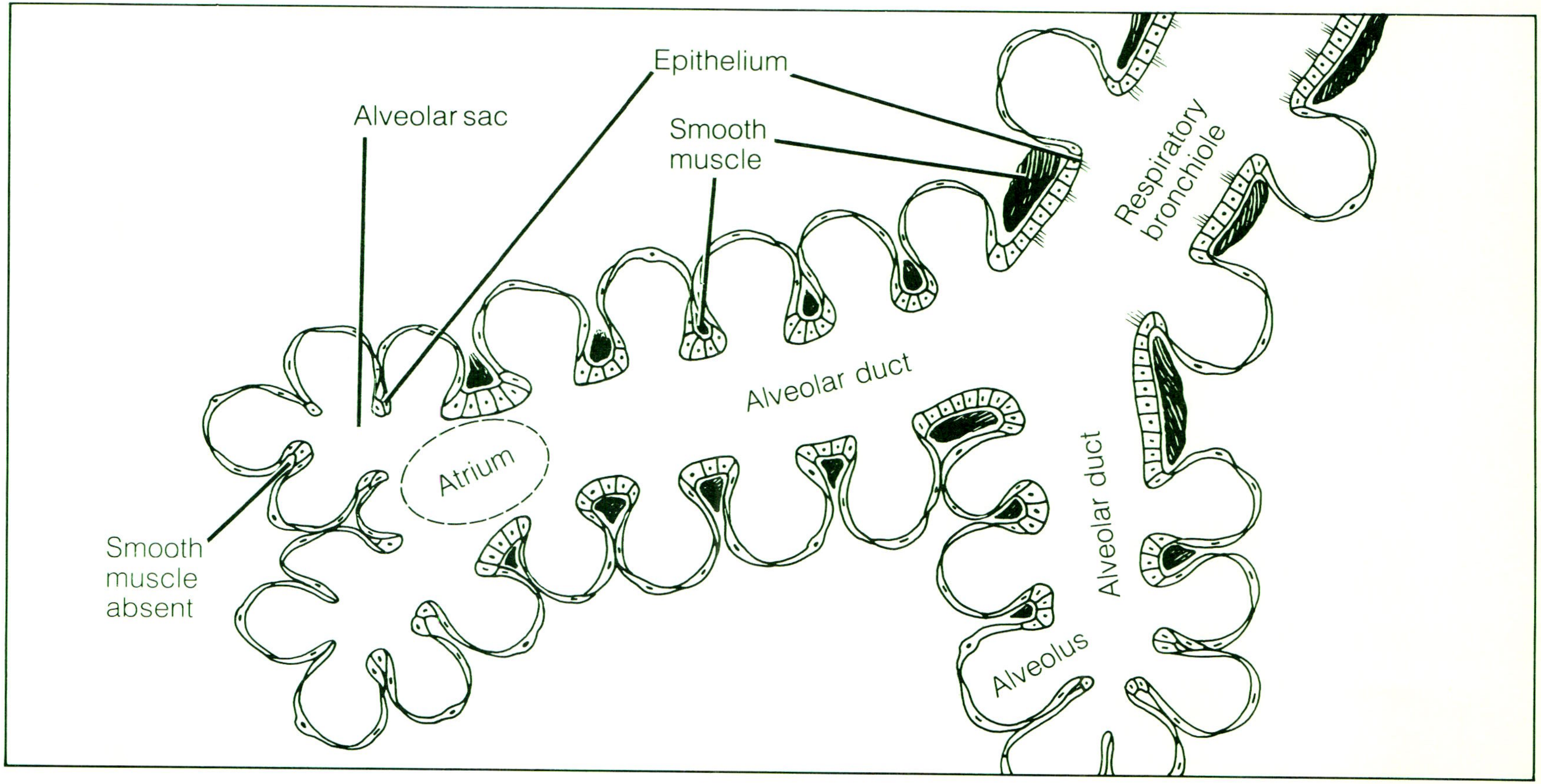

Figure 17-1. The respiratory portion of the respiratory tract. The major distinguishing feature of this portion of the tract is the presence of alveoli. Alveolar ducts can be distinguished from alveolar sacs by the presence of smooth muscle fibers in the walls of the former and their absence in the walls of the latter.

Table 17-1. Distinguishing features of respiratory tract components.

Tract Components			Wall Layers				
			Epithelium	**Lamina Propria**	**Glands**	**Skeletal Connective Tissue**	**Muscle**
Conducting portion (no alveoli)	Nasal cavity	Vestibule	Keratinized stratified squamous to nonkeratinized stratified squamous to respiratory epithelium.	Hair follicles.	Bowman's glands.	Bone/ cartilage.	None.
		Fossa		Venous sinuses.			
	Nasopharynx			Lymphoid nodules.	Mucous and serous glands (mostly mucous).	None.	Skeletal.
	Larynx		Respiratory epithelium and nonkeratinized stratified squamous over true vocal cords.	Gradual decrease in thickness and increase in number of elastic fibers.		Large hyaline cartilage rings and small elastic cartilages.	Skeletal in vocalis muscle and around cartilages.
	Trachea		Respiratory epithelium.			C-shaped hyaline cartilage rings.	Smooth in trachealis muscle.
	Bronchi: primary, secondary, tertiary		Gradual decrease in height, cilia, and goblet cells.			Complete rings in primary, plates of cartilage in smaller bronchi.	Several layers of circular smooth muscle.
	Bronchioles		Simple columnar with cilia and goblet cells.		None.	None.	Decreasing numbers of smooth muscle cells.
	Terminal bronchioles		Simple cuboidal, some cells ciliated, no goblet cells.				
Respiratory portion (alveoli present)	Respiratory bronchioles		Low cuboidal, with few cilia; no goblet cells.				
	Alveolar ducts and sacs		Some low cuboidal cells; no cilia.				Few smooth muscle cells.
	Alveoli		Mostly simple squamous (type I); some low cuboidal (type II) in septa.	Interstitium rich in capillaries and elastic fibers.			No muscle.

1. Respiratory epithelium

a. General features The epithelium lining most of the tract is ciliated pseudostratified columnar with goblet cells; it is generally referred to as respiratory epithelium. As the respiratory tract undergoes successive branching and its luminal diameter decreases, the epithelium gradually drops in height, and loses first goblet cells and then cilia as it approaches the alveoli.

b. Epithelial cell types

(1) Ciliated columnar cells Each of these cells, which predominate in the tract, has about 300 motile cilia (see Chapter 3) on its apical surface; there are associated basal bodies in the apical cytoplasm.

(2) Mucous goblet cells These cells, whose structure was described in Chapter 4, are the second most numerous type. They secrete the mucus that covers the epithelium and traps and removes bacteria and other particles from inspired air. Cilia projecting from columnar cells sweep the contaminated mucus toward the mouth for disposal.

(3) Brush cells Also columnar, these cells lack cilia; they often have abundant apical microvilli. Two types are present: One resembles an immature cell and apparently serves to replace dead ciliated or goblet cells. The other has nerve endings on its basal surface and appears to be a sensory receptor.

(4) Basal cells These small round cells lie on the basal lamina but do not reach the lumen. They appear to be stem cells that can replace the other cell types.

(5) Small granule cells These cells resemble basal cells, but they contain many small cytoplasmic granules and exhibit DNES activity (see Chapter 4).

c. Metaplasia This refers to the change in tissue organization or type undergone by epithelia in response to changes in the physical or chemical environment. For example, a smoker's respiratory epithelium typically develops more goblet cells in response to high pollutant levels and fewer ciliated cells in response to carbon monoxide. These changes, which are reversible, frequently cause congestion of the smaller airways.

2. Lamina propria Consisting of loose connective tissue, the lamina propria contains mucous glands in the upper tract (from the nasal cavity to the bronchi). Its elastic fiber content increases toward the alveoli. Skeletal connective tissue support begins as cartilage and bone in the nasal cavity and becomes cartilage only in the larynx. It gradually decreases, disappearing at the level of the bronchioles.

3. Smooth muscle This begins in the trachea, where it joins the open ends of the C-shaped tracheal cartilages (VI). In the bronchi, many layers of smooth muscle cells encircle the walls in a spiral. From this point, the thickness of the muscle layer gradually decreases until it disappears at the level of the alveolar ducts.

II. NASAL CAVITY.

This cavity is divided by the **nasal septum** into 2 bilaterally symmetric cavities that open to the exterior through the **nares** (nostrils). Each cavity consists of 2 chambers–a **vestibule** and a **nasal fossa**—which differ in position, size, and wall structure.

A. Vestibule:

The smaller, wider, anterior chamber of each side, it lies just behind the nares. The medial septum and lateral walls are supported by cartilage, and the epithelial lining is a continuation of the epidermis (see Chapter 18) that covers the nose. Just inside, the epithelium is keratinized, containing many sebaceous and sweat glands as well as thick short hairs called **vibrissae,** which filter large particles from inspired air. Deeper in the vestibule, the epithelium changes from keratinized to nonkeratinized stratified squamous and then to respiratory epithelium just before entering the nasal fossa.

B. Nasal Fossa:

This is the larger, narrower, and more posterior chamber on each side. Here the septum and lateral walls are lined by respiratory epithelium. They are supported by the bone of the skull and contain mucous glands and venous sinuses in the lamina propria.

Three curved bony shelves, termed **conchae,** or **turbinate bones,** project into each fossa from its lateral wall. These help warm and moisten the air by increasing the mucosal surface area and forming a system of baffles that cause turbulence and slow the air flow through the cavity. Alternating from side to side every 20–30 minutes, venous plexuses (**swell bodies**) in the conchal mucosa engorge with blood, causing it to swell. This action restricts air flow, directing it through the other side of the nose, and thus helps prevent overdrying of the mucosal surface. Arterial vessels in the fossa walls create a countercurrent system that warms air by directing blood flow from posterior to anterior (opposite to the flow of inspired air) in a series of small arches. Specialized olfactory epithelium (see Chapter 24) is present in the roof of each fossa.

III. PARANASAL SINUSES.

These are dilated cavities in the frontal, maxillary, ethmoid, and sphenoid bones around the nose and eyes. Their thin respiratory epithelial lining has few goblet cells and is bound tightly to the periosteum of the surrounding bones by a lamina propria that contains a few small mucous glands. Mucus produced here drains into the nasal fossa through small openings that are protected by the conchae.

IV. NASOPHARYNX.

The upper part of the pharynx (see Chapter 15), the nasopharynx is a broad single cavity overlying the soft palate. It is continuous anteriorly with the nasal fossae and inferiorly with the oral part of the pharynx (**oropharynx**). The walls, lined by respiratory epithelium, are supported by bone and skeletal muscle.

V. LARYNX.

A bilaterally symmetric tube, the larynx lies in the neck between the base of the oropharynx and the trachea. During swallowing, its opening is protected by the epiglottis. Its walls, supported by several laryngeal cartilages in the lamina propria, contain skeletal muscle and house the vocal apparatus.

A. Epiglottis:

This flap of tissue extends toward the oropharynx from the anterior border of the larynx. It is covered on its superior surface by nonkeratinized stratified squamous epithelium and on its inferior surface by respiratory epithelium. The lamina propria contains a few mucous glands and a small plate of elastic cartilage. During swallowing, the backward motion of the tongue forces the epiglottis over the laryngeal opening, directing food away from the airway and into the esophagus. After swallowing, the elastic cartilage helps to reopen and maintain the airway.

B. Laryngeal Cartilages:

Several cartilages frame the laryngeal lumen and serve as attachments for the skeletal muscles that control the vocal apparatus. The larger thyroid, cricoid, and most of the paired arytenoid cartilages are hyaline, while the smaller ones—the paired cuneiform and corniculate, the epiglottic, and the tips of the arytenoids—are elastic.

C. Vocal Apparatus:

The broad part of the larynx, below the epiglottis and surrounded by the thyroid cartilage, contains 2 bilaterally symmetric pairs of mucosal folds.

1. False vocal cords (vestibular folds) These are the upper pair of folds in the larynx. They are covered by respiratory epithelium and contain serous glands whose ducts open mainly into the cleft that separates them from the lower pair of folds.

2. True vocal cords This lower pair of folds is covered by stratified squamous epithelium; each contains 2 major structures: a large bundle of elastic fibers that run front to back, called the **vocal ligament;** and a bundle of skeletal muscle that runs parallel to the ligament, called the **vocalis muscle.** Air forced through the larynx by the ventilating mechanism (I.A.1) causes the true cords to vibrate. The vocalis muscle regulates the tension of the cords, while other muscles control the shape and position of the laryngeal lumen. In this way, the laryngeal muscles control the pitch (frequency) and other aspects of the sounds produced by the vibrating cords. The cords also assist the epiglottis in preventing foreign objects from reaching the lungs; they close to build up pressure when coughing is required to dislodge materials blocking the airway.

VI. TRACHEA.

This 10-cm tube extends from the larynx to the primary bronchi. It is lined by respiratory epithelium, and its lamina propria contains mixed seromucous glands that open onto its lumen. Its most characteristic feature is the presence of 16–20 C-shaped cartilage rings whose open ends are directed posteriorly. The opening is bridged by a fibroelastic ligament that prevents overdistention as well as by smooth muscle bundles **(trachealis muscle)** that constrict the lumen and increase the force of air flow during coughing and forced expiration.

VII. BRONCHIAL TREE.

This begins where the trachea branches to form 2 primary bronchi, one of which penetrates the hilum of each lung. The hilum is also the site at which arteries and nerves enter and veins and lymphatic vessels exit the organ. These structures, together with the dense connective tissue that binds them, form the **pulmonary root.** The bronchial tree undergoes extensive branching within the lungs. The changes in wall structure that accompany the progress of the bronchial tree toward the alveoli (Table 17–1) occur gradually and not at sharp boundaries.

A. Primary Bronchi:

There are 2 primary bronchi, one entering each lung. Their histologic appearance is quite similar to that of the trachea, but their cartilage rings and spiral bands of smooth muscle completely encircle their respective lumens. The path of the right primary bronchus is more vertical than that of the left. As a result, foreign objects that reach the bronchi are more likely to lodge in the right side of the bronchial tree.

B. Secondary Bronchi:

These **lobar bronchi** are branches that arise directly from the primary bronchi; each supplies one pulmonary lobe. Since the right lung has 3 lobes and the left only 2, the right primary bronchus gives rise to 3 secondary bronchi and the left primary bronchus gives rise to 2. Their histologic structure is similar to that of the primary bronchi except that their supporting cartilages (and those of the smaller bronchi) are arranged as irregular plates, or islands, of cartilage, rather than as rings.

C. Tertiary Bronchi:

Arising directly from the secondary bronchi, which they resemble histologically, each of these **segmental bronchi** supplies one bronchopulmonary segment (**pulmonary lobule**). Although each lung has 10 such segments, the different number of secondary bronchi causes the tertiary branching pattern to differ between the right and left lungs. Except for a decrease in overall diameter, the histologic appearance of tertiary bronchi is identical to that of secondary bronchi. Tertiary bronchi may branch several times to form successively smaller branches that are considered bronchi as long as their walls contain cartilage and glands.

D. Bronchioles:

These are branches of the smallest bronchi. The largest bronchioles differ from the smallest bronchi only by the absence of cartilage and glands in their walls. Large bronchioles are lined by typical respiratory epithelium; as they branch further, the epithelial height and complexity decrease to simple ciliated columnar or cuboidal. Each bronchiole gives rise to 5–7 terminal bronchioles.

E. Terminal Bronchioles:

The smallest components of the conducting portion of the respiratory system, these are lined by ciliated cuboidal or columnar epithelium and have no goblet cells. (The elimination of goblet cells before the cilia in the lower reaches of the bronchial tree is important in preventing individuals from drowning in their own mucus.) The lining here also includes dome-shaped cilia-free **Clara cells,** whose cytoplasm contains glycogen granules, lateral and apical Golgi complexes, elongated mitochondria, and a few secretory granules. Although the function of these cells is unclear, they may be serous secretory cells substituting for mucous goblet cells at this level. Each terminal bronchiole branches to form 2 or more respiratory bronchioles.

F. Respiratory Bronchioles: These are the first part of the respiratory portion, with a cuboidal epithelial lining that resembles that of the terminal bronchioles but which is interrupted by thin-walled saccular evaginations called alveoli. The number of alveoli increases as the respiratory bronchioles proceed distally. As the alveoli increase in number, the cilia decrease until they disappear.

G. Alveolar Ducts: These are simply the distal extensions of the respiratory bronchioles where the alveoli are so dense that the wall consists almost entirely of these sacs, and the lining has been reduced to small knobs of smooth muscle covered by cilia-free simple cuboidal cells. The knobs appear to project into the elongated lumen of the duct, each resting atop a thin septum that separates adjacent alveoli. The alveolar duct can thus be likened to a long hallway with so many doorways leading to small rooms (alveoli), that the hallway (the alveolar duct) appears almost to lack walls.

H. Atria and Alveolar Sacs: Atria are the distal terminations of alveolar ducts. The arrangement is comparable to a long hallway (alveolar duct) leading to a rounded foyer (atrium). The foyer has small doorways leading to some small rooms (alveoli), but also has 2 or more larger doorways leading into short, dead-end hallways (alveolar sacs). The short hallways are also lined by small rooms (alveoli). Put simply, the difference between atria and alveolar sacs is that the atria open into alveolar ducts, alveoli, and alveolar sacs, while the alveolar sacs open only into alveoli and atria. Although these distinctions can be made fairly easily in sections cut longitudinally through the entire system of passageways beginning with the alveolar duct, such perfect cuts are relatively rare in standard slides of lung tissue. More often, the various components are cut in oblique or cross section, and only the openings to the alveoli are seen, making it hard to distinguish between the sacs and the atria. In such cases, the only useful clue is the size of the knobs that project into the passageways. Those projecting into alveolar sacs lack smooth muscle and are thus smaller than those projecting into either the atria or the alveolar ducts.

VIII. ALVEOLI. Occurring only in the respiratory portion (which their presence distinguishes from the conducting portion), these small (about 200 μm in diameter) sacs open into a respiratory bronchiole, an alveolar duct, an atrium, or an alveolar sac. They are separated from one another by thin walls termed interalveolar (or alveolar) septa.

A. Interalveolar Septa: The structural features of these septa, which are specialized for gas exchange, are critically important to respiratory function. The septa consist of 2 simple squamous epithelial layers with the **interstitium** sandwiched between them. The interstitium consists of continuous (nonfenestrated) capillaries embedded in an elastic connective tissue that includes elastic and collagen fibers, ground substance, fibroblasts, mast cells, macrophages, leukocytes, and contractile interstitial cells that contract in response to epinephrine and histamine. This elastic tissue is an important component of the ventilating mechanism. Gas exchange occurs between the air in the alveolar lumen and the blood in the interstitial capillaries.

1. Blood-air barrier This term refers to the structures that oxygen and CO_2 must cross to be exchanged. Varying from 0.1–1.5 μm in thickness, it includes the following layers:

a. The film of pulmonary surfactant on the alveolar surface;

b. The cytoplasm of the squamous epithelial (type I alveolar) cells;

c. The fused basal laminae sandwiched between the type I alveolar and capillary endothelial cells; and

d. The cytoplasm of the squamous endothelial cells lining the interstitial capillaries.

2. Alveolar pores Each septum may be interrupted by one or more pores from 10–15 μm in diameter. These connect adjacent alveoli and may help to equalize pressure and allow collateral air circulation thus maximizing the use of available alveoli when some small airways are blocked.

B. Alveolar Cell Types:

1. Type I cells Also called type I alveolar cells, type I pneumocytes, and squamous alveolar cells, these are squamous epithelial cells that make up 97% of the alveolar surfaces. They are specialized to serve as very thin (often only 25 nm in width) gas-permeable components of the blood-air barrier. Their organelles (eg, Golgi complex, endoplasmic reticulum, mitochondria) cluster around the nucleus. Much of the cytoplasm is thus unobstructed by organelles, except for the abundant small pinocytotic vesicles that are involved in the turnover of pulmonary surfactant and the removal of small particles from the alveolar surfaces. They attach to neighboring epithelial cells by desmosomes and occluding junctions. The latter reduce pleural effusion—leakage of tissue fluid into the alveolar lumen. Type I cells can be distinguished from the nearby capillary endothelial cells by their position bordering the alveolar lumen and by their slightly more rounded nuclei.

2. Type II cells These cells, which are also called type II alveolar cells, type II pneumocytes, great alveolar cells, and alveolar septal cells, cover the remaining 3% of the alveolar surface. They are interspersed among the type I cells, to which they attach by desmosomes and occluding junctions. Type II cells are roughly cuboidal with round nuclei; they occur most often in small groups at the angles where alveolar septal walls converge. At the electron microscope level, they contain many mitochondria and a well-developed Golgi complex, but they are mainly characterized by the presence of large (0.2 μm), membrane-limited **lamellar (multilamellar) bodies.** These structures, which exhibit many closely apposed concentric or parallel membranes (lamellae), contain phospholipids, glycosaminoglycans, and proteins. Type II cells are secretory cells. Their secretory product, pulmonary surfactant, is assembled and stored in the lamellar bodies, which also carry it to the apical cytoplasm. There, the bodies fuse with the apical plasma membrane and release surfactant onto the alveolar surface.

3. Alveolar macrophages Known also as dust cells, these large monocyte-derived representatives of the mononuclear phagocyte system are found both on the surface of alveolar septa and in the interstitium. Macrophages are important in removing any debris that escapes the mucus and cilia in the conducting portion of the system. They also phagocytose blood cells that enter the alveoli as a result of heart failure. These alveolar macrophages, which stain positively for iron pigment (hemosiderin), are thus designated heart failure cells.

C. Pulmonary Surfactant:

Continuously synthesized and secreted by type II alveolar cells onto the alveolar surfaces, pulmonary surfactant is removed from these surfaces by alveolar macrophages and by type I and II alveolar cells. Its composition and continuous turnover allow it to serve 2 major functions. Not only does it reduce surface tension in the alveoli, it is also thought to have some bactericidal effects, cleaning the alveolar surface and preventing bacterial invasion of the many capillaries in the septa. The surfactant forms a thin 2-layer film over the entire alveolar surface. The film consists of an aqueous basal layer (**hypophase**) composed mainly of protein, which is covered by a monomolecular film of phospholipid (mainly **dipalmitoyl lecithin**) whose fatty acid tails extend into the lumen. By reducing surface tension, the surfactant helps prevent collapse of the alveoli during expiration. It thus eases breathing by decreasing the force required to reopen the alveoli during the next inspiration. Because surfactant secretion begins in the last weeks of fetal development, premature infants often suffer a condition called **hyaline membrane disease,** evidenced by respiratory distress (labored breathing) caused by the lack of surfactant. Luckily, surfactant secretion can be induced by administering glucocorticoids, significantly improving the infant's condition and chances for survival.

D. Alveolar Lining Regeneration: Daily turnover of about 1% of the type II cells, whose mitotic progeny form both type I and type II cells, allows for normal alveolar lining renewal. When these lining cells are destroyed by inhaling toxic gases, replacements for both types of cells are similarly derived from the surviving type II cells.

IX. PULMONARY CIRCULATION

A. Blood Supply: The lungs have a dual blood supply: the functional (pulmonary) circulation and the systemic (nutrient) circulation. The 2 systems communicate with one another through extensive anastomoses near the capillary beds.

1. Functional circulation This is provided by the pulmonary arteries and veins.

a. Pulmonary arteries Arising from the heart's right ventricle as large-diameter elastic arteries, the pulmonary arteries branch and enter the lung at the pulmonary root (VII). They follow the branching pattern of the bronchial tree to carry oxygen-poor blood to the lungs' capillary beds for oxygenation. Smaller branches (less than 1 mm in diameter) are of the muscular type, with a definitive internal elastic lamina. Pulmonary arteries have a thin intima and thinner media than do other arteries of equal size.

b. Pulmonary veins These collect oxygenated blood from the capillaries of the lungs and return it to the left atrium of the heart for distribution through the aorta and its branches. The larger branches of these veins accompany the bronchi, but the smaller branches travel unaccompanied in the connective tissue septa that separate the bronchopulmonary segments (VII.C). The thin intima of these vessels differs from other veins in that it lacks valves and contains a rich elastic fiber network in its subendothelial layer. While the media is absent in vessels smaller than 100 μm, in larger vessels it contains both smooth muscle and elastic fibers. The adventitia is thicker than that of pulmonary arteries.

2. Systemic circulation This is provided by the bronchial arteries and veins.

a. Bronchial arteries Typical muscular arteries (Chapter 11) arising from the aorta or from intercostal arteries, these are always smaller than the accompanying branches of the pulmonary arteries. The bronchial arteries enter at the pulmonary root and follow the branching pattern of the bronchial tree to the level of the respiratory bronchioles. Here they anastomose with branches of the pulmonary artery. Branches of the bronchial arteries carry oxygen-rich blood to capillaries in the bronchi, bronchioles, interstitium, and pleura. The blood collects in submucosal venous plexuses in various parts of the bronchial tree before entering the bronchial veins.

b. Bronchial veins Histologically, these are typical small veins that carry blood from the submucosal bronchial venous plexuses and always accompany the bronchial tree. Bronchial veins following the larger bronchi empty into the azygous, hemiazygous, or posterior intercostal veins. Those associated with the smaller portions of the bronchial tree empty directly into branches of the pulmonary veins.

B. Lymphatic Drainage: The lungs' lymphatic vessels are divided into superficial and deep networks, both draining toward the lymph nodes near the hilum. Vessels of the deep network have few valves; they accompany either the bronchial tree or the pulmonary veins in the intersegmental connective tissue. Vessels of the superficial network, which have many valves, are found in the visceral pleura. Lymph in the superficial network travels to the hilar nodes through vessels that either traverse the pleural surface or penetrate the lung surface and empty into intersegmental vessels. Lymphatic vessels are notably absent from interalveolar septa; at this level, the rich capillary network is responsible for draining excess interstitial fluid.

X. INNERVATION. Autonomic motor and general sensory nerves penetrate the pulmonary root, accompanying the blood vessels and the bronchial tree. Sensory nerves, which carry poorly localized pain sensations, report the presence of irritants in the airway and are involved in the cough reflex. Parasympathetic motor fibers (branches of the vagus nerve) stimulate bronchial constriction, while sympathetic fibers cause bronchial dilation. Sympathomimetic drugs such as isoproterenol are used to stimulate bronchodilation during asthma attacks.

XI. THE PLEURA. This serous membrane has 2 layers, one covering the lungs **(visceral pleura)** and the other covering the internal wall of the thoracic cavity **(parietal pleura)**. Like the peritoneum and the pericardium, the pleura consists of a thin squamous mesothelium attached to the organ or wall by a thin layer of connective tissue that contains collagen and elastic fibers. Bordered by the mesothelial cells, the narrow pleural cavity lies between the parietal and visceral pleurae. The cavity normally contains only a thin film of lubricating fluid that (together with the smooth mesothelial surfaces) reduces the friction between the lung surfaces and thoracic walls that would otherwise accompany the respiratory movements. Certain diseases and wounds allow excess air or fluid to enter the pleural cavity, increasing its size and restricting respiratory movement. While small amounts of air and fluids can be absorbed, larger amounts may precipitate lung collapse and require medical intervention.

Study-Focusing Questions*

1. List the components of the ventilating mechanism and indicate those involved in inhalation, exhalation, or both (334).
2. Name the 2 principal portions of the respiratory tree and list the functions of each (334).
3. List, in order, the segments of the respiratory tract through which air passes during inspiration (334–335).
4. Name 3 ways in which inspired air is conditioned in the respiratory tract (enroute to the alveoli) to optimize gaseous exchange (334–335). Name the structure(s) associated with each type of conditioning.
5. Compare the right and left lungs in terms of the:
   a. Number of primary and secondary bronchi each receives (341)
   b. Number of lobes in each (341)
   c. Angle at which the primary bronchi enter (**HR**)
6. Describe the changes in abundance (increase or decrease) of the following components of the respiratory tract walls in order from the nose to the alveoli.
   a. Diameter of lumen (340–341)
   b. Thickness of walls (340–350)
   c. Height of epithelium (335)
   d. Number of cilia (**HR**)
   e. Number of goblet cells (335)
   f. Number of glands (335)
   g. Amount of elastic tissue (335)
   h. Amount of smooth muscle (335)
   i. Amount of bone (**HR**)
   j. Amount of cartilage (335)
   k. Size of individual cartilages (335)
   l. Number of alveoli (345)
7. At which level(s) of the respiratory tree do you find the transitions from:
   a. The conducting portion to the respiratory portion (334)
   b. Ciliated pseudostratified columnar to nonkeratinized stratified squamous—and back again (340)
   c. Ciliated pseudostratified columnar to simple ciliated columnar epithelium (335)

*The page references in this section refer to *Basic Histology*, 6th ed., Junqueira L, Carneiro J, Kelley R (editors), Appleton & Lange, 1989. **HR** (for Histology Review) is occasionally used instead of a page reference to indicate the information referred to can be found in this book.

d. Simple columnar to simple cuboidal epithelium (335)
e. Simple cuboidal to simple squamous epithelium (345)

8. At which level(s) of the respiratory tree are the following initially lost?
   a. Goblet cells (335)
   b. Cilia (344)
   c. Glands (335)
   d. Cartilage (335)
   e. Smooth muscle (344)
   f. Lymphatic capillaries (352)
9. At which level(s) of the respiratory tree are the following found?
   a. Vibrissae (334, 339)
   b. Swell bodies (339)
   c. Elastic cartilage (340)
   d. C-shaped cartilages (340)
   e. Platelike cartilage islands (341)
   f. Anastomoses between the nutrient (bronchial) and functional (pulmonary) vessels (352)
   g. Clara cells (342)
   h. First appearance of alveoli (343)
   i. Pulmonary surfactant (348)
   j. Type I cells (347–348)
   k. Type II cells (348)
10. What is the function of each of the following in the respiratory system?
   a. Conchae (339)
   b. Vibrissae (334, 339)
   c. Swell bodies (339)
   d. Epiglottis (340)
   e. Cilia (335)
   f. Small granule cell (335)
   g. Clara cell (342)
   h. Alveolar pores (351)
   i. Pulmonary surfactant (348)
   j. Type I cells (347–348)
   k. Type II cells (348)
   l. Alveolar macrophages (349)
11. Sketch a section through 3 alveoli (344, 345, 346) and include and label the following:
   a. Alveolar sac
   b. Type I cells
   c. Type II cells
   d. Alveolar macrophages
   e. Alveolar septum
   f. Interstitium
   g. Alveolar pore
   h. Capillaries
   i. Endothelial cells
   j. Fused basal laminae
   k. Surfactant
   l. Blood-air barrier
12. Compare the effects of sympathetic and parasympathetic stimulation on bronchial and vascular smooth muscle (352).
13. Describe the pleura in terms of structure, function, and location (352).

Multiple-Choice Questions

For questions 17–1 through 17–4, select the single best answer.

17–1. Which of the arrows in the photomicrograph in Fig 17–2 is in the lumen of a respiratory bronchiole?

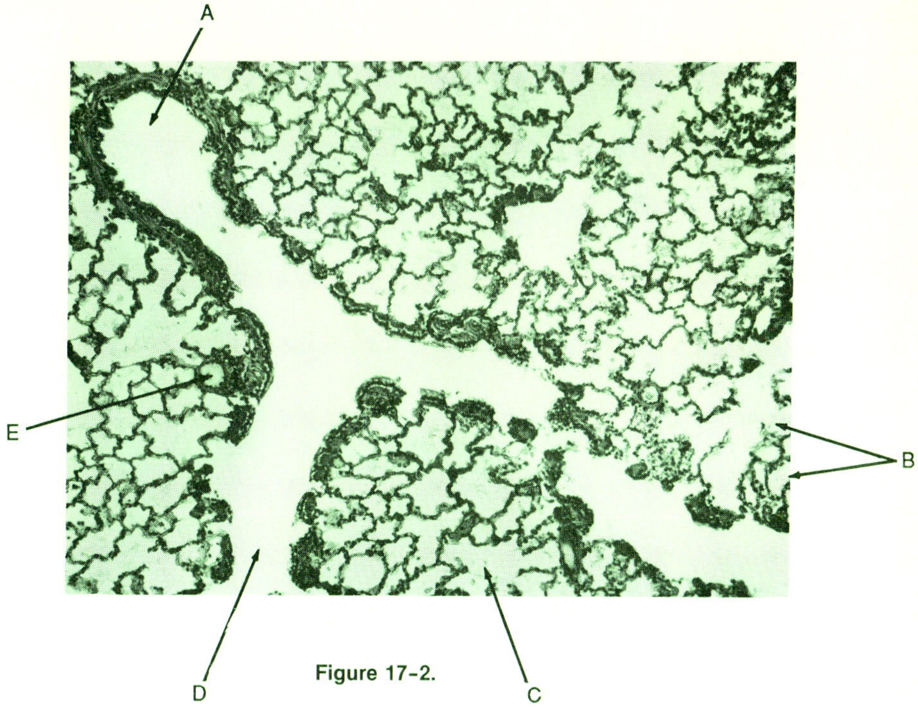

Figure 17-2.

17-2. The cell type shown in the electron micrograph in Fig 17-3 is a(n):
- **A.** Endothelial cell
- **B.** Goblet cell
- **C.** Alveolar macrophage
- **D.** Type I alveolar cell
- **E.** Type II alveolar (septal) cell

17-3. All the following show a decrease in amount from trachea to alveoli *except:*
- **A.** Cilia
- **B.** Elastic fibers
- **C.** Smooth muscle
- **D.** Cartilage
- **E.** Goblet cells

17-4. All the following are true of the visceral pleura *except:*
- **A.** It can be described as a serosa
- **B.** It is devoid of lymphatic vessels
- **C.** It includes a layer of simple squamous epithelium
- **D.** It contains abundant elastic fibers

MATCHING (questions 17-5 through 17-23): Each choice may be used once, more than once, or not at all.

Questions 17-5 through 17-17:

- **A.** Nasal cavity
- **B.** Nasopharynx
- **C.** Larynx
- **D.** Trachea
- **E.** Bronchi
- **F.** Bronchioles
- **G.** Terminal bronchioles
- **H.** Respiratory bronchioles
- **I.** Alveolar ducts
- **J.** Alveoli

17-5. Walls contain some elastic cartilage

17-6. First part of respiratory portion of respiratory tract

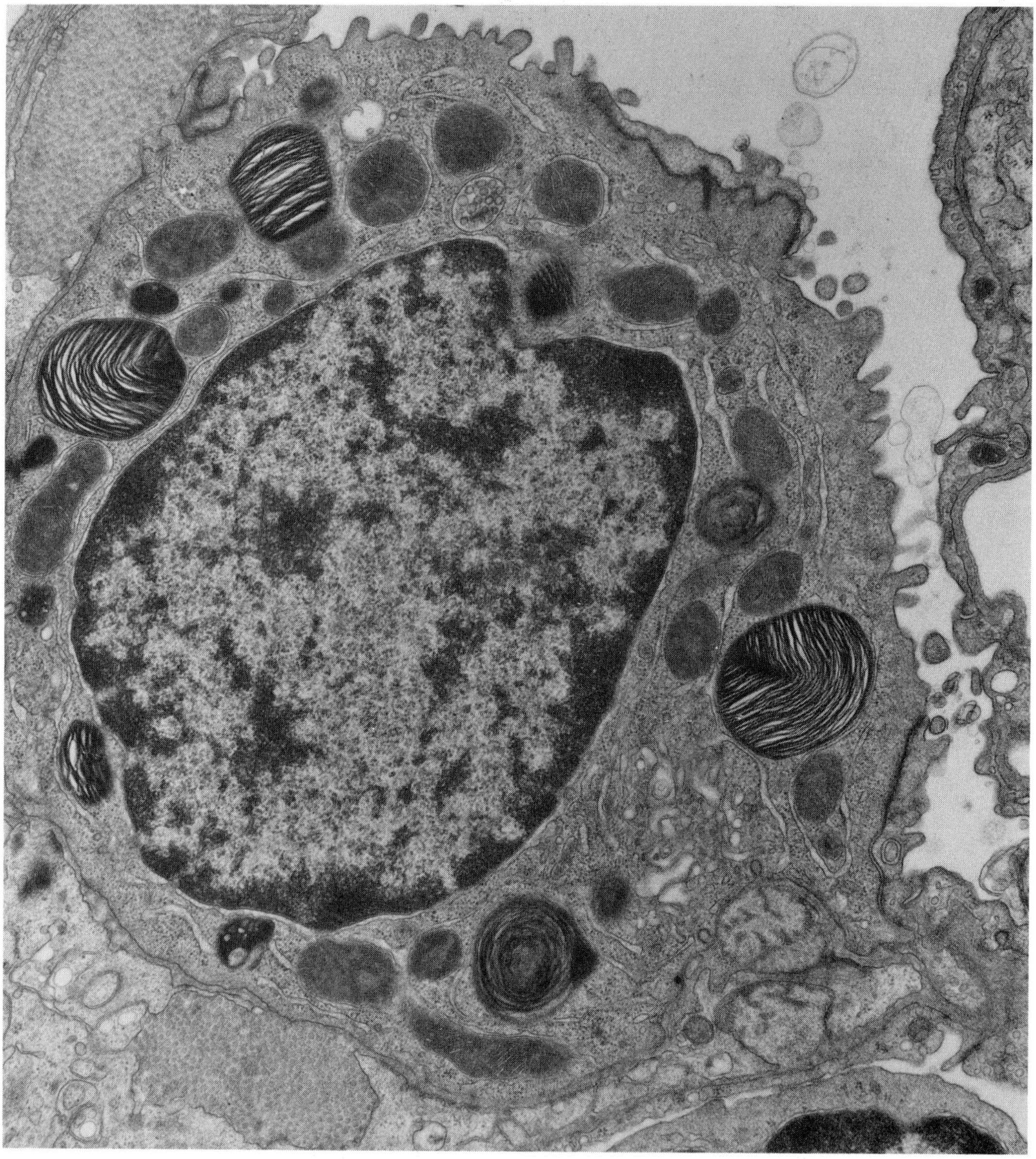

Figure 17-3.

17-7. Contain(s) swell bodies
17-8. C-shaped hyaline cartilages
17-9. Plate-like hyaline cartilages
17-10. Partly lined by nonkeratinized stratified squamous epithelium
17-11. First part of respiratory tract without cilia
17-12. First part of respiratory tract past trachea without cartilage
17-13. First part of respiratory tract without goblet cells
17-14. First part of respiratory tract without smooth muscle
17-15. Contain(s) vibrissae
17-16. Contain(s) pulmonary surfactant
17-17. Level at which anastomosis between the nutrient (bronchial) and functional (pulmonary) vessels occurs

Questions 17-18 through 17-23 use the letters in Fig 17-4.

17-18. Pulmonary surfactant
17-19. Fused basal laminae

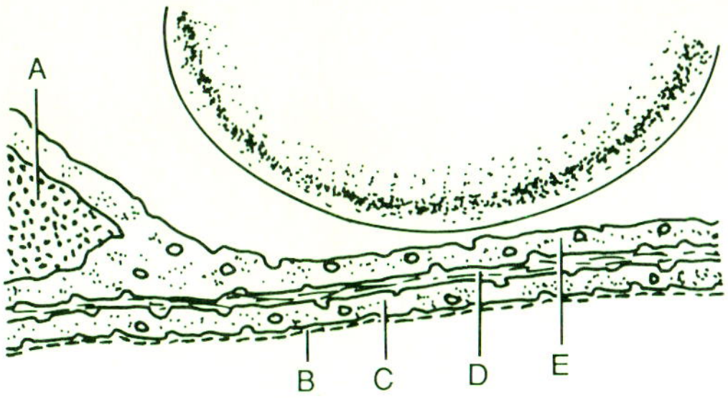

F. None of the above.

17-20. Nucleus of type II cell
17-21. Endothelial cytoplasm
17-22. Type I cell cytoplasm
17-23. Nucleus of type I cell

For questions 17-24 through 17-36, either, both or neither of the answers may be correct. Select

A if only A is correct
B if only B is correct
C if both A and B are correct
D if neither A nor B are correct

Question 17-24 through 17-30:

A. Right lung
B. Left lung
C. Both
D. Neither

17-24. Has 2 primary bronchi (per lung)
17-25. Has 2 secondary bronchi (per lung)
17-26. Has 3 secondary bronchi (per lung)
17-27. Receives the most vertical primary bronchus
17-28. Has 2 lobes
17-29. Has 3 lobes
17-30. Has 4 lobes

Questions 17-31 through 17-36:

A. Terminal bronchiole
B. Respiratory bronchiole
C. Both
D. Neither

17-31. Walls interrupted by alveoli
17-32. Lined by simple cuboidal epithelium
17-33. Cilia present
17-34. Goblet cells present
17-35. Smooth muscle present
17-36. Clara cells present

For questions 17-37 through 17-42, one, more than one, or all of the answers may be correct. Select

A if only (1), (2), and (3) are correct
B if only (1) and (3) are correct

C if only (2) and (4) are correct
D if only (4) is correct
E if all answers are correct

17–37. Portions of the respiratory tract lined by pseudostratified columnar epithelium include:
- **(1)** Trachea
- **(2)** Nasopharynx
- **(3)** Bronchi
- **(4)** Bronchioles

17–38. Structures that have a role in the conditioning of inspired air include:
- **(1)** Vibrissae
- **(2)** Nasal conchae
- **(3)** Goblet cells
- **(4)** Blood vessels

17–39. Clara cells:
- **(1)** Are found in terminal bronchioles
- **(2)** Appear to be secretory cells
- **(3)** May be taller than surrounding epithelial cells
- **(4)** Are ciliated

17–40. During inhalation:
- **(1)** The diaphragm contracts
- **(2)** The lumens of the bronchi and bronchioles increase in diameter
- **(3)** Some of the intercostal muscles contract
- **(4)** The elastic fibers contract

17–41. Alveolar pores:
- **(1)** Connect adjacent alveoli
- **(2)** Connect alveoli and terminal bronchioles
- **(3)** Allow air to enter alveoli whose tributary bronchioles are blocked
- **(4)** Close during inhalation

17–42. Pulmonary surfactant:
- **(1)** Is secreted by type II cells
- **(2)** Consists primarily of phospholipid
- **(3)** Reduces surface tension and helps prevent alveolar collapse
- **(4)** Has a bacericidal effect

18 Skin

Objectives

This chapter should help the student to:

- List the skin's functions and relate them to its structure.
- Name the 2 major components (layers) of skin and the basic tissue type that predominates in each.
- Name the 4 cell types commonly found in the epidermis and describe their structure, function, and location.
- Name the 5 layers of the epidermis of thick skin and describe the distinguishing structural features of each.
- Outline the steps in the processes of epidermal cell renewal and keratinization in relation to the epidermal layers.

- Compare thick and thin skin.
- Describe the steps in the synthesis and turnover of melanin granules.
- Name and compare the 2 layers of the dermis.
- Name and describe the layers of a hair follicle in both cross and longitudinal sections.
- Briefly describe the process of hair growth.
- Name and describe the important components of the nail complex.
- Briefly describe the process of nail growth.
- Describe the blood and nerve supply to the skin in terms of structure, location, and specialized function.
- Name and compare the 3 types of glands associated with the skin.
- Identify the type of skin, the named layers, keratinocytes, melanocytes, hair follicles and their layers, and type(s) of glands present in a slide or photomicrograph of a section of skin.

Synopsis

I. GENERAL FEATURES OF THE SKIN

A. General Functions: The skin is the largest and heaviest of the body's organs. It provides protection from microorganisms, toxic substances, dehydration, ultraviolet radiation, impact, and friction. It also acts as a sensory receptor and has a role in excretion, secretion, vitamin D metabolism, and the regulation of blood pressure and body temperature.

B. General Organization: Humans have skin (integument) of 2 types. **Thick skin,** restricted to the palms of the hands and soles of the feet, lacks hairs and has abundant sweat glands. **Thin skin,** which has hairs, covers the rest of the body. (The differences between thick and thin skin are detailed in section III.) Whether thick or thin, the skin consists of 2 distinct but tightly attached tissue layers, the epidermis and dermis, which are underlain by the hypodermis.

1. Epidermis The outer (superficial) layer of skin, composed of **keratinized stratified squamous epithelium,** derives from embryonic surface ectoderm. It is avascular, receiving nourishment from vessels in the underlying dermis. Its only innervation is by unencapsulated (free) nerve endings. The epidermal layer is further divided into 5 strata; these layers, in order from superficial to deep, are the stratum corneum, stratum lucidum, stratum granulosum, stratum spinosum, and stratum basale. The thickness of each of these layers differs in thick and thin skin (III).

2. Dermal-epidermal junction The stratum basale is underlain by a basement membrane connecting the epidermis and dermis. The junction has the appearance of zigzagging interdigitations between projections of the dermis—**dermal papillae**—and of the epidermis—**epidermal ridges.**

3. Dermis This inner (deeper) layer is a vascular connective tissue of mesodermal origin. It can be further divided into a superficial papillary layer and a deeper reticular layer. The papillary layer contains extensive capillary networks that nourish the epidermis. The reticular layer contains many arteriovenous anastomoses that help regulate blood pressure and body temperature. It is richly supplied with free nerve endings, a variety of encapsulated sensory receptors, and autonomic fibers, which control the vascular smooth muscle.

4. Hypodermis While not a part of the skin, this layer of loose connective and adipose tissue underlying the dermis flexibly binds the skin to deeper structures. Its thickness varies, depending on nutritional status, level of activity, body region, and gender. The hypodermis is also called the **subcutaneous fascia** and, where thick enough, the **panniculus adiposus.**

C. Structures Associated With the Skin: Glands (sebaceous and sweat), hairs, and nails arise from epidermal downgrowths into the dermis during embryonic development. These structures, which are mainly of epithelial origin, require epithelio-mesenchymal interactions between the epidermis and dermis for their formation and maintenance (V–VII).

II. DETAILED STRUCTURE OF THICK SKIN

A. Epidermis: The epidermis contains 2 major and 2 minor cell populations, each specialized for specific functions. Major populations include keratinocytes and melanocytes. Minor populations include Langerhans' cells and Merkel cells.

1. Keratinizing system **Keratinocytes** make up most of the epidermis. They participate in the continuous turnover of the skin surface by passing through 4 overlapping processes: cell renewal, or mitosis; differentiation, or keratinization; cell death; and exfoliation (the sloughing off of dead cells from the skin surface (Fig 18–1). The entire process, which takes 15–30 days, occurs in waves. A cell layer produced by a mitotic wave in the basal layer undergoes keratinization in synchrony. Each wave pushes the cell layers produced in earlier waves toward the surface. These layers from several waves, each at a different depth and step in the process, give a stratified appearance to vertical sections of the epidermis. The epidermis thus has 5 layers that are distinguished on the basis of the shape, staining properties, contents, and orientation of the keratinocytes they contain.

a. Stratum basale (stratum germinativum) This is a single layer of columnar basophilic keratinocytes, resting on the basal lamina that separates epidermis from dermis. These cells undergo intense mitotic activity and give rise to the keratinocytes in all other layers. They attach to their neighbors by **desmosomes** and to the basal lamina by **hemidesmosomes** (see Chapter 4). **Cytokeratin** intermediate filaments (**tonofilaments;** see Chapter 3) are important components of both junctions. The cytokeratin content increases as these cells move toward the stratum corneum, where it constitutes about 50% of their total protein. The basophilia of the basal layer is caused by ribosomes.

b. Stratum spinosum Lying above the stratum basale, this has several layers of large keratinocytes that are cuboidal or polygonal in its deeper layers and slightly flattened in the upper layer. **Tonofibrils** (tonofilament bundles) fill the cytoplasm, extend into the numerous cell processes that give these cells their spiny appearance, and insert into the desmosomes that attach the tips of these processes to those of adjacent cells. The mitotic rate here is slower than in the stratum basale. It should be noted that mitosis occurs only in the **malpighian layer,** which includes the stratum basale and stratum spinosum.

c. Stratum granulosum This lies above the stratum spinosum and consists of 3–5 layers of flattened polygonal (often diamond-shaped) cells that contain numerous membraneless **keratohyalin granules.** The intense basophilia of these granules is caused by their content of a highly phosphorylated histidine-rich precursor of the protein filaggrin. Cells in this layer also contain small ovoid or rodlike **lamellar granules.** These fuse with the plasma membrane and release their contents (glycosaminoglycans and phospholipids) into the intercellular spaces. This material may be important in sealing the deeper layers of the skin from the external environment.

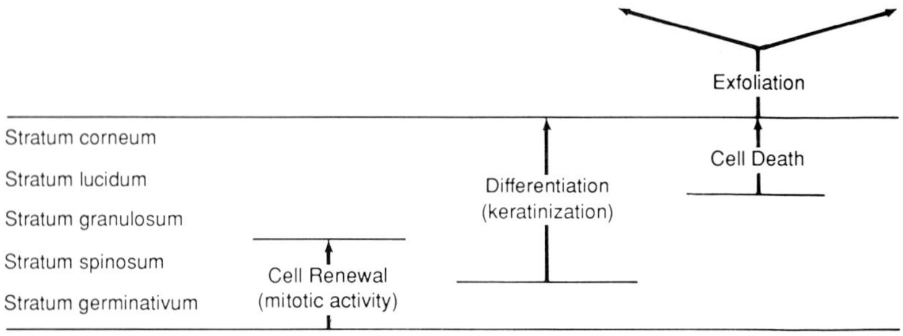

Figure 18–1. The keratinizing system of the epidermis.

d. Stratum lucidum Lying above the stratum granulosum, this layer is apparent only in thick skin. It is a narrow, acidophilic, translucent band of flattened keratinocytes whose nuclei, organelles, and intercellular borders are not visible. The cytoplasm contains dense cytokeratin aggregates embedded in an amorphous electron-dense matrix derived from the keratohyalin granules. This intracellular mixture of intermediate filaments and matrix constitutes the immature keratin that is sometimes termed **eleidin.**

e. Stratum corneum The outermost layer, this consists of 15–20 layers of dead, platelike enucleated keratinocytes with thickened plasma membranes. These cells, which represent the final stage of keratinization, are filled with mature keratin, a birefringent scleroprotein consisting of at least 6 polypeptides. The molecular weight of the polypeptides of mature keratin in the stratum corneum is higher than that of the polypeptides in the immature keratin of deeper, less-differentiated cells. Keratin's substructure includes tonofilament subunits formed by 3 coiled and intertwined polypeptide chains. Nine of these subunits coil together to form each 10-nm-thick intermediate filament. As they aggregate end to end, the tonofilament increases in length. Tonofilaments are embedded in and bound together by the amorphous matrix first found in keratohyalin granules. The dead cells are continuously sloughed (exfoliated) from the surface and replaced, through successive waves of mitosis and differentiation, by cells from the deeper layers.

2. Pigmentation system The color of skin is caused mainly by its content of the pigments melanin and carotene, the number of dermal blood vessels, and the color of the blood flowing through the vessels.

a. Melanin This is the term applied to a class of pigments that contribute to skin, eye, and hair color. Melanins, synthesized by **melanocytes,** include the dark brown pigment **eumelanin** found in the epidermis, the iris, and in brown and black hair; and the cysteine-containing pigment, **pheomelanin,** of red hair.

(1) Melanocytes These neural crest derivatives migrate into the developing epidermis during embryogenesis; although they are scattered among the keratinocytes of the stratum basale, they are not attached to them by desmosomes. They typically have round cell bodies, central nuclei, and long cytoplasmic processes that pass between the keratinocytes of the strata basale and spinosum and terminate in small indentations on the cell surfaces. Melanocytes, which make up 10–25% of this layer's cells, do not participate in keratinization. Their cytoplasm contains many mitochondria, a well-developed Golgi complex, short cisternae of the rough endoplasmic reticulum, and special membrane-lined organelles, **melanosomes,** in which melanin is synthesized. It should be noted that there is no difference in the number of melanocytes per unit area in the skins of dark- and light-skinned races. Differences in pigmentation are the result of differences in the normal rates of melanin synthesis, accumulation, and degradation.

(2) Melanin synthesis This involves the **tyrosinase-**mediated enzymatic conversion of **tyrosine** to **dopa (3,4-dihydroxyphenylalanine)** and of dopa to **dopaquinone.** Several additional steps are required to convert dopaquinone to melanin. In melanin-granule formation, tyrosinase is synthesized on ribosomes of the rough endoplasmic reticulum and transported to the Golgi complex. Membrane-limited **tyrosinase-**filled vesicles called melanosomes pinch off from the Golgi complex and accumulate in the Golgi region; they pass through 4 stages of development to become mature melanin granules:

(a) Stage I melanosomes These rounded vesicles exhibit tyrosinase activity associated with fine granular-to-filamentous material in the vesicle periphery. Melanin is not yet present.

(b) Stage II melanosomes The vesicles have become ovoid; they contain parallel filaments. The tyrosinase activity associated with these triggers the onset of melanin deposition on the filaments.

(c) Stage III melanosomes The same structure is seen here as in stage II, but the continued deposition of melanin has begun to obscure the parallel filaments.

(d) Stage IV melanosomes These are mature melanin granules (1 μm long, 0.4 μm in diameter) that are completely filled with melanin so that their ultrastructure is no longer visible.

(3) Factors in increased melanin synthesis

(a) Increased exposure to ultraviolet rays Such exposure to the sun not only darkens existing melanin but also speeds tyrosinase synthesis, increasing both the amount of melanin produced and the rate of production.

(b) Melanocyte-stimulating hormones These hormones, known as α- and β-MSH, which arise from the pituitary (see Chapter 20) and markedly enhance amphibian pigmentation, do not exist in free form in humans. Pituitary adrenocorticotropic hormone (ACTH), however, does contain a peptide sequence identical to α-MSH that is known to influence human pigmentation (see below).

(c) Addison's disease This involves the production of lower-than-normal levels of cortisol by the adrenal cortex (see Chapter 21). The pituitaries of affected patients release excessive ACTH in an attempt to stimulate the adrenals. The resulting stimulation of tyrosinase activity in the melanocytes leads to the hyperpigmentation that accompanies Addison's disease.

(4) Factors in decreased melanin synthesis

(a) Albinism This condition, in which no melanin pigment is produced, is most often caused by a genetic defect in tyrosinase synthesis and a consequent absence of tyrosinase activity. Melanocytes of affected individuals typically do contain melanosomes, but only up to stage II.

(b) Hydroquinone The active ingredient in some over-the-counter products that claim to remove "age spots," it inhibits melanin synthesis.

b. Fate of mature melanin granules Mature granules move from the Golgi region into the tips of the melanocytes' long cytoplasmic processes. They are then "injected" into the keratinocytes of the strata basale and spinosum in a process termed **cytocrine secretion.** (Keratinocytes, which act as melanin depots, usually contain more melanin than melanocytes do.) Melanin granules accumulate over the keratinocytes' nuclei, protecting the DNA within from the damaging effects of the sun's rays. Keratinocytes carry melanin with them as they move toward the skin surface. During keratinization, the granules, along with the keratinocytes' nuclei and organelles, are often digested by lysosomes.

c. Melanin function Certain of the sun's rays break apart the molecules in the skin, forming highly reactive free radicals. The cleavage of DNA by ionizing radiation or the recombination of normal DNA with other free radicals can change DNA structure, causing cell death or neoplastic transformation. The euchromatic DNA of dividing cells in the **malpighian layer** is most susceptible to these effects. Although melanin's darkness allows it to absorb some rays directly, its major protective effect is its ability to absorb the free radicals generated by ionizing radiation (with the granules thus acting like tiny free-radical sponges).

3. Langerhans' cells These star-shaped cells, which lack tonofilaments, are found mainly in the stratum spinosum (400–1000 cells/mm^2 of skin surface). They stain selectively with gold chloride and contain numerous rodlike or racket-shaped cytoplasmic granules (**Birbeck's granules**). They are thought to be antigen-presenting cells (see Chapter 14) that process and present to the lymphocytes any antigenic material that penetrates the skin's surface. Of mesodermal origin, they arise in bone marrow and belong to the mononuclear phagocyte system. Langerhans' cells are also found in oral and vaginal epithelium as well as in the thymus.

4. Merkel's cells Scattered among the cells of the stratum basale, these cells are most numerous in the thick skin (III.B). They resemble basal keratinocytes but have a clearer cytoplasm that contains many small dense granules. Free nerve endings form a disklike expansion (**Merkel's disk**) that covers the basal surface of each Merkel's cell. This arrangement suggests that the cells function as sensory mechanoreceptors, but other evidence suggests that they may have functions related to the diffuse neuroendocrine system.

B. Dermis: The dermis, which includes the hair follicles (found only in thin skin [V]) and sebaceous and sweat glands (VII), consists of 2 layers of vascular connective tissue that blend into one another at their common border.

1. Papillary layer This layer of loose connective tissue, rich in elastic fibers, lies directly beneath the epidermal basement membrane. Its projections—**dermal papillae**—interdigitate with the epidermal ridges, increasing the area of contact. Special collagen fibers, **anchoring fibrils**, extend from this layer into the epidermal basal lamina to reinforce the dermal-epidermal junction. The papillary layer contains a rich network of capillaries (IV.B) as well as an abundant supply of free nerve endings—some of which penetrate the epidermis. The tips of many dermal papillae contain encapsulated touch receptors called Meissner's corpuscles (see Chapter 24).

2. Reticular layer Lying beneath the papillary layer is a thicker layer composed of dense irregular connective tissue. Also richly vascularized, this layer contains many **arteriovenous anastomoses,** or **shunts** (IV.D), that control the amount of blood reaching the papillary capillaries and thus aid in regulating heat loss and blood pressure. The reticular layer also contains a rich supply of nerves with both free and encapsulated endings (eg, Pacinian corpuscles; see Chapter 24).

III. DIFFERENCES BETWEEN THICK AND THIN SKIN

A. Location: Thick skin is found only on the palms and the soles; thin skin covers the rest of the body surface.

B. Epidermis: While the epidermis of thin skin is essentially the same as that of thick skin, there are some important differences. The total thickness of thin skin is less than that of thick skin, the stratum corneum is also thinner, and the stratum lucidum is not apparent. The stratum granulosum of thin skin is thinner, and the stratum basale contains fewer Merkel's cells. In addition, thin skin typically lacks the surface pattern of ridges and grooves—**dermatoglyphics,** commonly known as fingerprints—that characterize thick skin.

C. Dermis: Like the epidermis, the dermal layers of thick and thin skin are the same, with certain exceptions. Thin skin, for example, contains fewer eccrine sweat glands and more sebaceous glands than does thick skin. Except for the glans penis, labia minora, clitoris, and the vermillion borders of the lips, the dermis of thin skin always contains hair follicles; that of thick skin does not. Elastic fibers are more abundant in thin skin and its dermal papillae contain fewer Meissner's corpuscles.

IV. BLOOD SUPPLY TO THE SKIN.

Although the epidermis is avascular, the skin still receives an extensive vascular supply through the dermal blood vessels, which can hold about 4.5% of the body's total blood volume.

A. Arterial Plexuses: One of the 2 arterial plexuses that provide the skin's blood supply lies at the border between the papillary and reticular layers of the dermis. The other lies at the border between the dermis and hypodermis. Both give rise to arterioles that feed the papillary capillaries.

B. Papillary Capillaries: The dermal papillae, which surround the epidermal ridges, contain a rich capillary network that provides oxygen and nutrients to the avascular epidermis.

C. Venous Plexuses: The capillary bed in each papilla drains, by a single venule, into one of 3 venous plexuses. Two of these lie in the same position as the arterial plexuses; the other lies between them in the middle of the reticular dermis.

D. Arteriovenous Anastomoses (Shunts): Within the dermal plexuses there are many anastomoses—direct connections—between the arteries and veins. Postganglionic autonomic fibers control the opening and closing of these shunts. When the shunts are closed, more blood flows through the papillary capillaries; when they are open, they direct blood away from the capillaries, increasing blood volume in the larger vessels—and thus increasing blood pressure. Opening the shunts also reduces the loss of body heat through the skin. Vascular smooth muscle in the plexuses thus helps control blood pressure and body temperature by regulating the amount of blood in the papillary capillaries.

V. HAIR.

Occurring only in thin skin, the color, size, shape, and distribution of hair vary according to such factors as race, age, sex, and body region. The structures in the skin that form hairs and maintain their growth are called **hair follicles.**

A. Hair and Follicle Development:

1. Follicles Early in the third month of human embryonic development, local epidermal thickenings form at the sites of future hairs, developing first on the eyebrows, chin, and upper lip, then over the rest of the thin skin. Cells at the base of each thickening invade the dermis, and a small **dermal papilla** invades the leading edge of the epidermal downgrowth. Interactions between the papilla and the invaginating epidermis induce the differentiation of the hair follicle. Hair begins to form in the **hair bulb** at the base of the hair follicle as a result of the keratinization of the bulb's epithelial cells. These cells are pushed toward the surface by the ongoing mitosis in the **germinal matrix** (hair bulb epithelium). Some epithelial cells in the lateral walls of the developing follicle divide, forming bulges that differentiate into sebaceous glands (VII.A).

2. Hairs By the fifth or sixth month of gestation, the fetus is covered by very fine hairs (**lanugo**). Just before birth, most of the lanugo is shed, except for the scalp, eyebrows, and eyelashes. A few months after birth, the remaining lanugo has been shed and replaced by coarser mature **terminal hairs;** the rest of the body is coverd with a coat of fine short hairs, called **vellus.** At puberty, coarse terminal hairs replace the vellus in specific body areas. The replacement is sex-dependent: in males, terminal hairs develop in the axilla and pubic regions, on the face, and to some extent, over the rest of the body. In females, they develop mainly in the axilla and the pubic regions.

B. Hair and Follicle Structure:

1. General features Hair follicles extend from the skin surface deep into the dermis or hypodermis. The follicle's broad base, or hair bulb, consists of a cap of rapidly dividing epithelial cells (the germinal matrix) overlying a dermal papilla that harbors the supply of nerves and blood. Cells from the germinal matrix become keratinized, forming the concentric layers of the hair shaft as they move toward the surface. Near the surface, distinct layers can be seen ensheathing the canal that contains the hair shaft.

2. Associated structures

a. Sebaceous glands Found near the neck of the epithelial sheath, these glands empty their secretions into the follicular canal. (See also VII.A.)

b. Arrector pili muscles These small bundles of smooth muscle fibers attach to the follicle's connective tissue sheath below the sebaceous glands. They extend obliquely toward the papillary dermis, where their other ends attach. When they contract, these muscles cause the hairs to stand upright, giving the appearance of gooseflesh. Contracting also squeezes the sebaceous glands, pushing their secretions into the neck of the follicular canal and out onto the surface of the skin.

3. Germinal matrix This cluster of epithelial cells capping the dermal papilla can be divided into 4 indistinct zones that are arranged concentrically around the papilla. The zone closest to the papilla resembles the stratum basale of the epidermis in both structure and function. It contains both columnar epidermal cells and the melanocytes that give the hair its color. This germinal layer gives rise to the poorly keratinized cells of the

medulla of the hair shaft and to the cells in the other 3 zones of the germinal matrix. Around the base of the bulb, this layer is continuous with the external root sheath that surrounds the entire bulb and shaft; near the surface, it is continuous with the stratum basale. Cells in the next concentric layer divide and differentiate to form the hair shaft's **cortex;** those in the next layer form the hair shaft's **cuticle.** The most peripheral layer of the germinal matrix forms the poorly keratinized cells of the internal root sheath.

4. Hair shaft layers These 3 concentric layers are formed by the germinal matrix (as just described). The cell borders are indistinct, however, and cross sections through hair follicles near the skin surface often do not show the cellular nature of the layers. In addition, the hair itself may be dislodged from the canal during tissue processing, leaving only the open space (**follicular canal**) that originally contained the shaft.

a. Medulla Forming the shaft's thin central core, the medulla is composed of poorly keratinized and often vacuolated cells.

b. Cortex This layer surrounds the medulla; it is composed of several layers of well-keratinized polygonal cells.

c. Cuticle This is the shaft's outermost layer. Within the bulb, its cells are cuboidal; farther up the shaft they become tall columnar, fill with keratin, and finally change their orientation to become a few layers of flattened highly-keratinized cells. These cells form the hard, shinglelike cuticle that covers the hair's outer surface.

5. Root sheaths The concentric sheaths surrounding the hair shaft are more clearly distinguished in the area between the bulb and the skin surface.

a. Internal root sheath The layer closest to the hair shaft, it extends only from the bulb to the level of the sebaceous gland ducts. At this point its soft keratin-filled cells are exfoliated into the follicular canal. There are 3 component layers:

(1) Cuticle of the internal root sheath This layer of flattened cells is separated from the cuticle of the hair shaft only by the follicular canal.

(2) Huxley's layer The middle layer of the internal root sheath consists of 1–3 layers of flattened cuboidal cells.

(3) Henle's layer The outermost layer of the internal root sheath, this translucent layer of flattened-to-cuboidal cells resembles the epidermal stratum lucidum.

b. External root sheath This surrounds the internal root sheath and is continuous with the epidermis. Above the level of the sebaceous glands, it includes all the layers of the epidermis. Below this level, it retains only the granulosum, spinosum, and basale. The granulosum is also lost toward the base of the follicle, leaving only the spinosum and basale, which become continuous with the layers of the germinal matrix.

c. Glassy membrane This is the thickened basal lamina underlying the stratum basale of the external root sheath and separating it from the surrounding connective tissue sheath.

d. Connective tissue sheath A layer of condensed connective tissue, this surrounds the entire follicle, including the bulb. It extends along the follicle to the surface where it blends into the looser papillary dermis.

C. Keratinization: Although both the hair and the epidermis contain keratin, there are differences in their keratinization. For example,

1. The keratin of the hair's cortex and cuticle is harder than that of the epidermis;

2. Keratinized hair cells remain tightly attached to one another, while those of skin are continuously sloughed;

3. Keratinization of the hair occurs intermittenly and is restricted to the bulb, while that of skin occurs continuously and over the entire surface; and

4. The keratinized epidermal cells are identical to one another, while those in hairs differ in structure and function depending on their position in the hair.

D. Hair Growth: Hair growth is not continuous but cycles through repeated growing and resting phases. In the growing phase, the proliferation and differentiation of cells in the germinal matrix cause the hair to elongate. In the resting phase, the germinal matrix becomes inactive and may atrophy. The hair detaches from the bulb, moving upward as the external root sheath retracts toward the surface. Eventually, the hair is shed. During the next growing phase, the lower part of the external root sheath grows downward again, either forming a new germinal matrix over the old papilla or stimulating formation of a new papilla. The bulb reforms and the next phase of the cycle—proliferation in the matrix and renewed hair growth—begins. Hair growth cycles do not occur synchronously in all body regions, but rather in patches, sometimes known as **growth in mosaic.** Several hormones, especially androgens, influence the pattern of terminal hair distribution and growth rate.

VI. NAILS.

These plates of highly keratinized cells are analogous to, but harder than, the stratum corneum.

A. Nail Development: The formation of the nails is similar to that of the hair, producing plates rather than cylinders.

1. At the end of the third month of embryonic development, a narrow plate of epidermis on the dorsal surface of the terminal phalange invades the underlying dermis of each finger and toe.

2. This invasion continues proximally, forming a furrow, called the **nail groove,** in the skin.

3. Epithelial cells beneath the groove proliferate to form the **nail matrix** whose composition and function are similar to those of the hair's germinal matrix. Continued proliferation in the nail matrix pushes the upper cells toward the surface.

4. The upper cells differentiate; they become highly keratinized and form the **nail plate.**

5. The developing nail plate is gradually pushed out of the groove by further cell proliferation and differentiation in the nail matrix. The forming plate slides distally on the dorsal surface of the digit, and the epidermis over which it slides becomes the **nail bed.**

B. Nail Complex Structure:

1. The nail plate (or nail) consists of 2 parts: the **nail body**—the visible part of the nail—and the **nail root**—the part hidden in the nail groove.

2. The nail and its supporting structures are surrounded by papillary dermis.

a. The **nail matrix** is a thickened region of epidermis containing proliferating cells in the layer that directly contacts the dermis, and keratinizing cells between this basal layer and the nail plate. The nail matrix surrounds the root of the nail plate, and extends beyond the nail groove.

b. The **nail bed** is located beneath the nail body, distal to the nail matrix. It consists of only the deeper epidermal strata, for which the nail serves as a stratum corneum.

c. The **eponychium** (or **cuticle**) is a thick keratinized layer extending from the upper surface of the nail groove over the most proximal portion of the nail body.

d. The **hyponychium** is a localized thickening of the stratum corneum that underlies the free (distal) end of the nail.

e. The **lunula** is the whitish, opaque, cresent-shaped region on the proximal part of the nail body, adjacent to the nail groove. Its distal border corresponds roughly to that of the underlying nail matrix.

VII. GLANDS OF THE SKIN

A. Sebaceous Glands:

1. Structure and location These exocrine glands are found in all thin skin, most often in association with hair follicles into which their ducts empty. In hairless thin skin, the glands open directly onto the skin surface. Their acinar secretory portions contain many large lipid-filled cells that have a foamy appearance. Sebaceous glands are most numerous in the skin of the face, forehead, and scalp.

2. Function The acinar cells of sebaceous glands fill with lipid droplets containing a mixture of triglycerides, waxes, squalene, and cholesterol and its esters. Their nuclei become pyknotic and the cells eventually burst, releasing their contents and other cell debris (together termed **sebum**) into the ducts. The entire cell is shed, a type of secretion known as **holocrine secretion.** The oily sebum moves through the ducts and into the hair follicle. It covers the hair and moves out onto the surface. Here, it lubricates the skin and may have some antibacterial or antifungal effects. The secretory activity of these glands, which begin functioning at puberty, is continuous and is increased by androgens.

B. Sweat Glands:

Two types of sweat glands, eccrine (or merocrine) and apocrine, are found in human skin. Both types develop as epidermal invaginations into the dermis and differ mainly in their size, distribution, and secretory products.

1. Eccrine sweat glands

a. Distribution The most numerous sweat glands in humans, these average about 3 million per individual. They are found in skin covering most of the body, except for the glans penis, the glans clitoridis, and the vermillion border of the lips. They are most abundant in thick skin, such as in the palms of the hands, where there are about 3000 per square inch.

b. Structure These are simple coiled tubular glands.

(1) Ducts The slightly coiled ducts are lined with simple-to-stratified cuboidal epithelium; their lining cells are smaller than those in the secretory portions and stain darker. Each duct opens directly onto the skin surface.

(2) Secretory portions These highly coiled parts of the sweat glands are located in deep reticular dermis or shallow hypodermis. Surrounding connective tissue condenses to form a sheath around the basal lamina, and there are numerous myoepithelial cells between the basal lamina and the secretory cells. The secretions are released via exocytosis (**merocrine secretion**). Secretory cells are larger and stain lighter than the duct-lining cells; 2 types are seen.

(a) Dark cells These pyramidal **mucoid cells** line most of the lumen of the secretory portion of the gland; their bases do not reach the basal lamina. They contain rodlike mitochondria, a well-developed Golgi complex, rough endoplasmic reticulum, many free ribosomes, and dark glycoprotein-containing granules.

(b) Clear cells Also pyramidal, these cells lack secretory granules, contain abundant glycogen, and surround the inner layer of dark cells. Their basal plasma membranes, which do contact the basal lamina, are highly infolded, suggesting that these cells are involved in ion and water transport.

c. Secretory product Eccrine sweat is a watery secretion whose main components (in addition to water) include sodium chloride, urea, ammonia, and uric acid. The glands thus assist in the excretion of byproducts of protein metabolism. In addition, evaporation of the water from the skin surface reduces the body temperature by cooling the blood in the papillary capillaries.

2. Apocrine sweat glands

a. Distribution Less numerous than the eccrine type, these glands occur mainly in the axilla, pubic and anal regions, and in the areolae of the breasts.

b. Structure Apocrine sweat glands, like the eccrine glands, are also simple coiled tubular glands, but they are generally larger.

(1) Ducts These coiled ducts are lined with low cuboidal epithelium and open into the hair follicles.

(2) Secretory portion Coiled and embedded in the dermis, each has a wide lumen lined by cuboidal-to-columnar cells. Myoepithelial cells are present between the secretory cells and the basal lamina.

c. Secretory product Apocrine sweat is a viscous, odorless fluid that, once secreted, acquires a distinctive odor as a result of bacterial degradation. The term *apocrine* derives from early evidence that the secretory cells of these glands released their apical cytoplasm along with the secretory product. Recent evidence, however, argues against apical shedding. Thus, while the secretory products of apocrine and eccrine sweat glands do differ, their mode of secretion—merocrine—is similar.

Study-Focusing Questions*

1. Name the 2 major layers of the skin (354) and compare them in terms of their:
   a. Thickness (354; 361)
   b. Vascularity (77, 362)
   c. Embryonic germ layer of origin (**HR**)
2. Describe the hypodermis in terms of its structure, function, and location (354, 362)
3. List the 4 cell types commonly found in the epidermis (354) and compare them in terms of their:
   a. Number (354, 359, 360, 361)
   b. Location (354, 359, 360, 361)
   c. Primary function (354, 359, 360, 361)
4. List the differences between thick and thin skin in terms of:
   a. The layers of the epidermis (358)
   b. The number of hair follicles (354, 362)
   c. The number of sweat glands (**HR**)
   d. The number of sebaceous glands (365)
   e. Their location in the body (354)
5. Beginning at the surface, list the 5 layers of the epidermis and compare the keratinocytes found in each layer in terms of (354–358):
   a. Their cell shape
   b. Their capacity for cell division
   c. Their staining properties
   d. The visibility of their nuclei and other organelles
6. Name the structures that specifically aid in binding the keratinocytes and melanocytes in the stratum basale to the underlying basal lamina (354, 359)
7. Name the embryonic cell type that forms melanocytes (359).
8. Name the enzyme found in melanocyte granules that is primarily responsible for melanin production (359).
9. Beginning with the synthesis of the enzyme named in the answer to question 8, list the steps in the production and maturation of melanin granules (359).
10. Describe how the melanin granules produced by melanocytes enter the keratinocytes (359).
11. Name 2 mechanisms responsible for the darkening of the skin after exposure to ultraviolet light (360).
12. Describe Langerhans' cells (360) in terms of:
    a. Their shape
    b. Their location (layer) in the epidermis

*The page references in this section refer to *Basic Histology,* 6th ed., Junqueira L, Carneiro J, Kelley R (editors), Appleton & Lange, 1989. **HR** (for Histology Review) is occasionally used instead of a page reference to indicate that the information referred to can be found in this book.

c. Their special staining properties
d. The shape(s) and name(s) of the granules they contain
e. Their location in the body, other than the epidermis
f. Their immune function

13. Describe Merkel's cells (361) in terms of:
    a. The type of skin (thick or thin) in which they are most abundant
    b. Their association with nerve endings
    c. Two of their possible functions
14. Name the 2 layers of the dermis (361–362) and compare them in terms of their:
    a. Primary tissue type
    b. Thickness
    c. Location in relation to the epidermis
15. Is hair growth continuous or discontinuous (362)?
16. Explain the expression *growth in mosaic* as it applies to hair (362).
17. Sketch a longitudinal section of a hair follicle (363, 364); include and label the following:
    a. Hair bulb
    b. Dermal papilla
    c. Germinal matrix
    d. Melanocytes
    e. Hair shaft
    f. Internal root sheath
    g. External root sheath
    h. Glassy membrane
    i. Connective tissue sheath
    j. Arrector pili muscle
18. Sketch a cross section through a hair follicle above the bulb (363); include and label the following:
    a. Medulla
    b. Cortex
    c. Cuticle
    d. Internal root sheath
    e. External root sheath
    f. Glassy membrane
    g. Connective tissue sheath
19. Above what level in the hair follicle is the internal root sheath no longer present (362)?
20. Compare the hardness of the keratin in hairs with that in the epidermis (364).
21. Sketch a longitudinal section of a fingertip through the nail (365); include and label the following:
    a. Root of the nail
    b. Eponychium
    c. Nail plate
    d. Nail matrix
    e. Nail bed
    f. Hyponychium
22. Of the components of the nail complex named in question 21, which is the only one that actually contributes cells to the growing nail (365)?
23. Describe sebaceous glands in terms of:
    a. The class of glands to which they belong, as determined by the shape of their adenomeres (tubular or acinar) (365)
    b. Their association with hair follicles (364, 365)
    c. Three places they occur without hair follicles (365)
    d. Their mode of secretion (merocrine, apocrine, or holocrine) (365)
    e. The name given to their secretion (365)
    f. The composition of their secretion (365)
24. Name the 2 types of sweat glands found in humans (366, 367) and compare them in terms of:
    a. The class of glands to which they belong as determined by the shape of their adenomeres (tubular or acinar)
    b. Their distribution in the skin

c. Their mode of secretion (merocrine, apocrine, or holocrine)
d. The composition of their secretion
e. Their innervation

25. Name the type of epithelium commonly found lining the ducts of sweat glands (366).
26. Sketch a vertical section through the skin (355), showing the boundaries of the epidermis, papillary dermis (don't forget the papillae), reticular dermis, and hypodermis. Indicate on this diagram the location of the 2 arterial plexuses, the papillary capillaries, the 3 venous plexuses, the origin of the lymphatic capillaries, and the 2 lymphatic plexuses (367).
27. Name the types of sensory receptors found in the:
    a. Epidermis (361, 367, 467)
    b. Dermal papillae (467)
    c. Reticular dermis (467)
    d. Papillae of hair follicles (467)
28. Name the components of the skin that have a role in the following functions:
    a. Protection from dehydration (354, 356)
    b. Protection from abrasion (355, 357)
    c. Protection from infection (355, 361)
    d. Protection from ultraviolet radiation (359)
    e. Regulation of blood pressure (367)
    f. Regulation of body temperature
    g. Sensory reception (367, 467)
    h. Excretion (366)

Multiple-Choice Questions

For questions 18–1 and 18–2, select the single best answer.

18–1. The functions of the skin include all of the following *except:*
- **A.** Thermoregulation
- **B.** Protection from ultraviolet radiation
- **C.** Sensation
- **D.** Production of vitamin C
- **E.** Protection from impact and friction

18–2. The arrector pili muscles:
- **A.** Are composed of bundles of myoepithelial cells
- **B.** May help push sebum onto the skin surface
- **C.** Have no effect on hair position in humans
- **D.** Attach directly to the external root sheath by desmosomes
- **E.** Contain capillary networks that nourish growing hairs

MATCHING (questions 18–3 through 18–41): Each choice may be used once, more than once, or not at all.

Questions 18–3 through 18–9:

- **A.** Epidermis
- **B.** Dermis
- **C.** Hypodermis
- **D.** All of the above
- **E.** A and B only
- **F.** B and C only

18–3. Derived primarily from mesoderm
18–4. Derived primarily from ectoderm
18–5. Part(s) of the skin
18–6. Contain(s) blood vessels
18–7. Contains the largest number of adipocytes
18–8. May contain hair bulbs

Questions 18–9 through 18–18:

A. Keratinocytes
B. Melanocytes
C. Langerhans' cell(s)
D. Merkel cell(s)

18–9. Most abundant in skin
18–10. Stellate (star-shaped) cells
18–11. Neural crest derivative(s)
18–12. Stain with gold chloride
18–13. Antigen-presenting cells
18–14. Contain Birbeck's granules
18–15. May have DNES functions
18–16. Intense tyrosinase activity
18–17. May be mechanoreceptors
18–18. Contain lamellar granules

Questions 18–19 through 18–27 (may have more than one correct answer):

A. Stratum corneum
B. Stratum spinosum
C. Stratum lucidum
D. Stratum basale
E. Stratum granulosum
F. None of the above

18–19. Contain(s) keratinocytes
18–20. Contain(s) melanocyte cell bodies
18–21. Site(s) of keratinocyte proliferation
18–22. Richest in keratohyalin granules
18–23. Keratinocyte organelles and nuclei not evident
18–24. Columnar keratinocytes
18–25. Squamous keratinocytes
18–26. Intensely eosinophilic
18–27. Hemidesmosomes present

Questions 18–28 through 18–35 use the letters in Fig 18–2.

18–28. Melanocytes
18–29. Medulla
18–30. Cortex
18–31. Papilla
18–32. Glassy membrane
18–33. Connective tissue sheath
18–34. Internal root sheath
18–35. External root sheath

Questions 18–36 through 18–41 use the letters in Fig 18–3.

18–36. Nail matrix
18–37. Nail root
18–38. Nail bed
18–39. Nail plate
18–40. Eponychium
18–41. Hyponychium

For questions 18–42 through 18–74, either, both, or neither of the answers may be correct. Select

A if only A is correct
B if only B is correct

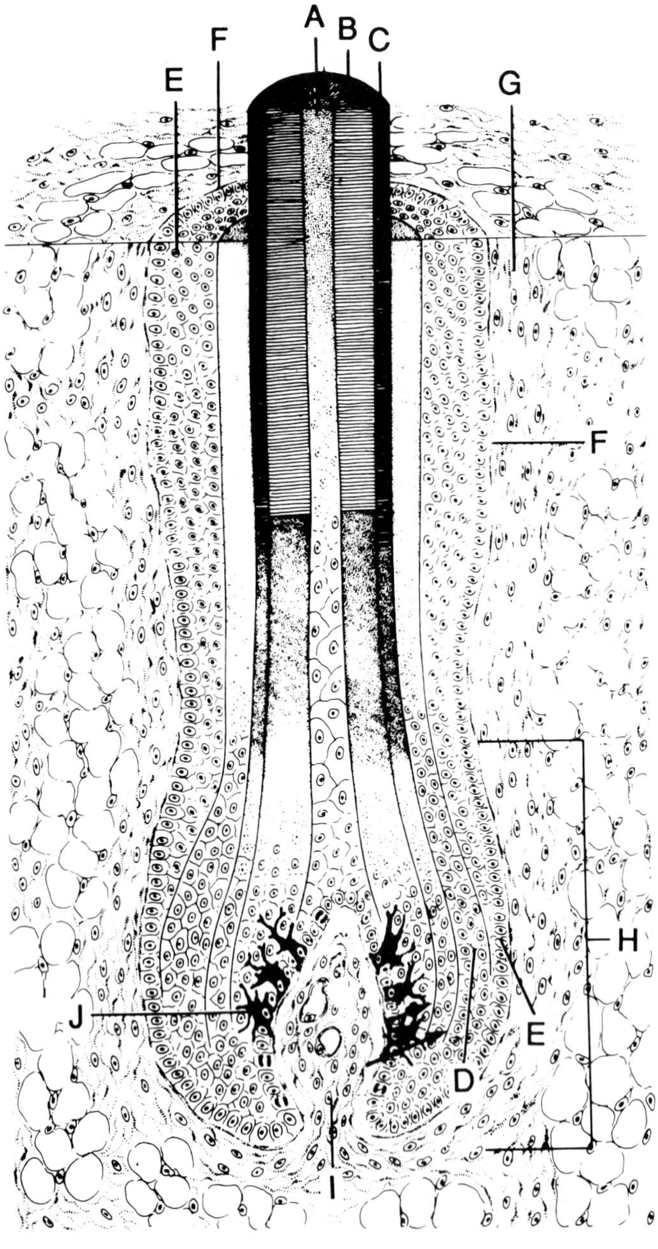

Figure 18-2.

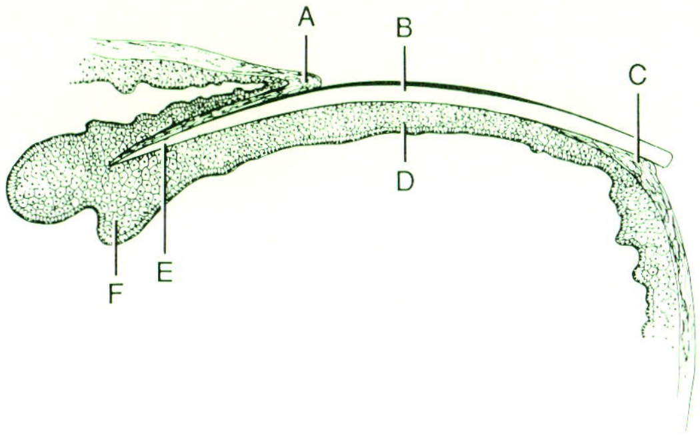

Figure 18-3.

C if both A and B are correct
D if neither A nor B is correct

Questions 18-42 through 18-49:

A. Thick skin
B. Thin skin
C. Both
D. Neither

18-42. Often lacks a definitive stratum lucidum
18-43. Palms and soles
18-44. Hairy skin
18-45. Often lacks a papillary dermis
18-46. More abundant sweat glands
18-47. Stratum granulosum may be incomplete
18-48. More abundant sebaceous glands
18-49. Scalp

Questions 18-50 through 18-56:

A. Keratohyalin granules
B. Lamellar granules
C. Both
D. Neither

18-50. Surrounded by a limiting membrane
18-51. Contain a phosphorylated histidine-rich protein
18-52. Contents released to extracellular spaces
18-53. Contents include phospholipids
18-54. Intensely basophilic
18-55. Found in the stratum granulosum
18-56. Contents help form a barrier to foreign materials

Questions 18-57 through 18-63:

A. Papillary dermis
B. Reticular dermis
C. Both
D. Neither

18-57. Dense irregular connective tissue
18-58. Dense regular connective tissue
18-59. Location of Meissner's corpuscles

18–60. Contains the capillaries that nourish the epidermis
18–61. Loose connective tissue
18–62. Thicker layer
18–63. Contain(s) blood vessels

Questions 18–64 through 18–74:

A. Eccrine sweat glands
B. Sebaceous glands
C. Both
D. Neither

18–64. Have coiled tubular adenomeres
18–65. Have acinar adenomeres
18–66. Exocrine glands
18–67. Ducts usually empty into hair follicles
18–68. Release only their apical cytoplasm during secretion
18–69. Holocrine secretion
18–70. Secrete by exocytosis (merocrine)
18–71. Oily-to-waxy secretion
18–72. Contain dark cells and clear cells
18–73. Pale-staining, foamy appearance
18–74. Rate of secretion controlled by circulating androgens

For questions 18–75 through 18–80, one, more than one, or all of the answers may be correct. Select

A if only (1), (2), and (3) are correct
B if only (1) and (3) are correct
C if only (2) and (4) are correct
D if only (4) is correct
E if all answers are correct

18–75. Structures that have a role in maintaining the integrity of the skin during abrasion include:
(1) Desmosomes
(2) Anchoring fibrils
(3) Hemidesmosomes
(4) Dermal papillae

18–76. Skin-associated regions that exhibit a relatively high rate of mitosis include the:
(1) Stratum germinativum
(2) Nail matrix
(3) Germinal matrix of hair bulbs
(4) Stratum granulosum

18–77. The basic tissue types found in the skin include:
(1) Epithelium
(2) Nerve
(3) Connective tissue
(4) Muscle

18–78. Hair growth:
(1) Cannot occur once the papilla of the bulb is destroyed
(2) Occurs in patches
(3) Is strongly influenced by circulating androgens
(4) Occurs continuously

18–79. Of the many functions served by the skin, those partly or completely provided by components of the dermis include:
(1) Protection from dehydration
(2) Thermoregulation
(3) Protection from ultraviolet radiation
(4) Regulation of blood pressure

18–80. Significant sites of arteriovenous anastomoses in the skin include the border(s) between the:
(1) Papillary and reticular dermis
(2) Dermis and epidermis
(3) Dermis and hypodermis
(4) Epidermis and basal lamina

Urinary System 19

Objectives

This chapter should help the student to:

- List the parts and functions of the urinary system and describe the roles of each organ.
- Identify and describe the substructures of the kidney as seen grossly in frontal section.
- Compare the kidney cortex and medulla in terms of structure and function.
- Name and describe the structure and function of each component of a nephron.
- Name the components and describe the function of the juxtaglomerular apparatus.
- Trace the circulation of blood through the kidney.
- Describe the ultrastructure of the filtration barrier of the renal corpuscle.
- Trace the flow of fluid from Bowman's space to a minor calyx, naming, in order, the tubules through which it flows and describing any changes in fluid composition that occur in each tubule segment.
- Compare the roles of ADH and aldosterone in renal function.
- Describe the structure of the walls of the calyces, renal pelvis, ureters, and urinary bladder.
- Name the parts of the male urethra and the epithelium found lining each part.
- Compare the urethras of males and females.
- Name and describe the sphincters that control the flow of urine through the urethra.
- Compare the countercurrent exchange system with the countercurrent multiplier system of the kidney.
- Differentiate between cortex and medulla and identify all of the vascular and tubular components as well as the components of the renal corpuscles and juxtaglomerular apparatus in a slide or photomicrograph of the kidney.
- Identify the components of the glomerular filtration barrier in a diagram or electron micrograph of a renal corpuscle.
- Identify the ureter, urinary bladder, and the parts of the urethra in histologic sections.

Synopsis

I. GENERAL FEATURES OF THE URINARY SYSTEM

A. Components of the System: The urinary system includes the kidneys and the urinary tract.

1. Kidneys These paired, bean-shaped, retroperitoneal organs are located in the posterior wall of the abdominal cavity.

a. Structural and functional subdivisions When sliced in the frontal plane (Fig 19–1), each kidney shows a dark-staining outer **cortex** and a light-staining inner **medulla** that partly surrounds the **renal hilum.** The hilum consists of a space, the **renal sinus,** that contains the larger renal blood vessels, the **renal pelvis,** and adipose tissue. Each human kidney consists of several pyramid-shaped subunits—**renal lobes**—whose bases lie in the cortex and whose apices lie in the medulla. The apices are cupped by **minor calyces** that collect and empty the urine from each lobe into the larger **major calyces.** These in turn empty into the single, funnel-shaped renal pelvis, which is continuous with the **ureter.** Each lobe consists of numerous **renal lobules,** each containing hundreds of **nephrons.** These are largely tubular structures that filter the blood, modify the filtrate to form urine, and empty into a series of **collecting tubules and ducts** which converge on the medulla and empty into the minor calyces.

b. Blood supply Because the kidneys are blood-filtering organs, their blood supply is crucial to their function. A pair of **renal arteries**—one to each kidney—branches from the aorta in the upper abdomen. Each artery undergoes successive branching to feed specialized capillary beds in both the cortex (**glomeruli** and **peritubular capillaries**) and medulla (**vasa recta**). Knowledge of the renal artery's branching pattern within the kidney is important. It aids in understanding how the blood reaches the capillaries that play specific and crucial roles in renal function. In addition, the structure, route, and location of the branches provide clues to the way in which the structural and functional subdivisions are arranged.

2. Urinary tract The structure of the **ureters, urinary bladder,** and **urethra,** which constitute the urinary tract, is described mainly in terms of their wall structure. Except for certain portions of the urethra, the lumen of the tract is characteristically lined by transitional epithelium.

B. General Functions of the System: The kidneys filter metabolic wastes from the blood; regulate the ion, salt, and water concentrations of the fluids that bathe the body's tissues; and produce renin and erythropoietin. The collection of raw filtrate from the blood in the glomerular capillaries is only the first step in urine production. This is followed by the reabsorption of important ions, small proteins, nutrients, and much of the water present. These are returned to the blood in the peritubular capillaries and

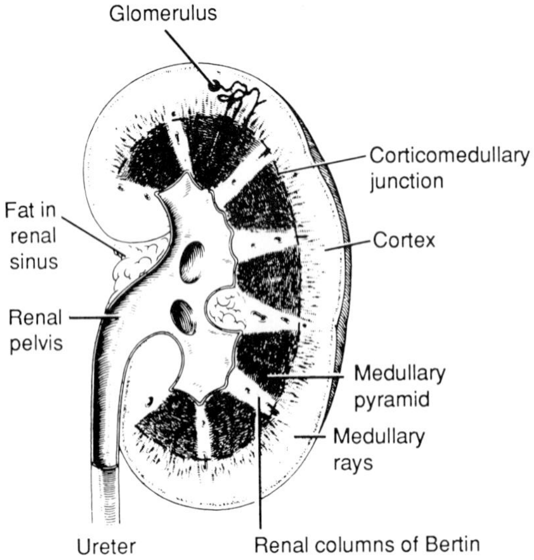

Figure 19–1. The general organization of the kidney.

vasa recta in precise proportions. The portion of the raw filtrate that is not reabsorbed constitutes the urine; it is carried by the ureters from the kidneys to the urinary bladder where it is temporarily stored and later released through the urethra.

II. KIDNEYS

A. General Organization:

The kidneys, which measure about 11 × 6 cm, are bean-shaped retroperitoneal organs encapsulated by dense connective tissue and surrounded by adipose tissue. Several components can be distinguished without the aid of a microscope:

1. Renal sinus This medial concavity of each kidney contains the renal pelvis, the entering and exiting blood vessels and nerves, and adipose tissue.

2. Hilum This consists of the renal sinus and its contents.

3. Cortex The kidney's dark-staining outer region, the cortex underlies the capsule. It contains the renal corpuscles, proximal and distal convoluted tubules, peritubular capillaries, and medullary rays.

4. Medulla This is the kidney's light-staining inner region, which partly surrounds the renal sinus. It consists of 10–18 medullary pyramids whose bases abut the cortex and whose apices (renal papillae) point inward, toward the renal sinus. It also contains the collecting ducts, loops of Henle, and vasa recta. Each renal papilla, perforated by openings of the collecting ducts, is cradled by a minor calyx into which the ducts empty. Several minor calyces empty into a major calyx. The major calyces empty into the renal pelvis, which in turn drains into the ureter.

5. Medullary rays These fingerlike extensions of medullary tissue that enter the cortex comprise clusters of collecting tubules and ducts. One medullary ray lies at the center of each renal lobule.

6. Renal lobes Each human kidney has 8–18 lobes, the kidney's largest subdivisions. Each lobe, which consists of a **medullary pyramid** and its associated cortex, contains numerous renal lobules.

7. Renal lobules Each of these subdivisions of the lobes consists of a central medullary ray and all the nephrons that empty into its collecting tubules. The borders between adjacent renal lobules are marked by interlobular arteries and veins.

B. Nephrons:

Nephrons are the basic functional subunits of the kidney. Each nephron includes a renal corpuscle, a proximal convoluted tubule, a loop of Henle, and a distal convoluted tubule.

1. Renal corpuscle As the blood-filtering unit of the nephron, each renal corpuscle consists of a glomerulus covered by Bowman's capsule. Together these structures form the filtration barrier. Each corpuscle has both a urinary and a vascular pole.

a. Glomerulus This is a small tuft of fenestrated capillaries whose fenestrae are covered by thin diaphragms. Modified smooth muscle cells, **mesangial cells,** lie between the capillary loops.

b. Bowman's capsule is a double-walled epithelial chamber. Its inner wall, or **visceral layer,** consists of **podocytes.** These cells have interdigitating foot processes **(pedicels)** that grasp the glomerular capillaries like fingers around a broom handle, and adhere tightly to the fused capillary-podocyte basal lamina. The outer wall—the **parietal layer**—is simple squamous epithelium. The chamber between the visceral and parietal layers is known as the **urinary** or **Bowman's space.**

c. Filtration barrier Consisting of the structures that separate the capillary lumen from the urinary space, the filtration barrier includes (1) the diaphragm-covered capillary fenestrations, (2) the fused basal laminae of the capillary endothelial cells and podocytes, and (3) the diaphragm-covered filtration slits that lie between the interdigitating pedicels.

d. Vascular pole This side of the corpuscle is where the afferent arterioles that feed the glomerular capillaries enter and the efferent arterioles that drain them leave. It lies opposite the urinary pole.

e. Urinary pole This side of the corpuscle is where the proximal convoluted tubule exits.

f. Filtration mechanism Blood is delivered to the glomerulus by the **afferent arteriole.** Arterial pressure forces fluid from the blood through the filtration barrier and into the urinary space. Each component of the barrier (fenestrae, diaphragms, basal lamina, filtration slits) aids in limiting the passage of blood components by size, thus preventing blood cells and large proteins from entering the urinary space. Molecules trapped in the basal lamina are periodically removed by the mesangial cells. A reduced volume of blood leaves the glomerulus via the **efferent arteriole,** and the raw filtrate in the urinary space enters the proximal convoluted tubule for further processing.

2. Proximal convoluted tubule An epithelial tube that begins at the urinary pole of the renal corpuscle, its lining is simple low columnar-to-cuboidal epithelium. The lining cells have abundant long microvilli. Together they form a **brush border** that partly obscures the lumen and increases the surface area available for absorption. The lining cells absorb about 85% of the sodium from the filtrate; a similar amount of water follows passively. All the glucose (unless present in great excess) and amino acids are reabsorbed by facilitated transport (see Chapter 3) and small proteins are reabsorbed by pinocytosis. The many mitochondria required for the energy-intensive absorptive function make the lining cells acidophilic. The convoluted part of the proximal tubule empties into its straight portion (also called the thick descending limb of the loop of Henle), which has a similar epithelium and function.

3. Loop of Henle

a. Structure Henle's loop, a U-shaped epithelial tube, includes thick and thin descending limbs, and thin and thick ascending limbs. It extends from the proximal convoluted tubule in the cortex, dips into the medulla, and returns to the cortex, where it empties into the distal convoluted tubule. The abrupt transition from thick to thin in both arms of the U is the result of changes from low columnar-to-cuboidal to squamous and back to cuboidal epithelium. The change in the luminal diameter is less dramatic than that in the external diameter.

b. Function A prerequisite for the production of hypertonic urine, the loop acts as a **countercurrent multiplier** to establish an osmotic gradient in the interstitial fluid of the medulla. **Hypertonic** (concentrated) and **hypotonic** (dilute) are relative terms. The point of reference assumed here is the tonicity of normal tissue fluid or blood **(isotonic)**. The medullary interstitium, for example, is approximately isotonic near the corticomedullary junction and gradually becomes most hypertonic near the tips of the medullary papillae. The descending and ascending portions of the loop of Henle play an important role in establishing and maintaining this osmotic gradient.

(1) Descending portion The first part of Henle's loop, it plays a passive role in making the medullary interstitium hypertonic and helps maintain the gradient. The filtrate entering the descending part of the thin loop is isotonic, but the removal of salt, nutrients, and water in the proximal tubule causes a reduction in volume from its raw state in the urinary space. Although the descending portion of the loop is permeable to water, it is impermeable to salt. As the fluid in its lumen passes deeper into the hypertonic medulla, it loses water to the interstitium and gradually becomes more hypertonic. Its tonicity equilibrates with the hypertonic interstitium, peaking at the bottom of the U as it enters the ascending portion.

(2) Ascending portion Two functional properties of the lining epithelium give this part of Henle's loop a more active role.

(a) Cells in the thick ascending portion constantly pump chloride ions from the filtrate into the interstitial fluid around the tubules. Sodium passively follows the chloride, increasing the salt concentration (and tonicity [osmolarity]) in the interstitium.

(b) Because this part of the loop is impermeable to water, the water in the filtrate cannot follow the salt into the interstitium and dilute it. As the filtrate ascends toward the distal convoluted tubule in the cortex, the removal of chloride and sodium (but not water) by the cells lining this portion of the loop causes the fluid in its lumen to gradually become isotonic or hypotonic. (The importance of the osmotic gradient to the production of hypertonic urine will become clearer after considering the events occurring in the collecting ducts that pass through the medulla enroute to the calyces.)

4. Distal convoluted tubule This final segment of the nephron lies in the cortex. Its epithelial lining is low cuboidal, with no brush border, making its lumen appear wider. Its lining cells are more basophilic than are those lining the proximal convoluted tubules. The lateral cell boundaries are indistinct as a result of their extensive lateral membrane interdigitations with their neighbors. The distal tubule epithelium forms a disk of tightly packed columnar cells called a **macula densa** at the point near the vascular pole of a renal corpuscle where it contacts an afferent arteriole. This disk may monitor the osmolarity of the fluid in the tubule lumen; the osmolarity of the fluid delivered by the loop of Henle changes little here. The distal convoluted tubule makes final adjustments of the salt, water, and acid balance. The presence of **aldosterone** causes the lining cells to remove more sodium and add phosphate to the fluid. The cells may further adjust the pH by secreting hydrogen and ammonium ions into the lumen.

5. Cortical and juxtamedullary nephrons Renal corpuscles are found throughout the cortex. While most of these belong to the cortical nephrons, the 15% closest to the medulla belong to the juxtamedullary nephrons. The latter group has short thick descending limbs and longer thin limbs that extend deeper into the medulla. The juxtamedullary nephrons bear the primary responsibility for setting up the osmotic gradient in the medulla.

C. Collecting Tubules and Ducts:

1. Structure These differ from the nephrons in their embryonic origin and can be easily distinguished from the proximal and distal tubules in sections. Their blocklike lining cells have distinct intercellular borders; they are cuboidal in the smaller tubules and columnar in the larger ducts of the medulla. Because their cytoplasm stains poorly, the cells appear to be clear or white.

2. Function The cortical collecting tubules receive hypotonic or isotonic urine from the nephrons and empty it into larger collecting ducts. These leave the cortex in medullary rays and enter the medulla, increasing in size until they open into a minor calyx through the tips of papillae. The medullary collecting ducts play the final role in forming hypertonic urine. Under the influence of **antidiuretic hormone (ADH** or vasopressin) they become permeable to water. As they pass through the osmotic gradient of the medulla, water diffuses passively from their lumens into the hypertonic medullary interstitium, causing the osmolarity of the fluid in their lumens to equilibrate with that of the interstitium; only a small volume of hypertonic urine is released. Without ADH, however, the collecting ducts remain impermeable to water and a larger amount of hypotonic or isotonic urine is produced.

D. Juxtaglomerular Apparatus:

Located near the vascular pole of a renal corpuscle at the point of contact between a distal convoluted tubule and an afferent arteriole, this includes **juxtaglomerular (JG) cells, a macula densa,** and **polkissen (extraglomerular mesangial) cells.** The JG cells, modified smooth muscle cells in the wall of the afferent arteriole, exhibit a typical secretory ultrastructure and numerous PAS-positive cytoplasmic granules. Although the influence of the macula densa on the JG cells is poorly understood, below-normal blood volume, blood pressure, or levels of blood sodium causes the JG cells to secrete renin. This enzyme cleaves plasma **angiotensinogen** to produce **angiotensin I,** which is converted to its active form, **angiotensin II,** by enzymes in the lungs. Angiotensin II, a vasoconstrictor, increases blood pressure and stimulates aldosterone production by the adrenal cortex, thereby increasing chloride and sodium reabsorption by the distal tubule. The sodium and chloride enter the blood in the peritubular capillaries and water follows, increasing blood volume and pressure. Increased blood pressure distends the afferent arterioles, stretching the JG cells and halting renin secretion. Polkissen cell function is unknown.

E. Blood Supply and Circulation: The arteries described below are accompanied by similarly named veins.

1. Each kidney receives a **renal artery**—a branch from the abdominal aorta.

2. Anterior and **posterior branches** arise from the renal artery before it reaches the renal hilum.

3. Interlobar arteries arise from the anterior and posterior branches in the renal hilum and penetrate the medulla between the medullary pyramids.

4. Arcuate arteries arise from the interlobar arteries and course along the arched border between the cortex and medulla.

5. Interlobular arteries arise at right angles from the arcuates; they penetrate the cortex between the medullary rays and lie at the borders between neighboring renal lobules.

6. Many **afferent arterioles** arise from each interlobular artery. Each afferent arteriole supplies a glomerulus (II.B.1.a).

7. An **efferent arteriole** carries blood away from the glomerulus.

a. Efferent arterioles of **cortical nephrons** branch to form a profusion of **peritubular capillaries** that carry absorbed products away from the proximal and distal tubules and converge to form the **stellate veins** of the peripheral cortex. These drain into the interlobular veins.

b. Efferent arterioles of **juxtamedullary nephrons** give rise to numerous straight capillary loops—vasa recta—that descend into the medulla.

8. Vasa recta arise mainly from the efferent arterioles of the juxtamedullary nephrons; some may arise from the arcuate artery. The descending parts of the vasa recta carry isotonic blood into the medulla. The blood loses water and picks up sodium as it passes deeper into the medulla. Unlike the loop of Henle, the ascending parts of the vasa recta are just as permeable to salt and water as are its descending parts. As the blood ascends through the gradient, it loses the salt it gained and regains the water lost during the descent. The blood carried away from the medulla is thus once again isotonic. The passive exchange of salt and water between the vasa recta and the interstitium is known as the **countercurrent exchange** mechanism. It is important in maintaining the osmotic gradient set up by the countercurrent multiplier system of Henle's loop. Blood in the ascending portions of these vessels drains into interlobular veins and exits through the veins that accompany the larger arteries.

F. Summary of Renal Function: An organized system of arteries carries blood to the glomeruli of the renal corpuscles. Each corpuscle acts as both filter and funnel, collecting raw filtrate and directing it to the proximal convoluted tubule where glucose, amino acids, small proteins, and 85% of the sodium and water are reabsorbed. The remaining fluid enters the loop of Henle, which sets up a hypertonic osmotic gradient in the medulla. The fluid leaves the loop and enters the distal convoluted tubule. Here, aided by the juxtaglomerular apparatus and aldosterone, the salt, ion, and water balance between the blood and urine are adjusted. The urine then exits the nephron through the collecting ducts, which pass back through the medulla. ADH renders the medullary collecting ducts permeable to water, allowing the water to flow out of the lumens of the collecting ducts and into the medullary interstitium. This results in the release of hypertonic urine into the minor calyx.

III. RENAL CALYCES & RENAL PELVIS.

The walls of each renal calyx and pelvis are composed of mucosa, muscularis, and adventitia; no submucosa is present. The mucosa, consisting of typical urinary (transitional) epithelium (see Chapter 4), is connected to an underlying helical meshwork of smooth muscle (muscularis) by a connective tissue lamina propria of variable density. The epithelium forms an osmotic barrier that protects the surrounding tissues from the hypertonic urine and the urine from dilution. The adventitia blends into the adipose tissue contained in the renal sinus.

IV. URETERS. These carry urine from the renal pelvis to the urinary bladder. While the lumen is narrower than that of the renal pelvis, the wall structure is similar, including the lining of transitional epithelium. The ureter wall thickens and the muscle cells change from a helical to a longitudinal array near the bladder before it fans out in the bladder wall to form the superficial and deep trigones of the bladder.

V. URINARY BLADDER. A distensible muscular sac lined by transitional epithelium, its walls are similar to those of the ureter, pelvis, and calyces but have a thicker muscularis. The smooth muscle fibers in this layer run in many directions; except near the opening into the urethra, they are not organized into layers. Here they form an involuntary **internal sphincter.**

VI. URETHRA. This differs in length, epithelium, and function in males and females.

A. Male Urethra: Longer than the female urethra, this conducts both urine and seminal fluid; it has 3 main parts:

1. **Prostatic portion** The most proximal part of the male urethra, it exits directly from the neck of the urinary bladder. It is surrounded by the prostate gland (see Chapter 22) and is lined by transitional epithelium. This portion receives the prostatic and ejaculatory ducts and empties into the membranous portion.

2. **Membranous portion** This is the shortest segment. It is encircled by the skeletal muscle of the membranelike urogenital diaphragm, whose fibers form a voluntary **external sphincter.** This portion of the urethra is lined by pseudostratified columnar epithelium and empties into the cavernous portion.

3. **Cavernous portion** Passing through the corpus cavernosum urethrae (**corpus spongiosum**) of the penis (see Chapter 22), this part of the male urethra is divided into **bulbous** and **pendulous** parts. Within the glans, near the tip of the penis, the urethral lumen widens to form the **fossa navicularis.** The epithelium changes here from pseudostratified columnar to stratified squamous. The urethra opens at the end of the penis through the **urethral meatus.** Numerous **glands of Littre** empty mucous secretions into the lumen all along the urethra; they are more numerous in the pendulous part.

B. Female Urethra: Shorter than the male urethra, this carries only urine. It is lined by stratified squamous epithelium and has patches of pseudostratified columnar. Midway along its path from the bladder to the exterior, it is surrounded by a voluntary external sphincter that is formed by the urogenital diaphragm.

Study-Focusing Questions*

1. Name the paired and unpaired organs of the urinary system (368).
2. List the general functions of the urinary system (368).
3. Sketch a frontal section of the kidney (369) and label the following:
   a. Capsule (368, 370)
   b. Cortex (368, 369)
   c. Medulla (368, 369)
   d. Medullary pyramids (368, 369)
   e. Medullary rays (368, 369)

*The page references in this section refer to *Basic Histology,* 6th ed., Junqueira L, Carneiro J, Kelley R (editors), Appleton & Lange, 1989. **HR** (for Histology Review) is occasionally used instead of a page reference to indicate that the information referred to can be found in this book.

   f. Renal columns of Bertin (368, 369)
   g. Major calyx (368, 369)
   h. Minor calyx (368, 369)
   i. Renal papilla (368, 369)
   j. Renal pelvis (368, 369)
   k. Renal sinus (368, 369)
   l. Hilum (368)
   m. Renal artery and vein (368, 381)
   n. Interlobar artery and vein (381, 385)
   o. Arcuate artery and vein (381, 385)
   p. Interlobular artery and vein (381, 385)
   q. Renal lobe (368)
   r. Renal lobule (368)

4. Name, in order, the major components of a nephron (368).

5. Sketch a nephron, label the components named in the answer to question 4, and show which components lie in the cortex and which in the medulla (368, 369).

6. Sketch a renal corpuscle (371) and label the following:
   a. Glomerulus (368–371)
   b. Bowman's capsule (368, 370, 371)
      (1) Visceral layer (podocytes) (369, 371)
      (2) Parietal layer (368–369, 371)
   c. Urinary space (368, 371)
   d. Afferent and efferent arterioles (368, 370, 371)
   e. Vascular pole (368, 371)
   f. Urinary pole (368, 371)
   g. Proximal convoluted tubule (368, 369, 370, 371)
   h. Mesangial cells (372, 373, 377)

7. Sketch the ultrastructure of a limited region of the glomerular filtration barrier (376) and label the following:
   a. Glomerular capillary lumen (374, 376, 377)
   b. Glomerular capillary endothelial cell (374, 376)
   c. Endothelial fenestrae (374, 376)
   c. Endothelial fenestrae (374, 376)
   d. Fused endothelial cell-podocyte basal laminae (374, 376)
   e. Secondary processes of podocytes (pedicels) (374, 376)
   f. Filtration slits (374, 376)
   g. Diaphragms covering filtration slits (376)
   h. Urinary space (376)

8. Describe a possible function for the mesangial cells in maintaining the integrity of the filtration barrier (373).

9. Compare the proximal and distal convoluted tubules in terms of:
   a. Their location in the kidney (375)
   b. Their epithelial lining
      (1) Height of epithelium (372, 373, 378, 379)
      (2) Presence of microvilli (372, 373, 375, 379)
      (3) Number of mitochondria (375, 378, 379)
      (4) Acidophilia (375, 378)
      (5) Basal membrane interdigitations (375, 378, 379)
      (6) Lateral membrane interdigitations (375, 378, 379)
   c. Their overall diameter (375, 378)
   d. The substances absorbed from or secreted into filtrate (382–383)

10. What is the general function of the loop of Henle (384)?

11. Compare the ascending and descending limbs of the loop of Henle in terms of:
   a. The presence of a thick portion that resembles the proximal convoluted tubule (374, 379)
   b. The presence of a thick portion that resembles the distal convoluted tubule (374, 379)
   c. The epithelial lining of the thin portions (374–375, 379)
   d. Which is freely permeable to water (384)
   e. Which is impermeable to water (384)

12. Compare cortical and juxtamedullary nephrons in terms of the:
   a. Predominant type (percentage of total) (375)

  b. Greater importance in establishing medullary hypertonicity (375)
  c. Length of their thin loops (375)
13. Compare the collecting tubules and ducts with the convoluted tubules in terms of:
  a. Their location (368, 369)
  b. Their epithelia
    (1) Variation in epithelial height (378)
    (2) Cytoplasmic staining intensity (378)
    (3) Visibility of intercellular borders (378)
14. Describe the juxtaglomerular apparatus in terms of:
  a. Its location (371, 380, 383)
  b. Its 3 named components (371, 380)
  c. The component(s) found in the wall of the afferent arteriole (371, 380)
  d. The component(s) found in the wall of the distal convoluted tubule (371, 380)
  e. The cell type responsible for the production of renin (380)
15. Trace the flow of blood from the renal arteries to the glomerular capillaries, giving, in order, the names of the arterial vessels (370, 381–383).
16. Compare the paths taken by blood leaving the cortical and the juxtamedullary glomeruli on its way to the renal vein. (***Hint:*** one path includes peritubular capillaries and stellate veins; the other includes the vasa recta (370, 381–383).
17. Compare the vasa recta with the thin loops of Henle from juxtamedullary nephrons in terms of:
  a. Their location (375, 381, 382)
  b. Their contents (381)
  c. The epithelial type and thickness (375, 379, 381–382)
  d. Which performs a countercurrent multiplier function (386)
  e. Which performs a countercurrent exchange function (387)
18. Compare aldosterone and ADH in terms of:
  a. Their sites of synthesis and secretion (387)
  b. The stimuli for their secretion (380, 387)
  c. Their sites of action in the kidney (380, 386, 387)
  d. Their role in kidney function (387–388)
19. Beginning with the stimulus for the production of renin, diagram the cascade that produces angiotensin II and explain its role in renal function (380, 381).
20. Trace the flow of fluid from the urinary (Bowman's) space to a minor calyx, naming, in order, the tubules through which it flows. Describe any changes in fluid composition (substances added or removed) and osmolarity (tonicity) that occur in each tubule segment (382–387).
21. Describe the structural features of the walls of the renal calyces, renal pelvis, ureters, and urinary bladder in terms of:
  a. The composition of the mucosa (including epithelial type and lamina propria) (387)
  b. The presence of submucosa (387)
  c. The orientation of smooth muscle fibers in the muscularis (388)
22. Name—in order from bladder to exterior—the parts of the male urethra and the epithelial type found lining each part (388–389).
23. Compare the urethras of males and females in terms of length, function, and epithelial lining (388–389).
24. Compare the internal and external urinary sphincters in terms of:
  a. Their location (389)
  b. Their muscle type and fiber orientation (389)
  c. Whether each is voluntary or involuntary (389)

Multiple-Choice Questions

For questions 19–1 through 19–5, select the single best answer.

19–1. The structure indicated by the letter A in the photomicrograph in Fig 19–2 is:
  A. The parietal layer of Bowman's capsule
  B. A macula adherens

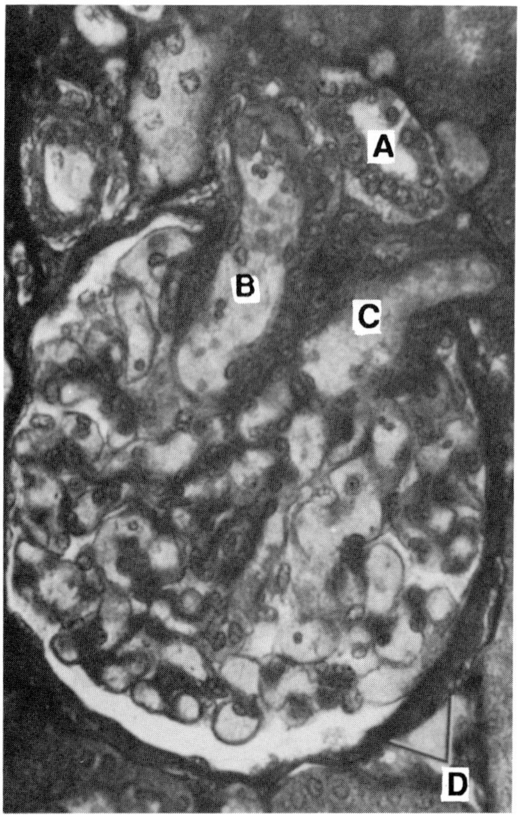

Figure 19-2.

C. A podocyte
D. A brush border
E. A macula densa

19-2. A renal lobule includes:
A. A renal pyramid and the associated cortex
B. A medullary ray and all the nephrons that empty into it
C. A renal pyramid and all the nephrons that empty into it
D. An interlobular artery and all the nephrons it supplies
E. None of the above

19-3. Blood in the arcuate arteries flows next into the:
A. Afferent arteriole(s)
B. Glomerular capillaries
C. Interlobular arteries
D. Interlobar arteries
E. Stellate veins

19-4. The type of epithelium found lining most of the urinary passages and bladder is:
A. Pseudostratified columnar
B. Simple columnar
C. Stratified squamous
D. Simple squamous
E. Transitional

19-5. Collections of cortical tissue found between the medullary pyramids are called:
A. Medullary rays
B. Renal columns of Bertin
C. Interlobular cortex
D. None of the above

MATCHING (questions 19–6 through 19–72): Each choice may be used once, more than once, or not at all.

Questions 19–6 through 19–13 use the letters in Fig 19–3.

19–6. Thick descending limb of loop of Henle
19–7. Thick ascending limb of loop of Henle
19–8. Thin limb of loop of Henle
19–9. Proximal convoluted tubule
19–10. Distal convoluted tubule
19–11. Distal convoluted tubule
19–12. Collecting tubule
19–13. Collecting duct

Questions 19–14 through 19–19 use the letters in Fig 19–4:

19–14. Primary process of podocyte
19–15. Secondary process of podocyte (pedicel)
19–16. Cell body of podocyte

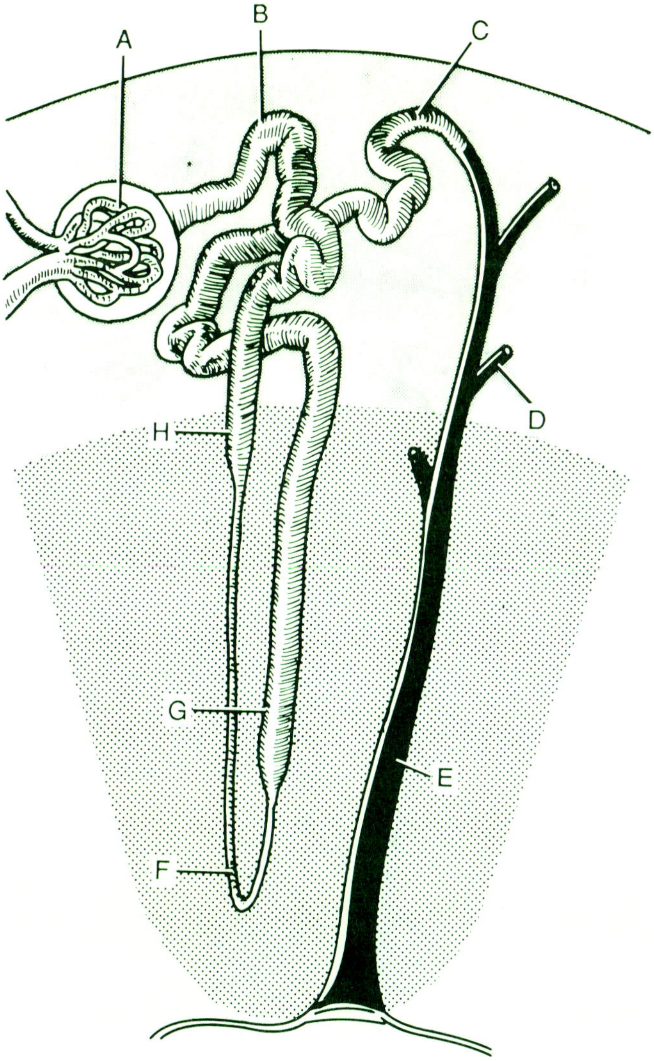

Figure 19–3.

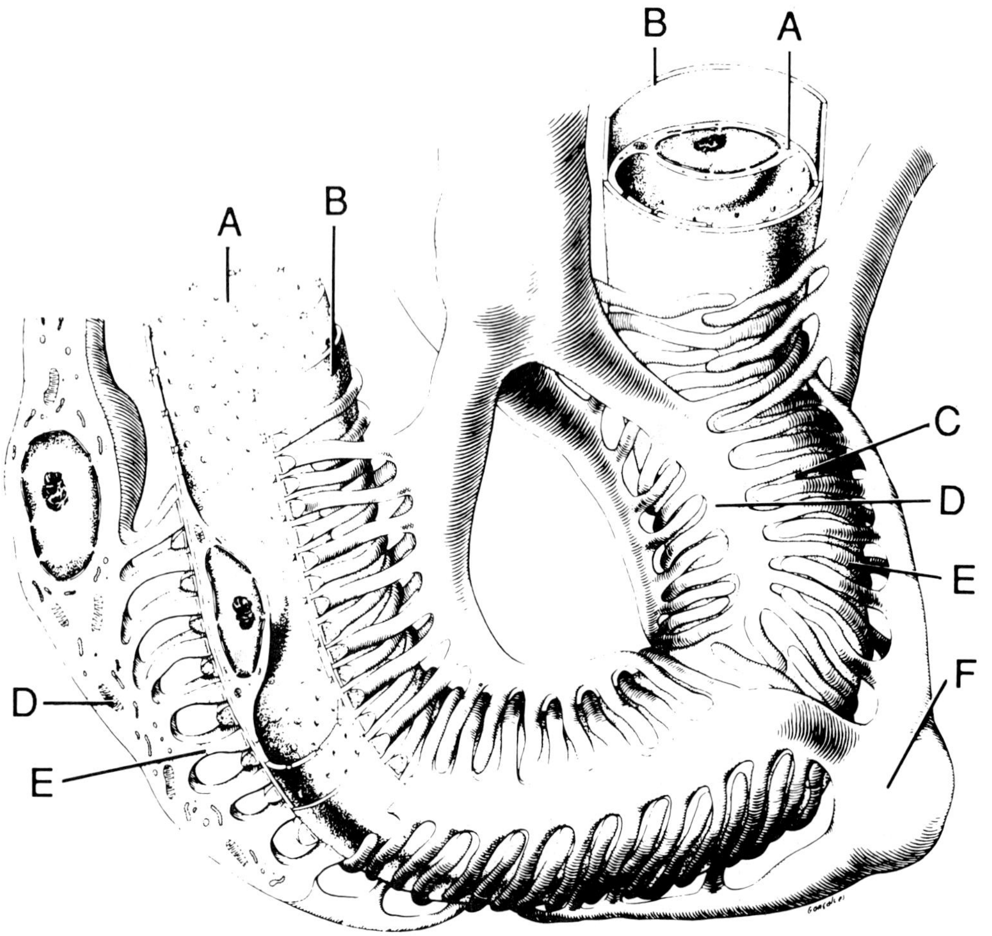

Figure 19-4.

19-17. Fused endothelium-podocyte basal lamina
19-18. Glomerular capillary endothelial cell
19-19. Filtration slit

Questions 19-20 through 19-30 use the letters in Fig 19-5:

19-20. Vascular pole
19-21. Urinary pole
19-22. Macula densa
19-23. Juxtaglomerular cells
19-24. Afferent arteriole
19-25. Efferent arteriole
19-26. Visceral layer of Bowman's capsule
19-27. Parietal layer of Bowman's capsule
19-28. Proximal convoluted tubule
19-29. Distal convoluted tubule
19-30. Microvilli

Questions 19-31 through 19-33 use the letters in Fig 19-6:

19-31. Podocyte
19-32. Mesangial cell
19-33. Glomerular capillary endothelial cell

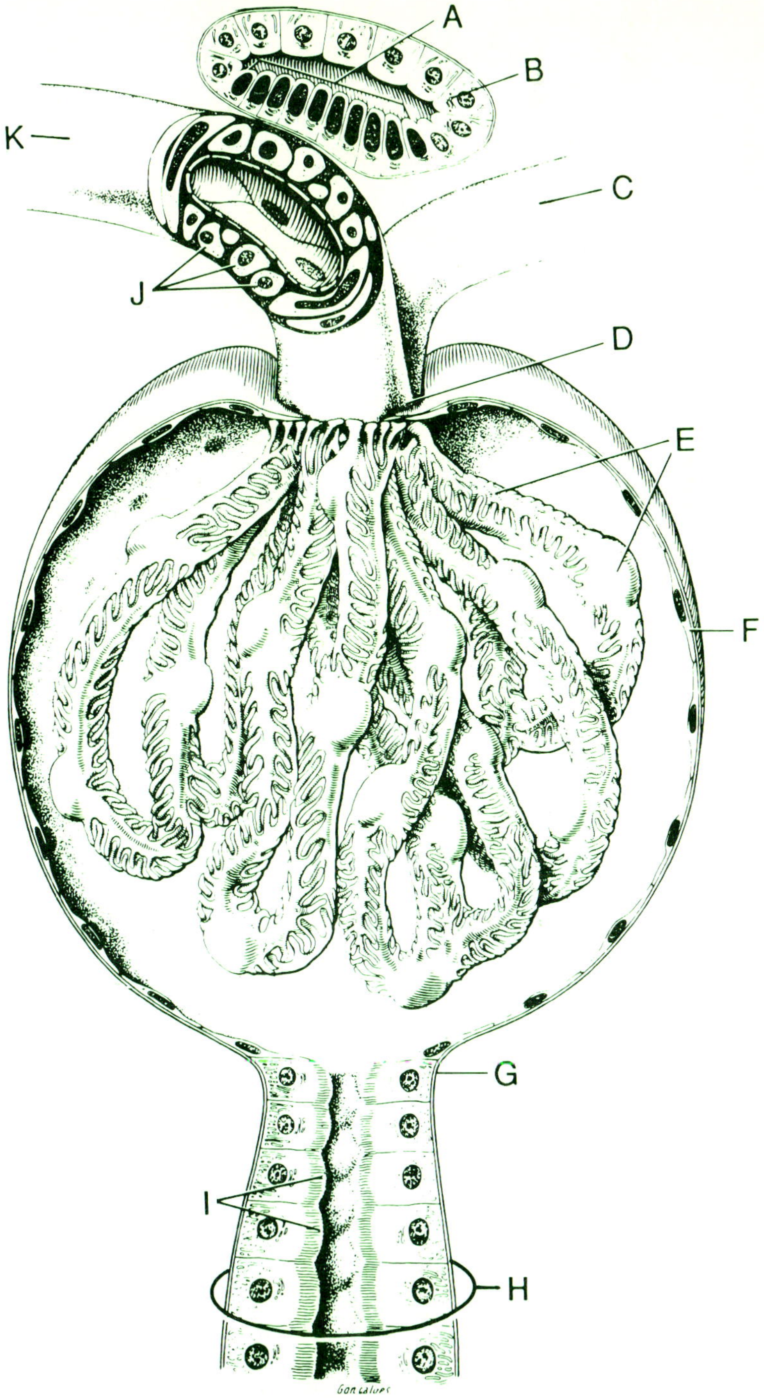

Figure 19-5.

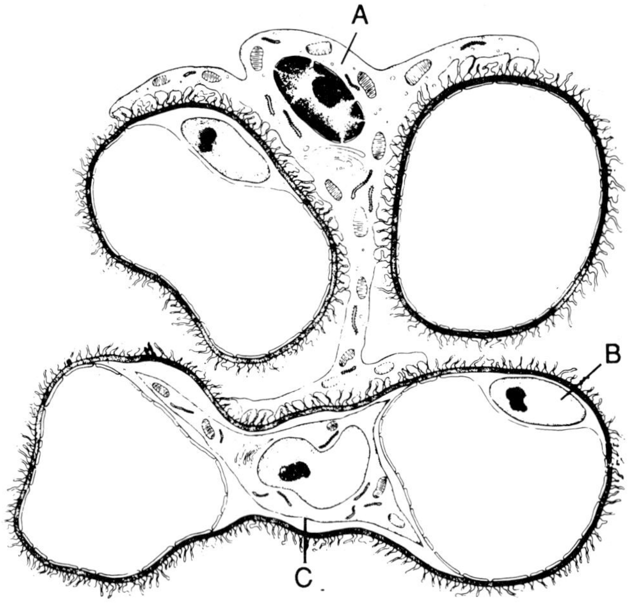

Figure 19-6.

Questions 19-34 through 19-39 use the letters in Fig 19-7:

19-34. Epithelial cell from thin loop of Henle
19-35. Epithelial cell from proximal convoluted tubule
19-36. Epithelial cell from distal convoluted tubule
19-37. Epithelial cell from collecting tubule or duct
19-38. Epithelial cell from ascending thick limb of loop of Henle
19-39. Epithelial cell from descending thick limb of loop of Henle

Questions 19-40 through 19-45:

A. Polkissen cells (extraglomerular mesangial cells)
B. Juxtaglomerular cells
C. Podocytes
D. Mesangial cells
E. All of the above

19-40. Secrete renin
19-41. Located in renal cortex
19-42. Appear to phagocytose material trapped in basil lamina of filtration barrier
19-43. Modified smooth muscle cells in wall of afferent arteriole
19-44. Form visceral layer of Bowman's capsule
19-45. Component of juxtaglomerular apparatus with unknown function

Questions 19-46 through 19-55:

A. Hypertonic
B. Hypotonic
C. Isotonic

19-46. Blood entering the glomerular capillaries
19-47. Fluid in the urinary space
19-48. Fluid in the proximal tubule
19-49. Fluid in the curve of Henle's loop

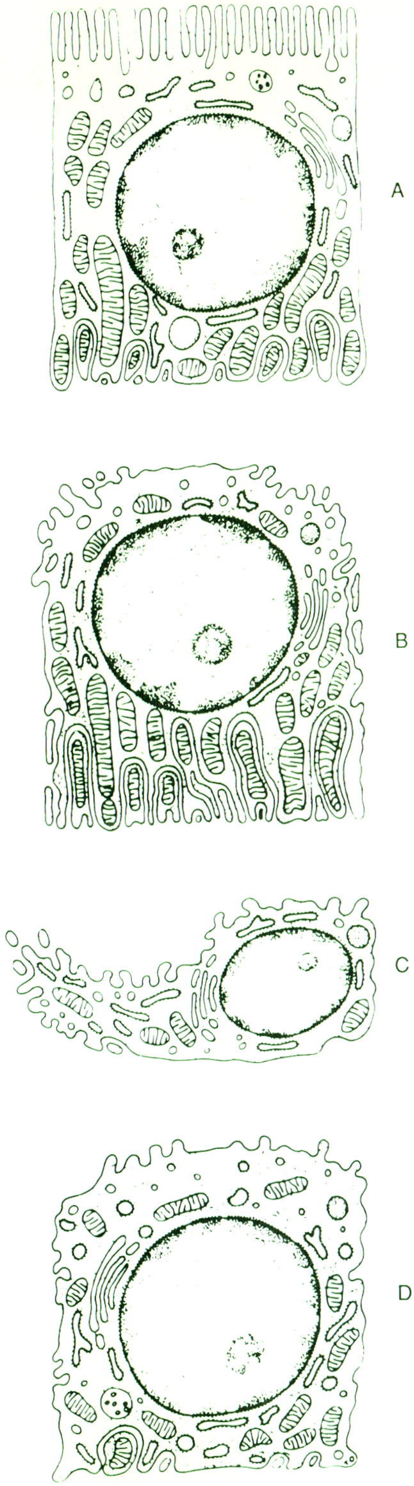

Figure 19-7.

19-50. Fluid in the curve of the vasa recta
19-51. Fluid in the ascending thick limb of Henle's loop as it leaves the medulla
19-52. Fluid in the medullary interstitium
19-53. Fluid entering the collecting tubules
19-54. Urine produced under the influence of ADH
19-55. Urine produced in the absence of ADH

Questions 19–56 through 19–72:

A. Simple squamous
B. Stratified squamous
C. Simple cuboidal
D. Simple columnar
E. Pseudostratified columnar
F. Transitional

19–56. Urinary bladder
19–57. Parietal layer of Bowman's capsule
19–58. Glomerular capillaries
19–59. Proximal tubule
19–60. Distal tubule
19–61. Thin loop of Henle
19–62. Collecting tubules
19–63. Papillary ducts
19–64. Minor calyx
19–65. Major calyx
19–66. Renal pelvis
19–67. Ureters
19–68. Prostatic urethra
19–69. Membraneous urethra
19–70. Penile (cavernous) urethra—proximal to fossa navicularis
19–71. Penile (cavernous) urethra—distal to fossa navicularis
19–72. Female urethra

For questions 19–73 through 19–124, either, both, or neither of the answers may be correct. Select

A if only A is correct
B if only B is correct
C if both A and B are correct
D if neither A nor B is correct

Questions 19–73 through 19–82:

A. Proximal tubule
B. Distal tubule
C. Both
D. Neither

19–73. Forms macula densa
19–74. Lining is similar to thin loop of Henle
19–75. Brush border
19–76. Convoluted portion lies in cortex
19–77. Actively removes sodium from filtrate
19–78. Actively removes chloride from filtrate
19–79. Removes glucose and amino acids from filtrate
19–80. Removes small proteins from filtrate by pinocytosis
19–81. Site of action of aldosterone
19–82. Lining cells are more acidophilic

Questions 19–83 through 19–97:

A. Renal cortex
B. Renal medulla
C. Both
D. Neither

19–83. Closer to capsule
19–84. Closer to renal sinus

19–85. Contains renal corpuscles
19–86. Contains papillary ducts
19–87. Location of medullary rays
19–88. Darker-staining region
19–89. Contains peritubular capillaries
19–90. Contains more vasa recta
19–91. Contains more thin loops of juxtamedullary nephrons
19–92. Contains stellate veins
19–93. Renal pyramids
19–94. Renal lobes
19–95. Renal lobules
19–96. Hypertonic interstitium
19–97. Isotonic interstitium

Questions 19–98 through 19–103:

A. Thin loop of Henle
B. Vasa recta
C. Both
D. Neither

19–98. Countercurrent exchange system
19–99. Countercurrent multiplier system
19–100. Form(s) a portion of the juxtaglomerular apparatus
19–101. Ascending portion impermeable to water
19–102. Lined by simple squamous epithelium
19–103. Permeability to water determined by presence or absence of antidiuretic hormone (ADH)

Questions 19–104 through 19–109:

A. Aldosterone
B. ADH
C. Both
D. Neither

19–104. Enzyme that cleaves angiotensinogen
19–105. Released from neurohypophysis (posterior pituitary)
19–106. Synthesized by the adrenal cortex
19–107. Synthesis stimulated by angiotensin II
19–108. Increases permeability of medullary collecting ducts to water
19–109. Stimulates chloride and sodium reabsorption by distal tubule

Questions 19–110 through 19–116:

A. Cortical nephrons
B. Juxtamedullary nephrons
C. Both
D. Neither

19–110. Associated efferent arterioles supply vasa recta
19–111. Associated efferent arterioles supply peritubular capillaries
19–112. More numerous
19–113. Long thin loops of Henle extending deep into medulla
19–114. Have shorter thick descending limbs of loop of Henle
19–115. Have proximal convoluted tubules located in cortex
19–116. Primarily responsible for establishing osmotic gradient in renal medulla

Questions 19–117 through 19–124:

A. Internal urinary sphincter
B. External urinary sphincter

C. Both
D. Neither

19–117. Surrounds membranous urethra
19–118. Surrounds bladder neck
19–119. Surrounds female urethra midway along its length
19–120. Smooth muscle
19–121. Skeletal muscle
19–122. Portion of urogenital diaphragm
19–123. Voluntary
19–124. Involuntary

For questions 19–125 through 19–127, one, more than one, or all of the answers may be correct. Select

A if only (1), (2), and (3) are correct
B if only (1) and (3) are correct
C if only (2) and (4) are correct
D if only (4) is correct
E if all answers are correct

19–125. Structural features of the epithelial cells lining the collecting ducts and tubules include:
(1) Weak-staining cytoplasm
(2) Numerous apical microvilli
(3) Distinct intercellular borders
(4) Extensive basal membrane invaginations interdigitating with numerous mitochondria

19–126. Structures found along the border between the renal cortex and medulla include the:
(1) Interlobular arteries and veins
(2) Medullary rays
(3) Interlobar arteries and veins
(4) Arcuate arteries and veins

19–127. The juxtaglomerular apparatus includes:
(1) Macula densa
(2) Polkissen cells
(3) Juxtaglomerular cells
(4) Podocytes

20 Pituitary & Hypothalamus

Objectives

This chapter should help the student to:

- Describe the location of the pituitary.
- Describe the embryonic origins of the pituitary.
- Name the divisions of the pituitary.
- Name the cell types found in each division of the pituitary and indicate any characteristic staining properties.

- List the hormones produced by the pituitary, indicating for each one the division and cell type responsible for its production as well as its target site.
- Describe the role of the hypothalamus in controlling pituitary function.
- Describe the blood supply to the pituitary and its role in pituitary function.
- Explain the role of negative feedback in controlling pituitary function.
- Distinguish between the neurohypophysis and the adenohypophysis and identify the cell types present in a slide or photomicrograph of the pituitary. Also locate and identify the pars anterior, pars tuberalis, pars intermedia, pars nervosa, infundibulum, Rathke's cysts, and the sinusoidal capillaries.

Synopsis

I. GENERAL FEATURES OF THE ENDOCRINE SYSTEM

A. Components of the System: The endocrine system includes several endocrine organs (eg, adenohypophysis, thyroid gland, adrenal gland), islands of endocrine tissue in exocrine glands (eg, islets of Langerhans), and some isolated endocrine cells (eg, cells with DNES functions in the mucosa of the digestive tract).

B. Origin: Endocrine glands are ductless glands that develop as invaginations of epithelial surfaces, such as oral ectoderm or gut endoderm, and eventually pinch off, losing contact with the parent epithelium.

C. Microscopic Structure: Endocrine glands typically contain numerous secretory cells arranged as cords, clumps, or hollow follicles that are in direct contact with capillaries or sinusoids.

D. Secretions: Endocrine cells release their secretions—typically hormones—into the bloodstream. Other products that are released into the bloodstream instead of into ducts (eg, enzymes, serum albumin), however, are also sometimes considered endocrine secretions. Hormones are molecules with specific regulatory effects on a particular target cell, tissue, or organ that is often located at a distance from the gland. Hormones can elicit specific and dramatic effects at very low concentrations, and they directly or indirectly affect all tissues; many are essential to the preservation of the internal steady-state environment. They play a crucial role in regulating the metabolism of carbohydrates, proteins, and lipids; the mineral and water balance in body fluids; growth; sex-related differences in body shape and sexual function; and (to some extent) behavior, temperament, and emotions.

1. Peptide hormones These proteins, glycoproteins, or short peptides bind to specific receptors on the target cell surface. They often stimulate the production of intracellular second messengers, such as cyclic AMP in the target cells.

2. Steroid hormones These lipid-soluble hormones easily cross the target cell's plasma membranes and thus directly affect cell function. They bind to specific binding proteins in the cytoplasm that transport them to other sites, including the nucleus, within the cell.

E. Neuroendocrine System: The complex, interrelated functions of the human body's cells, tissues, and organs are controlled and coordinated by 2 overlapping systems: the nervous system (discussed in Chapter 9) and the endocrine system (discussed here and in Chapters 21–23). Increasingly, these are considered parts of a single neuroendocrine system. Once called the master gland for its ability to control secretion by other glands, the **pituitary (hypophysis)** is now seen more as a focal connection between the endocrine and nervous systems. The secretory activities of its 2 parts, the adenohypophysis and the neurohypophysis, are both controlled by a nearby part of the brain, the **hypothalamus.** Hypothalamic activity is controlled by neural connections with other parts of the nervous system and by negative feedback from the hormones produced by the pituitary's target cells. Pituitary-related diseases present primarily as the effects of hypersecretion or hyposecretion of pituitary hormones; they may be caused by lesions of the pituitary, its target organs, or the hypothalamus.

II. GENERAL ORGANIZATION & EMBRYONIC ORIGINS OF THE PITUITARY.

The pituitary gland has 2 major divisions, the anterior adenohypophysis and the posterior neurohypophysis, that differ in embryonic origin as well as structure and function (Table 20–1).

A. Adenohypophysis:

1. Origin The adenohypophysis arises as an upward evagination of the ectoderm lining the primitive oral cavity. It contacts and fuses with the neurohypophyseal downgrowth.

2. General structure The adenohypophysis is composed of cords of glandular epithelial cells that are separated by the numerous sinusoidal capillaries of the secondary capillary plexus. It is not directly innervated by hypothalamic nerves.

3. Subdivisions The **pars distalis (pars anterior)** is the largest subdivision of the pituitary. The **pars tuberalis,** the superior extension of the pars distalis, forms a partial sleeve around the infundibulum of the neurohypophysis. The **pars intermedia** is a narrow band of adenohypophyseal tissue that borders the neurohypophysis. These divisions and their functions are discussed in detail in section III.

B. Neurohypophysis:

1. Origin The neurohypophysis arises as a downgrowth of the neural ectoderm of the hypothalamus and is therefore actually a part of the brain.

2. General structure The neurohypophysis contains abundant axons whose cell bodies are located mainly in the supraoptic and paraventricular nuclei of the hypothalamus.

3. Subdivisions The **infundibulum** consists of the **infundibular stem (neural stalk)** and the **median eminence.** The stem carries axons from the hypothalamus to the pars nervosa and contains the capillary loops of the primary capillary plexus. The median eminence of the **tuber cinereum** forms the floor of the hypothalamus. The **pars nervosa (infundibular process)** is the expanded lobe of the neurohypophysis; it contains axon terminals and numerous capillaries.

III. ADENOHYPOPHYSIS.

Each secretory cell in the adenohypophysis synthesizes and stores one of the following hormones: follicle-stimulating hormone (FSH), thyrotropin (thyroid-stimulating hormone; TSH), luteinizing hormone (LH), adrenocorticotropic hormone (ACTH), growth hormone (GH), and prolactin. The release of these hormones, which control the secretory activities of a variety of other glands, is regulated by specific releasing or inhibiting hormones that are produced by the hypothalamus and delivered to the adenohypophysis by the blood in the hypophyseal portal system.

A. Pars Distalis:

1. Chromophobes Because these cells stain poorly, they appear clear or white in tissue sections. Together, the 3 subpopulations of chromophobes make up about 50% of the epithelial cells in the pars anterior. They include:

a. The undifferentiated nonsecretory cells, which may be stem cells;

b. The partly degranulated chromophilic cells, which contain sparse granules; and

Table 20-1. Source, Target, and Effect of the Major Pituitary Hormones

Pituitary Source						
Region	**Cell Type**		**Hormone**	**Primary Target(s)**	**Direct Effects**	**Secondary Targets and Indirect Effects**
Pars distalis and tuberalis	Acidophils	Somatotropes	Growth, hormone (GH), somatotropic hormone (STH), somatotropin.	Liver.	Increases somatomedin secretion.	Stimulate most cells (especially epiphyseal chondrocytes) to increase growth rate; cause increased breakdown, & decreased synthesis of triglycerides in adipocytes and other cells; increase blood glucose and fatty acid; increase somatostatin secretion by hypothalamus and decreases GHRH levels
				Epiphyseal cartilage		
		Mammotropes	Prolactin, lactogenic hormone, luteotropic hormone (LTH).	Mammary gland.	Stimulate milk secretion.	Increase dopamine secretion by hypothalamus, inhibiting prolactin secretion; decrease prolactin-releasing factor (PRF) secretion.
				Brain.	Increase maternal behavior.	
				Corpus luteum.	Maintain progesterone secretion.	
	Basophils	Gonadotropes	Follicle-stimulating hormone (FSH).	Ovarian follicles.	Promotes follicle development.	Inhibits secretion of gonadotropin-releasing hormone (GnRH) by hypothalamic neurons.
				Seminiferous tubules.	Stimulates spermatogenesis.	
			Luteinizing hormone (LH), interstitial cell stimulating hormone (ICSH).	Ovarian follicles.	Stimulate follicle maturation, ovulation.	
				Corpus luteum.	Stimulate development, progesterone secretion.	
				Interstitial cells of testis.	Maintain cells, stimulate testosterone secretion.	
		Corticotropes	Adrenocorticotropic hormone (ACTH), corticotropin.	Zona fasciculata of adrenal cortex.	Stimulate synthesis and secretion of glucocorticoids.	Stimulate aldosterone production by zona glomerulosa of adrenal cortex; inhibit secretion of corticotropin-releasing hormone (CRH) by hypothalamic neurons.
				Zona reticularis of adrenal cortex.	Stimulate synthesis and secretion of adrenal androgens.	
		Thyrotropes	Thyroid-stimulating hormone (TSH).	Thyroid follicular cells.	Stimulates synthesis and release of thyroxine (T_4) and triiodothyronine (T_3).	Increases metabolic rate in most cells; inhibits production of TSH by pituitary thyrotropes.
Pars intermedia	Basophilic cells	Melanotropes	Melanocyte-stimulating hormone (MSH).	Melanocytes.	Increase melanin production, darkens existing melanin.	

Table 20-1. Source, Target, and Effect of the Major Pituitary Hormones

Pituitary Source		Hormone	Primary Target(s)	Direct Effects	Secondary Targets and Indirect Effects
Region	**Cell Type**				
Pars nervosa	Hypothalamic neuron cell bodies (primarily in the supraoptic nuculeus)	Antidiuretic hormone (ADH), or arginine vasopressin.	Collecting ducts of kidneys.	Absorption of water, production of hypertonic urine.	Increase or maintain blood volume, decrease salinity and solute concentration in blood; increase blood pressure.
			Vascular smooth muscle.	Vasoconstriction.	
	Hypothalamic neuron cell bodies (in both supraoptic and paraventricular nuclei)	Oxytocin.	Myoepithelial cells of mammary gland.	Cell contraction.	Milk ejection.
			Uterine smooth, muscle.	Cell contraction.	Induction of labor.

c. The follicular cells, the predominant chromophobe type, which form a stromal network that supports the other cells (chromophils). These stellate cells may have some phagocytic functions.

2. Chromophils Chromophils, the hormone-secreting cells of the adenohypophysis, stain intensely because of the abundant cytoplasmic secretory granules in which their hormones are stored. There is a specific cell type for each hormone. Usually larger than chromophobes, chromophils are subdivided into 2 classes:

a. Acidophils While these cells stain intensely with eosin and orange G, they do not stain with PAS. More abundant in the periphery of the gland, they are usually smaller than basophils and their granules are larger and more numerous. The acidophils include 2 major types of hormone-secreting cells: **Somatotropic cells,** which produce **growth hormone (GH, somatotropin),** and **mammotropic cells,** which produce **prolactin.** (A simple mnemonic device for remembering the hormones secreted by acidophils is *GPA*—*g*rowth hormone, *p*rolactin, *a*cidophils.)

b. Basophils These cells, which stain with hematoxylin and other basic dyes, are PAS-positive. More abundant in the core of the gland, they are usually larger than acidophils, with fewer and smaller granules. The 3 major types of hormone-producing basophils produce 4 major hormones. (A mnemonic for the hormones produced by basophils is *B-FLAT*—*B*asophils, *F*SH, *L*H, *A*CTH, *T*SH.)

(1) Each of the 2 types of **gonadotropic cells** produces a different gonadotropin. One produces **follicle-stimulating hormone (FSH);** the other produces **luteinizing hormone (LH;** called **interstitial cell-stimulating hormone [ICSH]** in males).

(2) Corticotropic cells produce **adrenocorticotropin (ACTH).**

(3) Thyrotropic cells produce **thyrotropin (thyroid-stimulating hormone, TSH).**

B. Pars Tuberalis: This is the funnel-shaped superior extension of the pars distalis that surrounds the infundibular stem. Its histologic features are similar to those of the pars distalis, but it contains mostly gonadotropes. The pars tuberalis contains many capillaries of the primary capillary plexus of the hypophyseal portal system.

C. Pars Intermedia: This is a band or wedge of adenohypophysis between the pars distalis and pars nervosa; it is rudimentary in humans. It contains **Rathke's cysts.** Small, irregular, colloid-containing cavities lined with cuboidal epithelium, these cysts are the remnants of Rathke's pouch. It also contains scattered clumps and cords of basophilic cells, or melanotropes, which secrete melanocyte-stimulating hormone (β-MSH).

D. Blood Supply and Hypophyseal Portal System:

1. Primary capillary plexus This profusion of capillaries is found in the upper infundibular stalk and lower median eminence; it extends into the pars tuberalis. The plexus receives blood from the anterior and posterior superior hypophyseal arteries (from the circle of Willis) and drains into the hypophyseal portal veins.

2. Hypophyseal portal veins These small veins and venules are located mainly in the middle and lower infundibular stalk and in portions of the pars tuberalis. They receive blood from the primary capillary plexus and carry it directly to the secondary capillary plexus in the pars distalis. Vessels carrying blood directly from one capillary plexus to another without returning to the general circulation are defined as portal vessels.

3. Secondary capillary plexus This rich capillary plexus located throughout the pars distalis also penetrates the pars tuberalis and pars intermedia. There are also some connections between this capillary bed and that in the pars nervosa. The capillaries between the clumps and cords of cells in the pars distalis belong to this plexus, which receives venous blood directly from the hypophyseal portal veins and arterial blood from the anterior inferior hypophyseal arteries. It is drained by the inferior hypophyseal veins into the internal jugulars.

E. Hypothalamic Releasing and Inhibiting Hormones: These small peptides are synthesized in the neuron (neurosecretory) cell bodies in the hypothalamic nuclei and are released by their axon terminals into the primary capillary plexus. They pass through the hypophyseal portal venules and into the secondary capillary plexus, from which they diffuse into the adenohypophysis to stimulate or inhibit the release of hormones by the acidophils and basophils.

1. Releasing hormones

a. Corticotropin-releasing hormone (CRH) is a 41-amino-acid peptide synthesized in the paraventricular nucleus; it stimulates the corticotropic cells to release ACTH.

b. Gonadotropin-releasing hormone (GnRH), a 10-amino-acid peptide synthesized in the preoptic and arcuate nuclei, stimulates the gonadotropic cells to release FSH and LH.

c. Thyrotropin-releasing hormone (TRH) is a 3-amino-acid peptide that stimulates the thyrotropic cells to release TSH (thyrotropin).

2. Inhibiting hormones

a. Somatostatin (GHIH [growth hormone-inhibiting hormone]) is a 14-amino-acid peptide synthesized in the suprachiasmatic nuclei that inhibits the somatotropic cells from releasing growth hormone (GH, somatotropin). It is also known to inhibit the secretion of glucagon, insulin, and other hormones associated with the gastrointestinal tract.

b. Dopamine (a prolactin-inhibiting hormone [PIH]), is a neurotransmitter synthesized in the arcuate nuclei that inhibits the mammotropic cells from releasing prolactin.

F. Summary of Adenohypophyseal Hormone Production:

1. Neurons of the hypothalamic nuclei synthesize releasing or inhibiting hormones and package them in neurosecretory vesicles.

2. The neurons transport the vesicles down axons in the **tuberoinfundibular** and **hypothalamohypophyseal tracts** to the axon terminals that surround the capillaries of the primary plexus.

3. Neural stimulation or hormonal feedback from the target organs of the adenohypophysis causes these nerves to fire an action potential that releases the appropriate releasing or inhibiting hormone from the axon terminals.

4. The releasing or inhibiting hormone then enters the primary capillary plexus and flows through the hypophyseal portal veins to the secondary capillary plexus.

5. There, the hormone diffuses out of the capillary lumen via the fenestrae and stimulates or inhibits the release of stored adenohypophyseal hormones from the acidophils or basophils.

6. The adenohypophyseal hormones enter the capillaries of the secondary plexus; they leave the adenohypophysis through the anterior inferior hypophyseal veins to enter the general circulation.

IV. NEUROHYPOPHYSIS.

The subdivisions of the neurohypophysis (outlined in II.B.3) all exhibit a similar microscopic structure. For the sake of brevity, the pars nervosa can be used in this discussion to represent the neurohypophysis. The neurohypophysis has 3 major structural components:

A. Axons of Neurosecretory Cells:

The neurohypophysis contains many unmyelinated axons whose cell bodies (soma) are located mainly in the **supraoptic and paraventricular nuclei** of the hypothalamus. Axons passing from these nuclei to the pars nervosa are together termed the hypothalamohypophyseal tract. The axons contain neurosecretory granules and exhibit large granule-filled dilations called **Herring bodies.** The neurosecretory materials in these granules, synthesized and packaged in the above-mentioned cell bodies, include the following products:

1. Neurohypophyseal hormones The hypothalamic neurons that terminate in the neurohypophysis release oxytocin and antidiuretic hormone around the capillaries in this part of the pituitary.

a. Oxytocin is a 9-amino-acid peptide synthesized mainly by cells of the paraventricular nucleus. It stimulates milk ejection by the mammary glands and stimulates the contraction of uterine smooth muscle during copulation and childbirth.

b. Antidiuretic hormone (ADH, arginine vasopressin) is a 9-amino-acid peptide synthesized mainly by cells in the supraoptic nucleus. It stimulates water resorption by the renal medullary collecting ducts (see Chapter 19) and contraction of vascular smooth muscle.

2. Neurophysin is a binding protein that complexes with neurohypophyseal hormones.

3. ATP (adenosine triphosphate). See Chapter 3 for a discussion.

B. Fenestrated Capillary Plexus:

Surrounding the axon terminals in the pars nervosa, these capillaries pick up the neurosecretory products and convey them to the general circulation.

C. Pituicytes:

These are highly branched glial cells whose processes surround and support the unmyelinated axons.

D. Summary of Neurohypophyseal Hormone Production:

1. Neurons of the supraoptic and paraventricular nuclei of the hypothalamus synthesize ADH and oxytocin, respectively.

2. The neurons package these hormones with neurophysin and ATP in neurosecretory vesicles.

3. The vesicles are transported by the neurons down axons in the hypothalamohypophyseal tracts to axon terminals among the capillaries of the pars nervosa.

4. Upon appropriate stimulation, these neurosecretory cells propagate an action potential along their axons, causing exocytosis of the vesicle contents at the axon terminals.

5. The released hormones enter the capillaries of the pars nervosa and leave the pituitary to enter the general circulation via the posterior inferior hypophyseal veins.

Study-Focusing Questions*

1. Describe the characteristics of an endocrine gland in terms of its:
  a. Embryonic origin (75, 76)
  b. Typical arrangement of secretory cells (76)
  c. Abundance of blood capillaries (76)
  d. Mode of release and transport of secretions (75, 390)
  e. Typical secretory product (390)

2. Describe hormones in terms of:
  a. The 2 basic types (chemical composition) (80)
  b. The relative distance and route taken between the secretory cell and the target site (80, 390)
  c. The relative amount needed to elicit a response from the target cell
  d. Their general function (390)

3. Describe the location of the pituitary (hypophysis) and its position with respect to the hypothalamus, sella turcica, and optic chiasm (390).

4. Name the 2 major divisions of the pituitary and compare them in terms of:
  a. Their embryonic origin (390, 391)
  b. Their basic microscopic structure (391, 398)
  c. Their connections with the hypothalamus (vascular versus neural) (396, 398)
  d. The major hormones released by each (393, 394, 397, 399)

5. Sketch the adult pituitary and hypothalamus and label the following (392–393):
  a. Adenohypophysis
  b. Neurohypophysis
  c. Hypothalamus
  d. Anterior lobe
  e. Posterior lobe
  f. Optic chiasm
  g. Pars distalis
  h. Pars tuberalis
  i. Pars intermedia
  j. Rathke's cysts
  k. Median eminence
  l. Infundibulum
  m. Pars nervosa
  n. Supraoptic nucleus
  o. Paraventricular nucleus
  p. Primary capillary plexus
  q. Secondary capillary plexus
  r. Hypophyseal portal veins

6. Name the 3 major parts of the adenohypophysis (390).

7. Name the 3 major types of parenchymal cells in the adenohypophysis, based on their staining properties, and give their approximate percentages (391–392).

8. Compare pituitary acidophils and basophils in terms of:
  a. Their staining properties–
    (1) Their affinity for acidic dyes such as eosin and orange G (392)
    (2) Their affinity for basic dyes such as hematoxylin and aniline blue (392)
    (3) With the PAS reaction (392)
  b. The hormones they secrete (393–395)

*The page references in this section refer to *Basic Histology,* 6th ed., Junqueira L, Carneiro J, Kelley R (editors), Appleton & Lange, 1989. **HR** (for Histology Review) is occasionally used instead of a page reference to indicate that the information referred to can be found in this book.

9. Name the primary target organs of (and their response to) the following hormones (394–397):
   a. FSH
   b. LH
   c. ICSH
   d. TSH
   e. Growth hormone
   f. Prolactin
   g. ACTH
10. Beginning with neural stimulation of the hypothalamus, trace the events leading to the secretion of the thyroid hormones T_3 and T_4 by the thyroid gland. Name, in order, the neural, endocrine, and vascular components involved (393, 398).
11. Name the major portions of the neurohypophysis (390).
12. Where are the cell bodies of the abundant unmyelinated axons of the pars nervosa found (398)?
13. Describe Herring bodies in terms of their contents and location (399).
14. List the contents of the neurosecretory vesicles in the axons of the pars nervosa (399).
15. Describe pituicytes in terms of structure and function (399).
16. Name the 2 major hormones released by the neurohypophysis, their target organs, and the effects they elicit (399).

Multiple-Choice Questions

For questions 20–1 and 20–2, select the single best answer.

20–1. All the following are true of endocrine glands *except* that they:
- **A.** May contain numerous secretory cells arranged as cords, clumps, or follicles
- **B.** Generally arise from epithelial surfaces during embryonic development
- **C.** Are typically highly vascular with abundant capillaries and sinusoids
- **D.** Have ducts that empty into connective tissues rather than onto epithelial surfaces
- **E.** Typically synthesize and secrete hormones

20–2. The portion of the pituitary indicated by the letter B in the photomicrograph shown in Fig 20–1 is the:
- **A.** Pars tuberalis
- **B.** Pars distalis
- **C.** Pars intermedia
- **D.** Pars nervosa
- **E.** Infundibulum

MATCHING (questions 20–3 through 20–30): Each choice may be used once, more than once, or not at all.

Questions 20–3 through 20–17 (more than one answer may be correct):

- **A.** ADH
- **B.** B-MSH
- **C.** CRH
- **D.** Dopamine
- **E.** Somatotropin
- **F.** FSH
- **G.** GnRH
- **H.** ACTH
- **I.** TSH
- **J.** Somatostatin
- **K.** Prolactin

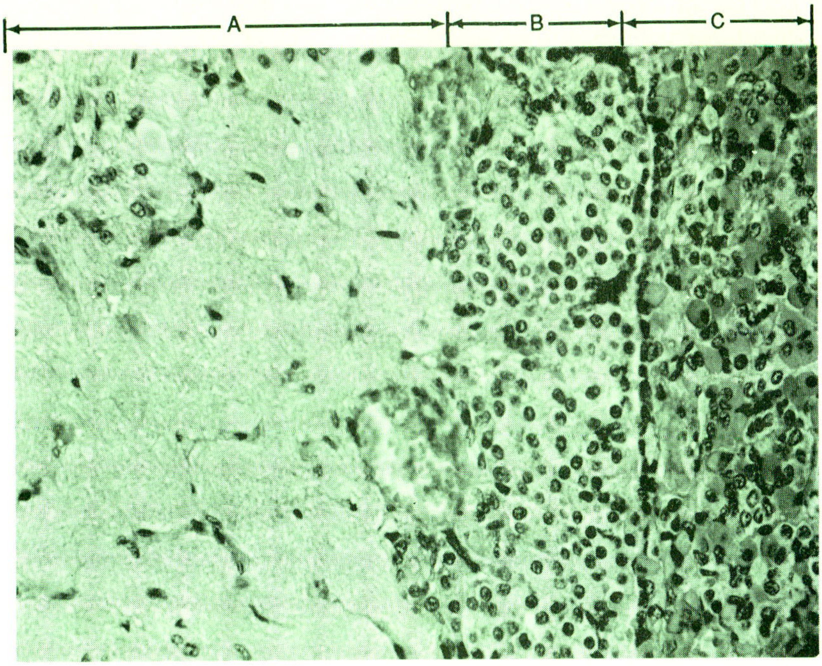

Figure 20-1.

L. LH/ICSH
M. TRH
N. Oxytocin
O. None of the above

20-3. Produced by cells whose cell bodies lie in the hypothalamic nuclei
20-4. Gonadotropins
20-5. Target is the renal collecting tubules
20-6. Targets include the myoepithelial cells of the mammary glands and uterine smooth muscle
20-7. Target is the adrenal cortex
20-8. Target is the secretory cells of the mammary glands
20-9. Secreted by the liver and kidneys
20-10. Carried to the target(s) by the hypophyseal portal system
20-11. Targets include both ovaries and testes
20-12. Acts directly on the thyroid gland
20-13. Inhibits prolactin synthesis
20-14. Target cells found in the adenohypophysis
20-15. Produced primarily in the supraoptic nucleus
20-16. Produced primarily in the paraventricular nucleus

Questions 20-17 through 20-34 use the letters in Fig 20-2.

20-17. Tuberoinfundibular tract
20-18. Rathke's cysts
20-19. Median eminence
20-20. Anterior lobe
20-21. Pars distalis
20-22. Pars nervosa
20-23. Pars intermedia
20-24. Hypothalamohypophyseal tract
20-25. Pars tuberalis

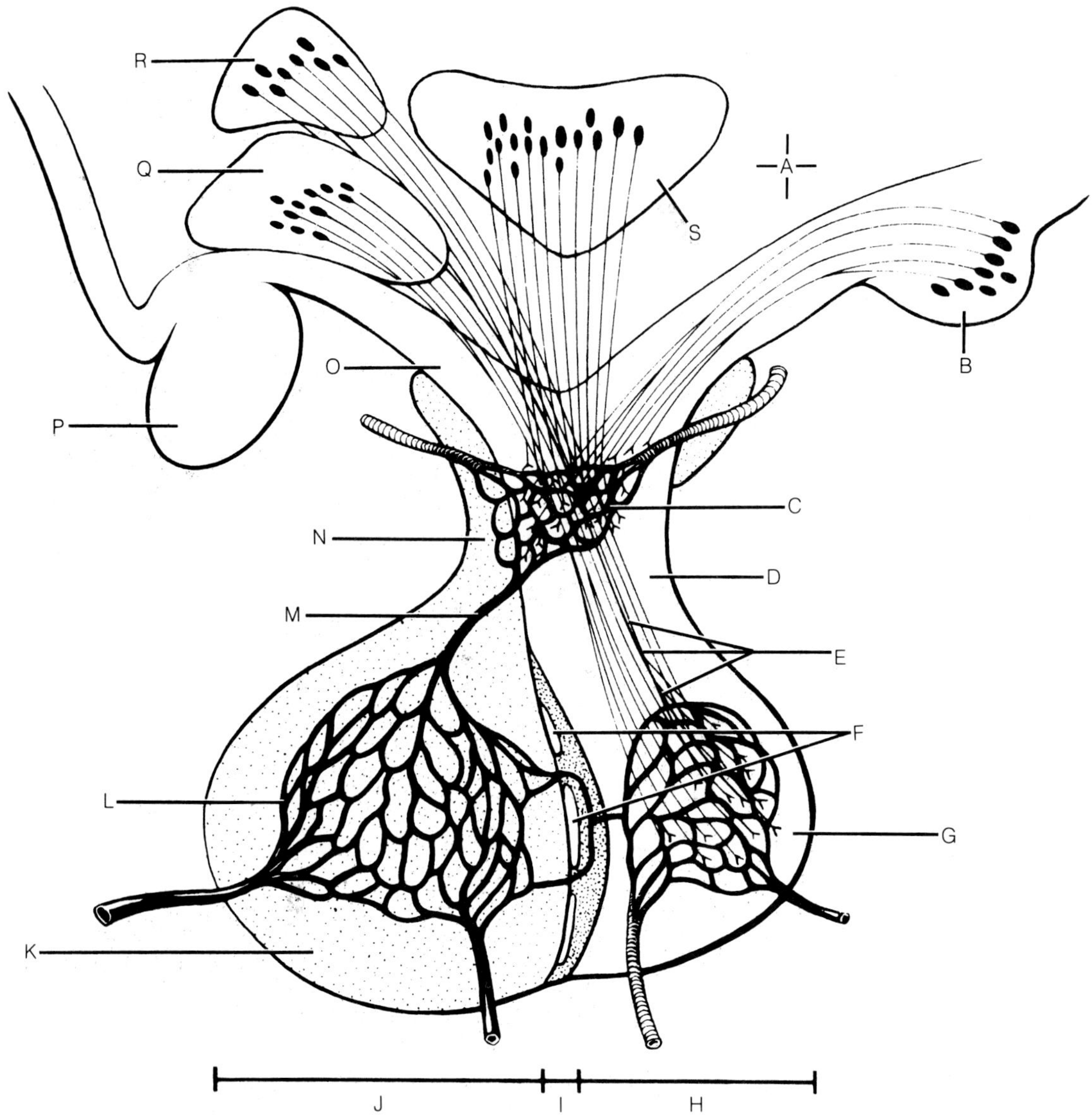

Figure 20-2.

20–26. Hypothalamic area
20–27. Infundibulum
20–28. Optic chiasm
20–29. Supraoptic nucleus
20–30. Paraventricular nucleus
20–31. Primary capillary plexus
20–32. Secondary capillary plexus
20–33. Hypophyseal portal vein
20–34. Posterior lobe

For questions 20–35 through 20–60, either, both, or neither of the answers may be correct. Select

A if only A is correct
B if only B is correct
C if both A and B are correct
D if neither A nor B is correct

Questions 20-35 through 20-45:

A. Acidophils
B. Basophils
C. Both
D. Neither

20-35. Stain with PAS technique
20-36. Secrete gonadotropins
20-37. Secrete prolactin
20-38. Secrete glycoproteins
20-39. Secrete somatotropin
20-40. Secrete somatomedin
20-41. Secrete ADH
20-42. Secrete ICSH
20-43. Secrete dopamine
20-44. Secrete ACTH
20-45. Secrete GnRH

Questions 20-46 through 20-60:

A. Adenohypophysis
B. Neurohypophysis
C. Both
D. Neither

20-46. Derived from oral ectoderm
20-47. Hormone production regulated by hypothalamus
20-48. Darker staining with standard techniques (eg, H&E)
20-49. Include(s) pars distalis
20-50. Include(s) pars tuberalis
20-51. Include(s) pars nervosa
20-52. Contain(s) chromophobes
20-53. Contain(s) chromophils
20-54. Contain(s) pituicytes
20-55. Contain(s) Herring bodies
20-56. Hormone production regulated by specific releasing and inhibiting factors
20-57. Hypothalamic influence mediated by hypophyseal portal system
20-58. Produces oxytocin
20-59. Innervated directly by axons of hypothalamic neurons
20-60. Innervated only by autonomic fibers of the carotid plexus

For questions 20-61 through 20-63, one, more than one, or all of the answers may be correct. Select

A if only (1), (2), and (3) are correct
B if only (1) and (3) are correct
C if only (2) and (4) are correct
D if only (4) is correct
E if all answers are correct

20-61. Hormones:
(1) Have specific regulatory effects on target cells
(2) Are produced by endocrine secretory cells
(3) Have significant effects at low concentrations
(4) Can function only very close to their site of secretion

20–62. The hypophyseal portal system:
(1) Includes the primary capillary plexus
(2) Carries releasing factors to the pars distalis
(3) Includes the secondary capillary plexus
(4) Picks up pituitary hormones and delivers them to the general circulation

20–63. Releasing and inhibiting hormones:
(1) Are produced only in the supraoptic and paraventricular nuclei
(2) Are released by axon terminals located near the primary capillary plexus
(3) Stimulate the synthesis and secretion of ADH and oxytocin
(4) May be small peptides composed of fewer than 50 amino acids.

21 Adrenals, Islets of Langerhans, Thyroid, Parathyroids, & Pineal Body

Objectives

This chapter should help the student to:

- Describe the location of the adrenal glands.
- Distinguish between the cortex and medulla of the adrenals in terms of their histologic structure, function, location, and embryonic origin.
- Describe the blood supply to the adrenals.
- Distinguish the 3 layers of the adrenal cortex in terms of each layer's histologic structure, the hormones secreted, and the layer's location.
- Compare the adult and fetal (provisional) adrenal cortices.
- Describe the roles of the pituitary, hypothalamus, and kidney in regulating adrenocortical hormone secretion.
- Describe the functional relationship between the adrenal medulla and the nervous system.
- Describe the role of adrenocortical hormones in regulating adrenomedullary function.
- Identify the capsule, cortex, zona glomerulosa, zona fasciculata, zona reticularis, medulla, chromaffin cells, and ganglion cells in a slide or photomicrograph of a section of the adrenal gland.
- Describe the size, staining properties, and distribution of the islets of Langerhans in the pancreas.
- Distinguish between the A (alpha), B (beta), D (delta), and F (PP) cells of the islets of Langerhans in terms of the hormones they secrete, their location in the islets, their relative numbers, the appearance of their granules, and any special staining properties.
- Describe the blood supply and innervation of the islets of Langerhans.
- Describe the role of the cells of the islets of Langerhans in regulating blood glucose levels.
- Identify the islets of Langerhans in a slide or photomicrograph of a section of the pancreas.
- Describe the location, shape, and embryonic origin of the thyroid gland.
- Describe the unique microscopic appearance of the thyroid gland.
- Describe the blood supply and innervation of the thyroid gland.
- Trace the steps in the synthesis, storage, and secretion of the hormones produced by the thryoid follicular cells, referring to the specific organelles that take part in the process.

- Describe the role of the pituitary gland and hypothalamus in the regulation of thyroid follicular activity.
- Describe the effects of thyroid hormones on their target tissues.
- Describe the structure, function, location, and embryonic origin of the C or parafollicular cells.
- Identify the thyroid follicles, follicular cells, basement membrane, colloid, capillaries, and parafollicular cells in a slide or photomicrograph of a section of the thyroid gland.
- Distinguish between an active and inactive thyroid gland on the basis of follicular morphologic characteristics.
- Describe the number, size, location, and embryonic origin of the parathyroid glands.
- Compare the 2 parenchymal cell types of the parathyroids (chief cells and oxyphil cells) in terms of their relative numbers and their appearance in light and electron microscopes.
- Describe the role of parathyroid hormone in controlling blood calcium and phosphate levels and the specific effects of this hormone on its target tissues.
- Describe the factor(s) that control(s) the secretory activity of the parathyroid glands.
- Compare parathyroid hormone and calcitonin in terms of their source and function.
- Identify the capsule, chief cells, and oxyphil cells in a slide or photomicrograph of a parathyroid gland.
- Describe the shape, location, and general histologic organization of the pineal gland.
- Compare the appearance in light and electron microscopes of the 2 major parenchymal cell types of the pineal (pinealocytes and astroglial cells).
- Describe the histologic appearance, chemical composition, and age-related changes of the corpora arenacea (brain sand).
- Describe the innervation and blood supply of the pineal.
- Name the most widely accepted function of the pineal.
- Describe the synthesis and function and the factors controlling the production of the pineal hormone, melatonin.
- Identify the pinealocytes, astroglial cells, and brain sand in a slide or photomicrograph of the pineal gland.

Synopsis

I. GENERAL FEATURES OF ENDOCRINE SECRETORY CELLS: STRUCTURE-FUNCTION RELATIONSHIPS.

Knowledge of a hormone's structure allows the prediction of the ultrastructure of the secretory cell that produces it. For example, cells that secrete steroid hormones contain abundant smooth endoplasmic reticulum, while those that secrete peptide hormones contain abundant rough endoplasmic reticulum. (Other general features of the structure and function of endocrine glands are described in Chapter 20.)

II. ADRENAL (SUPRARENAL) GLANDS.

Forming a cap over each kidney, these can be divided by embryonic origin, structure, and function into cortex and medulla.

A. Adrenal Cortex:

1. Embryonic origin The adrenal cortex is derived from coelomic intermediate mesoderm.

2. Structure in adults. Cells of the adrenal cortex have the characteristic structure of steroid-synthesizing cells (see Chapter 4). The cortex is divided into 3 layers, the zonae glomerulosa, fasciculata, and reticularis.

a. Zona glomerulosa The outermost cortical layer, it lies directly beneath the capsule and constitutes 15% of the adrenal volume. Its cells form arched clusters (glomeruli) surrounded by capillaries. The secretory cells of this layer produce **mineralocorticoids.**

b. Zona fasciculata The middle layer of the adrenal cortex, it constitutes 65% of the adrenal volume. Its cells form straight cords (fascicles) that run perpendicular to the organ surface. The cells in this layer produce **glucocorticoids** and some **adrenal androgens** upon appropriate stimulation.

c. Zona reticularis This is the innermost layer of the adrenal cortex and constitutes 7% of the adrenal volume. Its cells are arranged in irregular cords that form an anastomotic network (reticulum). While its cells resemble those in the fasciculata, they are smaller and more acidophilic. They contain fewer lipid droplets, more mitochondria, and numerous lipofuscin granules. The reticularis and fasciculata appear to constitute a single functional zone with the reticularis producing most of the glucocorticoids and adrenal androgens and the fasciculata representing a reserve zone to be called into action by prolonged stimulation.

3. Normal function The adrenal cortex produces 3 types of steroid hormones:

a. Mineralocorticoids Consisting mainly of **aldosterone,** these are produced by the zona glomerulosa in response to stimulation, primarily by angiotensin II but also to a lesser extent by ACTH. Aldosterone controls water and electrolyte balance mainly by stimulating sodium absorption by the distal renal tubules as well as through effects on the gastric mucosa and salivary glands.

b. Glucocorticoids Mainly **cortisol** and **corticosterone,** these are produced by the zona reticularis in response to ACTH and by the fasciculata in response to prolonged stimulation. Glucocorticoids control carbohydrate metabolism, especially by stimulating carbohydrate synthesis in the liver. They have the opposite effect in other tissues, catabolizing (degrading) carbohydrates to provide raw material for the liver. Glucocorticoids also suppress the immune response by decreasing the number of circulating lymphocytes and eosinophils.

c. Adrenal androgens These androgens, mainly **dehydroepiandrosterone,** are secreted in response to ACTH by the zona reticularis and, following prolonged stimulation, by the fasciculata. The masculinizing and anabolic effects of adrenal androgens are similar to those of testosterone but less potent.

4. Abnormal function

a. Hypersecretion **Cushing's syndrome** is an example of the hypersecretion of cortisol– and often of androgens. Its symptoms include truncal obesity, a round "moon face," high blood sugar, diabetes mellitus, hirsutism, amenorrhea, acne, and emotional lability. Hypersecretion of aldosterone (**Conn's syndrome,** for example) causes sodium and water retention, increasing the blood pressure (hypertension).

b. Hyposecretion Chronic hypofunction of the adrenal cortex (eg, **Addison's disease**) causes low levels of glucose, sodium, chloride, and bicarbonate and high levels of serum potassium. It results in weakness, nausea, weight loss, and elevated ACTH levels (the last causing hyperpigmentation). Without testicular androgens to compensate, decreased adrenal androgen synthesis in women may cause the loss of pubic and axillary hair.

5. Fetal, or provisional, cortex The thickest adrenal layer before birth, it is located between the medulla and the immature thin permanent cortex. It produces sulfated androgens that are activated by the placenta and enter the maternal circulation. After birth, the fetal cortex regresses, and the permanent cortex develops the 3 layers described above.

B. Adrenal Medulla:

1. Embryonic origin The adrenal medulla is derived from the neural crest.

2. Structure It contains 2 major cell types: chromaffin and ganglion cells.

a. Chromaffin cells Also known as **pheochromocytes,** these constitute the predominant medullary cell type; they are modified postganglionic sympathetic neurons that have lost their axons and dendrites. They contain large nuclei, abundant electron-dense secretory granules filled with catecholamines (epinephrine or norepinephrine), a well-developed Golgi complex, a few profiles of RER, and numerous oval mitochondria. Their secretory granules have a strong affinity for chromium-containing stains. Chromaffin cells synthesize and release their catecholamines upon neural stimulation, especially stress, mediated by preganglionic sympathetic neurons.

b. Ganglion cells The few parasympathetic ganglion cells present exhibit typical morphologic characteristics of autonomic ganglion cells (see Chapter 9).

3. Normal function For the adrenal medulla normal functions include the production of 2 types of catecholamines—epinephrine and norepinephrine—in response to preganglionic sympathetic stimulation (eg, stress). Both elevate blood glucose by stimulating glycogenolysis in the liver; they also increase the blood flow to the heart.

a. Epinephrine increases the heart rate and dilates blood vessels to the organs needed to combat or escape stress, such as cardiac and skeletal muscle. It dilates the bronchioles and constricts vessels in organs (eg, skin, digestive tract, kidneys) that are not essential in reacting to stress.

b. Norepinephrine constricts blood vessels in nonessential organs. By increasing peripheral resistance, it increases blood pressure and blood flow to the heart, brain, and skeletal muscle.

4. Abnormal function Hypersecreting chromaffin cell tumors (**pheochromocytomas**) cause a sustained stress response (especially hypertension) even in the absence of stress. Ganglion cell tumors (**neuroblastomas** and **ganglioneuromas**) are more common, especially in children, but their clinical manifestations vary.

C. Adrenal Blood Supply:

1. Main arteries There are 3 main arteries supplying each adrenal gland: the **superior suprarenal** from the inferior phrenic artery, the **middle suprarenal** from the aorta, and the **inferior suprarenal** from the renal **artery.** They penetrate the capsule separately, and their branches anastomose to form a subcapsular arterial plexus.

2. Subcapsular arterial plexus This gives rise to 3 groups of arteries:

a. The arteries of the capsule;

b. The arteries of the cortex, which branch to form the **cortical capillaries** that pass between the secretory cells and drain into the medullary capillaries; and

c. The arteries of the medulla, which pass through the cortex without branching until they reach the medulla, where they form the medullary capillaries.

3. Medullary capillaries, which receive a double blood supply from arteries of both the cortex and medulla, converge to form several medullary veins.

4. Medullary veins These converge to form a single large suprarenal vein.

5. Suprarenal vein Lying at the core of the medulla, this vein drains into the renal vein or directly into the inferior vena cava.

III. ISLETS OF LANGERHANS.

These small nests of endocrine cells distributed throughout the pancreas contain 4 major peptide hormone-secreting endocrine cell types:

A. A cells (alpha cells)

In response to low blood glucose, these cells secrete **glucagon,** the effects of which are opposite to those produced by insulin.

B. B cells (beta cells)

The most numerous cell type in the islets, these cells secrete **insulin** in response to high blood glucose. Insulin enhances glucose uptake by most cells, glycogen synthesis by hepatocytes, and triglyceride synthesis by adipocytes. B cell malfunction causes **diabetes mellitus,** a condition manifested as a great excess of blood glucose (**hyperglycemia**) that spills over into the urine (**glycosuria**). Hyperplasia and neoplasia of the B cells may result in **hyperinsulinism syndrome,** characterized by **hypoglycemia.**

C. D cells (delta cells) **Somatostatin,** which suppresses the release of insulin, glucagon, and growth hormone, is secreted by these cells. They may also secrete **gastrin,** which stimulates secretion by glands in the gastric mucosa. Zollinger-Ellison syndrome (gastrinoma) causes peptic ulcers through excessive acid secretion by parietal cells in the gastric mucosa. Somatostatinomas are rare tumors with complex effects.

D. F cells (PP cells) These cells secrete **pancreatic polypeptide,** which inhibits pancreatic exocrine secretion of enzymes and bicarbonate. It also causes relaxation of the gall bladder and decreases the secretion of bile.

IV. THYROID GLAND

Located in the neck, anterior to the larynx, the thyroid consists of 2 lobes connected by an isthmus. It is composed of numerous spheric follicles and is covered by a thin capsule that penetrates the parenchyma to form septa.

A. Thyroid Follicles: Each follicle consists of an outer simple epithelium of follicular cells enclosing a central lumen filled with **colloid.** The follicles, which vary in size, enlarge during stimulation.

B. Thyroid Follicular Cells:

1. Structure Thyroid follicular cells, which derive from endoderm, exhibit a typical peptide hormone-secreting cell ultrastructure. The cell height ranges from squamous in inactive glands to columnar during stimulation.

2. Normal function Thyroid follicular cells differ from other endocrine cells in that they store an intermediate form of their secretory product (**thyroglobulin**) extracellularly in colloid rather than internally in cytoplasmic granules. Stimulation by TSH (see Chapter 20), which generally follows an increased demand for energy, increases synthesis and secretion.

a. Synthesis and storage of thyroglobulin The steps required by this process are
(1) Synthesis of thyroglobulin protein, which contains many tyrosine residues, on the RER;
(2) Glycosylation of the protein in the ER and Golgi complex;
(3) Packaging in vesicles in the Golgi complex; and
(4) Fusion of the vesicles with the apical cell membrane, resulting in exocytosis of the thyroglobulin into the colloid in the lumen of the follicle.

b. Uptake and oxidation of iodide A molecular pump in the follicular cell's basal plasma membrane transfers circulating iodide into the cytoplasm. It is oxidized by peroxidase and then transferred to the cell's apex. Iodide uptake is also stimulated by TSH.

c. Iodination of thyroglobulin and formation of thyroid hormone Enzymes in the plasma membranes of the apical microvilli projecting into colloid catalyze the iodination of tyrosine residues in the thyroglobulin, a reaction that occurs at the microvillus-colloid interface. One iodide molecule is added to tyrosine, forming **monoiodotyrosine (MIT).** A second iodide molecule is then added to some tyrosine residues, forming **diiodotyrosine (DIT).** Coupling of the 2 iodinated tyrosines forms a thyronine molecule. Coupling 2 DIT molecules forms **tetraiodothyronine (thyroxine;** T_4), while coupling 1 MIT and 1 DIT forms triiodothyronine (T_3). Although T_4 makes up 90% of the thyroid hormones produced, it is not as potent as the less common T_3.

d. Thyroid hormone secretion Stimulation by TSH causes the follicular cells to pinocytose portions of the colloid, forming vesicles that contain iodinated thyroglobulin. These vesicles fuse with lysosomes containing enzymes that cleave the thyroglobulin.

The T_4 and T_3 released in this way diffuse out of the secondary lysosomes (see Chapter 3). They pass through the cytoplasm and cross the basal plasma membranes to reach the bloodstream.

e. Targets and effects of thyroid hormones T_3 and T_4 act on cells throughout the body to increase their basal metabolic rate (ie, the rate at which cells use glucose), promote cell growth, increase heart rate, raise body temperature, and generally enhance all energy-requiring cell functions. They also act on the TRH-secreting cells of the hypothalamus and the thyrotropes in the adenohypophysis to reduce TSH secretion (**negative feedback**).

3. Abnormal function

a. Hyperthyroidism The overproduction of thyroid hormone also known as thyrotoxicosis causes such symptoms as nervousness, palpitation, rapid pulse, muscular weakness, fatigue, weight loss with good appetite, excessive perspiration, intolerance of heat, and emotional lability. Hyperactive thyroid follicles that enlarge because of the increased height of the follicular epithelium and increased deposits of thyroglobulin cause a swelling of the thyroid gland known as **goiter.**

b. Hypothyroidism Termed **cretinism** in children and **myxedema** in adults, hypothyroidism causes poor glucose utilization. Its symptoms include lethargy, intolerance of cold, slowing of intellectual and motor skills, accumulation of glycosaminoglycans in the dermis (with consequent bloating), and sometimes weight gain. Since iodine is required for normal thyroid function, iodine-deficient diets reduce functional thyroxin production and often underlie cretinism and myxedema. Because uniodinated thyroxin caused by iodine deficiency cannot provide negative feedback on TSH production, follicular enlargement and goiter may accompany this type of hypothyroidism.

C. Parafollicular Cells (C cells): These are found in the thyroid gland, interspersed among the follicular cells or in clusters between the follicles. In humans, parafollicular cell cytoplasm stains poorly with standard stains and typically appears clear or white. Electron micrographs reveal numerous small secretory granules. C cells secrete **calcitonin** in response to high blood calcium. Calcitonin causes calcium uptake by cells and increased calcium deposition in bone, lowering the blood calcium levels.

V. PARATHYROID GLANDS. These 4 small glands, located on the posterior surface of the thyroid gland, are derived from the third and fourth pharyngeal pouches (endoderm). In adults, they are composed of 2 major parenchymal cell types, chief and oxyphil cells (which may be different forms of the same cell type).

A. Chief Cells: These are the most numerous of the parenchymal cells.

1. Structure These small (4–8 μm in diameter) polygonal cells exhibit typical peptide secretory cell ultrastructure; they contain abundant small secretory granules in their pale-staining cytoplasm.

2. Normal function Chief cells secrete **parathyroid hormone (PTH)** in response to low blood calcium levels. PTH increases blood calcium levels by acting at 3 target sites. In **bone,** PTH increases bone resorption. In the **kidney,** it increases phosphate excretion and calcium reabsorption and causes activation of a vitamin D precursor. In the **intestines,** PTH (perhaps by activating vitamin D) causes increased absorption of calcium from food by the intestinal mucosa.

3. Abnormal function

a. Hyperparathyroidism Excessive secretion of PTH elevates serum calcium (**hypercalcemia**) and decreases serum phosphate (**hypophosphatemia**). Its effects include increased urine calcium, abnormal deposits of calcium in the arteries and kidneys, and excessive loss of calcium from bones, resulting in **osteomalacia** and **osteitis fibrosa cystica.**

b. Hypoparathyroidism Insufficient secretion of PTH disrupts neuromuscular function. The resulting low blood calcium level leads to spontaneous and uncontrolled firing of action potentials. In peripheral nerves this may cause spastic muscle contraction, or **tetany.** The spontaneous firing of neurons in the brain may cause behavioral effects as well.

B. Oxyphil Cells: These are larger and less numerous than chief cells; their content of mitochondria makes them intensely acidophilic. Oxyphil function is not clearly understood.

VI. PINEAL BODY. This small conical organ (the epiphysis cerebri) is attached by a stalk to the roof of the diencephalon near the posterior aspect of the third ventricle. It is covered by pia mater, extensions of which penetrate the organ; these extensions carry blood vessels and form irregular septa. The pineal contains globular basophilic clusters of mineralized matrix known as **brain sand (corpora arenacea),** which increase in size and number with advancing age. The pineal's 2 major cell types are pinealocytes and astroglial cells.

A. Pinealocytes:

1. Structure These cells have large irregular nuclei with prominent nucleoli and pale basophilic cytoplasm. With the Del Rio Hortega silver stain, they exhibit long cytoplasmic processes that terminate as swellings in the septa near blood vessels. The role of pineal innervation (both sympathetic and through the stalk from the posterior commissure) is uncertain.

2. Normal function Pinealocytes secrete **melatonin.** Cyclic changes in plasma melatonin levels follow changes in environmental lighting, but the precise relationship is still unknown. Melatonin may both help establish circadian rhythms and have antigonadotropic effects that delay onset of sexual maturity until puberty. Other pineal secretions include arginine vasotocin and possibly additional substances that exert an antigonadotropic effect through the hypothalamohypophyseal axis.

3. Abnormal function Pineal lesions occur most often in young males and may cause either precocious or delayed sexual maturity. Because of their location, pineal tumors may restrict the flow of cerebrospinal fluid through the aqueduct of Sylvius, causing hydrocephalus and its accompanying symptoms.

B. Astroglial Cells: Also known as **interstitial cells,** these glia-like cells have elongated heterochromatic nuclei and long cytoplasmic processes that contain intermediate filaments. They are found around blood vessels and between clusters of pinealocytes.

Study-Focusing Questions*

1. Compare the adrenal cortex and medulla in terms of their embryonic origins (401).
2. Beginning with the 3 major arteries to the adrenal gland and ending with the venous drainage, trace the path taken by blood supplying the cells in the following areas:
   a. Adrenal capsule (401)
   b. Adrenal cortex (401)
   c. Adrenal medulla (***Hint:*** dual supply) (401)
3. Describe the endothelial lining of the medullary capillaries (fenestrated? with diaphragms?) (401).

*The page references in this section refer to *Basic Histology,* 6th ed., Junqueira L, Carneiro J, Kelley R (editors), Appleton & Lange, 1989. **HR** (for Histology Review) is occasionally used instead of a page reference to indicate that the information referred to can be found in this book.

4. Name, in order, the layers of the adrenal cortex, beginning with the layer closest to the capsule (401).

5. Compare the layers named in the answer to question 4 in terms of the:
  - **a.** Percentage of adrenal volume each occupies (402)
  - **b.** Typical structure of the steroid-secreting cells (88–89)
  - **c.** Shape and arrangement of the secretory cells (402–405)
  - **d.** Classes and specific examples of steroid hormones secreted by each layer (402–405)
  - **e.** Layer characterized by the presence of more lipofuscin pigment (404)

6. Compare glucocorticoids, mineralocorticoids, and adrenal androgens in terms of:
  - **a.** Their sites of synthesis (401, 405)
  - **b.** Their target organs and their effects on them (401, 405–406)
  - **c.** The factors that stimulate or inhibit their production (405–406)

7. Describe the fetal (provisional) cortex (406) in terms of:
  - **a.** Its size relative to the adult cortex
  - **b.** The number of layers
  - **c.** The age or time at which it begins involution
  - **d.** Its function

8. Name the 2 major cell types found in the adrenal medulla (406–407).

9. Name the 2 major catecholamines secreted by the parenchymal cells of the adrenal medulla (407–408)

10. Describe the role of the following in regulating the relative amount of epinephrine and norepinephrine secreted:
  - **a.** PNMT (**HR**)
  - **b.** Glucocorticoids (**HR**)
  - **c.** Dual blood supply to the medullary capillaries (**HR**)

11. Describe the factors leading to increased secretion of catecholamines by the adrenal medulla (408).

12. Describe the effects of increased catecholamine secretion (408).

13. Give the location of the islets of Langerhans (409).

14. Name the 4 major types of hormone-secreting cells in the islets and compare them in terms of:
  - **a.** Their location in the islets (409)
  - **b.** Their abundance (409–411)
  - **c.** Their secretory granules (409–411)
  - **d.** The hormone they produce (410)

15. Compare glucagon, insulin, somatostatin, and pancreatic polypeptide in terms of:
  - **a.** The cells that secrete them (410)
  - **b.** The factors that stimulate their secretion (410–411)
  - **c.** Their target organs and effects (410–411)

16. Describe the thyroid gland in terms of:
  - **a.** Its location (411)
  - **b.** The number of its lobes (411–412)
  - **c.** Its embryonic origin (411)
  - **d.** The hormones it secretes (411, 412)

17. Sketch a cross section through 3 adjacent thyroid follicles and the intervening tissue (414) and label the following:
  - **a.** Follicular (epithelial) cells (412, 414)
  - **b.** Basal lamina (412, 414, 417)
  - **c.** Colloid (412, 414, 417)
  - **d.** Capillaries (412, 414, 417)
  - **e.** Parafollicular cells (412, 414, 417)

18. On the drawing made for question 17, show the site of:
  - **a.** Stored thyroglobulin (413, 414, 417)
  - **b.** Iodination of tyrosine residues (416, 417)
  - **c.** Iodide oxidation (414, 417)
  - **d.** Thyroglobulin synthesis (414, 417)
  - **e.** Calcitonin synthesis (412)
  - **f.** Iodide pump (414, 417)
  - **g.** Cleavage of T_3 and T_4 from iodinated thyroglobulin (416, 417)
  - **h.** Release of T_3 and T_4 from follicular cells (416, 417)

19. Describe the effects of TSH on the thyroid follicles in terms of the:
    a. Size and shape of the follicular cell (412, 414)
    b. Diameter of the follicle (412, 414)
    c. Synthesis of thyroglobulin (412, 414)
    d. Uptake of iodide (414)
    e. Pinocytosis of colloid (416)
    f. Production of thyroxine (416)
20. List the steps in the synthesis and storage of thyroglobulin, naming all intra- and extracellular components involved (414–416).
21. List the steps in the iodination of the tyrosine residues of thyroglobulin, beginning with the uptake of iodide and ending with the condensation of MIT and DIT to form T_3 and T_4. Name the intracellular and extracellular components involved (414–416).
22. Beginning with the uptake of iodinated thyroglobulin, list the steps leading to the release of T_3 and T_4 from the follicular cell and name the organelles involved in each step (416).
23. Describe parafollicular cells in terms of:
    a. Their characteristic staining properties (412)
    b. Their location (412, 415)
    c. The hormone they secrete (412)
    d. The factor(s) that stimulate their secretion (413)
    e. The targets and effects of their hormones (413)
24. Describe the parathyroid glands in terms of:
    a. Their numbers (416)
    b. Their dimensions (416)
    c. Their usual location (416)
    d. Their embryonic origin (which pharyngeal pouches) (416–418)
    e. Their alternate location (416)
    f. The major hormone they produce (419)
25. Name the 2 major parenchymal cells types in the human parathyroids (419) and compare them in terms of:
    a. The number found in the gland
    b. Their diameters
    c. Their staining properties
    d. Their secretory products
    e. The number of mitochondria they contain
26. What is the normal calcium concentration in human plasma (419)?
27. Describe parathyroid hormone in terms of:
    a. The cell type that secretes it (419)
    b. The stimulus for hormone secretion (419)
    c. Its effect on blood calcium levels (419)
    d. Its effect on blood phosphate levels (419)
    e. Its 3 main target sites and the effects at each site (419)
    f. The effect of high blood calcium levels on the hormone's secretion (419)
    g. The hormone whose effect on blood calcium levels is opposite that of parathyroid hormone (419)
    h. The known effects of other hormones or nerves on parathyroid hormone secretion (419)
28. Describe the pineal body in terms of:
    a. Its shape and dimensions (419)
    b. Its location (419)
    c. Its vascular connective tissue covering (419)
    d. Its 2 principal cell types (419)
    e. The calcified bodies that are found between the cells and increase in number with age (421)
    f. The 2 known sources of its innervation (421)
    g. The major (best-characterized) hormone secreted (419)
    h. The indirect evidence that it may affect gonadal function (421)
29. Compare pinealocytes (419) with astroglial cells (419–421) in terms of:
    a. The size, shape, and staining intensity of their nuclei
    b. The presence of long cytoplasmic processes
    c. Their location in relation to blood vessels

Multiple-Choice Questions

For the questions 21–1 through 21–5, select the single best answer.

21–1. The cell shown in the electron micrograph in Fig 21–1 is most likely
- **A.** Peptide hormone-secreting cell
- **B.** Neuron cell body
- **C.** Pancreatic B (beta) cell
- **D.** Steroid hormone-secreting cell
- **E.** Astroglial cell

21–2. The rounded group of cells indicated by an arrow in the photomicrograph in Fig 21–2 is a(n):
- **A.** Thyroid follicle
- **B.** Pancreatic islet of Langerhans
- **C.** Collection of astroglial cells in the pineal body
- **D.** Adrenal medulla
- **E.** Glomerulus

21–3. The organ shown in the photomicrograph in Fig 21–3 is the:
- **A.** Thyroid gland
- **B.** Islets of Langerhans
- **C.** Pineal body
- **D.** Adrenal gland
- **E.** Parathyroid gland

21–4. The organ shown in the photomicrograph in Fig 21–4 is the:
- **A.** Thyroid gland
- **B.** Islets of Langerhans
- **C.** Pineal body
- **D.** Adrenal gland
- **E.** Parathyroid gland

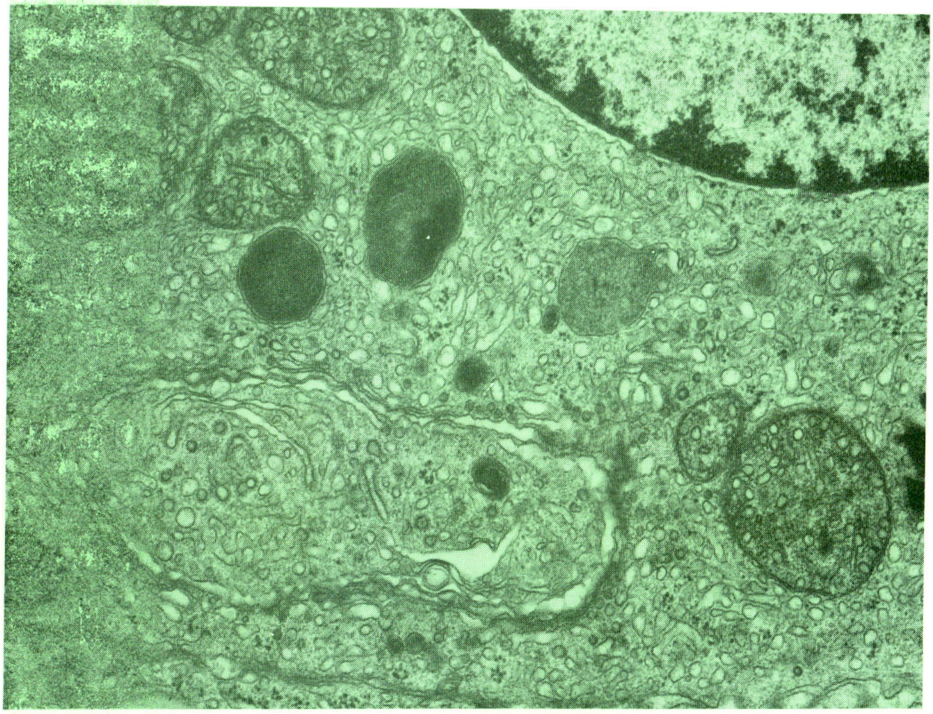

Figure 21–1.

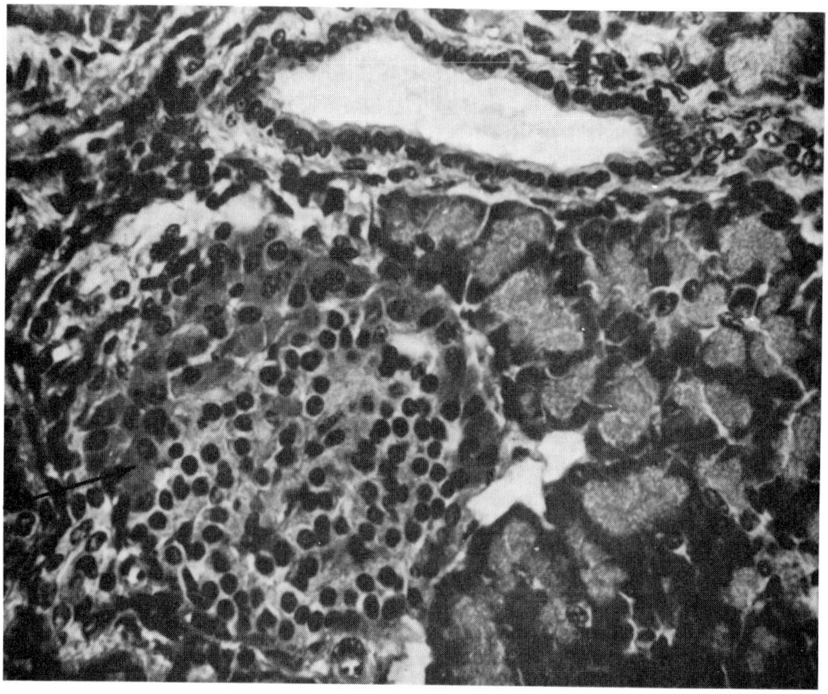

Figure 21-2.

21-5. The double blood supply to the adrenal medulla empties into its capillaries directly from the:
- **A.** Cortical and medullary veins
- **B.** Cortical capillaries and medullary arteries
- **C.** Superior and inferior suprarenal arteries
- **D.** Middle and inferior suprarenal arteries
- **E.** Subcapsular arterial plexus and suprarenal vein

MATCHING (questions 21-6 through 21-43): Each choice may be used once, more than once, or not at all.

Questions 21-6 through 21-13 use the letters in Fig 21-5:

21-6. Zona fasciculata
21-7. Capsule
21-8. Zona glomerulosa
21-9. Zona reticularis
21-10. Site(s) of aldosterone synthesis

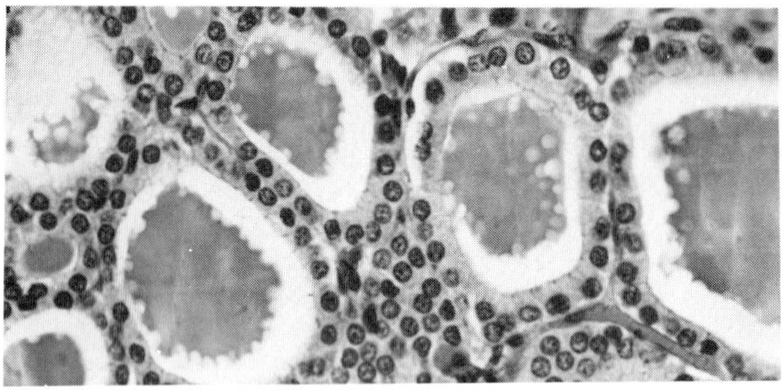

Figure 21-3.

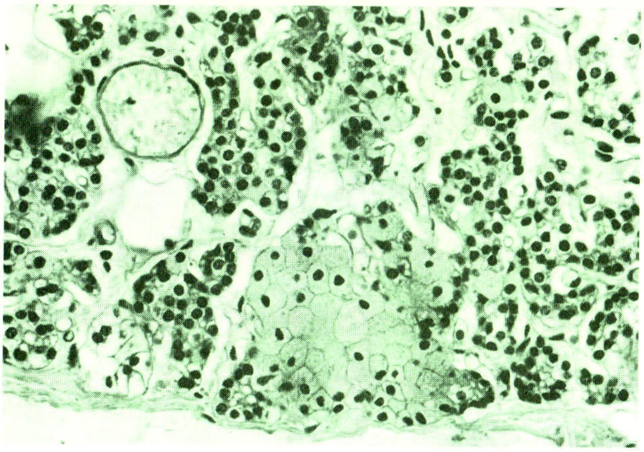

Figure 21-4.

21-11. Site(s) of androgen synthesis
21-12. Site(s) of glucocorticoid synthesis
21-13. Layer(s) responsive to ACTH stimulation

Questions 21-14 through 21-37 (may have more than one correct answer):

A. Aldosterone
B. Corticosterone
C. Dehydroepiandrosterone
D. Epinephrine
E. Norepinephrine
F. Glucagon
G. Insulin
H. Somatostatin
I. Pancreatic polypeptide
J. Thyroxin
K. Calcitonin
L. Parathyroid hormone
M. Melatonin

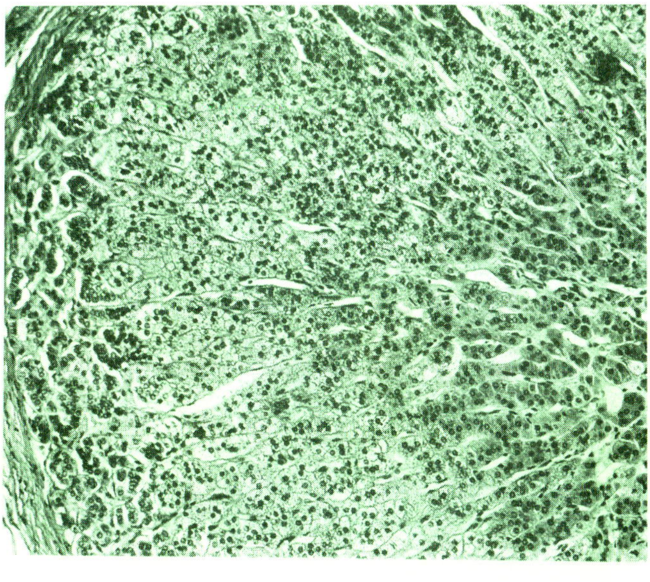

Figure 21-5.

21–14. Glucocorticoid(s)
21–15. Mineralocorticoid(s)
21–16. Androgen(s)
21–17. Steroid hormone(s)
21–18. Peptide hormone(s)
21–19. Catecholamine(s)
21–20. Synthesized and secreted by cells in the pancreas
21–21. Synthesized and secreted by cells in the thyroid gland
21–22. Synthesized and secreted by cells in the parathyroids
21–23. Synthesized and secreted by cells in the pineal body
21–24. Synthesized and secreted by cells in the adrenal glands
21–25. Produced in response to stimulation by pituitary hormones
21–26. Produced in response to elevated blood calcium levels
21–27. Produced in response to angiotensin II
21–28. Produced in response to stress
21–29. Produced in response to decreased blood calcium levels
21–30. Produced in response to increased blood sugar levels
21–31. Produced in response to decreased blood sugar levels
21–32. Production influenced by external visual stimuli
21–33. Storage form stored extracellularly
21–34. Storage form complexed with zinc
21–35. Increases basal metabolic rate
21–36. Decreases exocrine secretions of pancreas and liver
21–37. Increases absorption of salt by distal tubules

Questions 21–38 through 21–43:

A. A (alpha) cells
B. B (beta) cells
C. C (parafollicular) cells
D. D (delta) cells
E. F cells
F. None of the above

21–38. Produce insulin
21–39. Produce glucagon
21–40. Produce calcitonin
21–41. Produce somatostatin
21–42. Produce pancreatic polypeptide
21–43. Located in thyroid gland

For questions 21–44 through 21–59, either, both or neither of the answers may be correct. Select

A if only A is correct
B if only B is correct
C if both A and B are correct
D if neither A nor B is correct

Questions 21–44 through 21–50:

A. Steroid hormone-secreting cells
B. Peptide hormone-secreting cells
C. Both
D. Neither

21–44. Abundant smooth endoplasmic reticulum
21–45. Abundant rough endoplasmic reticulum
21–46. Abundant cytoplasmic lipid
21–47. Well-developed Golgi complex
21–48. Secretory granules

21-49. More basophilic
21-50. Mitochondria with tubular cristae

Questions 21-51 through 21-55:

A. Adrenal cortex
B. Adrenal medulla
C. Both
D. Neither

21-51. Produce(s) steroid hormones
21-52. Produce(s) catecholamines
21-53. Derived from neural crest
21-54. Derived from mesoderm
21-55. Contains chromaffin cells

Questions 21-56 through 21-59:

A. Calcitonin
B. Parathyroid hormone
C. Both
D. Neither

21-56. Increases bone resorption
21-57. Lowers blood calcium and increases osteogenesis
21-58. Below-normal concentrations in blood cause tetany
21-59. Diminishes absorption of phosphate in renal tubules

For questions 21-60 through 21-66, one, more than one, or all of the answers may be correct. Select

A if only (1), (2), and (3) are correct
B if only (1) and (3) are correct
C if only (2) and (4) are correct
D if only (4) is correct
E if all answers are correct

21-60. Glucocorticoids:
(1) Include cortisone and corticosterone
(2) Enhance the immune response
(3) Are produced in response to stimulation by ACTH
(4) Are produced primarily by the zona glomerulosa
21-61. Values that increase in response to catecholamine secretion include the:
(1) Blood glucose
(2) Blood pressure
(3) Heart rate
(4) Blood flow to skin
21-62. The fetal (provisional) cortex:
(1) Begins its involution at puberty
(2) Is located between the permanent cortex and medulla
(3) Has cells arranged in hollow follicles
(4) Secretes sulfate conjugates of adrenal androgens
21-63. Chromaffin cells:
(1) Produce epinephrine
(2) Produce norepinephrine
(3) Increase their rate of secretion in response to sympathetic stimulation
(4) May be found in sites other than the adrenal medulla
21-64. The colloid stored within a thyroid follicle:
(1) Contains the stored forms of both T_3 and T_4
(2) Is produced by the parafollicular cells
(3) Contains a relatively high concentration of iodine

(4) Is composed of numerous thyroglobulin-containing membrane-bound vesicles

21–65. Oxyphil cells:
- **(1)** Are larger than parathyroid chief cells
- **(2)** Contain abundant mitochondria
- **(3)** Are acidophilic
- **(4)** Contain abundant secretory granules

21–66. Brain sand:
- **(1)** Is found only in diseased pineal bodies
- **(2)** Contains calcium
- **(3)** Is intensely acidophilic
- **(4)** Can be used as a landmark by radiologists

22 Male Reproductive System

Objectives

This chapter should help the student to:

- Name and give the location of the various glands, ducts, and external genitalia of the male reproductive system.
- Describe the general organization of the components of the testis (coverings, septa, mediastinum, seminiferous tubules, intratesticular ducts) as they appear in a midsaggital section.
- Describe the embryonic origin of the male germ cells (spermatogonia) and their structural and positional changes in the walls of the seminiferous tubules during spermatogenesis.
- Know the number of chromosomes and amount of DNA found in the cells of the spermatogenic lineage at each step in spermatogenesis.
- Distinguish between spermatogenesis, spermatocytogenesis, and spermiogenesis.
- Describe the structure, function, location, and embryonic origin of the Sertoli (supporting) cells.
- Describe the composition, location, and probable function of the blood-testis barrier.
- Describe the structure (as viewed through light and electron microscopes), function, and location of the interstitial (Leydig) cells of the testes.
- Describe the function of temperature and the roles of the pituitary and the cells within the testis itself in the regulation of spermatogenesis.
- Trace the path of the spermatozoa from the seminiferous tubules through the intratesticular and excretory genital ducts. Describe the differences in duct wall structure and changes in the composition of the semen that occur in each portion of the pathway.
- Compare the seminal vesicles, prostate, and bulbourethral (Cowper's) glands in terms of general organization, epithelial lining, secretory products, and the point(s) at which their secretions enter the excretory pathway.
- Name the 3 erectile bodies found in the human penis. Describe their relative positions, and indicate which of them contains the urethra and forms the glans.
- Describe the histologic composition and appearance of erectile tissue.
- Describe the blood supply to the erectile tissue of the penis and the factors that control the functional transition from flaccid to erect and erect to flaccid.

Synopsis

I. GENERAL FEATURES OF THE MALE REPRODUCTIVE SYSTEM. This system consists of the external genitalia and a series of glands and ducts that produce and transport the male gametes (spermatozoa) and the seminal fluid. Together the seminal fluid and spermatozoa constitute the semen.

A. Glands: The glands of this system include the paired testes and several accessory glands.

1. Testes These are the male gonads, located in the scrotum; they are the primary glands of this system, with both exocrine and endocrine functions.

a. Exocrine component This part of the testes includes the seminiferous tubules, where spermatozoa are produced (spermatogenesis), and the intratesticular genital ducts. The seminiferous tubules deliver their exocrine products into these ducts for transport from the testes through a set of excretory genital ducts.

b. Endocrine component This consists of nests of testosterone-secreting interstitial cells in the connective tissue between the seminiferous tubules.

2. Accessory glands Located along the excretory genital duct system, these include the seminal vesicles, prostate glands, bulbourethral glands, and glands of Littre.

a. Seminal vesicles These are paired glands whose secretions increase the volume of the seminal fluid and raise its pH. They also add fructose, providing a source of nourishment and energy for the gametes.

b. Prostate gland More fluid, rich in citric acid (another nutrient) and acid phosphatase, is added by this gland.

c. Bulbourethral glands and **glands of Littre** These mucous glands help to lubricate the distal part of the duct system.

B. Ducts: The ducts of the male reproductive system are described in terms of their location, number, length, diameter, wall structure, and related functions.

1. Intratesticular ducts Located within the testes, these are continuous with the seminiferous tubules and include the tubuli recti, rete testis, and ductuli efferentes.

2. Excretory genital ducts These are located outside the testes and include the ductus epididymis, ductus, or vas, deferens, ejaculatory duct, and urethra. In these larger ducts the secretions of the testes and the accessory glands combine to form the semen.

C. External Genitalia: These include the penis and scrotum. The penis contains the most distal element of the duct system, the penile urethra. The scrotum contains the testes. The histology and reproductive function of the penis are covered with emphasis on erectile tissue, blood flow, and autonomic innervation.

II. TESTES

A. Embryonic Origin: Primordial germ cells, originating from yolk sac endoderm, migrate into the dorsal wall of the abdominal cavity and invade the mesoderm of the genital ridge, where they collect to form the primitive sex cords. The primordial germ cells form the spermatogonia, and the mesoderm forms the Sertoli cells, interstitial cells, and the connective tissue between the cords. The solid sex cords form seminiferous tubules, developing central lumens and anastomosing with adjacent cords. Later, the seminiferous tubules anastomose with remnants of the mesonephric tubules and the excretory duct system. The entire developing testis becomes encapsulated by connective tissue, separates from the dorsal wall, and descends into the scrotum.

B. General Organization:

1. External coverings

a. Tunica vaginalis This is a double-layered mesothelial sac that covers the anterior surface of each testis. This extension of the peritoneum is picked up during the descent of the testes into the scrotum.

b. Tunica albuginea This dense fibrous connective tissue capsule thickens along the posterior surface to form the **mediastinum testis.**

2. Internal structure

a. Septa These are extensions of the tunica albuginea that penetrate each testis and divide it into about 250 compartments, or lobules.

b. Lobules Each lobule includes 1–4 epithelial seminiferous tubules (the exocrine component) and loose vascular connective tissue that lies between the tubules and contains discrete clumps of testosterone-secreting interstitial cells of Leydig (the endocrine component).

C. Seminiferous Tubules:

1. General structure Each long (40–70 cm) narrow (0.2 mm) tubule is highly convoluted and packed into a small space. The walls of each tubule, from the exterior to the lumen, are composed of the following 3 layers:

a. The **tunica propria** is a thin tunic of fibrous connective tissue comprising several layers of fibroblasts. The innermost layer, which includes myoid cells that resemble smooth muscle cells, attaches to the basal lamina.

b. A well-defined **basal lamina** lies between the tunica propria and the seminiferous epithelium.

c. The stratified seminiferous epithelium is composed of 2 cell lineages: spermatogenic cells and supportive (Sertoli) cells.

2. Spermatogenic cells Deriving from embryonic yolk sac endoderm, these cells undergo spermatogenesis (II.D)—a multistep process of differentiation—that begins with the cells closest to the basal lamina (spermatogonia). The process ends with the release of spermatozoa into the tubule lumen. Cells at different steps in the process are identified according to their size, morphologic features of the nucleus, and position in the epithelium.

a. Spermatogonia are small round cells adjacent to the basal lamina. They are the least differentiated and are the only spermatogenic cell type present before puberty. They have a round nucleus with patchy heterochromatin. They are diploid for chromosome number (46, 2n), and diploid for DNA (2N) until stimulated to divide.

b. Primary spermatocytes are located closer to the lumen than are the spermatogonia. They are the largest germ cells present; each has a large round nucleus with dark strands of heterochromatin that resemble tangled string. They are usually seen in the prophase of meiosis I, the longest phase of meiosis (up to 22 days); they are also the most numerous germ cells present. They are diploid for chromosome number (46, 2n) and tetraploid for DNA (4N) in preparation for the first meiotic division.

c. Secondary spermatocytes are located closer to the lumen than are the primary spermatocytes. The product of the first meiotic division, they are about half the size of the primary spermatocytes that divide to form them. Secondary spermatocytes are rarely seen in histologic section because they undergo the second meiotic division almost immediately after formation. They are haploid for chromosome number (23, n) and diploid for DNA (2N).

d. Spermatids are products of the second meiotic division of secondary spermatocytes and are located next to the lumen. Spermatids are small cells with dark heterochromatic nuclei. They may exhibit a range of nuclear morphologic features, depending upon the stage of spermiogenesis. They are haploid for both chromosome number (23, n) and DNA (N).

e. Spermatozoa are located in the lumen. They are the result of spermiogenesis, the differentiation of spermatids (II.D). They are recognizable due to their large flagella (their structure is discussed in II.E). They are halpoid for both chromosome number (23, n) and DNA (N).

3. Supporting (Sertoli) cells These are derived from the mesoderm of the embryonic genital ridge.

a. Structure These elongated, branched, pyramidal epithelial cells extend from the basal lamina to the luminal surface of each seminiferous tubule. They exhibit deep cytoplasmic infoldings that surround the developing spermatogenic cells. Their large pale nuclei are usually ovoid and indented, each containing a prominent nucleolus. Sertoli cells have a well-developed smooth endoplasmic reticulum and Golgi complex, numerous mitochondria, and some rough endoplasmic reticulum. The margins of the cells are bound tightly to neighboring supporting cells by occluding junctions, forming continuous sheath around the tubule lumen.

b. Function The functions of the cells include

(1) Physical support for the spermatogenic cells, which are attached to one another by cytoplasmic bridges;

(2) Nutritional regulation of the spermatocytes, spermatids, and spermatozoa, which are isolated from the blood supply by the occluding junctions between the supporting cells. Spermatozoa therefore depend on these cells to mediate the exchange of nutrients and metabolites with the blood;

(3) Protection from autoimmune attack by immunoglobulins in the blood;

(4) Phagocytosis of residual bodies shed by the maturing spermatozoa; and

(5) Secretion of fluid for sperm transport; **androgen-binding protein (ABP),** which combines with the testosterone produced by interstitial cells and is released into the tubule lumen (ABP secretion increases in response to increased levels of FSH and testosterone); and inhibin, which acts on the pituitary to decrease FSH production. Although evidence is not conclusive, it is thought that they also secrete estrogen.

D. Spermatogenesis: This is the entire multistep process from spermatogonia through spermatozoa. It can be divided into 3 phases: spermatocytogenesis, meiosis, and spermiogenesis.

1. Spermatocytogenesis This is the production of primary spermatocytes from spermatogonia through a series of standard mitotic divisions. Daughter cells of early divisions form 2 types of spermatogonia, A and B. **Spermatogonia A** remain undifferentiated stem cells able to produce more A and B cells. **Spermatogonia B** may undergo further mitoses to form more spermatogonia B or enter meiosis to form primary spermatocytes.

2. Meiosis This process involves 2 successive cell divisions that yield 4 haploid spermatids from one diploid primary spermatocyte.

a. Meiosis I The first meiotic division involves the production of secondary spermatocytes from primary spermatocytes.

(1) During the **S phase** (DNA synthesis) prior to division, DNA doubles (as in mitosis), becoming tetraploid.

(2) During an extended **prophase,** the 23 pairs of homologous chromosomes (22 pairs of autosomes + XY) thicken by coiling. They pair up point-for-point (synapsis) and form bridges (chiasma) allowing the trading of DNA between paired chromosomes ("crossing over"). The nuclear membrane disintegrates late in prophase.

(3) During **metaphase,** the 23 pairs line up at the equatorial plate.

(4) During **anaphase,** the pairs separate, with one member of each pair moving toward the opposite pole.

(5) During **telophase,** the nuclear membranes reform in the daughter cells. Each of these secondary spermatocytes is now haploid, containing only one member of each homologous chromosome pair (22+X or 22+Y). The equatorial constriction tightens, but leaves the daughter cells connected by a narrow cytoplasmic bridge. Since DNA doubled prior to the first meiotic division, each secondary spermatocyte has a diploid amount of DNA.

b. Meiosis II The second meiotic division involves the production of spermatids from the secondary spermatocytes. During this division, the number of chromosomes in each cell remains the same (haploid), but the amount of DNA is halved (as during a standard mitosis), resulting in spermatids that are haploid for both the number of chromosomes and the amount of DNA.

3. Spermiogenesis This is the complex process of cytodifferentiation by which spermatids become spermatozoa. Because of the many structural changes involved, spermatids in various stages of this transformation exhibit stage-dependent variations in appearance. Spermiogenesis includes the following processes:

a. Acrosome formation Proacrosomal granules form in the Golgi complex and coalesce to form a large membrane-bound acrosomal vesicle that moves next to the nucleus and attaches to the nuclear envelope. The vesicle membrane spreads over the anterior surface of the nucleus, covering its anterior two-thirds and forming the **head cap.** The contents of the head cap are redistributed to form the mature acrosome (acrosomal cap), a large specialized lysosome. The contents of the acrosome are rich in carbohydrate and hydrolytic enzymes such as hyaluronidase, neuraminidase, acid phosphatase, and a trypsinlike protease.

b. Migration of the centrioles and formation of the flagellum The centrioles migrate to the posterior pole of the spermatid. A flagellum emerges from one, perpendicular to the cell surface, and forms the tail. The other centriole forms a collar around the base of the flagellum.

c. Shift of cytoplasm toward the flagellum The anterior plasma membrane now contacts the acrosome, and the excess cytoplasm forms a **residual body.**

d. Migration of mitochondria The mitochondria move toward the flagellum and form a spiral collar around the proximal part of the tail (the middle piece), concentrating themselves at the future site of high energy consumption. The fructose and citric acid in semen are important in sperm motility, serving as mitochondrial metabolites.

e. Condensation of nuclear chromatin The chromatin forms a dense mass with no visible substructure. The nucleus is surrounded by a cylindric band of microtubules associated with the posterior border of the acrosome (**manchette**). This causes flattening and elongation of the nucleus.

f. Sloughing of residual bodies When they are released into the tubule lumen, the spermatozoa release their residual cytoplasm. Much of this is phagocytosed by the supporting Sertoli cells.

E. Structure of Mature Spermatozoa:

1. Head In frontal view the head has an oval outline. On its side, it appears as a flat 4–5-μm-long and 2.5–3.5-μm-wide triangle with an anterior-directed apex (spearhead).

It is mostly nucleus, with the anterior two-thirds of the nucleus covered by the acrosome and the posterior region covered by the manchette.

2. Tail About 55 μm long and 0.5 μm thick, the tail is covered over its entire length by plasma membrane. It has 4 named parts:

a. Neck This includes the proximal centriole, connecting piece, capitulum, base of the flagellum, and an occasional mitochondrion.

b. Middle piece As the site of the mitochondrial sheath, the middle piece contains many mitochondria arranged end-to-end in a helix that makes about 15 turns around the flagellum. It is 5–7 μm long and 1 μm thick, with the annulus located at its posterior end. The flagellum in this region includes 9 outer dense fibers and 9 + 2 arrangement of microtubules at its core.

c. Principal piece This includes an outer fibrous sheath composed of dorsal and ventral longitudinal columns connected by circumferential ribs, with the flagellum at its core. Here the flagellum is composed of 7 outer dense fibers collected into 2 compartments and an inner 9 + 2 arrangement of microtubules.

d. End piece This portion of the tail lacks the fibrous sheath but otherwise has the same structure as the principal piece. As it tapers toward the tip, the 9 doublets dissociate to form 18 single microtubules.

F. Interstitial (Leydig) Cells: Derived from embryonic genital-ridge mesoderm, these cells secrete **testosterone.** They occur as highly vascularized nests of pale acidophilic cells in the connective tissue between the seminiferous tubules. Their large pale nuclei contain one or 2 prominent nucleoli. The cytoplasm contains the extensive smooth endoplasmic reticulum typical of steroid-secreting cells, a well-developed Golgi complex and lipid droplets.

G. Blood-Testis Barrier: Spermatogenesis involves the appearance of new sperm-specific proteins and glycoproteins on the differentiating spermatogenic cells. Since this process begins at puberty, well after development of the immune system, these surface molecules may be recognized as nonself antigens by the immune system. Without the protection of the blood-testis barrier, developing sperm would be damaged or destroyed by an autoimmune response. The barrier is formed by a continuous belt of junctional complexes joining the Sertoli cells at their lateral surfaces. It separates the seminiferous tubule lining into 2 functionally different compartments.

1. Basal compartment This small space between the basal lamina and the junctional belt is accessible to any blood-borne substance that can penetrate the basal lamina. This compartment houses the spermatogonia.

2. Adluminal compartment This compartment, which extends from the junctional belt inward to the center of the lumen, is inaccessible to blood-borne substances that are unable to pass the belt of junctional complexes. Only substances taken up by the supporting cells and passed on through their cytoplasm gain access to this privileged space.

III. DUCT SYSTEM.

Extending from the tubuli recti in the testis through the ejaculatory duct in the prostate and into the urethra, the duct system has roles in the maturation, storage, and transport of spermatozoa. All parts require adequate circulating testosterone for maintenance of normal function. The secretory epithelial lining provides spermatozoa with nutrients. Two complete sets of ducts (one per testis) empty into a common urethra.

A. Intratesticular Genital Ducts:

1. Tubuli recti (straight tubules) These connect the seminiferous tubules to the rete testis. The epithelium changes along their length. They begin with epithelium similar to that of the seminiferous tubules and gradually lose the spermatogenic cells until only

Sertoli cells are left in the short segment. It is replaced in the main segment by simple cuboidal epithelium supported by a dense connective tissue sheath.

2. Rete testis An anastomosing network of tubules lying in the mediastinum testis, the rete testis is lined by low cuboidal epithelium.

3. Ductuli efferentes (efferent ductules) There are from 10 to 20 4–6-mm long ducts connecting the rete testis with the epididymis. There is some smooth muscle in the walls, and the epithelium has alternating groups of simple cuboidal and ciliated columnar cells. The cuboidal cells absorb much of the fluid secreted by seminiferous tubules, while the cilia sweep the spermatozoa toward the epididymis. Together the ductules form the head of the epididymis, they converge to form a single ductus epididymis.

B. Excretory Genital Ducts:

1. Ductus epididymis This is a single, highly coiled 4–6-m long tube that comprises the body and tail of the epididymis. It is lined by pseudostratified columnar epithelium resting on a basal lamina. Its cells have abundant apical **stereocilia** (long, irregular, nonmotile microvilli) and secrete glycerophosphocholine (a possible capacitation inhibitor) and a glycoprotein of unknown function that binds to the spermatozoa. The epithelial cells also phagocytose and digest residual bodies sloughed off during spermatogenesis. A sheath of circular smooth muscle underlies the basal lamina, gradually thickening along the length of the tube. Peristaltic contractions of this muscle propel sperm toward the ductus deferens. Sperm move slowly through this long coiled tube, they are often seen in its lumen in tissue sections.

2. Ductus deferens (vas deferens) A single straight tube with thick muscular walls, it begins in the scrotum at the termination of the epididymis. It ascends within the spermatic cord through the inguinal canal into the abdomen, joining with the duct of the seminal vesicle in the pelvic cavity near the prostate. The lumen is narrowed by longitudinal mucosal folds. The lining is pseudostratified columnar epithelium, with fewer stereocilia than in the epididymis. The 3 layers of smooth muscle in the wall (inner and outer longitudinal, middle circular) are capable of powerful peristaltic contractions during ejaculation. The diameter of the duct increases near the termination to form the **ampulla,** which is characterized by a highly folded mucosa.

3. Ejaculatory duct This short duct, lined by pseudostratified columnar epithelium, is formed by the junction of the ductus deferens and the duct of the seminal vesicle. It penetrates the prostate to empty into the prostatic urethra.

4. Urethra The male urethra serves as a genitourinary passageway shared by the urinary and reproductive systems (its divisions, structure, and epithelial lining are described in Chapter 19).

IV. ACCESSORY GENITAL GLANDS

A. Seminal Vesicles: The paired seminal vesicles each consist of 2 highly coiled 15-cm-long tubes that develop as outgrowths of the ductus deferens. Their mucosa is highly folded, with primary, secondary, and tertiary branching patterns. The pseudostratified low columnar epithelium forms the secretory product. This is a thick, yellowish liquid that is rich in fructose; it also contains citrate, inositol, prostaglandins, and several proteins. Seminal vesicle secretions make up 70% of the human ejaculate. The smooth muscle underlying the lamina propria contracts during ejaculation. In each gland, the tubes converge to form a single duct that joins with the ductus deferens of each side to form the ejaculatory duct.

B. Prostate Gland: Located below the urinary bladder, the prostate surrounds the urethra at its origin from the bladder. It consists of 30–50 compound tubuloalveolar glands arranged in 3 concentric groups—mucosal, submucosal, and main—whose ducts empty independently into the urethra. The mucosa is folded, and the epithelium varies from tall cuboidal to pseudostratified columnar; it produces the secretory product, prostatic fluid, which is rich in citric acid and acid phosphatase. The fluid also contains amylase, fibrinolysin, and lipids. The entire gland is surrounded by a fibroelastic capsule containing smooth muscle that contracts during ejaculation, expelling the prostatic fluid into the urethra. Extensions of the capsule form smooth muscle-containing septa that penetrate the gland, divide it into indistinct lobes, and aid in expulsion of the prostatic fluid. Histologically, a characteristic feature of the prostate is the presence of **corpora amylacea** in the lumen of the gland. These small glycoprotein spheres become larger, more numerous, and calcified with age, but their significance is unknown.

C. Bulbourethral Glands (Cowper's glands): These paired spheric tubuloalveolar glands are 3–5 mm in diameter and are lined by cuboidal epithelium. Their ducts empty clear mucous secretions into the membranous urethra, where they act as a lubricant.

V. PENIS

A. General Organization: The penis consists of 3 cylindric bodies of spongy erectile tissue surrounded by a common loose connective tissue sheath and covered by hairless thin skin.

1. Corpora cavernosa Each of these 2 dorsally located erectile cylinders is penetrated by a deep artery and surrounded by a thick layer of dense fibrous connective tissue, the **tunica albuginea**.

2. Corpus spongiosum (corpus carvernosum urethrae) This single, smaller, ventrally located cylinder is surrounded by a somewhat thinner connective tissue sheath. Its expanded distal tip is termed the **glans penis.** The corpus spongiosum is penetrated along its length by the cavernous (penile) urethra, whose lumen is continuous with the exterior through an opening (the urethral meatus) in the glans.

3. Erectile tissue Within each of the cylinders is an irregularly arranged network of fibrous connective tissue trabeculae containing smooth muscle fibers. The trabeculae form the supporting framework between the numerous lacunae (vascular sinuses) that are lined by endothelium.

B. Blood Supply: The blood supply of the penis depends on its functional state.

1. Flaccid The peripheral dorsal arteries in the loose connective tissue sheath supply much of the arterial blood, which is drained by the superficial veins. In the flaccid state, arteriovenous shunts between the deep arteries in the corpora cavernosa and the superficial veins are open, and the branches of the deep arteries that feed the vascular spaces (the **helicine arteries**) are closed.

2. Erect In this condition, the arteriovenous shunt closes down. The deep arteries in the corpora cavernosa force blood through the dilated helicine arteries into the vascular spaces in the erectile tissue. The sudden filling of the lacunae may block the veins draining them. While the erectile tissue of the corpus spongiosum also fills, it does not become as rigid as the other 2 compartments.

C. Innervation: Parasympathetic stimulation causes erection by affecting the arteriovenous shunts and helicine arteries. The sympathetic discharge associated with ejaculation contributes to the subsequent decline of parasympathetic activity and the return of the penis to its flaccid state.

Study-Focusing Questions*

1. Draw a sketch of a sagittal section through a testis (423) and include and label the following components:
   a. Anterior surface
   b. Posterior surface
   c. Tunica albuginea (422, 423)
   d. Mediastinum testis (423)
   e. Interlobular fibrous septa (422, 423)
   f. Tunica vaginalis (422, 423)
   g. Testicular lobule (422, 423)
   h. Seminiferous tubules (422, 423)
   i. Tubuli recti (straight tubules) (422, 423)
   j. Rete testis (422, 423)
   k. Ductuli efferentes (422, 423)
2. How many of each of the structures named in question 1 are found in each testis (422, 423)?
3. Name, in order, the 3 layers of the wall of the seminiferous tubule, from the exterior to the lumen (422)
4. Name the 2 types of cells found in the germinal (seminiferous) epithelium (422).
5. Name, in order, the 3 phases of spermatogenesis (422) and compare them in terms of the:
   a. Cell type present at the beginning of each phase
   b. Cell type produced at the end of each phase
6. List the spermatogenic cell types in their order of appearance during spermatogenesis (422–427) and compare them in terms of:
   a. Their location in the germinal epithelium
   b. Their overall size (diameter)
   c. The appearance of their nuclei
   d. The number of chromosomes each contains
   e. The amount of DNA each contains
7. Describe the appearance, disappearance, changes, and movement of the following during spermiogenesis (424–427)
   a. Acrosome
   b. Centrioles
   c. Nucleus
   d. Manchette
   e. Mitochondria
   f. Residual bodies
8. Describe the contents and function of the acrosome (acrosomal cap) (425).
9. Describe the difference between spermatogonia A and B in terms of the cell type their progeny (daughter cells) become (422–423).
10. Describe Sertoli (supporting) cells in terms of:
    a. Their location (424, 427)
    b. Their shape and size (424, 427)
    c. The appearance of their nuclei (424, 427)
    d. Their 3 main functions (428)
11. Describe the blood-testis barrier (428, 433) in terms of:
    a. The cell type and cellular structures responsible for its formation
    b. Its location
    c. The contents of the basal and adluminal compartments it delineates
    d. Its function(s)
12. Describe the composition of the tissue found between the seminiferous tubules in the testicular lobules (431–432).

*The page references in this section refer to *Basic Histology,* 6th ed., Junqueira L, Carneiro J, Kelley R, (editors) Appleton & Lange, 1989. **HR** (for Histology Review) is occasionally used instead of a page reference to indicate that the information referred to can be found in this book.

13. Describe the interstitial (Leydig) cells (431–432) in terms of their:
    a. Location
    b. Shape
    c. Staining properties
    d. Primary function and the cellular organelle(s) involved
14. Name the cells primarily responsible for the production of the following and their major target sites and effects (in males):
    a. Testosterone (431–433)
    b. Androgen-binding protein (428, 433)
    c. Inhibin (431)
    d. FSH (431)
    e. LH
    f. Anti-Müllerian hormone (431)
15. Why is it important that the testes be maintained at a temperature below the core body temperature (432)?
16. What role do the following have in maintaining the optimal 35° C environment of the testes (432)?
    a. The scrotum
    b. The pampiniform plexus
    c. The cremaster muscle
17. Define cryptochidism (432) and describe its effect on:
    a. Spermatogenesis
    b. Testosterone production
18. List, in order, the 3 intratesticular ducts through which the spermatozoa pass after leaving the seminiferous tubules. Give the epithelial type found lining the lumen of each (479).
19. List, in order, the 3 excretory genital ducts (433) through which the spermatozoa pass on their way from the intratesticular ducts to the prostatic urethra and compare them in terms of:
    a. Their epithelial lining
    b. The amount and organization of smooth muscle in their walls
    c. The degree to which they coil
20. Compare stereocilia with true cilia in terms of the:
    a. Presence of basal bodies (434)
    b. Presence of microtubules at their core (434)
21. What is secreted by the cells lining the ductus epididymis (435)?
22. Compare the ampulla with the remainder of the ductus deferens in terms of their overall diameter and mucosal folds (435).
23. Compare the seminal vesicles, prostate gland, and bulbourethral glands in terms of:
    a. Their location and the point along the reproductive tract at which their ducts enter (423, 435–436)
    b. The composition of their secretory products (435–436)
    c. The epithelia lining their secretory portions (435–436)
    d. Their contribution to seminal fluid volume (435–436)
24. Describe the corpora amylacea (436) in terms of their location, biochemical composition, and change in number with age.
25. Sketch the penis in cross (423) and longitudinal (parasaggital) (437) section. Label the following in the sections indicated:
    a. Both cross and longitudinal sections
        (1) Corpus cavernosum penis
        (2) Corpus cavernosum urethra (corpus spongiosum)
        (3) Tunica albuginea
        (4) Urethra (pendulous)
        (5) Erectile tissue
        (6) Loose connective tissue
        (7) Skin
    b. Cross section only
        (1) Superficial and deep dorsal veins
        (2) Dorsal arteries
        (3) Deep arteries

c. Longitudinal section only
(1) Glans penis
(2) Fossa navicularis
(3) Prepuce

26. Describe the role(s) of the following in penile erection (438):
a. Parasympathetic innervation
b. The cavernous spaces (lacunae)
c. The helicine arteries
d. The arteriovenous shunts

Multiple-Choice Questions

For questions 22-1 through 22-5, select the single best answer.

22-1. The structure(s) shown in the photomicrograph in Fig 22-1 is/are the:
A. Seminiferous tubules
B. Ductus epididymis
C. Seminal vesicle
D. Ductus deferens
E. Tubuli recti

22-2. The structure(s) shown in the photomicrograph in Fig 22-2 is/are the:
A. Seminiferous tubules
B. Ductus epididymis
C. Seminal vesicle
D. Ductus deferens
E. Tubuli recti

22-3. The connective tissue sheath surrounding each seminiferous tubule is the:
A. Tunica albuginea
B. Septum
C. Tunica propria
D. Mediastinum testis
E. Tunica vaginalis

22-4. Spermatogonia are derived from:
A. Yolk sac endoderm

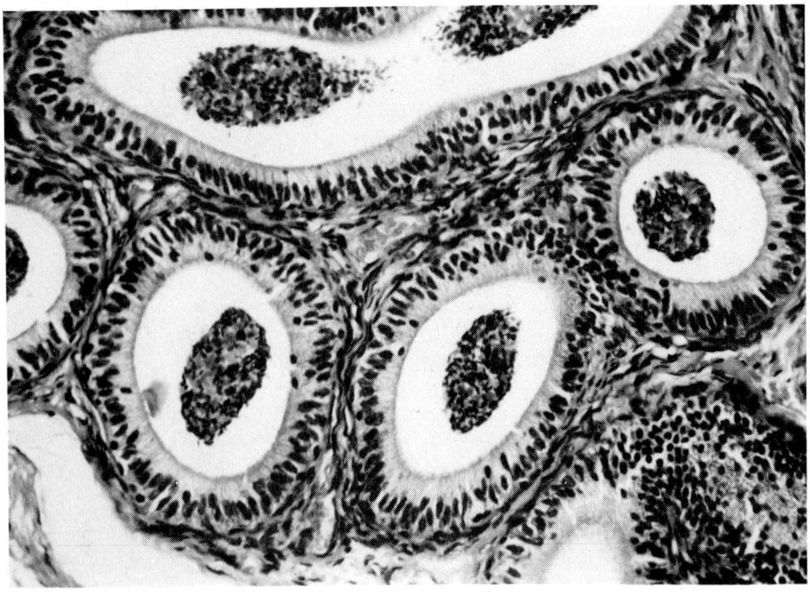

Figure 22-1.

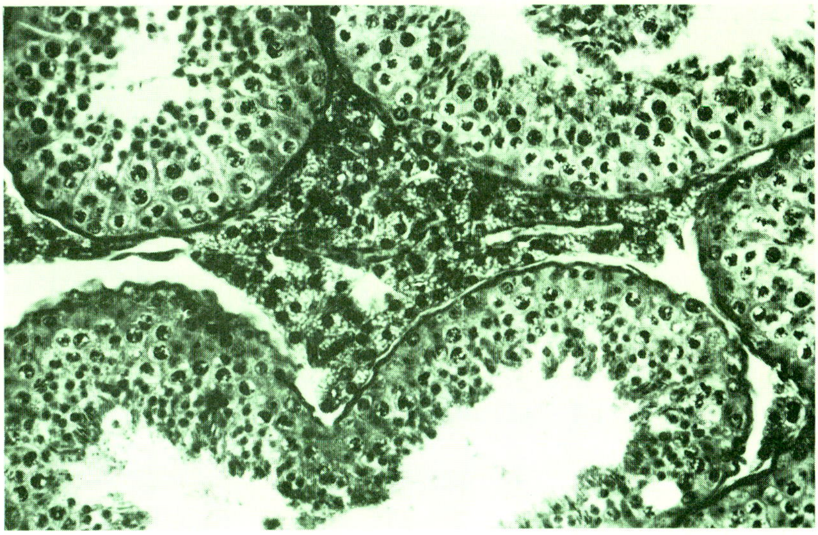

Figure 22-2.

B. Mesoderm in the genital ridge
C. The epithelial lining of the mesonephric tubules
D. Neural crest mesenchyme
E. Neural ectoderm

22-5. Spermiogenesis:
A. Occurs before puberty
B. Involves cytodifferentiation of spermatids
C. Includes spermatocytogenesis, meiosis, and spermatogenesis
D. Occurs in diploid cells
E. None of the above

MATCHING (questions 22-6 through 22-81): Each choice may be used once, more than once, or not at all.

Questions 22-6 through 22-24 use the letters in Fig 22-3.

22-6. Urinary bladder
22-7. Bulbourethral gland
22-8. Prostate
22-9. Seminal vesicle
22-10. Ductus deferens
22-11. Ampulla of ductus deferens
22-12. Ejaculatory duct
22-13. Penile urethra
22-14. Ductuli efferentes
22-15. Corpus cavernosum penis
22-16. Corpus cavernosum urethra
22-17. Ductus epididymis
22-18. Tubuli recti
22-19. Rete testis
22-20. Prepuce
22-21. Tunica vaginalis
22-22. Seminiferous tubules
22-23. Glans penis
22-24. Tunica albuginea

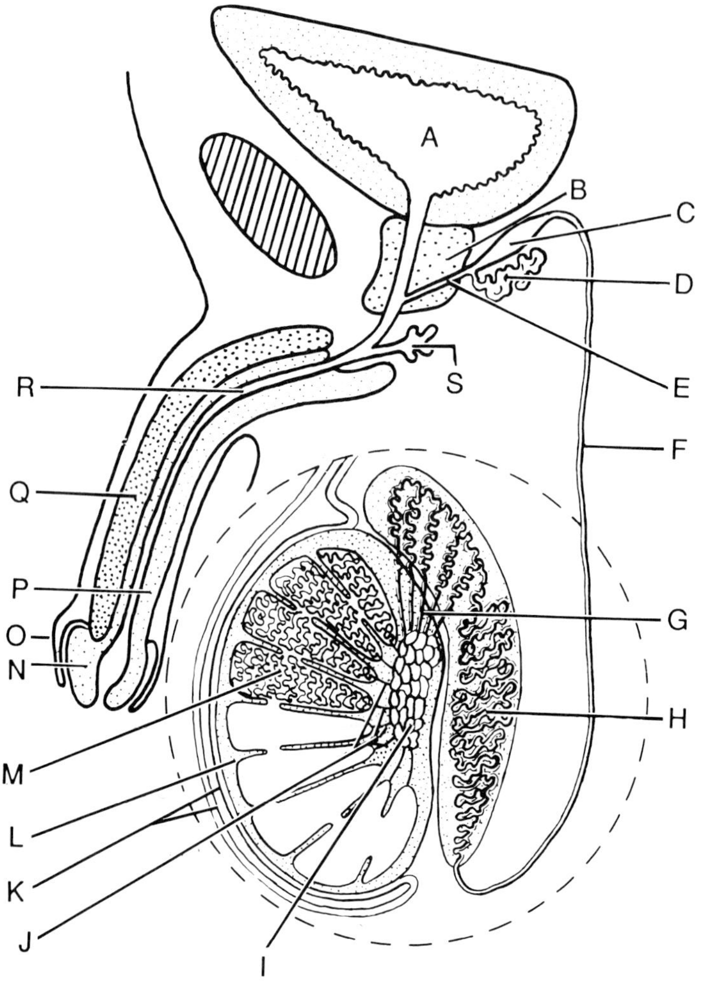

Figure 22-3.

Questions 22–25 through 22–37:

A. Spermatogonia
B. Primary spermatocytes
C. Secondary spermatocytes
D. Spermatids
E. Spermatozoa
F. Sertoli cells
G. Interstitial cells

22–25. Diploid (2n) chromosome number
22–26. Haploid (n) chromosome number
22–27. Usually seen in prophase of first meiotic division
22–28. Largest spermatogenic cell type
22–29. Only spermatogenic cell type present before puberty
22–30. Product of spermiogenesis
22–31. Product of spermatocytogenesis
22–32. Product of first meiotic division
22–33. Product of second meiotic division
22–34. Not a component of seminiferous epithelium
22–35. Derived from mesoderm in genital ridge

22-36. Rarely seen in histologic sections
22-37. Form the blood-testis barrier

Questions 22-38 through 22-46 use the letters in Fig 22-4.

22-38. Basal lamina
22-39. Myoid cells
22-40. Late spermatids
22-41. Early spermatids
22-42. Sertoli cell
22-43. Secondary spermatocyte
22-44. Primary spermatocyte
22-45. Spermatogonium
22-46. Interstitial cells

Questions 22-47 through 22-60:

A. Tubuli recti
B. Rete testis
C. Ductuli efferentes
D. Ductus epididymis
E. Ductus deferens
F. Ejaculatory duct
G. Prostatic urethra
H. Membranous urethra
I. Penile urethra

22-47. Single highly coiled duct
22-48. Number from 10 to 20
22-49. Located in mediastinum testis
22-50. Intratesticular genital ducts
22-51. Exhibits an ampulla near its termination

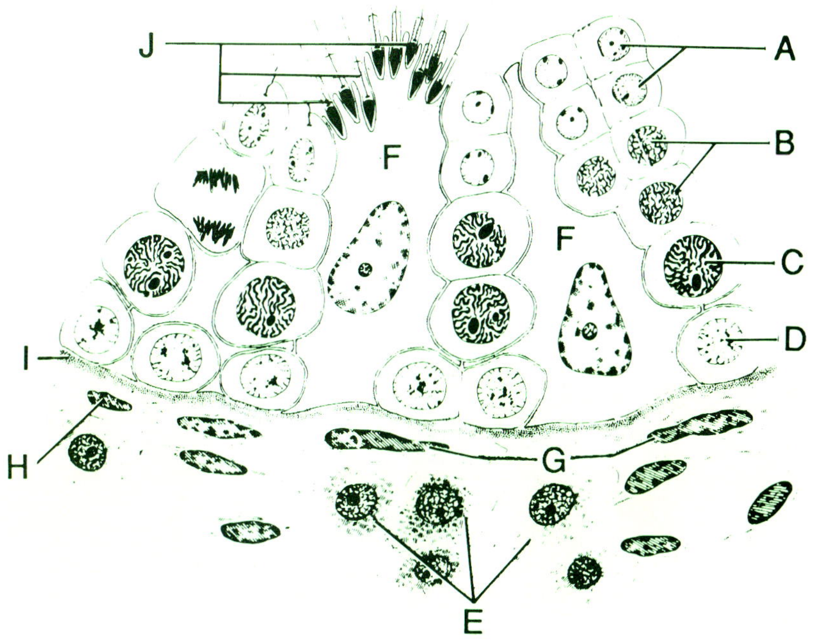

Figure 22-4.

22–52. Thickest muscular wall (3 layers)
22–53. Shortest portion of genitourinary tract
22–54. Second shortest portion of tract
22–55. Formed by junction of vas deferens and duct of seminal vesicle
22–56. Lined by pseudostratified columnar epithelium
22–57. Lining cells exhibit stereocilia
22–58. A portion of this duct is lined exclusively by Sertoli cells
22–59. Lined by alternating simple cuboidal and ciliated columnar epithelium
22–60. Lined by transitional epithelium

Questions 22–61 through 22–69 use the letters in Fig 22–5.

22–61. Tunica albuginea
22–62. Deep artery of the penis
22–63. Corpus cavernosum penis
22–64. Corpus cavernosum urethra
22–65. Urethra
22–66. Deep dorsal vein
22–67. Superficial dorsal vein
22–68. Dorsal arteries
22–69. Erectile tissue

Questions 22–70 through 22–81:

A. Testis
B. Seminal vesicles
C. Prostate gland
D. Bulbourethral glands
E. Glands of Littre

22–70. Common site of disease in older males
22–71. Secretions first enter reproductive tract in the urethra
22–72. Contains corpora amylacea

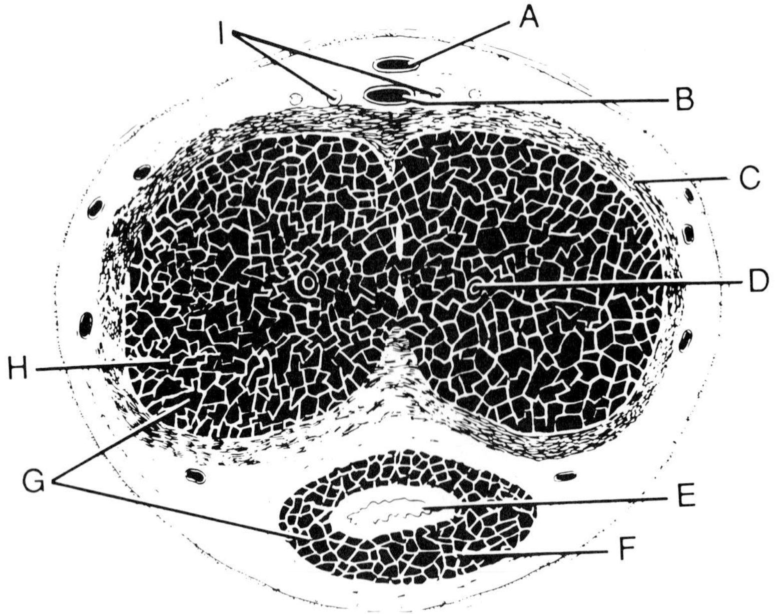

Figure 22–5.

22–73. Combined endocrine and exocrine functions
22–74. Secretes testosterone
22–75. Produces spermatozoa
22–76. Secretory product is rich in fructose
22–77. Secretory product is rich in acid phosphatase and citric acid
22–78. Produces 70% of ejaculate in humans
22–79. Secretes mucus
22–80. Secretions emptied directly into ejaculatory duct
22–81. Secretes inhibin

For questions 22–82 through 22–85, either, both or neither of the answers may be correct. Select

A if only A is correct
B if only B is correct
C if both A and B are correct
D if neither A nor B is correct

Questions 22–82 through 22–85:

A. Adluminal compartment
B. Basal compartment
C. Both
D. Neither

22–82. Contains spermatids
22–83. Contains spermatogonia
22–84. Contains Sertoli cells
22–85. Inaccessible to immune system

For questions 22–86 through 22–90, one, more than one, or all of the answers may be correct. Select

A if only (1), (2), and (3) are correct
B if only (1) and (3) are correct
C if only (2) and (4) are correct
D if only (4) is correct
E if all answers are correct

22–86. Functions of the Sertoli cells include:
(1) Physical support of the spermatogenic cells
(2) Phagocytosis of residual bodies
(3) Protection of spermatozoa from autoimmune attack
(4) Synthesis and secretion of androgen-binding protein

22–87. Interstitial (Leydig) cells:
(1) Secrete testosterone
(2) Have acidophilic cytoplasm
(3) Contain abundant smooth endoplasmic reticulum
(4) Are components of the seminiferous epithelium

22–88. Factors known to inhibit spermatogenesis include:
(1) Cryptorchidism
(2) LH
(3) Temperatures above 35°C
(4) Testosterone

22–89. Changes in the composition of seminal fluid that occur in the ductus epididymis include the:
(1) Addition of fructose
(2) Reduction in the number of residual bodies
(3) Release of acrosomal contents into fluid
(4) Addition of glycerophosphocholine

22–90. Erectile tissue:
(1) Is found in the corpus cavernosum penis
(2) Contains many endothelial cell-lined vascular spaces
(3) Is found in the corpus cavernosum urethra
(4) Fills with blood in response to stimulation by postganglionic sympathetic neurons

23 Female Reproductive System

Objectives

This chapter should help the student to:

- Name and describe the location and positional relationships between the internal organs and the external genitalia of the female reproductive system.
- Describe the location of the coverings, cortex, medulla, and follicles of the ovary as they appear in a longitudinal section.
- Describe the embryonic origin of the female germ cells (oogonia) and the changes they undergo during oogenesis.
- Describe the structural changes that accompany the successive stages of ovarian follicle maturation.
- Describe the process of ovulation.
- Describe the formation of the corpus luteum.
- Describe the role of FSH and LH in the activation and maturation of ovarian follicles and in ovulation.
- Name the cells responsible for the production of estrogen and progesterone and describe the conditions under which they are produced.
- Describe the role(s) of estrogen and progesterone in modulating the production of FSH and LH by the pituitary.
- Identify the following in a slide or photomicrograph of a section through an ovary: germinal epithelium, tunica albuginea, cortex, medulla, primordial follicles, primary follicles, secondary follicles, mature follicles, atretic follicles, oocytes, granulosa cells, theca interna, theca externa, antrum, cumulus oophorus, corona radiata, zona pellucida, corpus luteum, corpus albicans, granulosa lutein cells, theca lutein cells, and interstitial cells.
- Name and compare the wall structure of the segments of the oviduct.
- Describe the oviduct's structural features and functional activities that help to recover and transport the ovum after ovulation.
- Distinguish between the infundibulum, ampulla, isthmus, and interstitial (intramural) portion in a slide or photomicrograph of an oviduct and identify the mucosa, muscularis, serosa, ciliated cells, and nonciliated secretory (peg) cells.
- Describe the boundaries of the fundus, body, and cervix of the uterus and indicate which is covered by a serosa, by an adventitia, or by neither.
- Describe the thickness, location, and composition of the myometrium.
- Describe the changes in the myometrium during and after pregnancy.
- Describe the location, structure, and blood supply of the endometrium.
- Describe the changes in endometrial structure that accompany the phases of the menstrual cycle.
- Correlate cyclic changes in the endometrium with events occurring in the ovary and with changing levels of pituitary and ovarian hormones.

- Compare the structure of the wall of the cervix with that of the fundus and body of the uterus.
- Describe the effects of progesterone on the cervical secretions.
- Identify the following from a slide or photomicrograph of a section through the fundus or body of the cervix: the phase of the menstrual cycle, the endometrium, myometrium, serosa or adventitia, functionalis, basalis, endometrial glands, straight arteries, and coiled arteries.
- Identify the cervical glands, simple columnar epithelium, stratified squamous epithelium, internal os, cervical canal, and external os in a slide or photomicrograph of a section through the uterine cervix.
- Describe the changes in the embryo's structure and location and the usual amount of time elapsed between fertilization and implantation.
- Distinguish between zygote, morula, and blastocyst.
- Name the parts of the blastocyst and indicate which form the embryo and which form the fetal part of the placenta.
- Describe the process of implantation, including changes in both the embryo and the endometrium.
- Distinguish between the 3 named regions of the decidua.
- Distinguish between primary, secondary, and tertiary chorionic villi.
- Distinguish between the fetal and maternal parts of the placenta in terms of structure and function.
- Name the layers of the placental barrier.
- Identify the following in a slide or photomicrograph of an implanted blastocyst or early embryo: chorion, syncytiotrophoblast, cytotrophoblast, extraembryonic mesenchyme, inner cell mass, decidua capsularis and basalis, uterine glands, maternal lacunae, and primary, secondary, or tertiary chorionic villi.
- Describe the structure of the 3 layers of the vaginal wall.
- Describe the effect of estrogen on the vaginal epithelium.
- Describe the innervation of the vagina.
- From a slide or photomicrograph, distinguish the microscopic structure of the vaginal wall from that of the esophagus in terms of mucosal glands and orientation of smooth muscle in the muscularis.
- Name the parts of the vulva and describe their structure and innervation.
- Describe the histologic structure of the mammary glands in the prepubertal state, in adult women, during pregnancy, and during lactation.
- Describe the cellular synthesis and secretion of the various components of milk by the epithelial cells of the mammary gland alveoli.
- Name the hormone(s) responsible for breast growth, activation and maintenance of lactation, and milk ejection.
- Identify the functional state of a mammary gland (prepubertal, resting adult, pregnant, or lactating) from a slide or photomicrograph.
- Identify the secretory cells, alveoli, lactiferous ducts, lactiferous sinuses, connective tissue, adipocytes, and plasma cells in a slide or photomicrograph of a mammary gland.

Synopsis

I. GENERAL FEATURES OF THE FEMALE REPRODUCTIVE SYSTEM

A. Components of the System: This system includes the ovaries, uterine tubes (oviducts), uterus, vagina, and the external genitalia.

1. Ovaries These are the female gonads. They contain follicles that promote the development of the eggs (ova) they contain; they also produce estrogen. After a mature ovum is released, the remaining components of the follicle form a corpus luteum that produces both estrogen and progesterone.

2. Uterine tubes These oviducts capture the released ovum, serve as the primary site of fertilization, and convey the ovum (whether fertilized or unfertilized) to the uterus.

3. Uterus This is lined by a mucosa (endometrium) that undergoes cyclic structural changes controlled by the ovarian hormones. These changes prepare the uterus for its role as the site of implantation and nourishment of the fertilized ovum.

4. Vagina This tubelike organ helps to direct the spermatozoa through the cervical os, the narrow opening in the base of the uterus. The fluid in the vaginal lumen increases sperm motility. Under the influence of estrogen, the vaginal epithelium thickens and its cells accumulate glycogen, which is released into the lumen during exfoliation.

5. External genitalia These include the clitoris and labia minora and majora; they contain numerous nerve endings that play a role in sexual arousal.

B. Cyclic Changes: Between **menarche** (first menses) and **menopause,** cyclic changes occur, roughly every 28 days, in the structure and activity of each organ, especially the ovaries and uterus. The coordinated timing of these changes, crucial to normal reproductive function, is controlled mainly by the pituitary gonadotropins FSH and LH. These hormones directly affect the ovaries, modulating follicular growth and development as well as ovarian hormone production. Ovarian hormones (estrogen and progesterone) control the menstrual cycle (ie, the cyclic changes occurring in the uterine lining) and influence the production of pituitary gonadotropins through negative feedback.

C. Early Embryonic Development: Selected aspects of early embryonic development are described in this chapter as they relate to the structure and function of the female reproductive system. These include fertilization, preimplantation embryonic development, implantation, and the formation and functions of the placenta.

D. Mammary Glands: Because the mammary glands also undergo histologic changes related to the reproductive cycle, pregnancy, and pituitary and ovarian hormones, they are also covered in this chapter.

II. OVARIES

A. General Organization: The ovaries are paired almond-shaped organs ($3 \times 1.5 \times 1$ cm) that are attached by the mesovarium to the broad ligaments. They lie in the pelvic cavity.

1. Coverings Although the ovaries' outermost covering is called the **germinal epithelium,** it does not form oocytes, as the name suggests. It consists of a layer of simple cuboidal epithelium derived from the peritoneum. The inner covering, the **tunica albuginea,** consists of a dense connective tissue layer lying between the germinal epithelium and the ovarian cortex.

2. Internal structure Each ovary has a peripheral **cortex** and a central **medulla.** The cortex harbors most of the oocyte-containing ovarian follicles embedded in connective tissue **(stroma).** The medulla consists of stroma containing a rich vascular bed.

B. OVARIAN FOLLICLES: Each follicle consists of an oocyte surrounded by one or more layers of follicular (granulosa) cells. The ovarian cortex contains follicles at various stages of development.

1. Primordial follicles The earliest stage of follicular development, these inactive follicles are the only ones present prior to puberty, and constitute the majority thereafter. Each consists of a primary oocyte (most in the diplotene stage of meiosis I prophase) surrounded by one layer of flattened follicular cells.

2. Growing follicles Growth of the follicles is stimulated by pituitary FSH. The oocyte enlarges to a maximum diameter of 125–150 μm. The follicular epithelium becomes cuboidal and proliferates to become stratified (multilaminar) epithelium. The stromal connective tissue immediately surrounding the follicle differentiates, becoming the steroid hormone-producing **theca folliculi.**

a. Primary follicles These follicles consist of a primary oocyte surrounded by single or multiple layers of follicular cells. They have no antrum.

(1) Unilaminar primary follicles These consist of a single layer of cuboidal follicular cells surrounding an oocyte. At this stage, the glycoprotein-rich **zona pellucida** begins to form between the oocyte and the follicular cells.

(2) Multilaminar primary follicles These have multiple layers of follicular cells surrounding an oocyte. During this stage, the zona pellucida thickens and the **theca folliculi** begins to form.

b. Secondary follicles During this stage, cavities filled with fluid **(liquor folliculi)** appear between the follicular cells, gradually coalescing to form a single large cavity, or **antrum.** The theca folliculi forms 2 layers: the **theca interna**, containing a rich vascular network and steroid-secreting cuboidal cells with abundant smooth endoplasmic reticulum; and the **theca externa,** consisting primarily of vascular connective tissue.

3. Mature (graafian) follicles These are distinguished from late secondary follicles mainly by their large size (2.5 cm in diameter). In this stage, which immediately precedes ovulation, the antrum increases greatly in size. The oocyte is displaced to one side of the follicle, it is surrounded by a few layers of follicular cells **(corona radiata)** and rests on a pedestal of follicular cells **(cumulus oophorus)**.

4. Atretic follicles Although about 400,000 follicles are normally present at birth, only about 450 develop to maturity. About 99% become atretic (ie, they degenerate through autolysis) at various stages of development. Atresia of the primordial follicles leaves a space that is immediately filled by the stroma; as a result, no vestiges of atretic primordial follicles are seen in adult ovaries. The autolytic remnants of the larger primary and secondary follicles are removed by macrophages and replaced, by the stromal cells, with a wavy collagenous scar. The scar is gradually removed and remodeled into normal stromal tissue. Some thecal cells from the atretic follicles may remain, becoming interstitial cells that actively secrete steroids, especially androgens.

C. Origin and Maturation of Oocytes: Yolk sac endoderm gives rise to **primordial germ cells,** which migrate to the genital ridges from which the ovaries develop. The germ cells are surrounded by the flattened follicular cells of primordial follicles; they enter the first meiotic division and become arrested in prophase. At this point, they are termed **primary oocytes** (comparable to primary spermatocytes; see Chapter 22). The first meiotic division, which is completed just before ovulation, involves equal division of the chromatin but unequal division of the cytoplasm between the resulting **secondary oocytes.** The secondary oocyte that retains almost all the cytoplasm is the ovum; the other is termed the **first polar body.** Once formed, but still prior to ovulation, the ovum begins the second meiotic division, which halts in metaphase until fertilization occurs. At fertilization, the second meiotic division is completed and the **second polar body** is formed. The fertilized ovum is called the **zygote.**

D. Ovulation: Normally occurring about the 14th day of an idealized 28-day cycle, ovulation involves the rupture of a mature follicle and the release of the ovum. It is preceded and stimulated by a surge in LH production by the pituitary. The volume of the liquor folliculi in the antrum increases. The ovum and its surrounding corona radiata detach from the cumulus oophorus and float in the antrum. The stroma thins, possibly because of collagenase activity, and becomes ischemic between the preovulatory follicle and the surface of the ovary, indicating the site of imminent rupture, or **stigma.** Upon rupture, the ovum, with its corona radiata intact, is expelled by the ovary and captured by the uterine tube. If it is not fertilized within 24 hours, the ovum degenerates.

E. Corpus Luteum: This temporary endocrine gland is formed by the remnants of the follicle after ovulation.

1. Formation After ovulation, the follicle collapses and the granulosal lining is thrown into folds; a small amount of bleeding from the rupture may result in a central clot. Cells in the granulosa layer and theca interna enlarge and take on the appearance of steroid-secreting cells. The **granulosa lutein** cells are large pale-staining progesterone-secreting cells derived from the granulosa cells. The **theca lutein cells,** which secrete estrogen, are smaller, darker-staining cells derived from the cells of the theca interna.

2. Corpus luteum of menstruation If fertilization does not occur, the corpus luteum degenerates after about 14 days.

3. Corpus luteum of pregnancy If fertilization does occur, the corpus luteum enlarges. It is maintained for 6 months; although it gradually declines, it persists until the end of the pregnancy. In addition to estrogen and progesterone, the cells of this structure secrete **relaxin,** a polypeptide hormone that loosens the connective tissue attachment of the symphysis pubis, allowing the pelvic opening to enlarge during parturition.

4. Corpus albicans This dense connective tissue scar that replaces a degenerated corpus luteum is larger for a corpus luteum of pregnancy than for that of menstruation. Like the atretic follicles, it is eventually removed by macrophages.

F. Hormones and Ovarian Function: Pituitary FSH stimulates follicular growth during the first half of the cycle. The growing follicles produce estrogen, whose high midcycle level exerts negative feedback on FSH production. This stimulates a surge in the production of pituitary LH which controls final maturation of the follicle, stimulates ovulation, and controls the formation and maintenance of the corpus luteum. The corpus luteum produces both estrogen and progesterone. Progesterone inhibits LH production, causing the corpus luteum to degenerate after about 14 days unless fertilization occurs. If the ovum is fertilized and implants in the uterus, **chorionic gonadotropin** produced by the developing placenta maintains the corpus luteum in the absence of LH.

III. UTERINE TUBES.

Also called oviducts and fallopian tubes, these are paired 12-cm-long muscular tubes. The lumen of each is proximally continuous with the uterine cavity. Each tube extends from the uterus toward an ovary, with the distal end opening into the peritoneal cavity near the ovary.

A. Function: The uterine tube moves close to the ovary before ovulation and captures the ovum after ovulation. It provides a suitable environment for, and is the most common site of, fertilization and transports the zygote (or unfertilized ovum) to the uterus.

B. Uterine Tube Segments: Beginning proximal (ie, closest) to the uterus, the 4 segments are:

1. The **pars interstitialis** (or intramural portion), the segment that penetrates the uterine wall. It contains the fewest mucosal folds, and the myometrium contributes to its muscularis;

2. The **isthmus**, the narrow segment adjacent to the uterine wall, containing few mucosal folds;

3. The **ampulla,** the wide middle segment, which contains extensive branched mucosal folds and is the most common site of fertilization; and

4. The **infundibulum,** the funnel-shaped most distal segment, which opens near the ovary. Fingerlike extensions of its mucosal folds **(fimbriae)** project from the opening toward the ovary.

C. Wall Structure: The wall of the uterine tube has 3 layers.

1. Mucosa This includes the lamina propria and the lining epithelium. The folds of this layer are largest and most numerous in the ampulla; they decrease in size and number toward the uterus. The lining is a simple columnar epithelium that exhibits 2 major cell types:

a. Ciliated columnar cells The cilia on the apical surfaces of these cells beat in waves. While most beat toward the uterus and thus aid in egg transport, some beat toward the ovary and aid in sperm transport.

b. Peg cells These are shorter mucus-secreting cells interspersed among the cilitated cells. The film they produce is propelled toward the uterus by cilia, helping transport the ovum and hindering bacterial access to the peritoneal cavity.

2. Muscularis This layer exhibits inner circular and outer longitudinal layers. Its wave-like contractions move the ovum toward the uterus.

3. Serosa The outer covering of the tubes consists of visceral peritoneum.

IV. UTERUS.

A pear-shaped muscular organ in the pelvic cavity, this organ is the site of implantation and development of the early embryo.

A. Parts:

The uterus is grossly divided into 3 regions. The **body,** or **corpus,** is its large, round middle region. The **fundus** is the extension of the body above the point of entry of the uterine tubes. The neck, or **cervix,** is the narrow, inferior extension of the uterus into the vaginal canal.

B. Uterine Wall Structure.

In the fundus and body, this consists of 3 layers: the endometrium, myometrium, and serosa or adventitia.

1. Myometrium The muscularis of the uterus, it is the thickest tunic, consisting of 4 poorly defined layers of smooth muscle. The middle layers contain the abundant arcuate arteries that supply the endometrium. The smooth muscle of the myometrium grows extensively during pregnancy, involving both hypertrophy and hyperplasia. At birth, a surge of pituitary oxytocin induces the forceful myometrial contractions responsible for the expulsion of the fetus.

2. Endometrium The uterine mucosa, this layer consists of simple columnar epithelium supported by a lamina propria. Simple tubular glands extend from the surface into the lamina propria; their lining is continuous with the surface. The endometrium, which receives a double supply of blood, is divided into 2 regions:

a. Stratum functionale Also called the **pars functionalis,** this is the superficial temporary layer. It is responsive to ovarian hormones and undergoes cyclic thickening and shedding. This layer is further subdivided by some into a superficial **zona compacta** and a deeper **zona spongiosa.**

b. Stratum basale This thinner, deeper, permanent layer contains the basal portions of the endometrial glands and is retained during menstruation. It is the epithelial cells lining these glands that divide and cover the raw surface exposed during menstruation.

c. Blood supply Paired **uterine arteries** branch to form the **arcuate arteries** located in the middle of the myometrium. The arcuates give rise to 2 sets of arteries: **straight arteries** to the stratum basale and **coiled arteries** to the functionalis. The double blood supply to the endometrium is important in the cyclic shedding of the functionale: The coiled arteries are lost, while the straight arteries are retained.

3. Serosa and Adventitia These are the outer connective tissue coverings of the uterus. The fundus is covered by a cap of serosa, and the body is surrounded by an adventitia of loose connective tissue.

C. Menstrual Cycle:

The endometrium undergoes cyclic changes controlled by the ovarian hormones estrogen and progesterone. Ovarian hormone production is in turn controlled by the pituitary hormones FSH and LH and is related to follicular growth, to ovulation, and to the formation and degeneration of the corpus luteum. An average 28-day cycle is assumed in the description of the 3 phases below; the onset of menstrual bleeding is usually taken as day 1 of the cycle.

1. Menstrual phase This occupies the first 3–5 days of the cycle.

a. Endometrial changes The decline in ovarian progesterone production (caused by the degeneration of the corpus luteum of menstruation) causes intermittent constriction of the coiled arteries. This results in ischemia, degeneration, and shedding of the functionalis. Fragments of functionalis tissue along with blood and uterine fluid are discharged through the vagina as menstrual fluid. Because the straight arteries supplying the basale do not react to the hormonal changes, the basale remains intact.

b. Correlated ovarian changes In the absence of chorionic gonadotropin from an implanted embryo, the corpus luteum degenerates and progesterone production ceases.

2. Proliferative (or follicular) phase This phase occupies days 4–6 to day 14 of the cycle.

a. Endometrial changes Under the influence of increasing estrogen levels (and in preparation for possible implantation), the endometrium is regenerated from the remaining basale. As the functionalis thickens, the glands increase in length, remaining relatively straight.

b. Correlated ovarian changes Under the influence of pituitary FSH, the follicles grow and produce estrogen. The LH surge on day 14 induces ovulation and supports the formation of the corpus luteum.

3. Secretory (luteal) phase This stage occupies day 14 to day 28.

a. Endometrial changes The influence of progesterone from the developing corpus luteum causes growing of the glands, dilation of their lumens with secretions, edema of the connective tissue, and the resultant continuing thickening of the endometrium. The glands become highly coiled, exhibiting a sawtooth appearance in longitudinal section, and increase their secretion of glycoproteins (nutrients for the embryo before implantation). The coiled arteries elongate and grow closer to the luminal surface. By day 20 of the cycle, the endometrium is maximally prepared to receive an implanting embryo. Without implantation, the cycle begins again.

b. Correlated ovarian changes Pituitary LH supports the development of the corpus luteum. The granulosa lutein cells begin producing progesterone, and theca lutein cells produce estrogen. At the end of this phase, without chorionic gonadotropin from an implanted embryo, the corpus luteum degenerates and progesterone production ceases.

D. Uterine Cervix: The external surface of the cervix or neck of the uterus bulges into the vaginal canal. Its wall is composed primarily of dense connective tissue and includes only a small amount of smooth muscle. The mucosa has a tall simple columnar epithelium and highly branched cervical glands lining the internal surface (cervical canal). Stratified squamous epithelium covers its external (vaginal) surface. Although the cervical mucosa is not shed during menstruation, cyclic changes do occur in the amount and viscosity of the cervical secretions. At ovulation, for example, watery secretions permit penetration by sperm; in the luteal phase and during pregnancy, the secretions are abundant and viscous. Cervical dilation preceding parturition is due to intense collagenase activity in the cervical wall.

V. FERTILIZATION.

This occurs at the **ampullaristhmic junction** in the uterine tube when sperm penetrate the corona radiata, then the zona pellucida. Only one sperm head fuses with the plasma membrane of the ovum (**oolemma**). This event stimulates the completion of the second meiotic division of the ovum, and the second polar body is expelled. Finally, the haploid male and female pronuclei fuse to form the diploid nucleus of the zygote.

VI. PREIMPLANTATION DEVELOPMENT.

The zygote undergoes several rounds of mitosis to become a solid ball of cells, or **morula,** as it moves along the oviduct toward the uterus.

A cavity forms at the center of the embryo, which is now called a **blastocyst.** By this stage (the fourth day after fertilization), the embryo has entered the uterus. The blastomeres—the cells of the blastocyst—form 2 layers: a peripheral trophoblast, which will form the fetal part of the placenta, and a disk of cells (the inner cell mass), which will form the embryo, bulging into the cavity. After reaching the uterine lumen, the blastocyst floats free for 2–3 days before implantation. The zona pellucida dissipates at this time, allowing the trophoblast cells to contact the endometrium directly.

VII. IMPLANTATION

A. Decidual Reaction: Upon implantation, the penetration of the uterine epithelium by the early embryo, the endometrium undergoes changes referred to as the decidual reaction (the pregnant endometrium is now termed the **decidua**). During this reaction, the endometrium thickens and its stromal cells enlarge to become **decidual cells,** which secrete prolactin. The decidual reaction helps to prevent invasion of the trophoblast beyond the endometrium (a condition termed **placenta increta** or **percreta**). The decidua's 3 parts are:

1. The **decidua basalis,** the portion underlying the implantation site and forming the maternal part of the placenta;

2. The **decidua capsularis,** the portion overlying the implanted embryo and separating it from the uterine cavity; and

3. The **decidua parietalis,** the remainder of the endometrium, ie, the portion not in direct contact with the embryo.

B. Blastocyst Activity:

1. Trophoblast The trophoblast cells attach to the endometrium, divide rapidly, and differentiate into 2 layers. The **syncytiotrophoblast,** the highly invasive outer layer, consists of multiple nuclei in a single large cytoplasm. It is formed by the fusion of mononucleated cells from the underlying layer, the **cytotrophoblast.** The trophoblast erodes the uterine epithelium, allowing the embryo to invade the stroma. By day 9 after fertilization, the embryo is completely embedded in the endometrium and is surrounded by a trophoblastic shell. This type of implantation, in which the embryo becomes completely buried in the endometrium, is termed **interstitial implantation.**

2. Inner cell mass: The inner cell mass forms a bilaminar disk **(blastodisc),** which becomes the embryo itself, and a shell of extraembryonic mesoderm that lines the inner surface of the trophoblast. The blastodisc is separated from the extraembryonic mesoderm by a cavity, the **extraembryonic coelom.** The future embryo is thus separated from the endometrium by a 3-layered shell, or chorion.

3. Chorion This includes the syncytiotrophoblast, the cytotrophoblast and extraembryonic mesoderm. The chorion's 2 regions are:

a. The **chorion frondosum,** the portion adjacent to the decidua basalis, which forms the fetal part of the placenta; and

b. The **chorion laeve,** the portion adjacent to the decidua capsularis. Midway through pregnancy, this layer fuses with the decidua parietalis on the opposite side of the uterus, obliterating the uterine cavity.

VIII. PLACENTA.

This is a temporary organ whose formation begins during implantation. It is composed of both embryonic (chorion frondosum) and maternal (decidua basalis) tissues. The placenta transfers maternal nutrients and oxygen to the embryo, cleanses the fetal blood, and secretes hormones.

A. Steps in Placental Development (Placentation):

1. Lacunae The invading syncytiotrophoblast surrounds and delineates numerous islands of endometrial tissue containing blood vessels. Enzymes secreted by the syncytiotrophoblast lyse the maternal tissue, leaving spaces (lacunae) and rupturing blood vessels. The ruptured vessels fill the lacunae with maternal blood.

2. Primary villi These are solid cords that grow outward into the lacunae. Primary villi are composed of syncytiotrophoblast and cytotrophoblast.

3. Secondary villi The underlying extraembryonic mesenchyme invades the primary villi, forming secondary villi composed of syncytiotrophoblast, cytotrophoblast, and a core of extraembryonic mesenchyme.

4. Tertiary villi The extraembryonic mesenchyme in the secondary villi differentiates into blood vessels that will later establish connections with the umbilical vessels. Tertiary villi are thus composed of the syncytiotrophoblast, cytotrophoblast, and extraembryonic mesenchyme of the secondary villi, with blood vessels in their cores.

B. Placental Functions:

1. Transfer of nutrients and wastes By the twenty-third day of gestation, the fetal blood begins to circulate through the tertiary villi. Nutrients from the maternal blood in the lacunae reach the fetal circulation by passing through the syncytiotrophoblast; the cytotrophoblast, which later disappears after all the cells fuse with the syncytiotrophoblast; the basal lamina of the trophoblast; the extraembryonic mesenchyme; the basement membrane of the endothelial cells of the vessels in the tertiary villi; and the fetal endothelial cells. These 6 layers constitute the **placental barrier,** which permits only selected substances to cross to and from the maternal and fetal circulation. The boundary between fetal and maternal tissues is further marked by fibrinoid, a layer of the products of necrosis. This may form a nonantigenic barrier, which might explain maternal tolerance of fetal antigens (and vice versa).

2. Secretion of placental hormones The placenta secretes chorionic gonadotropin, chorionic thyrotropin, chorionic corticotropin; estrogens; progesterone; prolactin; and placental lactogen.

IX. VAGINA.

This muscular tube extends from the cervix to the external genitalia. Its walls lack glands, and vaginal lubrication involves secretions produced by the cervical and Bartholin's glands and the smaller mucous glands in the vestibule. The vaginal walls have 3 layers:

A. Mucosa:

This layer consists of stratified squamous epithelium, rich in glycogen, and supported by a lamina propria that contains abundant elastic fibers. Bacterial metabolism of glycogen from the lining cells exfoliated into the vaginal lumen results in the accumulation of lactic acid and causes the typically low pH of the vagina. The extensive capillary plexus in the lamina propria is the source of much of the fluid that seeps into the lumen during sexual stimulation. The vaginal mucosa contains few sensory nerve endings.

B. Muscularis:

Consisting mainly of longitudinal smooth muscle, the muscularis includes some circular fibers near the mucosa.

C. Adventitia:

This is the outer dense connective tissue sheath of the vagina. It is rich in elastic fibers and contains an extensive venous plexus; bundles of nerve fibers and clusters of neurons are also present.

X. EXTERNAL GENITALIA (VULVA). This area is richly innervated with Meissner's and pacinian corpuscles along with free nerve endings. The external genitalia include the following components:

A. Clitoris: A homologue of the dorsal part of the penis, it consists of 2 small erectile corpora cavernosa that end in a **glans clitoridis.** It is surrounded by a **prepuce** and covered by stratified squamous epithelium.

B. Vestibule: This receives the openings of the vagina and the urethra. It is lined by stratified squamous epithelium and includes 2 types of glands:

a. **Bartholin's glands (glandulae vestibulares majores)** are 2 large tubuloalveolar mucous glands on opposite sides of the vestibule. They are analogous to the bulbourethral (Cowper's) glands in males.

b. The **vestibular glands (glandulae vestibulares minores)** are smaller and more numerous mucous glands scattered around the vestibule, with the greater number near the urethra and clitoris. These are analogous to the glands of Littre in males.

C. Labia Minora: These are folds of skin with a core of spongy connective tissue covered by stratified squamous epithelium. They have a thin keratinized layer on their surfaces and while they contain sweat and sebaceous glands on both their surfaces, there are no hairs.

D. Labia Majora: These folds of skin have a core of subcutaneous fat and a thin layer of muscle. The inner surface of each is similar to that of the labia minora; the outer surface has more keratin and contains coarse hairs. Both surfaces contain numerous sebaceous and sweat glands.

XI. MAMMARY GLANDS. These accessory glands of the skin are specialized to secrete milk. Each of these compound tubuloalveolar glands contains 15–25 lobes, separated by both adipose and dense connective tissues. Each lobe empties through a **lactiferous duct,** which exhibits a terminal expansion, or **lactiferous sinus**, before opening independently on the surface of the richly innervated **nipple.** The extensive changes undergone by these glands are correlated with age and the functional state of the reproductive system.

A. Embryonic Development: **Milk lines,** paired ventral thickenings of the epidermis that run from forelimb to hindlimb, appear at 6 weeks. The caudal portions of these regress early. During the second trimester, 15–25 epithelial invaginations develop along these lines on each side of the thoracic region. These constitute the future lactiferous ducts. The remainder of the milk lines normally degenerates. Mammary secretion in newborns (under the influence of placental and maternal hormones) is common.

B. Prepubertal Mammary Gland: This nonfunctional gland is composed of lactiferous sinuses and ducts. The small nipple is surrounded by a lightly pigmented **areola.**

C. Changes During Puberty: The female breasts enlarge as a result of the accumulation of adipose and collagenous connective tissue, and the nipples become more prominent. Increased production of ovarian estrogen stimulates fat deposition and the proliferation—increased length, diameter, and branching—of the lactiferous ducts.

D. Adult Gland (resting): The basic subunits of the gland, the lobules develop as a result of growth during puberty. The lobules are separated from each other by loose interlobular connective tissue, and few secretory alveoli are present. Most of the lobules consist of several blind-ended **intralobular ducts,** these are lined by cuboidal epithelium that rests on a basal lamina and are surrounded by a discontinous layer of myoepithelial cells. All the intralobular ducts from one lobule empty into a single terminal **interlobular duct,** which leads to a larger lactiferous duct. The lactiferous ducts are lined by cuboidal-to-columnar epithelium, overlying a layer of densely packed, spindle-shaped, longitudinally oriented **myoepithelial cells** that separates the epithelium from its basal lamina. The lactiferous ducts empty through the stratified squamous-lined lactiferous sinuses. Minor changes occur during the menstrual cycle. The estrogen peak at ovulation induces further proliferation of the ducts, which can cause premenstrual breast enlargement, attended by transient edema and tenderness.

E. Adult Gland (during Pregnancy): The influence of several hormones, including estrogen, progesterone, prolactin, and human placental lactogen causes intense proliferation of the ducts and the growth of alveoli at their ends, enlarging the breasts. The terminal epithelium of the intralobular ducts proliferates and differentiates into milk-secreting cells, resulting in the formation of numerous secretory alveoli within the lobules. During pregnancy, the mammary alveolar cells are characterized by basal nuclei that are surrounded by rough endoplasmic reticulum, a supranuclear Golgi complex, scattered mitochondria, lysosomes, milk protein-containing secretory vesicles, and a few apical fat droplets. The alveolar cells and their basal lamina are separated by the myoepithelial cells. Late in pregnancy, the number of plasma cells in the interlobular connective tissue increases. These cells produce secretory IgA that is added to the mammary secretions (especially colostrum) and confers passive immunity on the newborn. Although the glands are well developed during pregnancy, secretions are not found in their lumens until late in the pregnancy, when they contain colostrum (protein-rich first milk), or during lactation, when they contain the actual lipid-rich milk.

F. Lactating Gland: With the loss of the placenta at birth, estrogen and progesterone levels decrease and prolactin levels increase. The major change in histologic appearance of the glands from pregnant glands is the accumulation of milk in the alveolar lumens and their accompanying dilation. The secretory cells reduce in height from low columnar to low cuboidal, and there are numerous fat droplets containing neutral triglycerides in their cytoplasm. During secretion, the fat droplets acquire a membrane from the cell apex **(apocrine secretion)**. Increased numbers of secretory vesicles containing milk proteins appear in the cytoplasm and are released via **merocrine secretion.**

1. Milk composition Milk typically comprises 4% lipids; 1.5% proteins (caseins, lactalbumin, IgA), 7% lactose (disaccharide of glucose and galactose), and 87.5% water.

2. Maintenance of lactation The sensory stimulus of suckling inhibits dopamine (or prolactin-inhibiting hormone) secretion by the hypothalamus. This increases the release of prolactin from the anterior pituitary, which in turn stimulates milk production in the mammary glands. With weaning—the cessation of suckling—prolactin levels fall and the alveoli degenerate.

3. Milk ejection reflex The sensory stimulus of suckling causes **oxytocin** synthesis in the hypothalamus. The release of oxytocin by the posterior pituitary stimulates myoepithelial cell contraction, ejecting milk from the alveoli into the lactiferous ducts.

G. Senile Involution: After menopause, the secretory portions, ducts, and adipose and interlobular connective tissues in the breasts atrophy.

Study-Focusing Questions*

1. List the paired and unpaired organs of the female reproductive system (439) and sketch a diagram showing their positional relationships (439).
2. Sketch a cross section of an ovary (440) and label the following:
   a. Germinal epithelium
   b. Tunica albuginea
   c. Cortex
   d. Medulla
   e. Ovarian follicles
3. Name, in order, the stages of follicular development, from primordial to mature (graafian) (440–441).
4. Differentiate between primordial and unilaminar primary follicles in terms of the height of the follicular epithelium (440, 441).
5. Differentiate between unilaminar and multilaminar primary follicles in terms of the number of layers of follicular cells surrounding the oocyte (440, 441).
6. Differentiate between primary and secondary follicles in terms of the presence of an antrum (440, 441).
7. Sketch a mature (graafian) follicle (441) and label the following (487):
   a. Theca externa
   b. Theca interna
   c. Antrum
   d. Liquor folliculi
   e. Follicular (granulosa) cells
   f. Oocyte
   g. Cumulus oophorus
   h. Corona radiata
8. Describe the following aspects of ovulation:
   a. Assuming menses begins on day 1 of an ideal 28-day menstrual cycle, on which day does ovulation occur (441)?
   b. Name the pituitary hormone whose production surges just before ovulation (441).
   c. Name the components of the mature follicle that are carried with the ovum, and those that are left behind after ovulation (442, 444).
9. Sketch a corpus luteum in cross section (440, 446) and indicate the location of the following:
   a. Fibrin clot or connective tissue core (if present)
   b. Granulosa lutein cells
   c. Theca lutein cells
   d. Surrounding stroma
10. Compare the corpus luteum of menstruation with the corpus luteum of pregnancy in terms of:
    a. The length of time they persist (444)
    b. The hormones they secrete (444)
    c. The hormone(s) that stimulate their formation and maintain their functional activity (444)
    d. Their size (446)
11. Name the hormones that have the following functions:
    a. Stimulate(s) follicle growth, oocyte maturation, and estogen production (459)
    b. Stimulate(s) ovulation (441)
    c. Stimulate(s) formation of the corpus luteum (459)
    d. Maintain(s) the corpus luteum of menstruation and stimulate(s) progesterone production (459)

*The page references in this section refer to *Basic Histology,* 6th ed., Junqueira L, Carneiro J, Kelley R (editors), Appleton & Lange, 1989. **HR** (for Histology Review) is occasionally used instead of a page reference to indicate that the information referred to can be found in this book.

- e. Maintain(s) the corpus luteum of pregnancy (444)
- f. Inhibit(s) FSH production and stimulate(s) LH production (459)
- g. Inhibit(s) LH production (444, 459)

12. Compare atretic follicles (443–444) and corpora albicans (446) in terms of:
    - a. Which degenerating ovarian structures they represent
    - b. Their size
    - c. The 2 types of each
    - d. The predominant tissue type(s) of which they are composed
    - e. Their persistance
13. Name the 4 segments into which each oviduct is divided and compare the segments (446) in terms of:
    - a. Their location in relation to the uterus and ovaries
    - b. Their luminal diameter
    - c. The size of their mucosal folds
    - d. The most common site of fertilization (447)
14. Name the 2 epithelial cell types found lining the lumen of the uterine tubes and compare them in terms of their height, apical specializations, and secretory activity (446).
15. Describe 3 ways in which the structure and function of the uterine tubes assist in ensuring safe passage of the ovum from the ovaries to the uterus (446–447).
16. On the diagram drawn for question 1, label and show the boundaries of the 3 parts of the uterus (447).
17. Name the 3 basic layers of the uterine wall (447).
18. Describe the myometrium (448) in terms of:
    - a. The type of muscle fibers it contains
    - b. The location(s) and name(s) of its major vessels
    - c. The 2 mechanisms responsible for its increased muscle mass during pregnancy
    - d. Its response to oxytocin during copulation and childbirth (400)
19. Name the 2 layers of the endometrium (448) and differentiate them in terms of which:
    - a. Includes the uterine epithelium (448)
    - b. Undergoes cyclic thickening and shedding (448)
    - c. Remains unchanged during the menstrual cycle (448)
    - d. Is more responsive to ovarian hormones (448)
    - e. Contains the portions of the endometrial glands that serve as the source of the epithelial cells that recover the uterine surface after menstruation (448)
    - f. Contains straight arteries (449)
    - g. Contains coiled arteries (449)
20. Compare the proliferative, secretory, and menstrual phases of the menstrual cycle (449–450) in terms of the:
    - a. Thickness of the functionalis
    - b. Appearance of the endometrial glands in histologic section
    - c. Degree of coiling of coiled arteries and their proximity to the epithelial surface
21. Draw a saggital section of the uterine cervix (455) and indicate the location of the simple columnar and stratified squamous epithelia (450) and the cervical glands (451, 455).
22. Describe fertilization in terms of:
    - a. The site where it usually occurs (447)
    - b. Whether it occurs before or after production of the second polar body by the ovum (444)
    - c. The change in chromosome number between the unfertilized and fertilized ovum (444)
    - d. The name applied to the fertilized ovum (444)
23. Distinguish between a zygote, a morula, and a blastocyst (452) in terms of:
    - a. Their size
    - b. The number of their cells
    - c. The size of their individual cells
    - d. The presence of a fluid-filled cavity
    - e. The stage at which the embryo reaches the uterus
    - f. The stage at which the inner cell mass and trophoblast initially form

g. The stage at which the zona pellucida disappears, allowing direct contact between the embryo and the uterine wall and leading to implantation

24. In general terms, name the structures that are formed by the inner cell mass and by the trophoblast (452).
25. Distinguish between the syncytiotrophoblast and the cytotrophoblast in terms of location and structure (452). Which disappears during later development (456)?
26. Describe decidual cells (457) in terms of structure, function, location, and origin.
27. Distinguish between the decidua basalis, decidua capsularis, and decidua parietalis in terms of location (452).
28. Distinguish between the chorion frondosum and chorion laeve in terms of their location (454).
29. Describe the formation of the lacunae (452) of the developing placenta in terms of:
    a. How these cavities in the endometrium originate
    b. How they become filled with maternal blood
    c. The tissue that forms their lining
30. Name the types of chorionic villi (452–454) and distinguish between them on the basis of the presence of the following:
    a. Syncytiotrophoblast
    b. Cytotrophoblast
    c. Extraembryonic mesenchyme
    d. Fetal blood vessels
31. Distinguish between the fetal (456–457) and maternal (458) parts of the placenta in terms of the:
    a. Specific structures (and regions) from which they originate
    b. Hormones they secrete (452, 458)
    c. Location of fibrinoid (454)
32. Draw a sketch of a chorionic villus extending into a lacuna (456) and label the 6 layers of the placental barrier (457–458) present during early pregnancy. Which of these layers is absent in late pregnancy (456)?
33. Name the 3 layers that form the wall of the vagina and describe the type of tissue(s) found in each layer (458).
34. Explain the usually acidic pH of the vagina and the increase of fluid in the vagina during sexual stimulation despite the fact that the vaginal wall has no glands (458).
35. List the components of the vulva and the structures that border the vestibule (459).
36. Compare the glandulae vestibulares majores (Bartholin's glands) with the glandulae vestibulares minores in terms of size, number, location, and secretory product (459).
37. Compare the clitoris and the penis (459) in terms of:
    a. Their embryonic origin
    b. Their size
    c. The presence of a glans and prepuce
    d. The number of erectile bodies
    e. Their epithelial covering
38. Compare the labia majora and labia minora (459) in terms of their location and the:
    a. Thickness of the stratum corneum on external and internal surfaces
    b. Presence of sweat and sebaceous glands
    c. Presence of coarse hairs
    d. Presence of smooth muscle
    e. Amount of their adipose tissue
39. Compare the innervation of the external genitalia (459) with that of the vagina (458).
40. Compare the prepubertal, resting adult, pregnant, lactating, and senile mammary glands (461–464) in terms of the presence and amounts of the:
    a. Lactiferous sinuses and ducts (461–464)
    b. Plasma cells (462)
    c. Adipose tissue (461, 465)
    d. Lobules (462)
    e. Alveoli (463)
    f. Fat droplets and secretory vesicles in alveolar cells (462, 463)
    g. Alveolar lumens distended with secretory product (milk) (compare micrographs on 462 and 463)

41. Compare the mechanism of secretion of milk proteins with that of milk lipids (463–464).

42. List the steps in the milk ejection reflex and name the structures involved in each step (464).

43. Describe the role of the plasma cells (462) and colostrum (464) in conferring passive immunity on the newborn.

44. Make a time line covering the period of the ideal 28-day menstrual cycle. Set day 1 as the first day of menstruation and indicate at which point, or over what periods in the cycle, the following events occur:
  - **a.** Uterus (449–450, 459)
    - **(1)** Menstrual phase
    - **(2)** Proliferative phase
    - **(3)** Secretory phase
  - **b.** Ovaries (440–446, 459)
    - **(1)** Follicular growth
    - **(2)** Degeneration of corpus luteum of menstruation
    - **(3)** Estrogen production
    - **(4)** Ovulation
    - **(5)** Progesterone production
    - **(6)** Corpus luteum forms
  - **c.** Pregnancy
    - **(1)** Fertilization (444)
    - **(2)** Entry of blastocyst into uterus (452)
    - **(3)** Implantation (452)
  - **d.** Pituitary (444, 448)
    - **(1)** FSH production
    - **(2)** LH surge

45. Name the cells that produce the following:
  - **a.** Relaxin (444)
  - **b.** Estrogen (444, 458, 459)
  - **c.** Follicle-stimulating hormone (459)
  - **d.** Luteinizing hormone (459)
  - **e.** Progesterone (444, 458)
  - **f.** Prolactin (393–394)
  - **g.** Oxytocin (464)
  - **h.** Androgens (444)
  - **i.** Chorionic gonadotropin (458)
  - **j.** Human placental lactogen (458)

Multiple-Choice Questions

For questions 23–1 through 23–8, select the single best answer.

23–1. The stage in ovarian follicle development that immediately follows the multilaminar primary follicle is the:
  - **A.** Unilaminar primary follicle
  - **B.** Secondary follicle
  - **C.** Primordial follicle
  - **D.** Corpus albicans
  - **E.** Graafian follicle

23–2. The section of endometrium shown in Fig 23–1 was taken from a uterus during which phase of the menstrual cycle?
  - **A.** Menstrual phase
  - **B.** Proliferative phase
  - **C.** Secretory phase
  - **D.** Follicular phase
  - **E.** None of the above

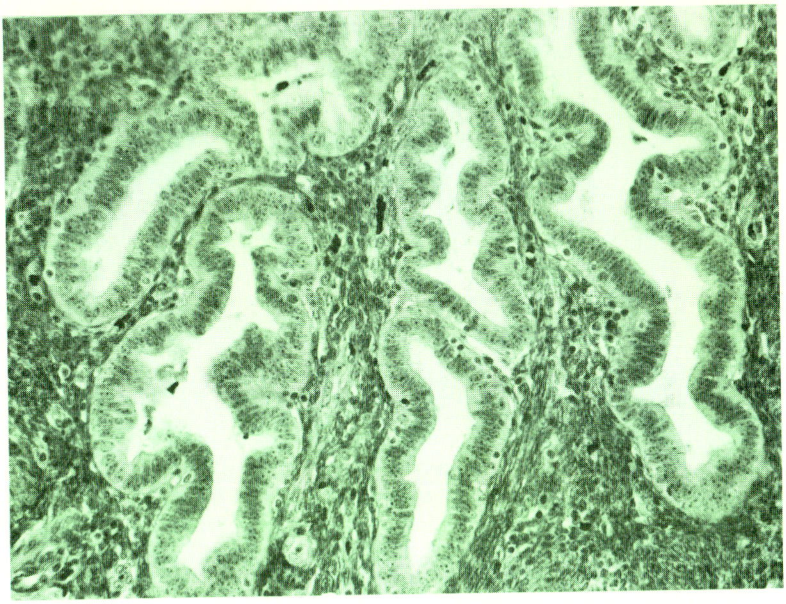

Figure 23-1.

23-3. The epithelial type shown in Fig 23-2 characteristically lines which female reproductive organ?
  A. Uterus
  B. Vagina
  C. Ovary
  D. Uterine tubes
  E. All of the above

23-4. The placenta is formed by the:
  A. Decidua basalis and the chorion laeve
  B. Decidua parietalis and the chorion frondosum
  C. Decidua capsularis and the chorion laeve
  D. Decidua parietalis and the chorion laeve
  E. Decidua basalis and the chorion frondosum

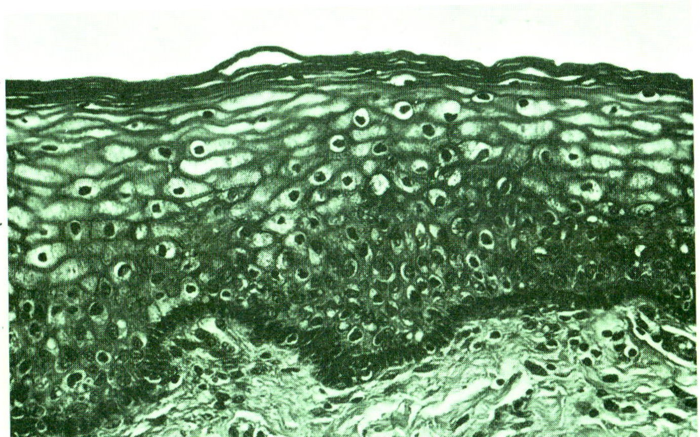

Figure 23-2.

23–5. The photomicrograph shown in Fig 23–3 is a cross section of the:
- **A.** Uterine cervix
- **B.** Body of the uterus
- **C.** Pars interstitialis of the uterine tube
- **D.** Ampulla of the uterine tube
- **E.** Isthmus of the uterine tube

23–6. The photomicrograph in Fig 23–4 depicts:
- **A.** A chorionic villus
- **B.** A uterine gland
- **C.** A mucosal fold of the uterine tube
- **D.** Fimbriae
- **E.** A vaginal gland

23–7. Secondary chorionic villi differ from primary chorionic villi in that they:
- **A.** Include the syncytiotrophoblast
- **B.** Include the cytotrophoblast
- **C.** Lack the cytotrophoblast
- **D.** Include the extraembryonic mesenchyme
- **E.** Lack fetal blood vessels

23–8. The acidic pH of the vaginal lumen is due primarily to:
- **A.** Bacterial conversion of the glycogen from exfoliated cells into lactic acid
- **B.** Bacterial conversion of mucus secreted by the vaginal glands into lactic acid
- **C.** Secretion of acid mucopolysaccharides by glands in the vaginal walls
- **D.** Secretion of HCl by cells in the vaginal glands
- **E.** Acidic secretions from the uterine glands entering the vagina through the cervix

MATCHING (questions 23–9 through 23–89): Each choice may be used once, more than once, or not at all.

Questions 23–9 through 23–14 use the letters in Fig 23–5.

23–9. Cervix
23–10. Vagina
23–11. Fimbriae
23–12. Uterine tube
23–13. Uterus
23–14. Ovary

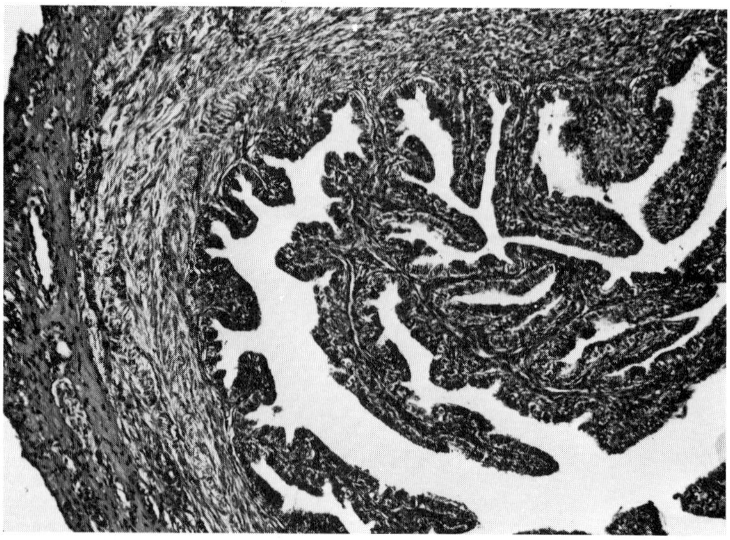

Figure 23–3.

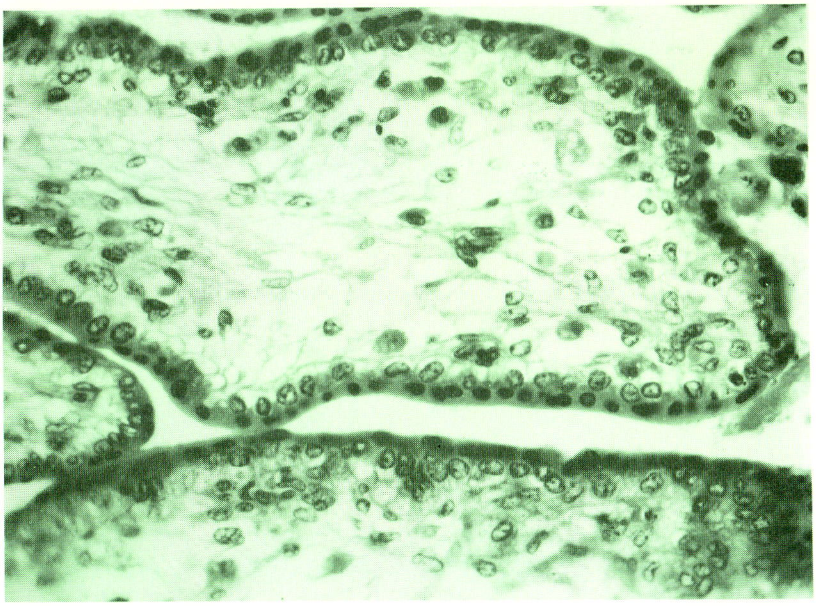

Figure 23-4.

Questions 23-15 through 23-22 use the letters in Fig 23-6.

23-15. Graafian follicle
23-16. Primordial follicle
23-17. Secondary follicle
23-18. Primary follicle
23-19. Corpus luteum
23-20. Atretic follicle
23-21. Medulla
23-22. Cortex

Questions 23-23 through 23-30 use the letters in Fig 23-7.

23-23. Oocyte nucleus
23-24. Cumulus oophorus
23-25. Corona radiata

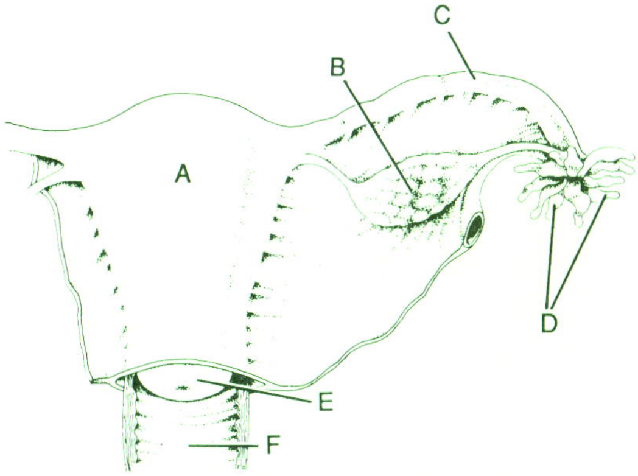

Figure 23-5.

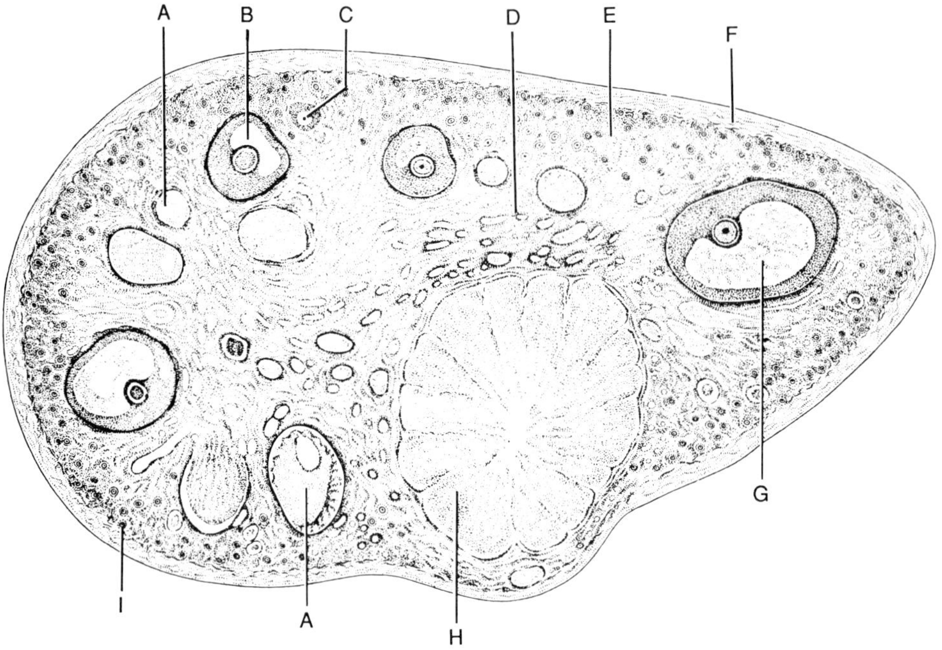

Figure 23-6.

23–26. Theca interna
23–27. Theca externa
23–28. Membrana granulosa
23–29. Oocyte
23–30. Antrum

Questions 23–31 through 23–40 use the letters in Fig 23–8.

23–31. Extraembryonic mesenchyme
23–32. Syncytiotrophoblast
23–33. Cytotrophoblast
23–34. Lacunae
23–35. Inner cell mass
23–36. Amniotic cavity

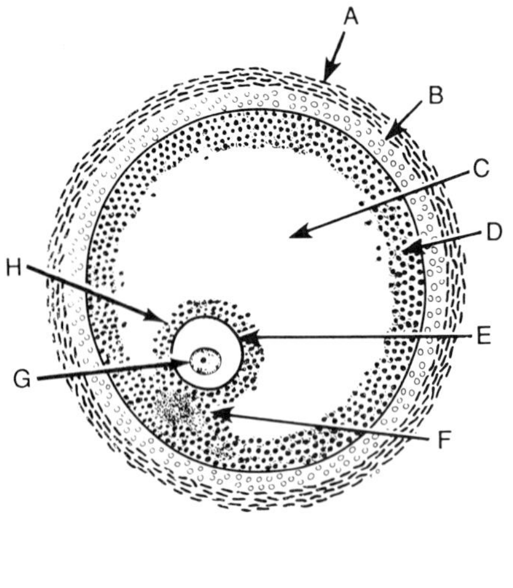

Figure 23-7.

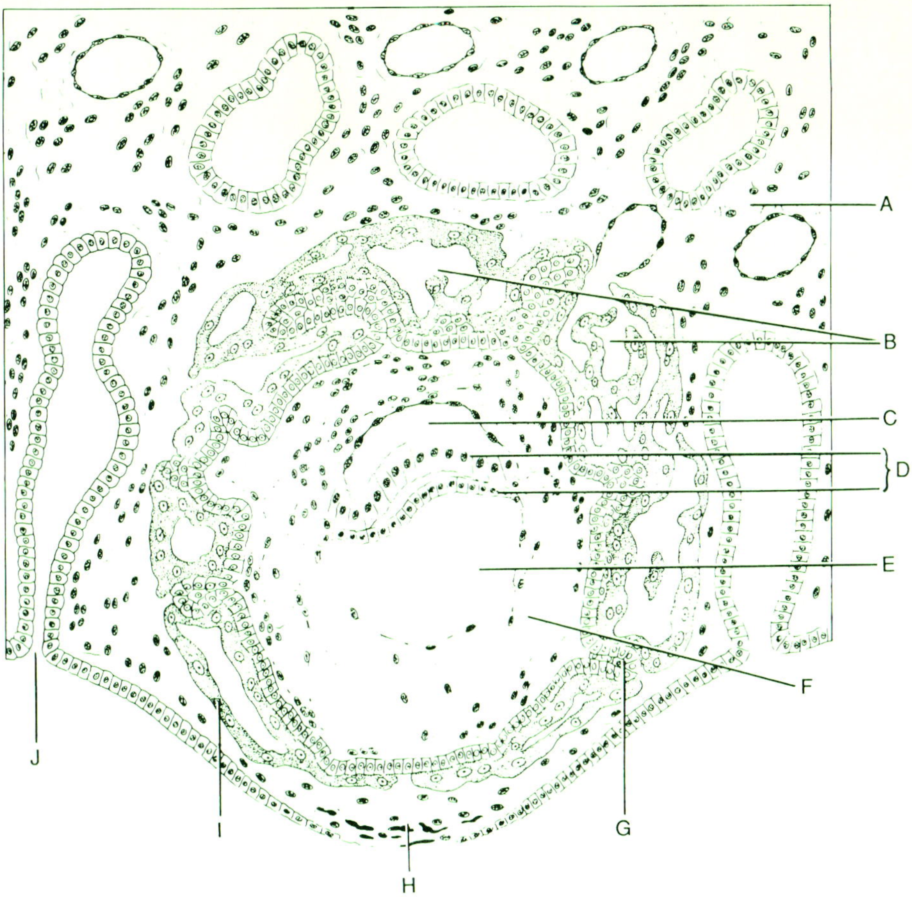

Figure 23-8.

23-37. Vitelline sac
23-38. Uterine gland
23-39. Decidua capsularis
23-40. Decidua basalis

Questions 23-41 through 23-49 use the letters in Fig 23-9.

23-41. Decidua capsularis
23-42. Decidua parietalis
23-43. Decidua basalis
23-44. Vitelline sac
23-45. Umbilical cord
23-46. Amniotic cavity
23-47. Uterine cavity
23-48. Myometrium
23-49. Cervical plug

Questions 23-50 through 23-58:

A. Morula
B. Blastula

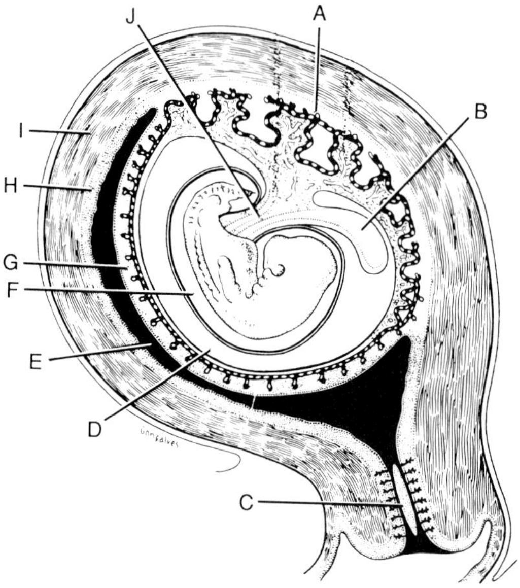

Figure 23-9.

C. Zygote
D. All of the above
E. None of the above

23–50. Solid ball of cells
23–51. Cell(s) are haploid
23–52. Single cell
23–53. Largest cell(s)
23–54. Stage at which zona pellucida disappears
23–55. Smallest cell(s)
23–56. Greatest number of cells
23–57. Contains an inner cell mass
23–58. Contain(s) a fluid-filled cavity

Questions 23–59 through 23–75 use the letters in Fig 23–10.

For the menstrual cycle time line shown in this figure, indicate which letter best corresponds to the activities below.

23–59. Secretory phase
23–60. Menstrual phase
23–61. Proliferative phase
23–62. Ovulation
23–63. Growth of ovarian follicle
23–64. Development of corpus luteum
23–65. Degeneration of corpus luteum of menstruation

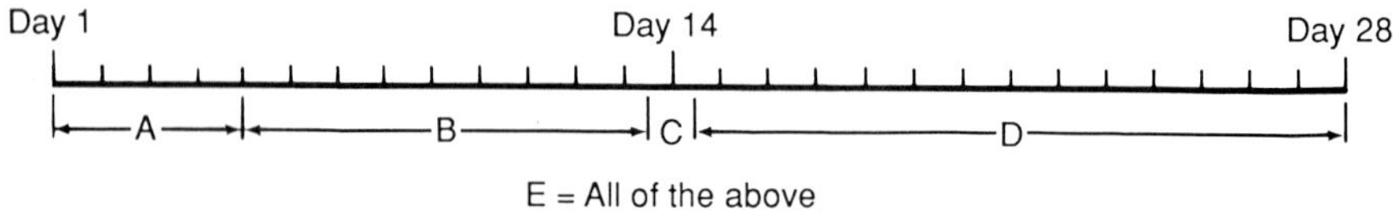

Figure 23-10.

23–66. Sloughing of stratum functionalis
23–67. Coiling of endometrial glands
23–68. Production of estrogen
23–69. Production of progesterone
23–70. Production of LH
23–71. Production of FSH
23–72. Period during which fertilization and implantation occur
23–73. Endometrium at its thinnest
23–74. Endometrium at its thickest
23–75. Stratum basale is present

Questions 23–76 through 23–89:

A. Estrogen
B. Progesterone
C. Ovarian androgens
D. Prolactin
E. FSH
F. LH
G. Relaxin
H. Oxytocin
I. Chorionic gonadotropin
J. Human placental lactogen
K. None of the above

23–76. Pituitary hormone that stimulates growth of follicles and oocytes
23–77. Pituitary hormone that stimulates ovulation
23–78. Produced by the syncytiotrophoblast
23–79. Involved in milk ejection reflex
23–80. Produced by interstitial cells
23–81. Produced by corpus albicans
23–82. Inhibits FSH production
23–83. Inhibits LH production
23–84. Stimulates LH production
23–85. Ovarian hormone whose secretion is stimulated by FSH
23–86. Ovarian hormone whose secretion is stimulated by LH
23–87. Characteristic product of granulosa lutein cells
23–88. Stimulates milk secretion
23–89. Secreted only by the corpus luteum of pregnancy

For questions 23–90 through 23–127, either, both or neither of the answers may be correct. Select

A if only A is correct
B if only B is correct
C if both A and B are correct
D if neither A nor B is correct

Questions 23–90 through 23–95:

A. Corpus luteum of pregnancy
B. Corpus luteum of menstruation
C. Both
D. Neither

23–90. Persists longer
23–91. Secretes progesterone
23–92. Secretes estrogen
23–93. Maintained primarily by pituitary LH
23–94. Maintained primarily by chorionic gonadotropin
23–95. Smaller

Questions 23-96 through 23-101:

A. Atretic follicles
B. Corpora albicans
C. Both
D. Neither

23-96. Remnants of degenerating ovarian follicles
23-97. Remnants of degenerating corpora lutea
23-98. May appear as collagenous scar(s)
23-99. Eventually removed by macrophages and replaced by stroma
23-100. Occur in larger numbers
23-101. May leave interstitial cells behind after degeneration

Questions 23-102 through 243-108:

A. Isthmus of uterine tube
B. Ampulla of uterine tube
C. Both
D. Neither

23-102. Closer to uterus
23-103. Larger mucosal folds
23-104. Contain(s) ciliated cells
23-105. Contains mucus-secreting peg cells
23-106. Wider lumen
23-107. Covered by serosa
23-108. Contain(s) smooth muscle in walls

Questions 23-109 through 23-116:

A. Functionale
B. Basale
C. Both
D. Neither

23-109. Includes the uterine epithelium
23-110. Includes connective tissue
23-111. Undergoes cyclic thickening and shedding
23-112. Changes little during menstrual cycle
23-113. More responsive to ovarian hormones
23-114. Contains cells that proliferate to recover uterine surface after menstruation
23-115. Contains the straight arteries
23-116. Contains the coiled arteries

Questions 23-117 through 23-123:

A. Syncytiotrophoblast
B. Cytotrophoblast
C. Both
D. Neither

23-117. Multinucleated mass formed by cell fusion
23-118. Component(s) of the placental barrier during early pregnancy
23-119. Component(s) of the placental barrier during late pregnancy
23-120. Lines lacunae
23-121. Formed by the trophoblast
23-122. Formed by the extraembryonic mesenchyme
23-123. May be found in contact with fibrinoid material

Questions 23–124 through 23–127 use the letters in Fig 23–11.

A. Fig 23–11A
B. Fig 23–11B
C. Both
D. Neither

23–124. Prepubertal mammary gland
23–125. Lactating mammary gland
23–126. Mammary gland in pregnancy
23–127. Senile mammary gland

For questions 23–128 through 23–137, one, more than one, or all of the asnwers may be correct. Select

A if only (1), (2), and (3) are correct
B if only (1) and (3) are correct
C if only (2) and (4) are correct
D if only (4) is correct
E if all answers are correct

23–128. Changes in ovarian follicle structure that accompany growth and maturation include
(1) Increased size of the antrum
(2) Increased size of the follicle
(3) Increased number of follicular (granulosa) cells
(4) Disappearance of the theca interna

23–129. Primary oocytes:
(1) Arise from division of the cells in the germinal epithelium
(2) Are diploid

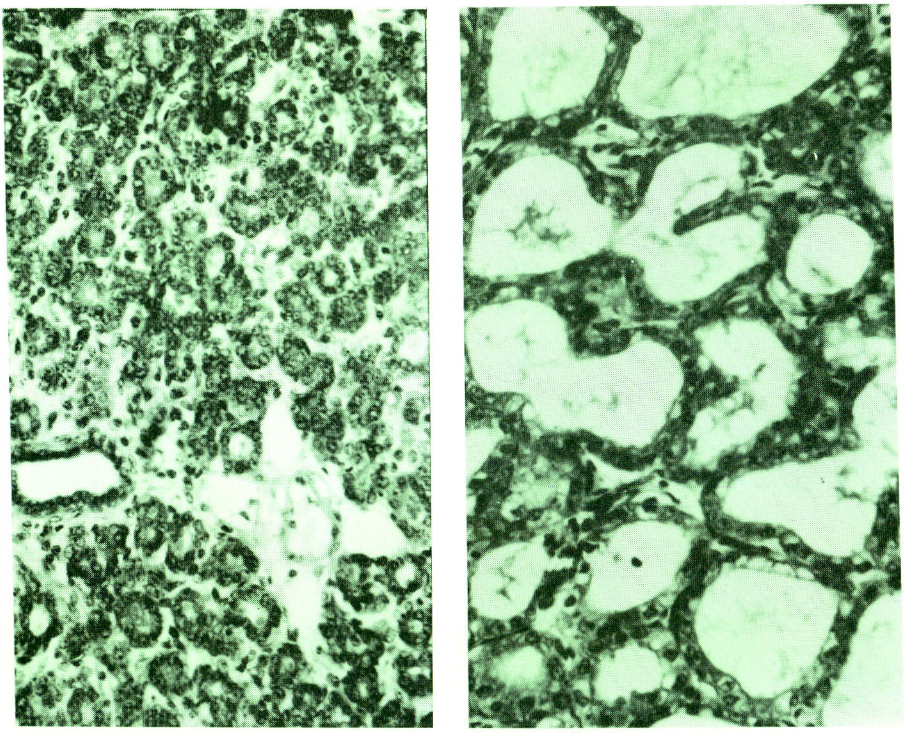

Figure 23–11.

(3) Are haploid
(4) Are derived from embryonic yolk sac endoderm

23–130. Components of the ovarian follicle that accompany the ovum during ovulation include the:
(1) Zona pellucida
(2) Theca interna
(3) Corona radiata
(4) Membrana granulosa

23–131. Granulosa lutein cells:
(1) Are large and pale-staining
(2) Contain abundant smooth endoplasmic reticulum
(3) Secrete progesterone
(4) Are derived from the cells of the theca interna

23–132. The myometrium:
(1) Increases in mass during pregnancy by hyperplasia (cell division)
(2) Increases in mass during pregnancy by hypertrophy (cell growth)
(3) Contracts in response to stimulation by oxytocin
(4) Contains the arcuate arteries

23–133. Fertilization:
(1) Usually occurs at the ampullaristhmic junction
(2) Occurs after the production of the second polar body
(3) Results in the formation of a zygote
(4) Usually occurs 3–5 days after ovulation

23–134. The inner cell mass:
(1) Is formed by the cytotrophoblast
(2) Forms the fetal part of the placenta
(3) Is first evident during the zygote stage
(4) Gives rise to the embryo

23–135. Decidual cells:
(1) Differentiate from endometrial stromal cells
(2) Appear before implantation
(3) Secrete prolactin
(4) Are formed by extraembryonic mesenchyme

23–136. Secretory mechanisms involved in milk production include:
(1) Holocrine secretion
(2) Merocrine secretion
(3) Cytocrine secretion
(4) Apocrine secretion

23–137. Colostrum:
(1) Contains primarily lipids
(2) Is released immediately following birth
(3) Is an incomplete form of milk produced only by hormonally deficient mothers
(4) Contains antibodies produced by plasma cells in the interlobular connective tissue of the mammary gland

Sense Organs

24

Objectives

This chapter should help the student to:

- Know the various classifications of sensory receptors and list the receptors that fit into each class.
- Know the structure, function, location, regenerative capacity, and mode of transduction of a stimulus into a neuronal action potential for the following receptors: free nerve endings, Merkel's corpuscles, Meissner's corpuscles, pacinian corpuscles, Ruffini's endings, muscle spindles, Golgi tendon organs, taste buds, olfactory epithelium, the eye, and the ear (vestibulocochlear apparatus).
- Locate and recognize the type(s) of receptors present in a side or photomicrograph of an organ or tissue by its microscopic structure.
- Identify the components of the receptor organs (eg, cells, spaces, capsule) from a slide, diagram, or photomicrograph.
- Relate the microscopic structure of each type of receptor to the sensory modality to which it responds.

Synopsis

I. GENERAL FEATURES OF THE SENSE ORGANS. Sense organs respond to stimuli by generating action potentials in their associated sensory (**afferent**) nerve cell process (sensory fiber). The signals are carried to the central nervous system for integration, allowing reflex (automatic) or conscious reactions to environmental changes. Sensory fibers usually carry signals for only one type (modality) of sensation, such as pain, touch, or temperature.

A. Classification of Receptors: Receptors can be classified by their relationship to the nervous system, by stimulus-sensitivity, and by the presence or absence of a capsule.

1. Relationship between the receptor and the nervous system

a. Neuronal receptors The sensory nerve ending receives the stimulus directly in these receptors. The stimulus partially depolarizes the nerve ending (this is a **generator potential**). The summation of several small generator potentials provides sufficient stimulus to reach threshold and fire an **action potential.** Examples of this type of receptor include cutaneous (skin) receptors and proprioceptors.

b. Epithelial receptors These are epithelial cells specialized to become depolarized—generate a **receptor potential**—in response to specific stimuli. The receptor potential causes the receptor cell to release neurotransmitters that then stimulate nearby sensory nerve endings. (The nerve endings are thus stimulated indirectly.) This mechanism is common in special sense organs, such as the rods and cones of the eye, and hair cells of the inner ear, and the sensory cells of the taste buds.

c. Neuroepithelial receptors These receptors are actually peripherally located neurons that receive a stimulus and carry the signal to the central nervous system along their own axons. The sensory cells of olfactory epithelium are the only mammalian example.

2. Adequate stimulus While receptors can be classified according to the stimulus to which they are most sensitive (ie, their adequate stimulus), they may also respond to other stimuli of higher intensity.

a. Mechanoreceptors respond to mechanical stimuli including:

(1) Touch, eg, free nerve endings, Merkel's corpuscles, Meissner's corpuscles, and encapsulated end-bulbs;

(2) Pressure, eg, free nerve endings, Meissner's corpuscles, pacinian corpuscles, and Ruffini corpuscles; and

(3) Vibration, eg, the above receptors plus those of the inner ear.

b. Thermoreceptors respond to temperature changes. Most of these are free nerve endings. Some with expanded tips have been identified as cold receptors; although Krause end-bulbs may also be cold receptors, this conclusion is still disputed. No specialized nerve endings have yet been identified as warmth receptors; those that are known are free nerve endings.

c. Nociceptors Free nerve endings that respond to noxious stimuli, ie, pain, these usually occur near epithelial surfaces such as the epidermis, the lining of the digestive tract, and the larger blood vessels. They are abundant in the cornea. There are no pain receptors in the brain except those associated with the blood vessels.

d. Chemoreceptors respond to specific chemical changes in their environments. They include the taste buds, the olfactory epithelium, and the carotid and aortic bodies.

e. Proprioceptors These receptors, which respond to changes in body position, allow us to sense, for example, the positions of our limbs with our eyes closed. Examples include muscle spindles, Golgi tendon organs, and the vestibular apparatus of the inner ear. Some mechanoreceptors in the joint capsules (eg, Ruffini corpuscles, free nerve endings, some pacinian corpuscles) also respond to displacement and thus may contribute to proprioception.

f. Photoreceptors produce nerve impulses in response to light. In humans, they are restricted to the retina of the eye.

3. Presence or absence of a capsule Encapsulated receptors are separated from the surrounding tissue by a specialized connective tissue sheath (capsule). Free nerve endings lack a capsule.

B. Distribution: Sense organs are distributed in a way that maximizes detection of their adequate stimulus. Touch receptors, for example, occur in high concentrations in the fingertips. The **receptive field** is the body region in which an adequate stimulus evokes a response. Its size is related to the degree of branching of the dendritic end of an afferent neuron and the distribution of the branches. Generally, the higher the concentration of nerve endings in a given area, the greater the sensitivity is.

C. Adaptation: This reflects the speed with which receptors can recover and respond to repeated stimulation.

II. RECEPTORS FOR SUPERFICIAL & DEEP SENSATION

A. Free Nerve Endings: Numerous and widely distributed, these are the peripheral dendritic branches of sensory neurons. Also known as naked or unencapsulated receptors, they are generally branches of unmyelinated or lightly myelinated fibers that are found in bundles or plexuses beneath epithelia. As the fibers penetrate the epithelium, they lose their Schwann cell investment and branch extensively among the epithelial cells. Branches of one nerve ending may cover a wide area and overlap the territories of others. Although different free nerve endings receive input for differing sensory modalities (eg, pain, cold, warmth, touch or pressure), they exhibit no structural specializations that betray their exact function. The most numerous of the receptors in the skin, they also occur in the walls of the respiratory and digestive tracts and the larger vessels, where some free nerve endings monitor dilation and contraction. Others provide nociception (pain reception) for the body interior.

B. Merkel's Corpuscles: These unencapsulated touch receptors, located deep in the epidermis (see Chapter 18), respond to direct pressure and, perhaps due to desmosomal attachments, to indirect pressure. They are most abundant in the thick glabrous (hairless) skin of the palms of the hands and soles of the feet. They have 2 major components. One is a specialized epithelial cell called **Merkel's cell** in the epidermis. These cells have abundant dense-core cytoplasmic granules and are attached to the surrounding epidermal cells by many desmosomes. The second component, a specialized nerve ending, loses its Schwann cell sheath as it penetrates the epidermal basal lamina. Its free end forms a flattened disk (**Merkel's disk**) near the Merkel's cell. This disk contacts the Merkel's cell in synapselike junctions and is enveloped by cytoplasmic extensions. The cytoplasmic granules resemble those in cells with DNES functions, but they do not contain catecholamines. The neurotransmitter has not been identified.

C. Other Nerve Endings With Expanded Tips: These are found near unremarkable epithelial cells deep in the epidermis; some function as cold receptors, responding to local cooling of the skin.

D. Meissner's Corpuscles: Elongated ovoid mechanoreceptors, these are covered by a thin capsule and contain multiple stacked lamallae of flattened Schwann cells as well as some fibroblasts. One or more nerve endings may enter a corpuscle from its base and zigzag through the stack. Functioning as touch and superficial pressure receptors, they are commonly found in the dermal papillae of the skin (see Chapter 18) and are most numerous in the glabrous skin of the fingertips, palms, soles, nipples, etc.

E. Pacinian Corpuscles: These receptors are highly sensitive to pressure. They are found in the deep dermis and hypodermis of the skin, in the periosteum of bones and joint capsules, and in mesenteries. Each has a well-developed capsule consisting of multiple layers of flattened fibroblastlike cells that are separated by narrow fluid-filled spaces. Larger and rounder than Meissner's corpuscles, they resemble a sliced onion in tissue sections. The nerve retains its myelin for a short distance after entering the capsule at one pole. The unmyelinated portion penetrates the capsule's core, surrounded by a few layers of tightly packed flattened Schwann cells. The nerve ending terminates near the opposite pole, often giving off several blunt-tipped branches.

F. Ruffini's Corpuscles: These slowly adapting mechanoreceptors are common in the dermis, hypodermis, and joint capsule. They have very thin capsules surrounding a fluid-filled cavity that contains a fine meshwork of collagen fibers that penetrate the capsule to anchor it in the surrounding tissue. The single nerve ending loses its Schwann cell sheath as it enters the capsule. It then gives off many unmyelinated branches that weave around the collagen fibers and are stimulated by movement in the surrounding connective tissue.

G. End-Bulbs: These fluid-filled spheroid bulbs with thin capsules (eg, Krause's end-bulbs) contain many nerve endings that enter at one pole and branch internally. Relatively common, they vary greatly in size; most act as mechanoreceptors. The largest end-bulbs are seen in the connective tissue of the genitalia (genital corpuscles), while the smallest are found in the conjunctiva. Others occur in the subepithelial connective tissue of the mouth, nasal cavity, and peritoneum and in the connective tissue around joints and nerve trunks.

H. Carotid Sinus: See Chapter 11 for a discussion of this mechanoreceptor.

III. PROPRIOCEPTOR SYSTEM

A. Muscle Spindles: These are encapsulated fusiform (spindle-shaped, with a wide equator and tapered poles) proprioceptors that are embedded in striated muscles. The capsule consists of several circumferential layers of flattened fibroblasts. Muscles that are responsible for delicate and precise movements (eg, eye muscles) contain more spindles than do those responsible for gross postural adjustments (eg, gluteus maximus). Muscle spindles receive both sensory and motor innervation.

1. Intrafusal fibers These comprise a bundle of 2–20 specialized muscle fibers lying inside the capsule. Oriented parallel to the extrafusal fibers—the typical muscle fibers outside the capsule—the intrafusal fibers cross the spindle pole-to-pole and attach to the capsule at its poles. Near the spindle's equator, the intrafusal fibers are separated from the capsule by a fluid-filled capsular space that contains nerve endings and sparse collagen fibers. Intrafusal fibers are shorter and narrower than most extrafusal fibers. They are striated at their polar extremities and nonstriated at the dilated centers. The nonstriated region, which lies in the equatorial region of the spindle, contains the nuclei and lacks myofilaments; it is unable to contract. The 2 types of intrafusal fibers include:

a. Nuclear chain fibers, which are small, short, and numerous, with nuclei oriented in chains or rows; and

b. Nuclear bag fibers, which are larger, fewer in number (one or 2 per spindle), and longer: they may extend beyond the capsule. Their nonstriated centers are more dilated, and the nuclei in this baglike dilation occur in a cluster rather than a row.

2. Sensory innervation This is of 2 types:

a. Primary annulospiral endings A single fairly large myelinated sensory (afferent) fiber penetrates each muscle spindle, losing its myelin sheath near the intrafusal fiber bundle. The unmyelinated portion gives off several branches that form ringlike or spiral endings around the nuclear expansion of each intrafusal fiber and become embedded in folds of the intrafusal sarcolemma. These endings show dynamic sensitivity; ie, they are more sensitive to the initial stretching of muscle.

b. Secondary flower-spray and annulospiral endings These occur in most spindles. One or more small myelinated sensory nerves loses its myelin sheath as it branches within the spindle. The branches may end in rings and spirals like those of primary endings, or they may end in a flower-spray pattern, with a terminal expansion of each branch contacting the sarcolemma. They differ from primary endings by terminating mainly on the smaller nuclear chain fibers and by exhibiting static sensitivity; ie, they are more sensitive to prolonged stretching of muscle.

3. Motor innervation The motor supply to intrafusal fibers of the muscle spindle is carried by small myelinated motor (efferent) fibers whose cell bodies lie in the ventral horn of the spinal cord gray matter. These **gamma motor neurons** terminate in 2 types of endings on the sarcolemma of the striated polar portion of intrafusal fibers. Most of the endings received by nuclear bag fibers resemble motor end-plates (see Chapter 9), with small clusters of **boutons terminaux.** Most motor nerve endings on nuclear chain fibers come from diffusely branching fibers, they contact the sarcolemma as multiple **boutons en passage.** Impulses carried by the gamma motor neurons cause the intrafusal fibers to contract, stretching their nonstriated regions (where the primary and secondary sensory endings are located). The motor neurons heighten the spindles' sensitivity to stretching of the muscle in which it is located.

B. Golgi Tendon Organs: These encapsulated proprioceptors are located mainly near muscle-tendon junctions. Each is surrounded by a capsule of flattened fibroblasts and filled with several large collagen fiber bundles, some of which extend beyond the capsule and insert into the tendon. Some extrafusal muscle fibers may attach to the receptor's collagen bundles, allowing activation by either muscle stretching or contracting. Each receptor receives a single large myelinated sensory fiber that loses its myelination as it enters the capsule, giving off unmyelinated branches that run lengthwise through and between the organ's collagen bundles.

IV. CHEMORECEPTORS

A. Taste Buds: These are chemoreceptors found mainly on the dorsal surface of the tongue. They are found in smaller numbers on the oral surface of the soft palate and the laryngeal surface of the epiglottis. Lingual taste buds are embedded in **papillae,** small epithelial projections of the tongue's surface. **Fungiform** papillae carry taste buds on their apical surfaces, while **foliate** and **circumvallate** papillae carry them on their lateral surfaces. Some papillae are more sensitive to certain taste modalities than to others, and some may be sensitive to more than one of the basic tastes described for humans (sour/acid, bitter, sweet, and salty). No clear structure-function relationships have been described to account for the differences in sensitivity, however. Taste buds are ovoid, they lie beneath the epithelial surface, and they communicate with the oral cavity through a small opening called a **taste pore.** Chemicals in the oral cavity enter the taste pore to stimulate the taste receptors. The 5 types of cells that constitute the taste buds are all believed to be different stages in the life cycle of a single cell type that undergoes continuous turnover.

1. Type I **Dark supporting cells** are narrow columnar cells with apical microvilli and an elongated heterochromatic nucleus. The most numerous of the 5 types, these contain many mitochondria, fine filaments, electron-dense granules, free ribosomes, and abundant rough endoplasmic reticulum. Their membrane-bound granules release glycosaminoglycans into the taste pore. Although they lie between the sensory cells, they have no sensory innervation; they may represent an intermediate phase of differentiation between basal and sensory cells.

2. Type II **Light sensory cells** are broad columnar cells with apical microvilli and are the next most numerous. There are fewer filaments, abundant smooth endoplasmic reticulum and mitochondria, and a pale round basally located nucleus; the cell's base contacts unmyelinated sensory nerve endings. Chemical stimuli contacting the microvilli are converted to electrical impulses, transmitted to the nerve endings, and perceived as taste. Type II cells differ from type III cells in that they directly transmit receptor potentials to the sensory nerves through electrical synapses.

3. Type III **Sensory cells,** like type II cells, are columnar cells with apical microvilli. Chemical stimuli cause these cells to release neurotransmitters (chemical synapses), which in turn stimulate the sensory nerve endings that contact the cells on their basal and lateral surfaces. Each type III cell may be innervated by several afferent fibers.

4. Type IV **Basal cells** are located in the base of the taste bud. These polygonal cells, which may derive from type V cells, are the stem cells from which the sensory and supporting cells arise; they contain fewer and poorly developed organelles.

5. Type V **Perigemmal cells,** the crescent-shaped cells around the periphery of the taste bud, contain an elongated nucleus, filament bundles, and few organelles. They may enclose some nerve endings and give rise to the basal cells.

B. Olfactory Epithelium: The main chemoreceptor for the sense of smell (**olfaction**), this pseudostratified columnar epithelium forms a small part of the nasal cavity's epithelial lining. It is restricted to the upper surface of the **superior concha (turbinate bone)** and extends into the **sphenoethmoidal** recess. The epithelium has 3 types of cells, whose nuclei lie in rows at 3 different levels.

1. Olfactory cell These bipolar neurons derived from embryonic neuroepithelium are broad at the middle and narrow at the apex and base. Each exhibits a small apical expansion from which 6–20 long nonmotile cilia extend into the mucus lining the nasal cavity. Scented substances interact with the receptor sites of these specialized cilia to elicit a receptor potential; the tufts of cilia increase the surface area available for chemical-stimulus reception. The base of each olfactory cell tapers to form an axon hillock, from which arises the axon that carries the impulse to the brain. The large round pale nuclei of these cells lie in the middle row, below those of the supporting cells and above those of the basal cells.

2. Supporting cells These columnar cells are broader at their microvillus-covered apices than at their bases. Their pale nuclei lie in the broad subapical cytoplasm and form the top row of nuclei, between the epithelial surface and the row of sensory-cell nuclei. They contain both rough and smooth endoplasmic reticula, lysosomes, lipid droplets, and a reddish-brown pigment. This pigment gives the olfactory mucosa a dark yellow color that allows it to be distinguished from the surrounding respiratory epithelium. Supporting cells are attached to the neighboring olfactory cells by junctional complexes.

3. Basal cells These small conical cells lie at the base of the olfactory epithelium, their nuclei form the deepest of the 3 rows. Their narrow cell processes, which extend between the other cells of the olfactory epithelium are difficult to distinguish with the light microscope.

C. Carotid and Aortic Bodies: See Chapter 11 for a discussion of these chemoreceptors.

V. THE EYE.

The eye is a complex organ of vision that contains the retina and specialized structures to refine visual images before they reach the retina's photosensitive cells. The layered structure of the globe (eyeball) can be better understood in light of its embryonic origin.

A. Embryonic Development:

1. Tunica interna (retina) and lens The eye begins development as the **optic bulb,** or **optic vesicle,** a hollow bulbous outgrowth of the embryonic brain. As the outgrowth contacts the overlying surface ectoderm, 2 important events occur. The bulb induces the overlying ectoderm to thicken and form the **lens placode.** The portion of the bulb in contact with the ectoderm then invaginates to form the double-walled **optic cup.** This later forms the **tunica interna,** or **retina.** The cup's outer layer forms the **pigmented epithelium** of the retina, while the inner layer forms the photosensitive **neural retina.** The lens placode thickens further and then invaginates to form the **lens vesicle,** which later pinches off to form the lens. The newly formed lens lies in the oriface of the optic cup. The stalk connecting the optic cup to the brain becomes the **optic nerve.**

2. Tunica fibrosa and tunica vasculosa Mesenchymal tissue condenses around the tunica interna to form the globe's 2 outer tunics. The outer layer becomes the tunica fibrosa, between it and the tunica interna lies the tunica vasculosa.

B. The Tunics:

1. Tunica fibrosa The eye's outermost tunic, it has 2 major components. The anterior one-sixth forms the transparent cornea; the posterior five-sixths forms the opaque sclera. The junction between the cornea and sclera is termed the limbus.

a. Cornea This transparent 1-mm-thick disk of avascular tissue bulging from the front of the eye has 5 layers:

(1) Anterior epithelium This is the outermost layer. It consists of a thin (50 μm) nonkeratinized stratified squamous epithelium of 5–6 cell layers, richly supplied with sensitive free nerve endings.

(2) Bowman's membrane (anterior limiting lamina) This is a thickened (7–12 μm) basement membrane, consisting of ground substance and irregular bundles of fine reticular fibers. It contains no cells and represents the condensed outer layer of the stroma.

(3) Stroma (substantia propria) The core of the cornea, this constitutes about 90% of its thickness. It consists of several layers of collagen fiber bundles oriented parallel to those in the same layer and perpendicular to those in adjacent layers. Flattened fibroblasts and occasional lymphocytes are found between the fibrous layers.

(4) Descemet's membrane (posterior limiting membrane) This is a 5–10-μm thick basement membrane that differs from Bowman's membrane in both composition and position. It contains elastin, but no elastic fibers, and its atypical collagen fibers form a 3-dimensional network decorated with clusters of electron-dense granules.

(5) Corneal endothelium (posterior epithelium) This is a simple low cuboidal epithelium that lines the corneal disk's internal surface.

b. Limbus This is the highly vascularized ringlike junction between the cornea and the sclera. Its vascular network and the fluid in the anterior chamber nourish the avascular cornea. The corneal stroma near the limbus contains an irregular endothelium-lined channel, the **canal of Schlemm,** that drains fluid from the anterior chamber toward veins in the area of the limbus. Blockage of the canal can cause increased intraocular pressure and **glaucoma.**

c. Sclera This is the opaque white connective tissue covering of the posterior five-sixths of the eye. It is separated from the peripheral tissues and anchored in the orbit by dense connective tissue called **Tenon's capsule.** The space between the capsule and the sclera is called **Tenon's space.** The sclera is usually divided into 3 layers:

(1) Episclera This is the sclera's outermost layer. It consists of fibroelastic tissue through which the ocular muscle tendons pass to insert into the next layer.

(2) Substantia propria The sclera's thick middle layer consists of a dense mat of collagen fiber bundles and elastic fibers. The collagen fibers of the ocular muscle tendons insert into this layer and mingle with the scleral fibers. Numerous fibroblasts are scattered among the fibers.

(3) Lamina fusca This is the sclera's loose connective tissue inner layer. It contains many elastic fibers and the melanocytes that give the sclera's inner surface a brownish color. It is separated from the choroid only by the narrow perichoroidal space.

2. Tunica vasculosa (uvea) The middle tunic of the eye, this has 3 major components: the choroid (posterior), ciliary body, and iris (anterior).

a. Choroid Lying between the sclera and the retina's pigmented epithelium, the choroid is composed of 4 layers:

(1) The **suprachoroidal lamina** is the choroid's outermost layer. Its composition is similar to that of the sclera's lamina fusca, from which it is separated by the perichoroidal space.

(2) The **vascular lamina** consists of loose connective tissue, richly supplied with multiple whorllike veins. These converge and empty into 4 larger vortex veins that exit the back of the eye by penetrating the sclera.

(3) The **choriocapillary layer (choriocapillaris)** consists of a single thin layer of small fenestrated sinuses that are embedded in loose connective tissue.

(4) **Bruch's membrane,** the choroid's innermost layer, is the basement membrane of the retina's pigmented epithelium.

b. Ciliary body Extending forward from the choroid, this is a ringlike triangular thickening of the tunica vasculosa at the level of the lens. It contains the same layers as the choroid except for the choriocapillary layer. There are 2 structural specializations: the ciliary processes and the ciliary muscles.

(1) The **ciliary processes** are irregular outgrowths of the ciliary body extending toward the lens. These epithelium-covered connective tissue ridges serve as the origin of fibers of a circular ligament called the **zonule,** or **ligament of Zinn.** Zonule fibers insert into the lateral edge of the lens to hold it in place. The epithelial covering of these processes consists of 2 layers derived from the wall of the optic cup.

(a) The pigmented epithelium bordering the internal cavity of the eye is called the **ciliary epithelium.** It contains cells that exhibit the basal and lateral plasma membrane infoldings typical of ion- and water-transporting cells. Its cells secrete **aqueous humor,** which flows past the lens and through the pupil to fill the anterior chamber. From the anterior chamber, the aqueous humor penetrates the tissue near the limbus through a mazelike series of spaces until it reaches the canal of Schlemm. From here it passes to scleral veins in the limbic region as described above.

(b) The deeper epithelial layer, derived from the outer layer of the optic cup, consists of a pigmented simple columnar epithelium resting on a basal lamina.

(2) The **ciliary muscles** are bundles of smooth muscle fibers located around the periphery of the ciliary bodies near their junction with the sclera. Ciliary muscles are divided into 3 groups by muscle fiber direction. Contraction of all the groups of muscles pulls the ciliary body and choroid forward, releasing the tension exerted by the zonule fibers on the lens and allowing the lens to round up for near vision. Relaxation of all the groups leads to increased tension on the zonule fibers, flattening the lens for focusing on distant objects. Fine adjustments of individual muscles allow focusing on objects at intermediate distances.

c. **Iris** This structure gives the eye its characteristic color (brown, blue, etc) and controls the amount of light reaching the retina. Projecting as a flattened ring from the ciliary body, the iris extends in front of the lens and leaves a circular opening at its center, the **pupil.** The iris includes the most anterior extension of the tunica vasculosa and forms the border between the anterior and posterior chambers of the eye. The **anterior chamber** lies between the posterior surface of the cornea and the anterior surface of the iris; the **posterior chamber** lies between the posterior surface of the iris and the anterior surfaces of the lens and zonule.

(1) The **anterior surface** of the iris is a discontinuous layer of pigment cells and fibroblasts and has a rough appearance. The **stroma** is a poorly vascularized connective tissue that contains many fibroblasts and melanocytes. The **vascular stratum** lies between the stroma and the posterior epithelium; it contains many blood vessels. The **posterior surface** is smooth and heavily pigmented; it is continuous with the double layer of retinal epithelium that covers the ciliary processes.

(2) There are 2 sets of involuntary muscles:

(a) The **sphincter pupillae** is a ringlike collection of smooth muscle fibers in the pupillary margin of the iris. It contracts under **sympathetic** control and partly closes the pupillary opening.

(b) The **dilator pupillae** consists of fibers extending like the spokes of a wheel from the ciliary body to the pupillary margin. It contracts under **parasympathetic** control and widens the pupillary opening.

3. **Tunica interna, or retina** This derives from the optic cup and is considered an extension of the central nervous system. It is divided into anterior and posterior portions. The nonphotosensitive anterior portion forms part of the ciliary body and iris, while the posterior portion is a highly specialized photoreceptor. The junction between the photosensitive and nonphotosensitive portions of the retina is located behind the ciliary body and is termed the **ora serrata.** The posterior portion of the retina is itself divided into 2 distinct layers based on structure, function, and embryonic origin:

a. **Pigmented epithelium** This layer derives from the optic cup's outer wall. It contains abundant melanin and consists of a simple cuboidal epithelium resting on a thick elastic basement membrane (**Bruch's membrane**) that separates it from the choroid. The cells have many apical microvilli that embrace the outer segments of the rods and cones in the overlying neural retina. While not a photoreceptor, pigmented (or pigment) epithelium is important in vision. Its ability to absorb light that has passed through the retina's photosensitive layer reduces light scattering, ensuring that light stimulates the rods and cones only on its first pass through the neural retina. At the level of the electron microscope, pigment cells show basal plasma membrane infoldings and interdigitating mitochondria that are typical or ion- and water-transporting cells. These cells also phagocytose and degrade the flattened vesicles shed by the outer segments of the rod cells.

b. Neural retina This highly organized, exquisitely sensitive photoreceptive organ derives from the optic cup's inner wall. While retinal pigmented epithelium continues forward in the ciliary body and iris, the neural retina extends forward only to the ora serrata.

C. Cells of the Neural Retina:

Although 10 layers are distinguishable, only 3 major layers of retinal neurons are concerned with the reception and integration of visual signals and the transduction of visual information to the brain as nerve impulses. These are the **photoreceptive cells (rods and cones), bipolar cells,** and **ganglion cells.**

1. Rods and cones These can be compared in terms of their similarities and differences.

a. Similarities

(1) Both rods and cones are photoreceptive cells that are located deep in the retina, adjacent to the pigment-cell layer. Light must penetrate the more superficial layers of the neural retina to reach and stimulate them.

(2) They are both composed of 2 structurally different segments:

(a) The **outer segment,** the specialized, dendritic portion of each cell, is filled with a stack of flattened membrane-limited vesicles and contains the visual pigment molecules. The distal tip of this segment is embraced by the microvilli of the pigment epithelial cell.

(b) The **inner segment** is separated from the outer segment by a constriction. Basal bodies in the inner segment near this constriction give rise to 1–2 intracytoplasmic cilia that pass through the constriction into the outer segment. The inner segment is rich in polyribosomes and glycogen granules, the many mitochondria near the constriction provide the energy required for the visual process.

b. Differences

(1) Cell shape Rod cells are narrow elongated cells with long thin cylindric outer segments. Cone cells, however, tend to be plumper with shorter conical outer segments.

(2) Vesicles

(a) The membranes of the flattened vesicles in the rods are independent of, and entirely inside, the plasma membrane of the outer segments. The visual pigment, synthesized on polyribosomes, is incorporated into the membranes of small vesicles in the inner segment. These small vesicles move to the outer segment and fuse to form flattened vesicles. The vesicles, which are formed continuously, gradually move toward the apex of the outer segment, where they are shed and phagocytosed by pigmented epithelial cells.

(b) The flattened vesicles of the cones arise as invaginations of the outer segment's plasma membrane and are turned over more slowly than those in the rods.

(3) Cell number There are about 120 million rods but only about 6 million cones per retina.

(4) Visual pigment The globular protein **rhodopsin** is synthesized in the inner segment of the rods and becomes localized in the outer surfaces of the stacked vesicles in their outer segments. Rhodopsin is bleached by light, a photochemical reaction that initiates the visual process. The visual pigment in the cones is **iodopsin,** which is evenly distributed throughout their outer segments. Iodopsin is most sensitive to red light.

(5) Sensitivity Rods which are more sensitive to light, are responsible for vision in low light (night vision). They respond to slight differences in light intensity and shades of gray. Cones require more intense light (day vision); however, they permit greater visual acuity and are responsible for color vision.

2. Bipolar cells Lying in the middle of the neural retina, these cells constitute 2 populations of interneurons between the photoreceptors and the ganglion cells. They relay visual signals initiated in the photoreceptors to the ganglion cells.

a. Each diffuse bipolar cell synapses with ganglion cells and with 2 or more photoreceptors (mostly rods).

b. Each monosynaptic bipolar cell synapses with a single cone and a single ganglion cell. The visual acuity associated with the cones may be partly attributable to their more direct connections with the brain.

3. Ganglion cells These cells have large cell bodies and nuclei and lie close to the inner surface of the optic globe. Their dendrites establish synaptic contacts with bipolar cells, while their axons form a layer of nerve fibers that cover the inner surface of the retina and converge to form the fiber bundles of the optic nerve. Their long axons exit the eye via the optic nerve, carrying visual signals to the regions of the brain responsible for sight.

4. Other cell types The cells of the neural retina also include minor populations of neurons and important glial cells.

a. Neurons **Horizontal cells** have processes that terminate near the synapses between the photoreceptor and bipolar cells. The processes of **amacrine cells** terminate near the synapses between the bipolar and ganglion cells. Although horizontal and amacrine cell functions are obscure, they may involve signal integration prior to transmission to the brain.

b. Supporting cells include **astrocytes, microglia,** and a group of large, highly branched **Müller cells** that span the entire width of the neural retina and embrace the processes of various retinal neurons.

D. Layers of the Neural Retina: These can be described in terms of their location and composition. Beginning near the pigmented epithelium and moving toward the central cavity of the globe, the layers are:

1. The outer segments of the rods and cones;

2. The inner segments of the rods and cones;

3. The external limiting membrane, consisting of the outer processes of the Müller cells;

4. The external nuclear layer, consisting of the nuclei of the rods and cones;

5. The external plexiform layer, consisting of the processes of and synapses between the photoreceptors and bipolar cells;

6. The internal nuclear layer, consisting of the nuclei of the bipolar cells;

7. The internal plexiform layer, consisting of the processes of and synapses between the bipolar and ganglion cells;

8. The ganglion cell layer, consisting of the ganglion cell bodies;

9. The nerve fiber layer, consisting of the axonal processes of the ganglion cells that coverge to form the optic nerve; and

10. The inner limiting membrane, consisting of the inner processes of the Müller cells.

E. Fovea Centralis: The part of the neural retina directly opposite the center of the lens, the fovea lies at the center of a small spot, called the macula lutea because of its yellow color in the living state. Because the fovea contains the greatest concentration of cones, it is the part of the retina with the greatest visual acuity. The lateral displacement of all retinal layers except the photoreceptors makes it the thinnest part of the neural retina. It is devoid of blood vessels and derives nutrition from the underlying choriocapillary layer.

F. Optic Disk: Also known as the papilla, nerve head, and blind spot, this is the site where the ganglion cells' axons converge at the back of the eye and exit to form the optic nerve. It is devoid of photoreceptor cells and thus insensitive to light. Retinal vessels enter and exit the eye's interior through the center of the optic disk and then ramify in all directions over the retina's internal surface. Capillaries from smaller branches penetrate the inner layers of the retina except in the area of the fovea. The retina's outer layers are supplied by diffusion from vessels in the choriocapillaris.

G. Optic Nerve: This consists of the ganglion cell axons that converge and leave the eye at the optic disk. Once in the optic nerve, the axons acquire a myelin sheath from oligodendrocytes. As it leaves the eye, the optic nerve acquires a sheath of dura mater, which is continuous with the sclera, as well as arachnoid and pia mater. It contains the retinal artery and vein at its core.

H. Vitreous Body: The transparent, gellike substance that fills the large vitreous space between the lens and retina, this body consists mostly of water (about 99%) and hyaluronic acid. It also contains some collagenlike fibrils, mainly around the periphery, that form its capsule. Cells, which are rare, include a few macrophages and hyalocytes, stellate cells with oval nuclei that are responsible for fibril and hyaluronic acid production. During development, the central artery extends from the optic nerve head through the vitreous, reaching the lens as the **hyaloid artery.** This artery later degenerates, leaving behind the narrow cylindric **hyaloid canal.**

I. Lens: This is a transparent biconvex structure of epithelial origin. Nourished by the aqueous humor, it has neither innervation nor vascularization. The lens is suspended behind the pupil, between the posterior chamber and vitreous body, by the zonule fibers of the ciliary processes. Its elasticity allows it to be deformed by the ciliary muscles and return to its original shape. Changes in lens curvature permit focusing on near or far objects, a process termed **accommodation.** The lens has 3 major components:

1. Lens capsule This special elastic and transparent basal lamina covers the entire lens and prevents wandering cells from penetrating it. The capsule consists mainly of fine types III and IV collagen fibrils embedded in a homogeneous matrix that is rich in glycoproteins and sulfated glycosaminoglycans.

2. Subcapsular epithelium The cell height of this low cuboidal epithelium beneath the capsule on the anterior lens surface gradually increases to columnar near the lens equator, where cell division occurs. Its cells, which have few organelles, form the lens fibers.

3. Lens fibers These long, narrow, hexagonal, highly differentiated epithelial cells make up most of the lens. During differentiation, they lose their nuclei, fill with proteins called crystallins, and develop a variety of plasma membrane specializations, including junctional complexes and ridgelike processes.

J. Accesory Structures of the Eye:

1. Conjunctiva There are 2 parts to this structure: A thin nonkeratinized stratified squamous epithelium covers the sclera on the eye's anterior surface up to the cornea (**bulbar conjunctiva**), and a stratified columnar epithelium covers the inner surface of the eyelids (**palpebral conjunctiva**). The conjunctiva is underlain by a lamina propria of loose vascular connective tissue that contains many lymphocytes, macrophages, and plasma cells.

2. Eyelids (palpebrae) These skin folds are specialized to protect the eyes.

a. From the exterior inward, the 5 layers of the eyelids include:

(1) Thin skin, lacking hairs except at the free margin;

(2) Loose connective tissue containing slips of the **orbicularis oculi muscles** that close the eyes;

(3) Dense connective tissue, forming the **tarsal plate** that provides flexible support and harbors the specialized sebaceous **tarsal (meibomian) glands.** Each tarsal gland has a long central duct, which opens on the free margin of the lid. The oily secretion released by the ducts prevents the opposing lids from sticking together and forms a layer over the film of tears, slowing their evaporation;

(4) A lamina propria of loose connective tissue; and

(5) The palpebral conjunctiva, which covers the internal surface of the eyelids.

b. The free margin of each lid exhibits, in addition to the openings of the tarsal glands, a row of thick terminal hairs: the eyelashes. Many loosely coiled sweat glands **(glands of Moll)** lie between the small sebaceous **glands of Zeis** associated with each hair follicle.

c. Near the superior margin of the upper eyelid, the **levator palpebrae superioris muscle** inserts into the skin and the top of the tarsal plate, serving to elevate (open) the lid.

3. Lacrimal apparatus The 4 components of the lacrimal apparatus provide a continuous flow of tears to lubricate and protect the eyes.

a. Lacrimal glands These tear-secreting compound tubuloalveolar glands are located superolaterally, in the bony orbit of each eye. Each gland has several lobes that contain columnar secretory cells with pale-staining secretory granules. The secretory units are surrounded by myoepithelial cells and loose connective tissue. **Lysozyme** secreted by the glands helps protect the eyes from bacterial infection. Tears are released behind the upper eyelid and flow over the eye, wetting and lubricating its anterior surface. The excess is drained away through the **lacrimal puncta.**

b. Lacrimal puncta These are small, 0.5-mm holes, one in the free margin of each lid near the medial palpebral angle. Tears enter the puncta by capillary attraction and pass into the **lacrimal canaliculi** (about 8 mm long); these join to form a short duct that empties into the lacrimal sac. The pumping action of the orbicularis oculi muscles also aids the flow of tears.

c. Lacrimal sac This is a dilation of the lacrimal drainage system, located in the bony lacrimal fossa between the nose and medial angle of each eye, and opens inferiorly into the nasolacrimal duct. The flow of tears is aided by gravity.

d. Nasolacrimal duct Collected tears are carried by this duct from the lacrimal sac through the bony canal and into the nasal cavity through the inferior meatus.

VI. THE EAR.

The 3 major components of this collection of structures specialized for hearing and balance are known as the external, middle, and internal ears.

A. External Ear:

1. Auricle (pinna) This is a funnel-like plate of elastic cartilage sandwiched between 2 layers of skin. The skin contains modified apocrine sweat glands, the **ceruminous glands,** that produce a waxy secretion **(cerumen)**. The auricle collects and focuses sound waves toward the tubelike external auditory meatus.

2. External auditory meatus This is the canal leading to the tympanic membrane, which is surrounded by elastic cartilage along its outer third and by bone along its inner two-thirds. Sound waves gathered by the auricle are carried internally by the meatus and cause the tympanic membrane to vibrate.

3. Tympanic membrane This membrane—the eardrum—covers the internal opening of the meatus. The outer of its 3 layers is epidermis, the middle is dense connective tissue, and the inner is cuboidal epithelium.

B. Middle Ear:

This lies in a cavity in the temporal bone. Its connection with the auditory meatus is closed by the tympanic membrane. It communicates with the pharynx through the **auditory (eustachian) tube** and with air-filled cavities (mastoid air cells) in the temporal bone's mastoid processes. The auditory tube, which is surrounded by elastic cartilage, remains collapsed except during swallowing, when its walls separate and allow pressure in the middle ear cavity to equilibrate with the environmental pressure.

1. Windows The medial bony wall of the middle ear cavity has 2 membrane-covered openings, the oval and round windows, that lie at the border between the middle and the internal ears.

2. Auditory ossicles The main functional components of the middle ear are 3 uniquely shaped small bones that bridge the middle ear cavity from the tympanic membrane to the oval window membrane. The **malleus** (hammer), **incus** (anvil), and **stapes** (stirrup) refine and transmit vibrations from the tympanic membrane to the fluid in the internal ear. Small muscles attached to the ossicles prevent loud sounds from damaging the ear through excessive vibration.

3. Mucosa The middle ear has a simple squamous-to-cuboidal lining, containing occasional mucous or seromucous glandular cells. A thin lamina propria binds the lining tightly to the periosteum of the middle ear walls and ossicles. Near the auditory canal, the epithelium changes to the pseudostratified columnar that lines the canal and the portion of the pharynx into which it opens.

C. Internal Ear: Also called the labyrinth or vestibulocochlear apparatus, this consists of 2 types of mechanoreceptors, one concerned with hearing and the other with equilibrium.

1. Embryonic development This begins with one disklike ectodermal thickening **(otic placode)** on each side of the head. Each placode invaginates to form an **otic vesicle,** which undergoes further outpocketings to form a complex of interconnected chambers and canals, the **membranous labyrinth.** Once the basic chambers are formed, their epithelial lining differentiates further to form the various special cells and sensory organs described below. Mesenchyme condenses around the forming membranous labyrinth to form a shell called the **bony labyrinth.**

2. Bony labyrinth Consisting of 2 interconnected compartments, the vestibule and the cochlea, the bony labyrinth protects and supports the delicate membranous labyrinth. The cavity between the membranous and bony labyrinths is filled with a fluid called **perilymph.**

a. Vestibule An oblong cavity, the vestibule holds the membranous labyrinth components concerned with equilibrium (the utricle and saccule). Three thin semicircular canals, oriented in 3 distinct planes at right angles to each other, exit the vestibule via small openings and penetrate the surrounding temporal bone.

b. Cochlea This snailshell-like spiral canal houses the part of the membranous labyrinth concerned with hearing. The spiral's screwlike bony core, the **modiolus,** around which the canal makes 2.5–2.75 turns, houses a spiral collection of auditory nerve cell bodies, the **spiral ganglia.** The thread of the screwlike modiolus is a spiraling bony shelf, the **osseous spiral lamina,** which supports the special auditory epithelium (spiral organ of Corti).

3. Membranous labyrinth Lying within and conforming to the shape of the bony labyrinth, the membranous labyrinth's interconnected chambers and channels contain a fluid called **endolymph.** The walls are mainly simple squamous epithelium, small portions of this develop into a sensory epithelium in which the cells rise gradually to a more columnar shape. While they develop from successive outpocketings of the same otic vesicle and remain connected, the auditory and vestibular receptor organs are structurally and functionally distinct.

a. Vestibular portion This part of the internal ear is concerned with balance. It lies directly behind the tympanic membrane; each of its major divisions—the semicircular ducts, utricle, and saccule—has its own special sensory organ.

(1) Duct, utricle, and saccule

(a) The **3 semicircular ducts** are curved tubular evaginations of the utricle lying within the semicircular canals. As they leave the utricle, the superior, lateral, and posterior ducts begin as small dilations termed **ampullae.** At its termination, the lateral duct connects directly with the utricle. The superior and posterior ducts converge to form a single slightly wider duct, which then joins the utricle.

(b) The **utricle** is the largest membranous component of the vestibular system. This kidney-shaped sac connects with the semicircular canals through their ampullae, and with the saccule through the narrow **utriculosaccular duct.**

(c) The **saccule** is smaller and more spheric. It communicates with the utricle and endolymphatic duct through the utriculosaccular duct and with the cochlear duct through the short narrow **ductus reuniens.**

(d) The **endolymphatic duct** is a tubular evagination of the utriculosaccular duct, terminating in a blind-ended expansion called the **endolymphatic sac.** This sac is lined by tall columnar epithelium and surrounded by richly vascularized loose connective tissue. Duct and sac functions may include the production of, and removal of debris from, the endolymph.

(2) Vestibular sensory organs A small region of the wall of each major component of the membranous labyrinth contains specialized sensory cells.

(a) Cells Two major types of cells occur in the sensory areas:

***(i)* Hair cells** are the receptor cells. Each has several long microvilli (stereocilia) and a single true cilium extending from its apical surface. There are 2 types of hair cells: The goblet-shaped type I cells, surrounded by afferent nerve endings; and columnar type II cells, with both afferent and efferent nerve endings on their basal and lateral surfaces.

***(ii)* Supporting cells** are columnar, with basal nuclei and short apical microvilli. They lie between the receptor cells and produce the thick glycoprotein-rich **gelatinous layer** that covers the sensory epithelium and bulges into the membranous labyrinth's lumen.

(b) Maculae These are the sensory portions of the walls of the utricle and saccule. They are ovoid buttons of specialized epithelium covered by a gelatinous layer into which the sensory cells' microvilli and cilia extend. In the maculae of both the utricle and the saccule, small rocklike **otoliths** (statoliths), crystals of calcium carbonate and protein, cover the gelatinous layer. Changes in head position cause changes in endolymph flow, moving the otoliths. These movements are transmitted through the gelatinous layer, displacing the hair cells' cilia and microvilli and stimulating the associated nerve endings.

(c) Crista ampullaris This is the sensory region in each ampulla of the semicircular canals. Although the hair cells and supporting cells are similar to those in the maculae, they are arranged in transverse ridges (cristae) rather than buttonlike bulges (maculae). The conical gelatinous layer of a crista is termed the **cupula**; it lacks otoliths.

b. Auditory portion (cochlear duct) This part of the ear, conforms to the spiral cochlear chamber. The cochlear duct arises as an outpocketing of the saccule and contains the spiral organ of Corti.

(1) The cochlear duct uncoiled The auditory portion's general structure can be more easily understood if one pictures the cochlear contents removed from their bony canal and uncoiled. The cochlear duct then appears as a tube within a tube. The outer tube is lined by simple squamous epithelium that is bound tightly to the bony walls of the cochlea, and it contains perilymph. It begins at the oval window and ends at the round window. The upper half of the outer cavity (**scala vestibuli**) extends from the oval window to the apex of the spiral (**helicotrema**), while the lower half (**scala tympani**) extends from the helicotrema to the round window. Between these lies the cochlear duct, with its cavity (**scala media**) filled with endolymph.

(2) The cochlear duct in situ When these membranous structures are seen within the coiled cochlea, a section through a single turn of the cochlea appears as shown in Fig 24-30 (in *Basic Histology*). In situ, the cochlear duct appears triangular in profile and can be considered to have a roof, a lateral wall, and a floor.

(a) Roof This simple-squamous-lined membrane is known as the **vestibular (Reissner's) membrane.** It separates the scala vestibuli from the scala media and extends at an acute angle from the upper surface of the osseous spiral lamina to the outer bony wall of the cochlea.

(b) Lateral wall This part of the duct is formed mainly by the **stria vascularis,** an unusual partly stratified epithelium overlying a profusion of capillaries. The stria vascularis is thought to produce the endolymph that fills the cochlear duct.

(c) Floor This includes the spiral organ of Corti and the spiral lamina on which it rests. It separates the scala media from the scala tympani.

***(i)* Spiral lamina** This portion of the floor has both osseous and membranous parts. The osseus spiral lamina is the thread of the screwlike modiolus. The membranous spiral lamina extends from the edge of the thread across the cochlear canal to the spiral crest on the lateral wall. It includes a thin fibrous layer—the **basilar membrane**—at its core. Sensory cells of the spiral organ of Corti rest on the membranous portion.

***(ii)* Spiral organ of Corti** This complex structure is highly sensitive to vibration. It is anchored to the osseous spiral lamina by the **spiral limbus,** an epithelium-covered region of loose connective tissue. Extending from the limbus is a glycoprotein-rich flap, the **tectorial membrane.** The distal expansion of this membrane covers the sensory cells' apical surfaces much the way the gelatinous layer covers the maculae of the utricle and saccule. Bridging the space between the spiral limbus and the sensory cells, the tectorial membrane defines a channel termed the **internal spiral tunnel.** The spiral organ of Corti contains 2 major cell types, supporting and sensory cells.

***(a)* Supporting cells** A second channel that is smaller and triangular in profile lies just lateral to the internal spiral tunnel; it is known as the inner tunnel. The walls of the inner tunnel are formed by rows of supporting cells called **inner and outer pillar cells.** Pillar cells have broad bases containing their nuclei, and elongated cell bodies that contain tonofilament bundles.

***(b)* Sensory cells** As in the vestibular system, the sensory cells here are also called hair cells. **Inner hair cells** form a single row between the internal spiral tunnel and the inner tunnel. They are goblet-shaped, with apical stereocilia and a basal accumulation of mitochondria. The **outer hair cells** form 3 parallel rows lateral to the outer pillar cells and rest on columnar supporting cells called Deiter's cells. Outer hair cells are more columnar than the inner hair cells; they have basal nuclei and mitochondria. The 100 or so stereocilia of each outer hair cell are arranged in a V or W pattern and penetrate the cuticular plate, an apical expansion of the outer pillar cell. The tips of the stereocilia are covered by the tectorial membrane. Cochlear hair cells lack true cilia. They are innervated by the dendritic processes of bipolar neurons in the spiral ganglion. These processes pass from the ganglion in the modiolus through the connective tissue of the spiral limbus and basilar membrane to reach the hair cells.

4. Hearing Sound waves collected by the auricle traverse the auditory meatus and cause the tympanic membrane to vibrate. This vibration moves the ossicles, and movement of the stapes in the oval window transmits the vibrations to the perilymph in the scala vestibuli. The perilymph carries the vibrations from the scala vestibuli through the helicotrema and into the scale tympani. These vibrations in the perilymph cause the delicate membranous spiral lamina and the associated organ of Corti to move in relation to the tectorial membrane, displacing the hair cell stereocilia. Movement of the stereocilia then causes the generation of an action potential in the bipolar spiral ganglion cell processes. Neural signals generated in the cochlea are transmitted to the brain through the cochlear nerve (a collection of axons of the bipolar cells). Cochlear sensitivity is tonotopic—localized for sounds of different frequencies. The portion of the organ of Corti in the basal region of cochlea responds best to high-frequency sounds; that in the apical region responds best to low-frequency sounds.

Study-Focusing Questions*

1. Distinguish between a generator potential and a receptor potential in terms of the type of receptor in which each is formed (466).
2. List all the receptors that fall into the following categories and note which receptors overlap categories:
   a. Mechanoreceptors (466–467, 489)
   b. Chemoreceptors (466, 469–470, 223)
   c. Thermoreceptors (467)
   d. Photoreceptors (466, 479)
   e. Neuronal receptors (466)
   f. Epithelial (secondary) receptor cells (466)
   g. Neuroepithelial receptors (466)
   h. Proprioceptors (466, 467–469)
   i. Touch and pressure receptors (467)
   j. Warmth receptors (467)
   k. Pain receptors (nociceptors) (467)
   l. Cutaneous (skin) receptors (467)
3. List the types of sensations detected by free (unencapsulated) nerve endings (467).
4. Compare Meissner's corpuscles, Ruffini's endings, hair follicles, Merkel's corpuscles, and pacinian corpuscles (467) in terms of:
   a. The type of nerve fibers they contain
   b. The number of nerve fibers they contain
   c. The arrangement of their nerve fibers
   d. Their presence of a capsule
   e. The structure of the capsule, if present
   f. The sensory modality to which they are most sensitive
   g. Their location
5. Compare the intrafusal muscle fibers found in muscle spindles with extrafusal muscle fibers, in terms of their location in relation to the muscle spindle capsule (467).
6. Name the 2 types of intrafusal muscle fibers and compare them in terms of (467–469):
   a. Their diameter
   b. Their length
   c. The distribution of their nuclei
   d. The type(s) of sensory nerve endings they receive
7. Beginning with a sharp tap of the patellar tendon, list the sequence of events that produce the knee jerk reflex (469).
8. Compare muscle spindles with Golgi tendon organs in terms of function and the type of fibers (other than nerve fibers) found inside the capsule of the receptor (467–469).
9. List the types of receptors found in joint capsules. What is their function (469)?
10. Which sense organ in the head (besides the eye) contributes important information for proprioception (sense of equilibrium and position in space) (489)?
11. Name the 3 types of lingual papillae that harbor taste buds (469) and compare them in terms of:
    a. Their distribution on the tongue (469–470)
    b. The distribution of taste buds over their surfaces (**HR**)
12. Name the types of cells found in taste buds (469–470, **HR**) and compare them in terms of:
    a. Their shape
    b. Their cytoplasmic inclusions
    c. The presence of microvilli
    d. Their function
13. In what part of the nasal cavity is the olfactory epithelium located (470)?

*The page references in this section refer to *Basic Histology,* 6th ed., Junqueira L, Carneiro J, Kelley R (editors) Appleton & Lange, 1989. **HR** (for Histology Review) is occasionally used instead of a page reference to indicate that the information referred to can be found in this book.

14. Name 3 types of cells found in olfactory epithelium (470) and compare them in terms of:
    a. Their shape
    b. The positions of their nuclei
    c. The specializations of their apical surface (where applicable)
    d. Their function
15. Compare taste buds and olfactory epithelium in terms of:
    a. Their basic function
    b. The type of receptor cell (neuronal receptor, epithelial receptor, neuroepithelial receptor (466)
    c. The specializations of the receptor cell apical surface (470)
    d. The way they transmit their signals to the nervous system (generator or receptor potential) (466, 470)
16. Compare von Ebner's glands **(HR)** and Bowman's glands (470) in terms of:
    a. Their locations
    b. Their apparent function
    c. The type of secretion
17. List in order, the major steps in the embryonic development of the eye **(HR)**
18. Name the 3 compartments in the eye and give the boundaries of each (471, 474, 475)
19. Name, in order from outer to inner, the 3 basic tunics (or layers) that make up the globe of the eye (471); list the major components of each, in order from anterior to posterior (471–472, 473, 474, 479)
20. Describe the sclera in terms of:
    a. Its predominant tissue type (471)
    b. Its vascularity (472)
    c. The proportion of the eye it covers (471)
21. List, in order from anterior to posterior, the 5 layers of the cornea and describe the composition of each (472). Which layer is thickest?
22. Compare the sclera and cornea in terms of their:
    a. Transparency (471, 472)
    b. Blood supply and source of nourishment (472, 473)
    c. Amount of sensory innervation (472)
23. Beginning with its outer surface (attaching to the sclera) name, in order, the layers of the choroid and compare them in terms of the number and size of the blood vessels they contain (473).
24. What structure may be described as the ringlike triangular anterior thickening of the vascular layer of the eye (475)?
25. What is the function of the ciliary muscles (475, 478–479)?
26. How is the ciliary body attached to the lens (476, 478)?
27. Describe the site of production, the composition, and the circulatory route taken by the aqueous humor (476).
28. Name the 2 muscles found in the iris and compare them in terms of:
    a. Their cell type (477)
    b. The orientation of their fibers (477)
    c. The type of autonomic innervation that causes them to contract (477)
    d. The effect of their contraction on the amount of light entering the eye
29. What role does the heavy pigmentation of the vascular layer play in vision (477)?
30. Name, in order from outside to inside, the layers of the lens (216).
31. List some unusual characteristics of the cells referred to as "lens fibers" (478).
32. Choose the correct condition of the following structures when the eye is focusing on a near object (478–479).
    a. Ciliary muscles (contracted or relaxed)
    b. Lens shape (rounded or flattened)
33. Name the 2 layers of the retina and compare them in terms of:
    a. Their embryonic origin (479)
    b. Their location (inner or outer) (474, 479)
    c. Their tissue type (epithelium, connective tissue, muscle, nerve (479, 481)
    d. Their photosensitivity (481)
    e. Their phagocytic capacity (481, 483)
    f. Their melanin content (479–481)
    g. How far and in what form they extend anteriorly (480)
34. In the neural retina, although several layers can be distinguished histologically, only

3 layers of retinal nerve cells are involved in the reception and relay of visual signals to the brain. Name the cells in these 3 layers (481) and answer the following questions:

a. Which cells serve as the actual photoreceptors (481)?
b. In which order do the cells relay the signal (481)?
c. Which layer is first crossed by incoming light (482)?
d. Which cells contribute axons to the optic nerve (481, 482)?
e. Which cells can generate an action potential (486)?

35. Compare the rods and cones (482–483) in terms of:
a. Their shape
b. Their ability to function as photoreceptors (yes or no)
c. Their location in the retina
d. Their divisibility into outer and inner segments
e. Their physical association with the pigmented epithelium
f. The independence of their flattened vesicles from the plasma membrane
g. The phagocytosis of their flattened vesicles by the pigmented epithelial cells
h. The type of visual pigment they contain
i. The distribution of visual pigment in the outer segment
j. Their number in the human retina
k. Their visual acuity in bright and low light
l. Their sensitivity to shades of gray and color
m. Their association with monosynaptic bipolar cells
n. The sharpness of the images they form (acuity)

36. Name the types of neuroglia found in the neural retina (483).

37. Beginning with the tear layer on the surface of the cornea, list, in order, the entire series of layers, fluids, compartments, etc, through which light must pass in order to reach the outer segments of the rods and cones (474, 475, 482)

38. Beginning with the bleaching of the visual pigment by light, list the steps leading to the generation of an action potential by the ganglion cells (484–487)

39. Name the muscles involved in opening and closing the eyelids (palpebrae). Indicate which are voluntary and which are involuntary (488, **HR**).

40. Name the 3 types of glands found within the eyelids and compare them in terms of their secretions and where their ducts open (487, 488)

41. Describe the lacrimal gland in terms of:
a. Its location (487–488)
b. Its type (488)
c. The appearance of the glandular epithelium (488)
d. The composition of its secretion (tears) (489)

42. Trace the path of flow of tears over the eye and through the named components of the lacrimal apparatus (488–489). Why do people's noses "run" when they cry?

44. List the 3 major structural components of the external ear (489–490), the 5 of the middle ear (490), and the 2 of the inner ear (490) and name the major function of each component.

45. Name the 3 major regions of the bony labyrinth and the portions of the membranous labyrinth each contains (490).

46. Compare the perilymph and the endolymph (490) in terms of their:
a. Location
b. Composition
c. Site of production (492)

47. List the 4 divisions of the vestibular portion of the membranous labyrinth (489) and name the sensory organ located in each (491). Which division lacks a sensory organ (491)?

48. What is the name for the auditory portion of the membranous labyrinth (491–492)? Name the sensory organ it contains (490, 492).

49. Make a schematic drawing of what the contents of the cochlea would look like if they were removed and uncoiled (489) and show the location of the following:
a. Oval window
b. Scala vestibuli
c. Helicotrema
d. Scala tympani
e. Round window

f. Scala media (cochlear duct)
g. Perilymph
h. Endolymph
The overall appearance should resemble a narrow tube (cochlear duct) within a wider tube, with the scala vestibuli beginning at the oval window and extending to the helicotrema, and the scala tympani beginning at the helicotrema and ending at the round window.

50. In situ, the cochlear duct (scala media) has a triangular appearance (493). Name the structure(s) that form its roof, lateral wall, and floor.

51. Name the structures in the maculae (491) and in the crista ampullaris (492) that correspond to the following structures in the organ of Corti (493):
- **a.** Inner and outer hair cells
- **b.** Stereocilia
- **c.** Pillar cells
- **d.** Tectorial membrane

52. Compare the apex and the base of the organ of Corti in terms of the sound frequency to which each responds best (495).

53. Beginning with the act of lying down, list, in order, and naming all the structures of the vestibular apparatus that play a part, the sequence of events that lead to the relaying of a signal to the brain that the position of the head has changed (495).

54. Beginning with the entrance of a sound into the external ear, list, in order and naming all the involved cavities, moving bones, membranes, and cells, the sequence of events leading to the generation of an action potential by the bipolar spiral ganglion cells (495).

Multiple-Choice Questions

For questions 24–1 through 24–8 select the single best answer.

24–1. Which of the following receptors are unencapsulated?
- **A.** Pacinian corpuscles
- **B.** Muscle spindles
- **C.** Free nerve endings
- **D.** Golgi tendon organs
- **E.** Meissner's corpuscles

24–2. Muscle spindles contain all of the following *except*:
- **A.** Intrafusal fibers
- **B.** Nuclear chain fibers
- **C.** Extrafusal fibers
- **D.** Nuclear bag fibers
- **E.** Flower-spray endings

24–3. The thickest layer of the cornea is:
- **A.** Descemet's membrane
- **B.** The stroma
- **C.** The corneal endothelium
- **D.** The anterior epithelium
- **E.** Bowman's membrane

24–4. The junction between the cornea and the sclera is called the:
- **A.** Ora serrata
- **B.** Iris
- **C.** Ciliary body
- **D.** Limbus
- **E.** Episclera

24–5. The aqueous humor of the eye is produced by the:
- **A.** Canal of Schlemm
- **B.** Choriocapillary layer
- **C.** Endolymphatic sac
- **D.** Ciliary epithelium
- **E.** Stria vascularis

24–6. The structure that serves as the border between the anterior and posterior chambers of the eye is the:
- **A.** Iris
- **B.** Lens
- **C.** Zonule
- **D.** Ora serrata
- **E.** Vitreous body

24–7. The fovea of the eye:
- **A.** Is also known as the blind spot
- **B.** Is the region where the axons of the ganglion cells converge and leave the eye as the optic nerve
- **C.** Is the region where retinal veins converge to leave the eye
- **D.** Is the thinnest part of the neural retina
- **E.** Contains no photoreceptive cells

24–8. The receptors shown in the photomicrograph in Fig 24–1 are:
- **A.** Meissner's corpuscles
- **B.** Pacinian corpuscles
- **C.** Taste buds
- **D.** Free nerve endings
- **E.** Merkel's disks

MATCHING (questions 24–9 through 24–84): Each choice may be used once, more than once, or not at all.

Questions 24–9 through 24–22 (may have more than one correct answer):

- **A.** Mechanoreceptor
- **B.** Thermoreceptor

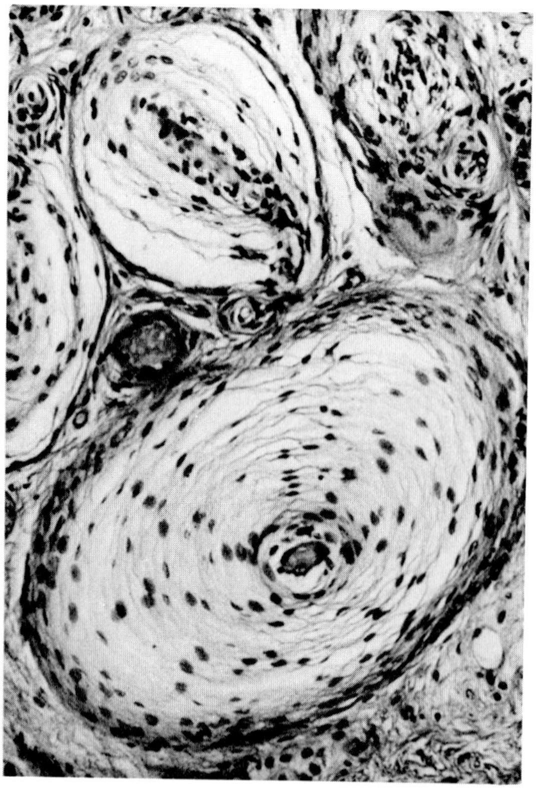

Figure 24–1.

C. Nociceptor
D. Proprioceptor
E. Photoreceptor
F. Chemoreceptor

24–9. Muscle spindle
24–10. Carotid body
24–11. Free nerve endings
24–12. Organ of Corti
24–13. Pain receptor
24–14. Golgi tendon organ
24–15. Olfactory epithelium
24–16. Macula of the saccule
24–17. Ruffini's endings
24–18. Meissner's corpuscle
24–19. Pacinian corpuscle
24–20. Merkel's corpuscle
24–21. Taste bud
24–22. Neural retina

Questions 24–23 through 24–38:

A. Tunica fibrosa (external layer)
B. Tunica vasculosa (middle layer)
C. Tunica interna (internal layer)
D. All of the above
E. None of the above

24–23. Retina
24–24. Uvea
24–25. Lens
24–26. Cornea
24–27. Choroid
24–28. Limbus
24–29. Globe
24–30. Ciliary body
24–31. Vitreous
24–32. Derived from optic vesicle
24–33. Derived from mesenchyme
24–34. Rods and cones
24–35. Fovea
24–36. Conjunctiva
24–37. Choriocapillary layer
24–38. Iris

Questions 24–39 through 24–46:

A. Bipolar cells
B. Ganglion cells
C. Horizontal cells
D. Amacrine cells
E. Müller cells

24–39. Carry visual signals to the brain
24–40. Glial cells
24–41. Classified as diffuse or monosynaptic
24–42. Large nuclei, located closest to the vitreous
24–43. Cell processes terminate near synapses between bipolar and ganglion cells
24–44. Cell processes terminate near synapses between photoreceptors and bipolar cells
24–45. Span the entire width of the neural retina
24–46. Nuclei located in the internal nuclear layer

Questions 24–47 through 24–51:

A. Bowman's membrane
B. Descemet's membrane
C. Bruch's membrane
D. None of the above

24–47. Innermost layer of the choroid
24–48. Posterior epithelium of the cornea
24–49. Contains elastin
24–50. Basement membrane of the pigmented epithelium
24–51. Anterior epithelium of the cornea

Questions 24–52 through 24–69 use the letters in Fig 24–2.

24–52. Tectorial membrane
24–53. Pillar cells
24–54. Spiral limbus
24–55. Inner hair (sensory) cells
24–56. Outer hair (sensory) cells

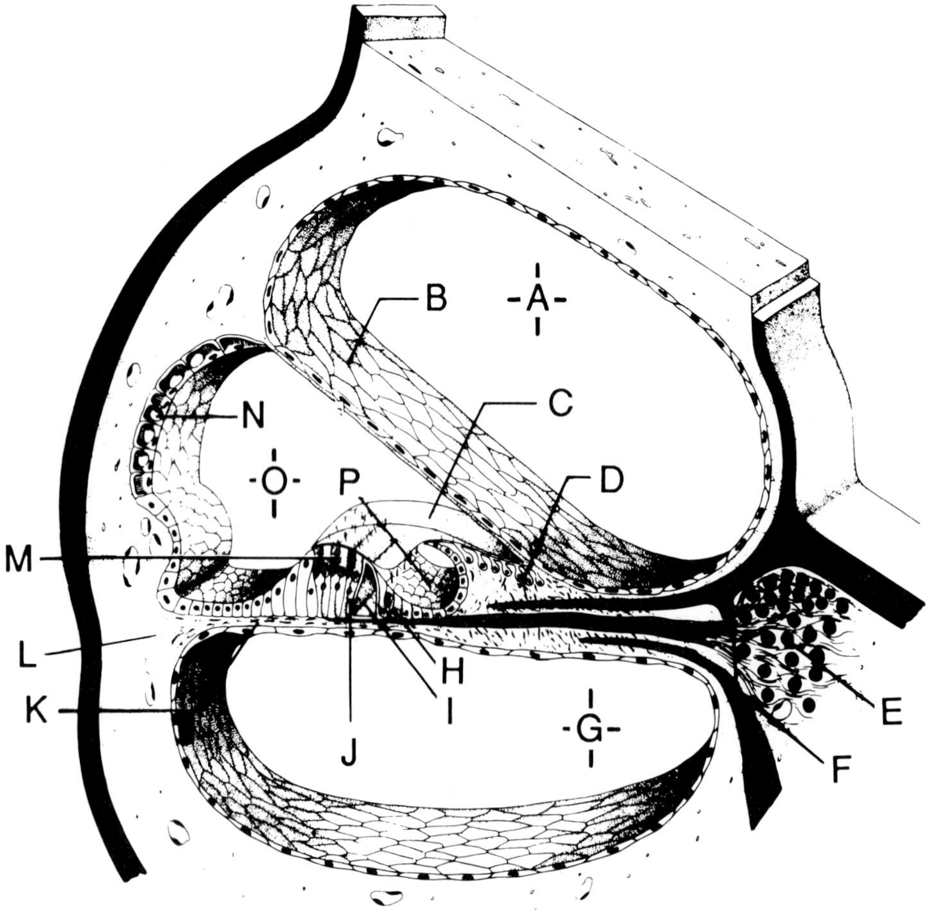

Figure 24–2.

24-57. Scala media
24-58. Scala tympani
24-59. Scala vestibuli
24-60. Osseous spiral lamina
24-61. Roof of cochlear duct
24-62. Contains endolymph
24-63. Stria vascularis
24-64. Basilar membrane
24-65. Lumen of cochlear duct
24-66. Internal spiral tunnel
24-67. Produces endolymph
24-68. Spiral ganglion
24-69. Spiral ligament (membranous spiral lamina)

Questions 24-70 through 24-84:

A. External ear
B. Middle ear
C. Internal (inner) ear
D. All of the above
E. None of the above

24-70. Communicate(s) with the pharynx through the eustachian tube
24-71. Include(s) the auricle
24-72. Also known as the labyrinth
24-73. Contain(s) the cochlea
24-74. Contain(s) the ossicles
24-75. Communicate(s) with the mastoid air cells
24-76. Include(s) the external auditory meatus
24-77. Include(s) the tympanic membrane
24-78. Include(s) the ceruminous glands
24-79. Contain(s) the vestibular apparatus
24-80. Contain(s) endolymph
24-81. Contain(s) perilymph
24-82. Include(s) the modiolus
24-83. Include(s) the semicircular canals
24-84. Contain(s) the organ of Corti

For questions 24-85 through 24-103, either, both, or neither of the answers may be correct. Select

A if only A is correct
B if only B is correct
C if both A and B are correct
D if neither A nor B is correct

Questions 24-85 through 24-91:

A. Sphincter pupillae muscle
B. Dilator pupillae muscle
C. Both
D. Neither

24-85. Under sympathetic control
24-86. Under parasympathetic control
24-87. Contract(s) in low light
24-88. Smooth muscle
24-89. Located in the pupillary margin of the iris
24-90. Contraction causes lens to flatten
24-91. Arranged like the spokes of a wheel

Questions 24–92 through 24–103:

A. Rod cells
B. Cone cells
C. Both
D. Neither

24–92. Photoreceptors
24–93. Lack(s) an outer segment
24–94. Flattened vesicles are independent of plasma membrane
24–95. Contain(s) iodopsin
24–96. Responsible for night vision
24–97. Greatest visual acuity
24–98. Absent from the fovea
24–99. Contain(s) intracytoplasmic cilia
24–100. Most abundant
24–101. Located in the layer of the retina adjacent to the pigmented epithelium
24–102. Contain(s) rhodopsin
24–103. Responsible for color vision

For questions 24–104 through 24–113, one, more than one, or all of the answers may be correct. Select

A if only (1), (2), and (3) are correct
B if only (1) and (3) are correct
C if only (2) and (4) are correct
D if only (4) is correct
E if all answers are correct

24–104. Golgi tendon organs:
(1) Are encapsulated
(2) Contain intrafusal muscle fibers
(3) Are found at muscle-tendon junctions
(4) Have both motor and sensory innervation

24–105. Type III cells of taste buds:
(1) Have apical microvilli
(2) Release neurotransmitters in response to chemical stimuli
(3) May be innervated by several sensory fibers
(4) Arise from basal cells

24–106. Olfactory (sensory) cells:
(1) Have a tuft of specialized cilia on their apical surfaces
(2) Are actually neurons
(3) House the middle row of nuclei in the olfactory epithelium
(4) Are distributed in the respiratory epithelium throughout the nasal cavity

24–107. The optic vesicle:
(1) Gives rise to the neural retina
(2) Gives rise to the pigmented epithelium
(3) Induces the formation of the lens placode
(4) Invaginates to form the lens vesicle

24–108. The cornea:
(1) Constitutes the anterior one-sixth of the tunica fibrosa (external layer)
(2) Is composed of 5 layers
(3) Is avascular
(4) Accounts for eye color

24–109. Contraction of the ciliary muscles:
(1) Is under involuntary control
(2) Is required for focusing on near objects
(3) Allows accommodation
(4) Pulls the ciliary body anteriorly

24–110. The pigmented epithelium of the retina:
(1) Rests on Bruch's membrane

(2) Continues anteriorly over the ciliary body and iris
(3) Is derived from the outer wall of the optic cup
(4) Phagocytoses flattened vesicles shed by the cone cells

24–111. Lens fibers:
(1) Are highly differentiated epithelium cells
(2) Lack nuclei
(3) Exhibit unusual ridgelike plasma membrane specializations
(4) Are composed of type III collagen

24–112. Tears:
(1) Are secreted by the meibomian glands
(2) Leave the eye surface through the lacrimal puncta
(3) Are secreted by the glands of Moll
(4) Contain lysozyme

24–113. The semicircular canals:
(1) Contain the cristae ampullares
(2) Emanate from the vestibule
(3) Contain no otoliths
(4) Are arranged in 3 planes perpendicular to one another

Answers to Multiple-Choice Questions

Chapter 1: Methods of Study*

Single Best Answer

1–1. A (5)
1–2. C (7)

Matching

1–3. E (1, 2, 3)
1–4. C (2–3)
1–5. A (1–2)
1–6. B (2–3)
1–7. A (1–2)
1–8. D (2–3)
1–9. B (2–3)
1–10. F (3)
1–11. B (9–10)
1–12. B (9)
1–13. D (14)
1–14. A (10, 13)
1–15. C (13–14)
1–16. D (14–16)
1–17. C (13)
1–18. B (9–10)
1–19. F (16)

Either, Both, or Neither

1–20. A (2)
1–21. B (3)
1–22. B (3)
1–23. C (10)
1–24. B (7)
1–25. C (1–3)

*The page references in this section refer to *Basic Histology,* 6th ed., Junqueira L, Carneiro J, Kelley R (editors) Appleton & Lange, 1989. **HR** (for Histology Review) is occasionally used instead of a page reference to indicate that the information referred to can be found in this book.

1–26. B (7)
1–27. A (**HR**)
1–28. B (**HR**)
1–29. B (8)
1–30. D (3)
1–31. C (3)
1–32. B (3)
1–33. B (3)

One, More Than One, or All

1–34. A (1)
1–35. B (12)
1–36. B (5, 8, 13)
1–37. E (10, 13)
1–38. B (1–2)

Chapter 2: Histochemistry & Cytochemistry*

Single Best Answer

2–1. B (18)
2–2. C (20)
2–3. D (24–26)

Matching

2–4. C (22–23)
2–5. A (20)
2–6. C (22–23)
2–7. E (19)
2–8. B (3)
2–9. D (24–25)
2–10. D (24–25)
2–11. D (3)

One, More Than One, or All

2–12. E (18–20)
2–13. A (19)
2–14. A (20, 25)
2–15. A (3, 19, 22)
2–16. A (26–27)

Chapter 3: The Cell*

Single Best Answer

3–1. D (51–52)
3–2. B (22–23, 40)
3–3. C (30–31)
3–4. E (43–48)
3–5. C (31, 32)
3–6. B (43)
3–7. D (48)
3–8. A (37)
3–9. B (60)
3–10. D (40, 42)
3–11. E (55)
3–12. D (41–43)
3–13. B (34)
3–14. D (41)
3–15. D (59)

Matching

3–16. A (34)
3–17. B (34)
3–18. C (35)
3–19. C (34)
3–20. A (34)
3–21. C (29, 34)

3-22. A (37)
3-23. B (40)
3-24. G (32-33)
3-25. H (53-56)
3-26. C (44)
3-27. J (46, 47)
3-28. F (46, 47)
3-29. I (51)
3-30. K (48-49)
3-31. D (50)
3-32. E (54, 56)
3-33. D (35)
3-34. B (35)
3-35. E (37)
3-36. C (33-34)
3-37. E (37)
3-38. G (38)
3-39. D (37)
3-40. G (38)
3-41. D (35, 36)
3-42. E (39)
3-43. C (35, 57)
3-44. A (31, 32)
3-45. A (38)
3-46. C (56)
3-47. B (30, 32)

Either, Both, or Neither

3-48. C (43-44, 46, 48)
3-49. B (48)
3-50. C (43)
3-51. A (43)
3-52. C (44-48)
3-53. B (48)
3-54. D (49)
3-55. A (46, 47)
3-56. A (44)
3-57. A (47)
3-58. A (43)
3-59. B (48)
3-60. A (47)
3-61. A (28, 30)
3-62. B (28, 30)
3-63. A (28, 30)
3-64. C (28, 30)
3-65. A (28, 30)
3-66. B (28, 30)

One, More Than One, or All

3-67. E (38)
3-68. E (30-33)
3-69. B (43, 48, 49)
3-70. E (45, 47, 60)
3-71. E (58-60)
3-72. C (40, 41)
3-73. C (35)
3-74. E (35, 56-57)
3-75. E (50-51)
3-76. E (53-55)
3-77. D (35, 57)

Chapter 4: Epithelial Cells & Tissues*

Single Best Answer

4-1. D (65)
4-2. C (73-74, 366)
4-3. B (69)
4-4. C (65, 74-75)
4-5. B (71)

Matching

4-6. A (73, 334)
4-7. C (73, 387)
4-8. E (72)
4-9. B (74, 335)
4-10. D (73)
4-11. F (73)
4-12. D (77)
4-13. G (77)
4-14. B (77)
4-15. C (77)
4-16. E (77)
4-17. F (77)
4-18. A (77)
4-19. B (81)

4-20. D (88-89)
4-21. C (86)
4-22. D (88-89)
4-23. A (79)
4-24. A (68)
4-25. B (68)
4-26. D (68, 70)
4-27. C (68, 71)
4-28. D (67, 68)
4-29. C (67)

Either, Both, or Neither

4-30. C (71-72)
4-31. B (71-72)
4-32. A (72-73)
4-33. A (72-73)
4-34. B (71-72)
4-35. A (72-73)
4-36. A (72)
4-37. B (71)
4-38. C (71-74)

One, More Than One, or All

4-39. A (64, 66, 78)
4-40. A (72, 74, 75)
4-41. B (67-68, 71)
4-42. C (72)
4-43. B (76-77)
4-44. B (76-77)
4-45. A (76-77)
4-46. E (66)

Chapter 5: Connective Tissue*

Single Best Answer

5-1. D (91)
5-2. B (104)
5-3. A (37, 96)
5-4. E (116)
5-5. A (91)
5-6. E (93)
5-7. C (100)
5-8. D (102)
5-9. B (117)

Matching

5-10. D (96)
5-11. C (96)
5-12. A (101)
5-13. E (113, 116)
5-14. D (110)
5-15. A (104)
5-16. C (108)
5-17. B (112-113, 115)
5-18. E (105)
5-19. C (109)
5-20. D (110)
5-21. A (104)

Either, Both, or Neither

5-22. B (98, 99)
5-23. B (98, 99)
5-24. C (98, 99)
5-25. D (96, 98, 99)

One, More Than One, or All

5-26. E (91, 119-120)
5-27. E (93, 98, 101, 104)
5-28. E (99)
5-29. E (118)
5-30. E (100-101, 113, 117-118)

Chapter 6: Adipose Tissue*

Single Best Answer

6–1. E (122–124)
6–2. B (123–124)

Matching

6–3. C (122)
6–4. A (123)
6–5. D (123)
6–6. A (123)
6–7. B (123)
6–8. C (122)
6–9. C (123)

Either, Both, or Neither

6–10. B (121)
6–11. A (121)
6–12. A (121)
6–13. A (121, 124)
6–14. C (121)
6–15. B (125)
6–16. A (122)
6–17. A (121, 125)
6–18. B (125)
6–19. B (125)
6–20. C (124, 125)
6–21. A (121)
6–22. B (125)

One, More Than One, or All

6–23. E (122–124)
6–24. B (123)
6–25. C (123)

Chapter 7: Cartilage*

Single Best Answer

7–1. D (127)
7–2. E (38, 130)
7–3. B (129)
7–4. C (127)
7–5. A (128)
7–6. C (131)
7–7. A (130)

Matching

7–8. A (127)
7–9. E (127, 132, 133)
7–10. C (135)
7–11. A (127)
7–12. C (133)
7–13. B (132)
7–14. A (127)
7–15. B (132)
7–16. C (135)
7–17. D (129, 132)
7–18. C (**HR**)
7–19. A (127)
7–20. D (131, **HR**)

Either, Both, or Neither

7-21. C (131-132)
7-22. A (131-132)
7-23. B (131-132)
7-24. A (131-132)
7-25. A (131-132)
7-26. D (131-132)

One, More Than One, or All

7-27. C (127, 130, 133)
7-28. A (130)
7-29. C (130)

Chapter 8: Bone*

Single Best Answer

8-1. D (140)
8-2. C (136)
8-3. C (**HR**)
8-4. A (143, 144)

Matching

8-5. A (137)
8-6. C (137)
8-7. D (137)
8-8. F (137)
8-9. B (137)
8-10. E (137)
8-11. F (137, 139, 142)
8-12. A (137)
8-13. B (137, 140)
8-14. A (137, 139, 156)
8-15. D (137, 150)
8-16. A (137)
8-17. B (137, 141)
8-18. B (140-141)
8-19. A (137)
8-20. B (137, 155)
8-21. B (137, 140)
8-22. C (136, 137)
8-23. D (145, 148)
8-24. A (137, 140)
8-25. B (137, 140)
8-26. E (140)
8-27. E (157)
8-28. D (157)
8-29. A (157)
8-30. B (157)
8-31. A (157)
8-32. D (157-158)
8-33. C (157)
8-34. D (157-158)

Either, Both, or Neither

8-35. B (142)
8-36. B (157)
8-37. B (142)
8-38. C (142)
8-39. A (142, 143)
8-40. D (142)
8-41. C (142)
8-42. C (142, 153-154)
8-43. A (143)
8-44. B (143)
8-45. A (143)
8-46. A (144)
8-47. B (144)
8-48. D (144)
8-49. A (143)
8-50. B (144)
8-51. A (144)
8-52. A (153-154)
8-53. B (145)
8-54. B (144)
8-55. A (144)
8-56. B (143, 144)
8-57. B (144)
8-58. B (144)
8-59. A (144)
8-60. A (145)
8-61. B (147)
8-62. B (147)
8-63. A (147)
8-64. B (148)
8-65. C (131, 145, 147)
8-66. C (145, 148)

8-67. B (148)
8-68. C (153)
8-69. B (**HR**)
8-70. C (145, 148)
8-71. B (155)
8-72. A (155)
8-73. C (154-155)
8-74. A (155)
8-75. A (155)
8-76. D (155)
8-77. A (155)
8-78. B (155)
8-79. A (155)
8-80. B (155)
8-81. A (155)

One, More Than One, or All

8-82. A (148, 151-153, 155-156)
8-83. E (141-142)
8-84. B (145, 146)
8-85. E (157-158)

Integrative Multiple-Choice Questions: Connective Tissues*

Single Best Answer

CT-1. B (125)
CT-2. C (120, 155)
CT-3. C (120, 155)
CT-4. C (103)
CT-5. D (133)

Matching

CT-6. F (113-117)
CT-7. D (127, 132-133)
CT-8. E (122)
CT-9. G (91)
CT-10. B (101)
CT-11. E (96, 98, 99, 100)
CT-12. A (142)
CT-13. B (95, 127)
CT-14. A (142)
CT-15. D (66, 95)
CT-16. C (95, 100)
CT-17. A (95, 116)
CT-18. C (100)
CT-19. A (133)
CT-20. E (95)
CT-21. B (Chemical designation for 3 type II α1 chains)
CT-22. B (95, 100)
CT-23. F (135)
CT-24. E (121-123)
CT-25. A (116-117)
CT-26. F (127)
CT-27. E (121)
CT-28. D (118)
CT-29. E (122)
CT-30. F (157)
CT-31. A (113)
CT-32. H (91)
CT-33. C (117-118)
CT-34. G (154)
CT-35. F (127)
CT-36. H (91, 115)
CT-37. C (130)
CT-38. E (91, 130)
CT-39. B (91, 130)
CT-40. D (130)
CT-41. A (93, 130)
CT-42. C (93, 130)

One, More Than One, or All

CT-43. C (105, 115, 140)
CT-44. E (104, 118, 130, 137)
CT-45. E (104, 118, 130, 137)
CT-46. A (106, 140, 235-236)

Chapter 9: Nerve Tissue*

Single Best Answer

9-1. C (164)
9-2. B (160)
9-3. D (160)
9-4. E (190–191)
9-5. C (187)
9-6. B (167–168, 182)
9-7. D (160–162, 164)

Matching

9-8. B (171)
9-9. E (172)
9-10. D (170)
9-11. C (170)
9-12. B (172, 176)
9-13. E (174–176)
9-14. F (187)
9-15. C, D (170)
9-16. A (171)
9-17. B **(HR)**
9-18. G (171)
9-19. A (190)
9-20. B (190)
9-21. C (190–191)
9-22. E (190–191)
9-23. A (190)
9-24. C (166)
9-25. E (166)
9-26. D (166)
9-27. B (166)
9-28. A (166)

Either, Both, or Neither

9-29. A (160)
9-30. B (160, 187)
9-31. C (176–178)
9-32. C (160)
9-33. A (160)
9-34. A (190)
9-35. B (176, 177)
9-36. B (172–173)
9-37. B (187)
9-38. A (171)
9-39. B (170)
9-40. C (170–171)
9-41. A (190)
9-42. B (189)
9-43. A (189)
9-44. B (189)
9-45. B (164–166)
9-46. D (164–166)
9-47. C (164–166)
9-48. E (164–166)
9-49. A (164–166)
9-50. A (164–166)
9-51. A (172–176)
9-52. B (161, 162)
9-53. A (164–166, 182)
9-54. A (164–166)
9-55. C (176–178)
9-56. A (176–178)
9-57. A (176–178)
9-58. C (176–178)
9-59. B (176–178)
9-60. B (176–178, 188)
9-61. A (176–178)
9-62. C (171, 172–176)
9-63. A (171, 172, 176)
9-64. A (182)
9-65. A (182)
9-66. A (173)
9-67. B (171, 176)
9-68. A (171, 172, 176)

One, More Than One, or All

9-69. A (163, 164, 185)
9-70. E (162, 164, 175, 176)
9-71. C (185, 186)
9-72. E (166–167, 182–183)
9-73. A (181)
9-74. E (160)
9-75. E (171, 190, 192)

Chapter 10: Muscle Tissue*

Single Best Answer

10–1. C (207)
10–2. E (199)
10–3. A (199, 200)
10–4. D (203–204)
10–5. D (201–204)
10–6. A (196–198)

Matching

10–7. B (198)
10–8. C (198)
10–9. F (197)
10–10. A (198)
10–11. G (198)
10–12. D (198)
10–13. E (198)
10–14. A (201, 202)
10–15. E (195, 198)
10–16. A (195)
10–17. D (195, 205)
10–18. B (195)
10–19. C (195)
10–20. C (195)
10–21. F (201, 207–208, 211)
10–22. C **(HR)**
10–23. B (207)
10–24. F (197, 207, 211)
10–25. F (197, 211)
10–26. A (202, 212, 227)
10–27. D (198, 208, 209)
10–28. E (194)
10–29. F (197, 207, 211)
10–30. B (194)
10–31. B (208)
10–32. D (194)
10–33. A (194)
10–34. F (195, 207, 209)
10–35. C (211)
10–36. B (207)
10–37. C (212)
10–38. D (197)
10–39. C **(HR)**
10–40. A (196, 207, 211)

Either, Both, or Neither

10–41. A (198)
10–42. B (198)
10–43. B (200)
10–44. B (200)
10–45. A (200)
10–46. A (200)
10–47. A (200)
10–48. D (199)
10–49. D (212)
10–50. A (198, 200)
10–51. B (196–198)
10–52. C (196–198)
10–53. A (196–198)
10–54. B (196–198)
10–55. A (196–198)
10–56. D (204, 206)
10–57. C (204, 206)
10–58. A (204, 206)
10–59. B (204, 206)
10–60. B (204, 206)
10–61. A (204, 206)
10–62. A (204, 206)

One, More Than One, or All

10–63. A (201–202)
10–64. A (200–201)
10–65. A (202–203)
10–66. B (202–203, 207)
10–67. B (212)

Integrative Multiple-Choice Questions: Basic Tissue Types*

Single Best Answer

BT-1. B (136)
BT-2. D (117)
BT-3. C (196)
BT-4. E (387)
BT-5. A (458)
BT-6. E (74, 139–140, 194, 207, 210)

Matching

BT-7. A (64, 91, 160, 194)
BT-8. B (115)
BT-9. C (160)
BT-10. D (75, 104, 194, 398)
BT-11. A (64)
BT-12. A (66, 77)
BT-13. B (104, 112)
BT-14. A (64)
BT-15. B (91)
BT-16. A (71–72)
BT-17. C (161, 164)
BT-18. D (49)
BT-19. A (78)

Either, Both, or Neither

BT-20. C (184, 212)
BT-21. C (40)
BT-22. C (176, 195)
BT-23. C (203–204)
BT-24. C (185, 202–203)

One, More Than One, or All

BT-25. B (78, 121, 130, 196)
BT-26. E (78, 125, 184, 202–203)

Chapter 11: Circulatory System*

Single Best Answer

11-1. D (217)
11-2. B (224)
11-3. D (225, **HR**)
11-4. B (227)
11-5. B (216)
11-6. B (220)
11-7. C (218)
11-8. D (218)
11-9. D (225)

Matching

11-10. B (226–227)
11-11. G (226–227)
11-12. D (226–227)
11-13. A (226–227)
11-14. F (226–227)
11-15. E (226–227)
11-16. C (226–227)
11-17. H (226–227)
11-18. F (226–227)
11-19. H (226–227)
11-20. E (226–227)
11-21. D (226–227)
11-22. G (226–227)

Either, Both, or Neither

11–23. C (214–215)
11–24. B (225)
11–25. A (221, 224)
11–26. B (224, 225)
11–27. A (214, 221)
11–28. B (225)
11–29. B (221)
11–30. C (220, 224)
11–31. C (215)
11–32. B (227)
11–33. A (221)
11–34. B (**HR**)
11–35. A (**HR**)
11–36. C (**HR**)
11–37. D (**HR**)
11–38. A (210)
11–39. A (226)
11–40. C (226)
11–41. B (227)
11–42. C (239, 273)
11–43. A (227)
11–44. B (217, 227)
11–45. D (**HR**)
11–46. A (227)
11–47. B (217, 227)

One, More Than One, or All

11–48. E (217)
11–49. C (214)
11–50. B (225–227)
11–51. E (214)
11–52. E (223–224)
11–53. E (219–220)
11–54. E (220)
11–55. E (227–228)

Chapter 12: Blood Cells*

Single Best Answer

12–1. C (229)
12–2. D (233)
12–3. E (**HR**)
12–4. C (243–244)
12–5. B (94–95, 229)
12–6. A (231)
12–7. D (238)
12–8. C (244)

Matching

12–9. A, B (233)
12–10. C, D, E (233)
12–11. A, B (233)
12–12. F (233)
12–13. D (232)
12–14. C (237, 238)
12–15. E (236)
12–16. F (229)
12–17. A (236, 237, 238, 241)
12–18. C (237)
12–19. A (240, 241)
12–20. B (241)
12–21. E (232)
12–22. D (239)
12–23. E (235)
12–24. F (233)
12–25. F (233)

Either, Both, or Neither

12–26. A (229, **HR**)
12–27. C (229, **HR**)
12–28. B (229, **HR**)
12–29. C (229, **HR**)

One, More Than One, or All

12–30. C (229)
12–31. A (231, 232, 233)
12–32. E (235, 236, 239, 240)
12–33. E (232–233)
12–34. B (240)

Chapter 13: Hematopoiesis*

Single Best Answer

13–1. C (245)
13–2. D (257)
13–3. C (245–246)
13–4. C (246)
13–5. A (248)
13–6. D (249)
13–7. B (253)
13–8. D (256)

Matching

13–9. B (249)
13–10. F (249)
13–11. F **(HR)**
13–12. F (249)
13–13. A (247)
13–14. C (250)
13–15. A (250)
13–16. B (252)
13–17. C (250, 253)
13–18. F (251)
13–19. D (253)
13–20. E (253)
13–21. D (246)
13–22. B (246)
13–23. A (246)
13–24. C (249–250)

Either, Both, or Neither

13–25. C (247, 248, 250–255)
13–26. C (247, 248, 250–255)
13–27. A (247, 248, 250–255)
13–28. D (247, 248, 250–255)
13–29. A (247, 248, 250–255)
13–30. C (247, 248, 250–255)
13–31. B (247, 248, 250–255)

One, More Than One, or All

13–32. B (259)
13–33. C (257)
13–34. D (247, 249–250)
13–35. A (247)
13–36. B (254–255)
13–37. B (256)

Chapter 14: Lymphoid System*

Single Best Answer

14–1. E (260, 263–265)
14–2. D (260)
14–3. C (263–265)
14–4. E (270, 273)

Matching

14-5. F (**HR**, 261)
14-6. E (**HR**, 261)
14-7. D (**HR**, 261)
14-8. C (**HR**, 261)
14-9. B (**HR**, 261)
14-10. A (**HR**, 261)
14-11. D (**HR**, 261)
14-12. C (**HR**, 261)
14-13. E (262, 271)
14-14. B (256)
14-15. D (273)
14-16. C (270, 271)
14-17. D (110, 111)
14-18. C (261)
14-19. A (261)
14-20. F (260)
14-21. C (261)
14-22. B (261)
14-23. A (261)
14-24. B (261)
14-25. E (261)
14-26. B, D (261)
14-27. E (261)
14-28. D (261)
14-29. B (280)
14-30. D (280)
14-31. A (280)
14-32. C (280)
14-33. B (280)
14-34. E (263, 271, 273-274)
14-35. F (263, 271, 277)
14-36. D (263, 271, 277)
14-37. B (273)
14-38. C (271)
14-39. F (271, 274)
14-40. D (262, 271, 273)
14-41. A (260)
14-42. F (260)
14-43. B (274)
14-44. F (271, 274)
14-45. C (271)
14-46. A (263)
14-47. C (266, 271)
14-48. B (277)

Either, Both, or Neither

14-49. C (261)
14-50. B (260)
14-51. A (260)
14-52. C (261-262)
14-53. B (261)
14-54. A (261-262, 269)

One, More Than One, or All

14-55. A (261-262)
14-56. E (260)
14-57. B (266)
14-58. E (110, 111, 261, 273, 277)
14-59. A (240, 277, 280)
14-60. A (240, 268)

Integrative Multiple-Choice Questions: Circulatory, Hematopoietic, & Lymphoid Systems*

Single Best Answer

CHL-1. C (194, 258, 262)
CHL-2. D (112, 254, 255, 273)
CHL-3. B (233)
CHL-4. D (253-255)

Matching

CHL-5. B (263)
CHL-6. C (238)
CHL-7. E (328)
CHL-8. I (246)
CHL-9. J (249)
CHL-10. G (235)
CHL-11. D (243)
CHL-12. H (225)
CHL-13. A (232-233)
CHL-14. F (260)

Either, Both, or Neither

CHL-15. A (240)
CHL-16. A (240, 273)
CHL-17. A (273)
CHL-18. B (273)
CHL-19. A (263)
CHL-20. C (261-262)
CHL-21. A (261-262)
CHL-22. B (260)
CHL-23. D (236)

One, More Than One, or All

CHL-24. D (240, 249, 253-255)
CHL-25. A (258-259)
CHL-26. B (259)
CHL-27. E (109, 237, 261)

Chapter 15: Digestive Tract*

Single Best Answer

15-1. B (285)
15-2. B (288-289)
15-3. D (288)
15-4. D (290)
15-5. B (292)
15-6. C (293)
15-7. D (297)
15-8. E (309)

Matching

15-9. A (284)
15-10. C (284)
15-11. D (284-285)
15-12. A (284)
15-13. B, D (284-285)
15-14. C (286)
15-15. D (286)
15-16. B (286)
15-17. E (286)
15-18. F (286)
15-19. A (286)
15-20. G (286)
15-21. H (286)
15-22. I (286)
15-23. F (289)
15-24. D (289)
15-25. A (289)
15-26. H (289)
15-27. D (289)
15-28. E (289)
15-29. G (289)
15-30. B (289)
15-31. A, B, D (288, 289)
15-32. H (289)
15-33. F (306)
15-34. B (295)
15-35. C (304)
15-36. A (295)
15-37. C (304)
15-38. A (294-295)
15-39. B (295)
15-40. C (304)
15-41. D (300)
15-42. E (300)
15-43. C (304)
15-44. A (294)
15-45. B (295)

Either, Both, or Neither

15-46. A (288)
15-47. B (288)
15-48. B (285, 288)
15-49. A (286)
15-50. A (286)
15-51. D (287)
15-52. A (289)
15-53. B (285)
15-54. C (290)
15-55. A (290)
15-56. D (282)
15-57. A **(HR)**
15-58. C (290)
15-59. B (290)
15-60. B (306)
15-61. A (297, 306)

15-62. B (306)
15-63. A (305)
15-64. B (309)
15-65. A (297, 306)
15-66. C (298, 306)
15-67. C (300, 304)
15-68. B (309)
15-69. C (298, 301, 306)

One, More Than One, or All

15-70. D (286, 287)
15-71. A (288-289)
15-72. A (292-297)
15-73. E (290, 297)
15-74. A (305, 307)
15-75. A (301, 302)
15-76. A (300)
15-77. A (298, 305-306)
15-78. A (309-310)

Chapter 16: Glands Associated With the Digestive Tract*

Single Best Answer

16-1. A (314)
16-2. C (315)
16-3. B (314)
16-4. C (318)
16-5. C (322)

Matching

16-6. D (311)
16-7. E (314)
16-8. A (312)
16-9. C (314)
16-10. B (312)
16-11. B (314)
16-12. A (**HR**)
16-13. D (75)
16-14. F (324)
16-15. E (324)
16-16. A (320)
16-17. A (318-321)
16-18. E (318-321)
16-19. B (324)
16-20. F (331, **HR**)
16-21. A (320)
16-22. A (318, 320, 324)
16-23. C (326)
16-24. C (325)

Either, Both, or Neither

16-25. A (86, 311, 312, 314)
16-26. B (86, 311, 312, 314)
16-27. A (311)
16-28. B (311)
16-29. B (311)
16-30. A (311)
16-31. A (311)
16-32. B (311)
16-33. A (314)
16-34. D (312)
16-35. A (312)
16-36. B (86)
16-37. C (312-315)
16-38. C (312, 315-316)
16-39. D (312, 315-316)
16-40. B (316)
16-41. B (315)
16-42. A (312, 315-316)
16-43. A (320-321)
16-44. B (320-321)
16-45. A (246, 279, 320)
16-46. C (320-323)
16-47. D (320-323)
16-48. A (321)
16-49. B (333)
16-50. B (316)
16-51. A (316)
16-52. C (304)
16-53. C (304, 316)

One, More Than One, or All

16–54. E (315)
16–55. C (312)
16–56. B (311, 312, 314)
16–57. B (86, 88, 311, 324 326)
16–58. B (316)
16–59. E (317)
16–60. E (320)
16–61. C (320)
16–62. A (331, 333)

Chapter 17: Respiratory System*

Single Best Answer

17–1. D (343)
17–2. E (347)
17–3. B (335)
17–4. B (352)

Matching

17–5. C (340)
17–6. H (334, 342)
17–7. A (339)
17–8. D (335, 340)
17–9. E (341)
17–10. C (340)
17–11. H or I (345)
17–12. F (341–342)
17–13. G (343)
17–14. I (344)
17–15. A (334, 339)
17–16. J (348)
17–17. H (352)
17–18. B (346)
17–19. D (346)
17–20. F (346)
17–21. E (346)
17–22. C (346)
17–23. A (346)

Either, Both, or Neither

17–24. D (334, 341)
17–25. B (341)
17–26. A (341)
17–27. A (**HR**)
17–28. B (341)
17–29. A (341)
17–30. D (341)
17–31. B (342)
17–32. C (342)
17–33. C (342)
17–34. A (342)
17–35. C (342)
17–36. A (342)

One, More Than One, or All

17–37. E (342)
17–38. E (334–335)
17–39. A (342)
17–40. A (352)
17–41. B (350)
17–42. E (348–349)

Chapter 18: Skin*

Single Best Answer

18–1. D (354)
18–2. B (364, **HR**)

Matching

18-3. (354)
18-4. (354)
18-5. E (354)
18-6. F (354, 362, 367)
18-7. C (354)
18-8. F (364, 365)
18-9. A (354)
18-10. C (360)
18-11. B (359)
18-12. C (360)
18-13. C (360)
18-14. C (360)
18-15. D (361)
18-16. B (359)
18-17. D (361)
18-18. A (357)
18-19. A, B, C, D (354-358)
18-20. D (358-359)
18-21. B, D (356)
18-22. E (356)
18-23. A, C (356)
18-24. D (354)
18-25. A, C (356)
18-26. C (356)
18-27. D (354)
18-28. J (363)
18-29. A (363)
18-30. B (363)
18-31. I (363)
18-32. F (363)
18-33. G (363)
18-34. D (363)
18-35. E (363)
18-36. F (365)
18-37. E (365)
18-38. D (365)
18-39. B (365)
18-40. A (365)
18-41. C (**HR**)

Either, Both, or Neither

18-42. B (356)
18-43. A (354)
18-44. B (354)
18-45. D (354)
18-46. A (**HR**)
18-47. B (**HR**)
18-48. A (364)
18-49. A (364)
18-50. B (356)
18-51. A (356)
18-52. B (356)
18-53. B (356)
18-54. A (356)
18-55. C (356)
18-56. B (356)
18-57. B (361)
18-58. D (361)
18-59. A (362, 467)
18-60. A (361)
18-61. A (361)
18-62. B (361)
18-63. C (361-362)
18-64. A (365-366)
18-65. B (365-366)
18-66. C (365-366)
18-67. B (75, 364, 365-366)
18-68. D (77, 367)
18-69. B (365-366)
18-70. A (365-366)
18-71. B (365-366)
18-72. A (366)
18-73. B (**HR**)
18-74. B (366)

One, More Than One, or All

18-75. E (354, 361)
18-76. B (354, 356, 362, 365)
18-77. E (354, 361, 362, 363)
18-78. A (362)
18-79. C (354, 362, 367)
18-80. B (362, 367)

Chapter 19: Urinary System*

Single Best Answer

19-1. E (382 or 383)
19-2. B (368)
19-3. C (381, 385)
19-4. E (387)
19-5. B (368)

Matching

19-6. H (369)
19-7. G (369)
19-8. F (369)
19-9. B (369)
19-10. C (369)
19-11. A (369)
19-12. D (369)
19-13. E (369)
19-14. D (374)
19-15. E (374)
19-16. F (374)
19-17. B (374)
19-18. A (374)
19-19. C (374)
19-20. D (371)
19-21. G (371)
19-22. A (371)
19-23. J (371)
19-24. K (371)
19-25. C (371)
19-26. E (371)
19-27. F (371)
19-28. H (371)
19-29. B (371)
19-30. I (371)
19-31. A (377)
19-32. C (377)
19-33. B (377)
19-34. C (379)
19-35. A (379)
19-36. B (379)
19-37. D (379)
19-38. B (379)
19-39. A (379)
19-40. B (380)
19-41. E (369, 373, 380)
19-42. D (373)
19-43. B (380)
19-44. C (368-369)
19-45. A (380)
19-46. C (Blood is isotonic by definition)
19-47. C (386)
19-48. C (386)
19-49. A (384, 386)
19-50. A (386, 387)
19-51. B (383-384, 386)
19-52. A (383-384, 386)
19-53. B (383-384, 386)
19-54. A (383-384, 386)
19-55. B (383-384, 386)
19-56. F (387)
19-57. A (368, 371)
19-58. A (372-374)
19-59. C or D (373)
19-60. C (375)
19-61. A (374-375)
19-62. C or D (378)
19-63. D (378)
19-64. F (387)
19-65. F (387)
19-66. F (387)
19-67. F (387)
19-68. F (389)
19-69. E (389)
19-70. E (389)
19-71. B (389)
19-72. E (389)

Either, Both, or Neither

19-73. B (371, 378)
19-74. D (379)
19-75. A (371, 373)
19-76. C (369, 370)
19-77. A (382-383)
19-78. B (384)
19-79. A (382-383)
19-80. A (382-383)
19-81. B (386-387)
19-82. A (373)
19-83. A (369, 370)
19-84. B (368, 369)
19-85. A (368, 369, 370, 371)
19-86. B (369, 378, 385)
19-87. A (368, 369, 379)
19-88. A **(HR)**
19-89. A (381-382)
19-90. B (385)
19-91. B (375)
19-92. A (382-383, 385)
19-93. B (368, 385)
19-94. C (368)
19-95. A (368)
19-96. B (384, 386, 387)
19-97. A (384, 386, 387)
19-98. B (387)
19-99. A (386)
19-100. D (380)
19-101. A (384)
19-102. C (374-375, 381)
19-103. D (384, 386, 387)
19-104. D (380)
19-105. B (386)
19-106. A (380-381)
19-107. A (380-381)
19-108. B (386-387)
19-109. A (384, 386)
19-110. B (381-382)
19-111. A (381-382)
19-112. A (375)

19–113. B (375)
19–114. B (375)
19–115. C (385)
19–116. B (375)
19–117. B (389)
19–118. A (388)
19–119. B (389)
19–120. A (388)
19–121. B (389)
19–122. B (**HR**)
19–123. B (389)
19–124. A (388)

One, More Than One, or All

19–125. B (373, 375, 378)
19–126. D (381–382, 385)
19–127. A (369, 380)

Chapter 20: Pituitary & Hypothalamus*

Single Best Answer

20–1. D (75–76, 390)
20–2. C (399)

Matching

20–3. A, C, D, G, J, M, N (396, 397, 398–399)
20–4. F, L (394)
20–5. A (400)
20–6. N (400)
20–7. H (396)
20–8. K (395, 397)
20–9. O (395)
20–10. C, D, G, J, M (390–391, 396)
20–11. F, L (395, 396, 397)
20–12. I (395)
20–13. D (396)
20–14. C, D, G, J, M (396)
20–15. A (399)
20–16. O (399)
20–17. B (**HR**)
20–18. F (392)
20–19. O (392)
20–20. J (392)
20–21. J (392)
20–22. G (392)
20–23. I (392)
20–24. S (398)
20–25. N (392)
20–26. A (392)
20–27. D (392)
20–28. P (392)
20–29. Q (392)
20–30. R (392)
20–31. C (393)
20–32. L (393)
20–33. M (393)
20–34. H (393)

Either, Both, or Neither

20–35. B (392)
20–36. B (394)
20–37. A (393)
20–38. B (392)
20–39. A (393)
20–40. D (395)
20–41. D (399–400)
20–42. B (394)
20–43. D (396)
20–44. B (394, **HR**)
20–45. D (396)
20–46. A (391)
20–47. C (396, 398–400)
20–48. A (399)
20–49. A (392)
20–50. A (392)
20–51. B (392)
20–52. A (391)
20–53. A (391–392)
20–54. B (399)
20–55. B (399)
20–56. A (396)
20–57. A (390–396)
20–58. B (399)
20–59. B (398–400)
20–60. A (391)

One, More Than One, or All

20–61. A (390)
20–62. E (390–391)
20–63. C (390–391, 396, 398–400)

Chapter 21: Adrenals, Islets of Langerhans, Thyroid, Parathyroids, & Pineal Body*

Single Best Answer

21–1. D (404)
21–2. B (409)
21–3. A (414)
21–4. E (418)
21–5. B (401, 402)

Matching

21–6. C (403)
21–7. A (403)
21–8. B (403)
21–9. D (403)
21–10. B (401)
21–11. C, D (401)
21–12. C, D (401)
21–13. B, C, D (405–407)
21–14. B (405)
21–15. A (406)
21–16. C (406)
21–17. A, B, C (405–406)
21–18. F, G, H, I, J, K, L (409–412, 419)
21–19. D, E (407)
21–20. F, G, H, I (409–411)
21–21. J, K (411–412)
21–22. L (419)
21–23. M (419)
21–24. A, B, C, D, E (405–408)
21–25. A, B,C, J (405–407, 412)
21–26. K (413)
21–27. A (380)
21–28. D, E (408)
21–29. L (419)
21–30. G (411)
21–31. F (410)
21–32. M (421)
21–33. J (413)
21–34. G (410)
21–35. J (411)
21–36. I (411)
21–37. A (380)
21–38. B (410)
21–39. A (410)
21–40. C (412)
21–41. D (410)
21–42. E (410)
21–43. C (412)

Either, Both, or Neither

21–44. A (88–89)
21–45. B (80–81)
21–46. A (88–89)
21–47. C (80–84, 88–89)
21–48. B (81)
21–49. B (81)
21–50. A (88–89)
21–51. A (402)
21–52. B (407)
21–53. B (406)
21–54. A (401)
21–55. B (407)
21–56. B (419)
21–57. A (419)
21–58. B (419)
21–59. B (419)

One, More Than One, or All

21–60. B (401, 405–406)
21–61. A (408, **HR**)
21–62. C (406)
21–63. E (407–408)
21–64. B (413–416)
21–65. A (419)
21–66. C (421)

Chapter 22: Male Reproductive System*

Single Best Answer

22-1. B (434)
22-2. A (423)
22-3. C (422)
22-4. A (**HR**)
22-5. B (422)

Matching

22-6. A (423)
22-7. S (423)
22-8. B (423)
22-9. D (423)
22-10. F (423)
22-11. C (423)
22-12. E (423)
22-13. R (423)
22-14. G (423)
22-15. Q (423)
22-16. P (423)
22-17. H (423)
22-18. J (423)
22-19. I (423)
22-20. O (423)
22-21. K (423)
22-22. M (423)
22-23. N (423)
22-24. L (423)
22-25. A, B, F, G (422-424)
22-26. C, D, E (422-424)
22-27. B (423)
22-28. B (424)
22-29. A (422)
22-30. E (422)
22-31. B (422)
22-32. C (424)
22-33. D (424)
22-34. G (422, 431)
22-35. F, G (**HR**)
22-36. C (424)
22-37. F (428)
22-38. I (424)
22-39. G (424)
22-40. J (424)
22-41. A (424)
22-42. F (424)
22-43. B (424)
22-44. C (424)
22-45. D (424)
22-46. E (424)
22-47. D (434)
22-48. C (433)
22-49. B (433)
22-50. A, B, C (433)
22-51. E (435)
22-52. E (435)
22-53. H (389)
22-54. F (**HR**)
22-55. F (435)
22-56. D, E, F, H, I (389, 434, 435)
22-57. D, E (434-435)
22-58. A (433)
22-59. C (433)
22-60. I (389)
22-61. C (437)
22-62. D (437)
22-63. H (437)
22-64. F (437)
22-65. E (437)
22-66. B (437)
22-67. A (437)
22-68. I (437)
22-69. G (437)
22-70. C (436)
22-71. C, D, E (389, 436)
22-72. C (436)
22-73. A (422)
22-74. A (422, 431)
22-75. A (422)
22-76. B (435)
22-77. C (436)
22-78. B (435)
22-79. D, E (389, 436)
22-80. B (423, 435)
22-81. A (431)

Either, Both, or Neither

22-82. A (428)
22-83. B (428)
22-84. C (428)
22-85. A (428, 433)

One, More Than One, or All

22-86. E (428, 433)
22-87. A (431-432)
22-88. B (432-433)
22-89. C (434-435)
22-90. A (436-438)

Chapter 23: Female Reproductive System*

Single Best Answer

23-1. B (441)
23-2. C (449, 451)
23-3. B (458)
23-4. E (454, 455)
23-5. D (446, 448)
23-6. A (457)
23-7. D (454)
23-8. A (458)

Matching

23-9. E (439)
23-10. F (439)
23-11. D (439)
23-12. C (439)
23-13. A (439)
23-14. B (439)
23-15. G (440)
23-16. I (440)
23-17. B (440)
23-18. C (440, 441)
23-19. H (440)
23-20. A (440)
23-21. D (440)
23-22. E (440)
23-23. G (441)
23-24. F (441)
23-25. H (441)
23-26. B (441)
23-27. A (441)
23-28. D (441)
23-29. E (441)
23-30. C (441)
23-31. F (454)
23-32. I (454)
23-33. G (454)
23-34. B (454)
23-35. D (454)
23-36. C (454)
23-37. E (454)
23-38. J (454)
23-39. H (454)
23-40. A (454)
23-41. G (455)
23-42. H (455)
23-43. A (455)
23-44. B (455)
23-45. J (455)
23-46. D (455)
23-47. E (455)
23-48. I (455)
23-49. C (455)
23-50. A (452)
23-51. E (444, **HR**)
23-52. C (444)
23-53. C (452)
23-54. B (452)
23-55. B (452)
23-56. B (452)
23-57. B (452)
23-58. B (452)
23-59. D (449)
23-60. A (449)
23-61. B (449)
23-62. C (441)
23-63. B (448)
23-64. D (444, 448)
23-65. A (444)
23-66. A (448-450)
23-67. D (449)
23-68. E (448)
23-69. D (444, 448)
23-70. E (441, 459)
23-71. B (444, 460)
23-72. D (441, 452)
23-73. A (448, 450)
23-74. D (448, 449)
23-75. E (448)
23-76. E (459)
23-77. F (459)
23-78. I, J (458)
23-79. H (464)
23-80. C (444)
23-81. K (446)
23-82. A (459)
23-83. B (459)
23-84. A (459)
23-85. A (459)
23-86. B (459)
23-87. B (459)
23-88. D, J (458, 459)
23-89. G (444)

Either, Both, or Neither

23–90. A (444)
23–91. C (444)
23–92. C (444)
23–93. B (444)
23–94. A (444)
23–95. A (444)
23–96. A (443–444)
23–97. B (446)
23–98. C (443–444, 446)
23–99. C (443–444, 446)
23–100. A (443–444)
23–101. A (444)
23–102. A (446)
23–103. B (446)
23–104. C (446)
23–105. C (446)
23–106. B (446)
23–107. C (446)
23–108. C (446)
23–109. A (448, 450–451)
23–110. C (448)
23–111. A (448, 449)
23–112. B (448, 449)
23–113. A (448, 449)
23–114. B (448, 449)
23–115. B (449)
23–116. A (449)
23–117. A (452)
23–118. C (456)
23–119. A (456)
23–120. A (452)
23–121. C (452)
23–122. D (452, 455)
23–123. A (454)
23–124. D (462, 463)
23–125. B (463)
23–126. A (462)
23–127. D (462, 463)

One, More Than One, or All

23–128. A (441)
23–129. C (444)
23–130. B (442)
23–131. A (444)
23–132. E (400, 448)
23–133. B (444, 447)
23–134. D (452)
23–135. B (454, 457)
23–136. C (463, 464)
23–137. C (464)

Chapter 24: Sense Organs*

Single Best Answer

24–1. C (467, 468)
24–2. C (467–468)
24–3. B (476)
24–4. D (473)
24–5. D (477)
24–6. A (474)
24–7. D (483, 487)
24–8. B (469)

Matching

24–9. A, D (466, 467)
24–10. F (223, 466)
24–11. A, B, C, D (467, 469)
24–12. A (466, 489, 492)
24–13. C (467)
24–14. A, D (466, 469)
24–15. F (470)
24–16. A (495)
24–17. A (466, 467)
24–18. A (466, 467)
24–19. A (466, 467)
24–20. A (466, 467)
24–21. F (469–470)
24–22. E (466, 479)
24–23. C (472, 479)
24–24. B (471, 473)
24–25. E (471, 474, 475)
24–26. A (471, 472–473)
24–27. B (471, 473)
24–28. A (473)
24–29. D (472–473)
24–30. B (472, 475)
24–31. E (472, 479)
24–32. C (479)
24–33. B, C (**HR**)
24–34. C (472, 481)
24–35. C (487)
24–36. E (472, 487)
24–37. B (472, 473)
24–38. B (472, 477)

24-39. B (481, 486)
24-40. E (483-484)
24-41. A (483)
24-42. B (475, 481, 482)
24-43. D (482, 483)
24-44. C (482, 483)
24-45. E (482, 483)
24-46. A (481)
24-47. C (473, 478)
24-48. D (472-473, 476)
24-49. B (**HR**)
24-50. C (479)
24-51. D (472-473, 476)
24-52. C (493)
24-53. J (493)
24-54. D (493)
24-55. H (493)
24-56. M (493)
24-57. O (493)
24-58. G (493)
24-59. A (493)
24-60. F (493)
24-61. B (493)
24-62. O (492, 493)
24-63. N (493)
24-64. K (493)
24-65. O (493)
24-66. P (493)
24-67. N (492, 493)
24-68. E (493)
24-69. L (493)
24-70. B (490)
24-71. A (489)
24-72. C (490)
24-73. C (490)
24-74. B (490)
24-75. B (490)
24-76. A (489)
24-77. A (490)
24-78. A (490)
24-79. C (490)
24-80. C (490)
24-81. C (490)
24-82. C (490)
24-83. C (491)
24-84. C (490)

Either, Both, or Neither

24-85. A (477)
24-86. B (477)
24-87. B (**HR**)
24-88. A (477)
24-89. A (477)
24-90. D (475, 478-479)
24-91. B (477)
24-92. C (481)
24-93. D (482)
24-94. A (482)
24-95. B (483)
24-96. A (482)
24-97. B (483)
24-98. A (487, **HR**)
24-99. C (483)
24-100. A (482, 483)
24-101. C (482)
24-102. A (482)
24-103. B (483, 485)

One, More Than One, or All

24-104. B (469)
24-105. E (470)
24-106. A (470, 471)
24-107. A (479)
24-108. A (472, 475, 476)
24-109. E (475, 478-479)
24-110. E (479, 483)
24-111. A (478)
24-112. C (487-489)
24-113. E (489, 491)

INDEX

NOTE: Page numbers in bold face type indicate a major discussion. A *t* following a page number indicates tabular material and an *i* following a page number indicates an illustration. Drugs are listed under their generic names. When a drug trade name is listed, the reader is referred to the generic drug name.

D

N

O

R

T